The Art and Science of Mental Health Nursing

Principles and Practice

Third Edition

Edited by Ian Norman and Iain Ryrie

Open University Press
McGraw-Hill Education
McGraw-Hill House
Shoppenhangers Road
Maidenhead
Berkshire
England
SL6 2QL

email: enquiries@openup.co.uk

world wide web: www.openup.co.uk

and Two Penn Plaza, New York, NY 10121–2289, USA
First published 2013

A catalogue record of this book is available from the British Library

ISBN-13: 978-0-33-524561-1 (pb)
ISBN-10: 0-33-524561-7 (pb)
eISBN: 978-0-33-524562-8

Library of Congress Cataloging-in-Publication Data
CIP data applied for

Typesetting and e-book compilations by
SR Nova Pvt Ltd., Bangalore, India

Printed by CPI Printers

Praise for This Book

"I am delighted to offer an enthusiastic endorsement for the 3rd edition of this important book. First produced in 2004, significant changes in the delivery of mental health services, our understanding of productive ways of working with a population in need and the importance of the services user perspective have all been readdressed in this most recent revised edition. The previous editions were very well received and this most recent version offers important revisions and added value to what was already a well founded and essential textbook for both students and qualified practitioners.

The book is cleverly structured, easily read and presented with clarity by the impressive range of contributing authors. The Editors and Authors are to be congratulated for this important updated edition.

I have little doubt that this 3rd edition will be as successful as the first and second. I see it as essential reading for students undertaking nursing undergraduate programs and it has value both for mental health and general nurse undergraduate programs. It also provides an important 'refresher' for those undertaking professional development and update courses. I feel able to recommend it with confidence to this broad audience."

Emeritus Professor Tony Butterworth CBE.
FMedSci, FRCN, FQNI, FRCPsych FRSA.
Interim Chair, NHS Institute for Innovation and Improvement Chair, Foundation of Nursing Studies.

"The 3rd Edition must succeed the 2nd as a core text for mental health nurse students and experienced nurses alike. This considerable feat is achieved, in no small part, by virtue that the Editors have a clear picture of what constitutes mental health nursing and have an insightful way of organizing this wonderful world of mental health nursing. The expertise of the contributors, and the guidance and advice offered in their contributions, ensures this text provides all qualified mental health nurses with an invaluable practical resource to be consulted on an on-going basis. This is a text which needs to be available in copious numbers in any library supporting a pre-registration nursing training, but also deserves a place in any productive clinical team delivering mental health nursing."

Simon McArdle, University of Greenwich, UK

"This book is certainly one of the key textbooks I would recommend to all mental health nursing students and practitioners in the UK. It captures both the 'art' and 'science' of our profession and this current edition articulates extremely well the service user perspective and changing policy context in which mental health nurses practice. The scope of the book is admirable and from a pedagogical perspective many of the chapters include 'applied case studies' or 'reflective thinking spaces' which illuminate and make real the often complex nature of mental health nursing."

Dr Andrew Clifton, Huddersfield University, UK

"An incredibly useful and insightful book for those working within the field of mental health, this 3rd edition deconstructs and discusses a variety of topical principles, practices and perspectives that underpin mental

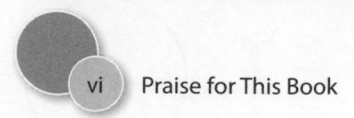

illness and mental health nursing. The structure and presentation of the subject matter allow the book to meet both current curriculum and workforce development needs for students and qualified staff. The further development and discussion around the areas of Service Development, Older Person, Therapeutic Relationship, Continuing Professional Development, Talking Therapies and Alternative Therapies were particularly useful and impressive."

Brian Bell, University of Wolverhampton, UK

"This is a contemporary text drawing on the practical aspects of what it is to be a Mental Health Nurse underpinned by the available evidence base. This 3rd edition builds upon earlier versions and situates the person as the focus. It reflects the contemporary context of Mental Health Nursing practice, which requires technical skills whilst engendering the message that the society we care for require compassionate nurses. I believe this balance is achieved through consideration of the art and science of Mental Health Nursing, and is packaged in a user friendly text which will be a reliable point of reference."

Dr Shelly Allen, University of Salford, UK

"Can one book draw together the collective knowledge of a profession that has evolved over the last century? The answer is "no", but Norman and Ryrie's *The Art and Science of Mental Health Nursing* probably gets as close to this as possible. This comprehensive third edition has more chapters, which are more succinct than the previous edition, with a detailed contents page that makes it easier to use as a reference book. Drawing on a wide variety of authors, the book is coherent and well-edited and underpinned by an optimistic, recovery-focused approach to mental health nursing.

The different parts to the book represent a range of conceptual approaches to understanding mental health nursing, which covers the material in an interesting and informative way. The frequent use of scenarios and "thinking spaces" encourages application of theory to practice and I will be recommending this as a core text within the mental health specific modules."

John Westhead, Staffordshire University, UK

"This book is a must have for anyone that studies within the mental health care setting. It highlights simple ideas while also giving a realistic and more complex notion of what mental health is. It brings to the forefront some issues that aren't normally discussed openly within society."

Nathan Hicks, Mental Health Nursing Student, Anglia Ruskin University

"As a newly qualified mental health practitioner, this book has influenced my approach to clinical practice with a determination to integrate theory and practice. Although, this has proven to be an impossible challenge at some times, adopting this book in the clinical environment will help me demonstrate a good understanding of the principles mental health nursing."

Jean-Louis Ayivor, Newly qualified Mental Heath Practitioner

"The 2nd edition of this book has been essential throughout all modules of my course and was a useful guide to dip into when my knowledge base was challenged in placement areas. This 3rd edition brings additional and up-to-date information which will see me through to the end of my training and beyond into practice as a qualified nurse."

Julie Sheen, Mental Health Nursing Student, University of Essex

Dedication

For Kay and Doris, from your boys

Brief Table of Contents

Detailed Table of Contents

Contributors

Anne Aiyegbusi, Deputy Director of Nursing, Specialist and Forensic Services, West London Mental Health NHS Trust and Visiting Fellow, Buckinghamshire New University, UK.

Ryan Askey-Jones, BABCP-accredited Cognitive Behavioural Therapist and Mental Health Nurse, Teacher of Mindfulness, UK.

Sally Askey-Jones, Tutor, Mental Health Department, Florence Nightingale School of Nursing & Midwifery, King's College London, UK.

Paul Calaminus, CAMHS Service Director, South London and Maudsley NHS Foundation Trust, UK.

Samantha Coster, Research Fellow, Florence Nightingale School of Nursing and Midwifery, King's College London, UK.

Crispin Day, Head, Centre for Parent and Child Support, South London and Maudsley NHS Foundation Trust and Head, CAMHS Health Services Research Unit, Department of Psychology, King's College London, UK.

Julie Dilallo, Consultant Nurse CAMHS, Oxleas NHS Foundation Trust, UK.

Graham Durcan, Associate Director, Criminal Justice Programme, Centre for Mental Health, and Senior Fellow, Institute of Mental Health, Nottingham, UK.

Megan Ellis, Programme Leader (The Helping Families Programme) and Deputy Head, Centre for Parent and Child Support, CAMHS National and Specialist Service, South London and Maudsley NHS Foundation Trust, UK.

Ann Gallagher, Reader in Nursing Ethics, Editor of *Nursing Ethics*, International Centre of Nursing Ethics, University of Surrey, Guildford, UK.

Lina Gega, Lecturer in Mental Health, Norwich Medical School, University of East Anglia, UK.

Sue Gurney, Mental Health Pathways Project Co-ordinator, Croydon Borough Team, NHS South West London, UK.

Cheryl Kipping, Consultant Nurse Dual Diagnosis, South London and Maudsley NHS Foundation Trust, London, UK.

Simon Lawton-Smith, Head of Policy, Mental Health Foundation, London, UK.

Alison I. Machin, Principal Lecturer, Pre-registration Nursing (Adult), Faculty of Health and Life Sciences, Northumbria University, Newcastle upon Tyne, UK.

Tony Machin, Programme Manager, Post Qualifying and Postgraduate Studies (Mental Health), Faculty of Health & Life Sciences, Northumbria University, Newcastle upon Tyne, UK.

Niall McCrae, Lecturer, Mental Health Department, Florence Nightingale School of Nursing and Midwifery, King's College London, UK.

Sandra Moran, Senior Lecturer, Pre-registration Nursing (Mental Health), Faculty of Health and Life Sciences, Northumbria University, Newcastle upon Tyne, UK.

David Morning, Senior Lecturer Mental Health, Faculty of Health and Life Science, Northumbria University, UK.

Ian P.S. Noonan, Lecturer, Mental Health Department, Florence Nightingale School of Nursing and Midwifery, King's College London, UK.

Ian Norman, Professor, Florence Nightingale School of Nursing and Midwifery, King's College London, UK.

Kingsley Norton, Consultant Psychiatrist in Psychotherapy, Head of Psychotherapy, John Conolly Wing, St Bernard's Hospital, Middlesex, UK.

Mary O'Toole, Lecturer in Mental Health Nursing, Faculty of Health, Education and Society, Plymouth University, UK.

Jane Padmore, Consultant Nurse, CAMHS, South London and Maudsley NHS Foundation Trust, UK.

Caroline Parker, Consultant Pharmacist, Central & North West London NHS Foundation Trust, UK.

Jean Penny, Visiting Professor of Healthcare Improvement, University of Derby and Faculty Member for Patient Safety and Quality Improvement, NHS Institute for Innovation and Improvement, UK.

Rachel Perkins, Consultant with the Implementing Recovery through Organizational Change, (ImROC) programme and Chair of Equality 2025 cross-government strategic advisory group on disability issues, London, UK.

Karen Pilkington, Senior Research Fellow, School of Life Sciences, University of Westminster, London, UK.

Hagen Rampes, Assistant Professor, Faculty of Medicine, Department of Psychiatry, University of Toronto and Staff Psychiatrist, Mood and Anxiety Disorders Program, Centre for Addiction and Mental Health, Toronto, Canada.

Julie Repper, Recovery Lead, Nottingham Healthcare Trust and Associate Professor, University of Nottingham, UK.

Charlotte Roberts, Ward Manager, Kent and Medway Adolescent Unit, South London and Maudsley NHS Foundation Trust, UK.

Debbie Robson, Programme Leader and Research Nurse in Medication Management, Section of Mental Health Nursing, Health Services and Population Research, Institute of Psychiatry, King's College London, UK.

Anthony Ross, Senior Lecturer Mental Health, Faculty of Health and Life Science, Northumbria University, UK.

Iain Ryrie, Statt Nurse, Elite Care Services, Southsea, Hampshire.

Jacqueline Sin, NIHR Research Fellow, Florence Nightingale School of Nursing and Midwifery King's College London, UK.

Susan Sookoo, Lecturer, Mental Health Department, Florence Nightingale School of Nursing and Midwifery King's College London, UK.

Simon Westrip, Senior Lecturer, Mental Health, Faculty of Health and Life Sciences, University of Northumbria, UK.

Helen Wilde, Lead Systemic Psychotherapist, Kent and Medway Adolescent Unit, South London and Maudsley Hospitals, UK.

Toby Williamson, Head of Development & Later Life, Mental Health Foundation, London, UK.

Preface

The first edition of this book, published in 2004, quickly became a best-seller and it is now an established core text for mental health nurse education programmes in the UK and beyond. This third edition has been revised substantially to incorporate changes to the policy context of mental health nursing, the legal framework of mental health care within the UK, advances in treatment, changes in the philosophy and principles of mental health and also in response to the many comments we have received from readers of the first two editions, who have pointed to aspects of mental health nursing which merit more attention.

Our aim, as in previous editions, has been to produce a comprehensive textbook that takes account of the diversity of mental health nursing as a practice discipline and the contemporary context in which nursing is practised. In so doing we have sought to avoid the tendency within academic nursing, and some other textbooks, to present a restrictive concept of mental health nursing as a uni-dimensional activity – typically as an 'art' concerned with nurses' therapeutic relationships with 'people' in distress, *or* as a 'science', concerned with evidence-based interventions that can be applied to good effect by nurses, often working in what might be seen as extended roles, to 'patients' with defined mental illness. The polarized views expressed by both artists and scientists within mental health nursing are becoming less relevant today than previously as the focus of mental health care changes towards an emphasis on promoting social inclusion and recovery, reducing social stigma and supporting principles such as choice. Thus, evidence-based practice and interventions are now framed within a recovery-oriented approach that emphasizes the central place of the person with mental health problems and the impact of services upon his or her life journey, rather than the place of the 'patient' within mental health services. In reality, practising nurses must be artists *and* scientists simultaneously and they need to find ways of integrating these elements while meeting policy directives and service users' demands. This book seeks to be a resource to practising nurses to help them meet this remit.

It seems to us that any contemporary account of mental health nursing as a practice discipline needs to establish its case within three broad parameters:

- professional diversity;
- national policy; and
- service user perspectives.

Professional diversity

We avoid aligning the discipline of mental health nursing to any one theoretical perspective but, rather, acknowledge the breadth and complexity of the perspectives upon which mental health nurses draw in their work. The title of this book reflects our aim, therefore, which is to provide an integrative account of the discipline that accommodates its many origins, influences and practices. To assist this process we introduce a schema in Chapters 1 and 2 which integrates explanatory models of mental health and illness, and which demonstrates each one's crucial, though partial, contribution to our understanding of the human condition. We contend that all mental health nursing, whatever its origin or theoretical basis, can be mapped onto this schema. Further, no one part of the schema is, itself, adequate to deal with people's changing needs in relation to mental health and mental illness.

National policy

The UK National Health Service (NHS) and social care provision have long been subject to government policy. As a consequence professionals who work in these organizations must be expected to adjust their practice to meet contemporary demands. Today mental health nurses have increasing levels of professional responsibility and autonomy, and in many settings lead the delivery of care.

The first edition of this book pre-empted the findings of the Chief Nursing Officer for England's (2006) review of mental health nursing in its call for mental health nurses to incorporate the principles of recovery into their work with service users and focus on improving their health outcomes.

The second edition, published in 2009, reflected moves internationally to widen the focus of mental health services from a concern with individuals suffering from mental disorder and their families, to improve the mental health of communities and populations as a whole. Looking to the future we anticipate that the demands of health promotion, for promoting healthy living and for reducing health inequalities, which many of us come across in our daily clinical work, will become more pressing. Our impression is that most mental health nurses have yet to find ways of incorporating this within their work and that the focus of nursing care remains treatment and care rather than primary or secondary prevention.

The third edition is published at a time when questions are being raised in the British media about the motivation and education of nurses (see e.g. Marrin 2009; Odone 2011; Phillips 2011) and enquiries and reports cite unacceptably low standards of nursing, particularly for older people with mental and physical health difficulties and other vulnerable patient groups – for example the Health Service Ombudsman's report (Abraham 2011); the Care Quality Commission (CQC) report (2011) and the forthcoming report of Robert Francis, QC, following the full public inquiry into the role of the commissioning, supervisory and regulatory bodies in the monitoring of Mid-Staffordshire Foundation NHS Trust.

There have been many such reports into cases of poor nursing, dating back to the enquiries into abuses at Ely and Normansfield Hospitals in the 1960s and 70s and beyond (Walshe and Higgins 2002) and so it is far from certain that nursing care standards are in decline, in spite of what media reports would have us believe. What is striking though is the public attention that these recent inquiries have received and our impression is that public confidence in nursing is at a low point.

Typically, inquiries that expose poor nursing are followed by a response from the UK government designed to promote care standards. Recent initiatives have been the Prime Minister's Commission (2010) (established by the outgoing Labour prime minister, Gordon Brown), the Nursing & Care Quality Forum (2012) and most recently a consultation document issued by the Chief Nurse for England and the Director of Nursing at the UK Department of Health (Cummings and Bennett 2012). This document acknowledges reports of unacceptable nursing care and identifies six values and behaviours (the so-called '6 Cs') which it says nurses exhibit when they are performing at their best: care, compassion, competence, communication, courage and commitment.

In the final chapter of this edition we make our own contribution to the quality of nursing debate by proposing a multi-factorial nursing care quality framework grounded in the literature and our clinical experience, which applies particularly to older people with mental health difficulties, but may have a wider application beyond this client group. If our framework of nursing care quality is consistent with the experience of readers we hope it will help to provide a platform for interventions and initiatives to improve the quality of nursing care.

Service user perspectives

An important tenet that underpins this textbook is our belief that mental health nursing is concerned primarily with helping people find meaning and purpose in their lives, and assisting them in the process of recovery. Nurses cannot do this adequately unless they (we) are prepared to hear

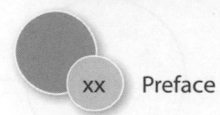

service users' accounts of their difficulties and appreciate their own preferences for a meaningful life. This fact is so central to understanding how mental health nurses can help that we have sought to make it explicit throughout the book, rather than confine it to a single chapter. Thus, each contributor incorporates user perspectives into their chapter. The terminology used to describe recipients of mental health services does however vary between contributors. There are chapters that use the term 'patient' and others that refer to 'service user' or to 'client'; these terms tell us something about the perspective that the contributor brings to bear on their work.

Following the introduction of the schema in Chapters 1 and 2, which is used to integrate explanatory models of mental health and illness, it follows that all perspectives are valid, though each is partial. We have, therefore, chosen not to standardize these terms (into service user, for example), but have allowed contributors to speak for themselves.

Content and organization

The book is divided into six parts. Part 1, 'Foundations', deals with the historical origins and contemporary basis of mental health nursing. Chapter 1 introduces a schema that provides an integrative account of the many and varied factors that influence our sense of mental health and well-being. In Chapter 2 the schema is used to explore a range of aetiological theories for understanding mental illness. Chapter 3 examines the origins and traditions of mental health nursing, Chapter 4 considers health promotion and Chapter 5 deals with recovery and social inclusion as a fundamental orientation for contemporary mental health care. In this part we include a chapter on improving mental health services (Chapter 6) and a new chapter which deals with nurses' continuing professional development (Chapter 7).

Part 2, 'Contexts', considers the policy context (Chapter 8) and the service context and organization of mental health services (Chapter 9). While most examples are drawn from the UK context, these chapters take a thematic approach to the key

social policy issues facing mental health nurses in their work and show how these are reflected in the organization of mental health services. Thus we have tried to produce a text that is not too parochial and which can cross geographical boundaries. Other chapters in this section cover the legal (Chapter 10) and ethical (Chapter 11) frameworks within which mental health nurses practice.

Part 3, 'Core procedures', covers the fundamental processes of mental health nursing care. The chapters here have a very practical orientation. They are concerned with the 'know-how' of mental health nursing, with the skills needed by nurses working in partnership with clients in any care setting. Chapter 12 deals with the engagement of clients in treatment and how best to work with them to identify and solve their problems. Chapter 13 considers the creation of the therapeutic environment within mental health nursing settings, and subsequent chapters consider assessment (Chapter 14), care planning (Chapter 15), admission and discharge (Chapter 16), assessment and management of risk of suicide and self-harm (Chapter 17) and of aggression and violence (Chapter 18).

Part 4 incorporates 12 chapters which cover the interventions which mental health nurses can draw upon in the course of their work. It includes chapters on self-management (Chapter 19), psychological interventions (Chapters 20, 21, 22 and 23), working with groups (Chapter 24) and families and carers (Chapter 25), pharmacological interventions and medication management (Chapters 26, 27 and 28), complementary and alternative therapies (Chapter 29) and promoting physical health (Chapter 30).

Part 5, 'Client groups', examines the major challenges confronting those who use mental health services and outlines evidence-based interventions available to the mental health nurse. Each of the 11 chapters in this section is oriented to a particular type or group of disorders that a person can experience (Chapters 31–41).

As discussed previously in Part 6 of this book we, together with our colleague Sam Coster, draw upon the research literature and our current clinical experience to propose that the causes of poor nursing, particularly for older people, are multifactorial, arising from the stressful demands of nursing older people who may be agitated, withdrawn or disorientated and have complex physical needs, in the context of perceived poor job control, low status care work and poor professional support.

Each chapter begins with an overview that outlines its scope and content and concludes with a set of bullet points to summarize the main points. An annotated bibliography at the end of each chapter points the reader towards more detailed reading. The chapters also include 'thinking spaces' which provide the reader with an opportunity for reflection and to consolidate what they have learned. Case studies are used within some chapters to illustrate the practical application of the material. Though written primarily for mental health nurses and nursing students the book aims also to provide a useful reference for other health care professionals, lay carers and for people with mental health difficulties.

We owe the success of his book to the authors of the individual chapters who have been chosen to reflect the many diverse professional perspectives within mental health care. All are experts in their field and in writing their chapter each was asked to draw upon their specialist knowledge and practice rather than try to relate their subject to a narrow definition of mental health nursing. Without the commitment and patience of each author, this book would not have been written. We are grateful to each of them for taking time out of their busy lives to produce their chapters. This book will have been successful if it goes some small way to helping mental health nurses become skilful, well-informed and sensitive practitioners who work confidently in the context of mental health services to promote mental health and in partnership with service users to help them regain control over their lives.

Ian Norman and Iain Ryrie
London, UK
September 2012

References

Abraham, A. (2011) *Care and Compassion*. London: Parliamentary and Health Service Ombudsman.

CNOE (Chief Nursing Officer England) (2006) *Review of Mental Health Nursing: from values to action*. London: DH.

CQC (Care Quality Commission) (2011) *Dignity and Nutrition Inspection Programme: National Overview*. London: CQC.

Cummings, J. and Bennett, V. (2012) *Developing the Culture of Compassionate Care: Creating a new vision for nurses, midwives and care-givers*. London: DH.

Marrin, M. (2009) *Fallen Angels: The nightmare nurses protected by silence*, available at: www.the-times.co.uk/tto/public/sitesearch.do?querystring=marrin&p=tto&pf=all&bl=on#http://www.thetimes.co.uk/tto/public/sitesearch.do?querystring=marrin&navigators=&from=20090101&to=20100101&p=tto&pf=all&bl=on&service=searchframe, accessed 26 September 2012.

Nursing & Care Quality Forum (2012) www.dh.gov.uk/health/2012/05/nursing-forum.

Odone, C. (2011) Sulky, lazy and patronising: finally, we admit the existence of the bad nurse, the NHS's dirty little secret, *Telegraph Online*, available at http://blogs.telegraph.co.uk/news/cristinaodone/100083415/sulky-lazy-and-patronisingfinally-we-admit-the-existence-of-the-bad-nurse-the-nhss-dirty-little-secret, accessed 26 September 2012.

Phillips, M. (2011) The moral crisis in nursing: voices from the wards, *Daily Mail*, 21 October, available at: http://melaniephillips.com/the-moral-crisis-in-nursing-voices-from-the-wards, accessed 26 September 2012.

Prime Minister's Commission on the Future of Nursing & Midwifery in England (2010) *Front Line Care*, available at: http://webarchive.national-archives.gov.uk/20100331110400/http:/cnm.independent.gov.uk, acessed 26 September 2012.

Walshe, K. and Higgins, J. (2002) The use and impact of inquiries in the NHS, *British Medical Journal*, 325(7369): 895–900.

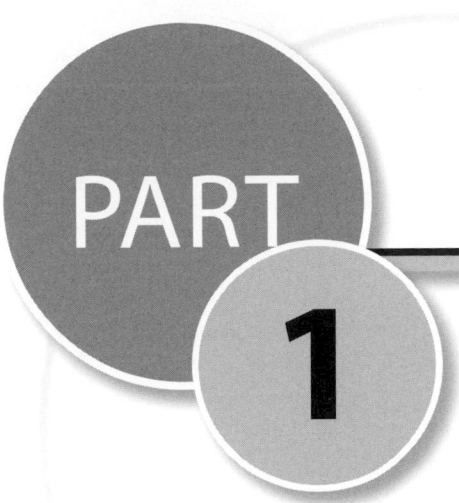

PART 1

Foundations

Chapter 1

Mental Health

Iain Ryrie and Ian Norman

No health without mental health (HM Government 2011)

1.1 Introduction

Whether you begin this book as a student nurse or a registered practitioner, the UK government's assertion sets a significant challenge for mental health nursing. It implies that physical health counts for little if people do not also enjoy mental health. Cardiovascular fitness or an immune system that provides protection from the common cold may be of little value to a person who is in the depths of depression or experiencing an acute episode of schizophrenia.

'No health without mental health' has a deeper meaning. Whatever we experience is both dependent on our mental faculties and contributes to our sense of mental health, since all of life is realized through mental processes. In its most rudimentary form, mental health is the culmination of everything that contributes to the experience of being human.

In this opening chapter we introduce a simple framework to map human experience and use it as a starting point for understanding mental health. We demonstrate how mental health arises from the integration of all that we experience and fluctuates as all things relative to it change. The emergence of mental health as a complex, integral phenomenon is clarified and its implications for the work of mental health nurses are explored. In summary this chapter covers:

- a framework for mental health;
- the nature of mental health;
- integral mental health;
- implications for nursing.

Thinking Space 1.1

Mental health can be conceptualized as a state of well-being in which the individual realizes his or her own abilities, can cope with the normal stresses of life, can work productively and fruitfully, and is able to make a contribution to his or her community. In this positive sense, mental health is the foundation for well-being and effective functioning for an individual and for a community.

(WHO 2007)

(Continued)

Read through the above definition of mental health a few times to familiarize yourself with its content and meaning. You will notice that the first sentence describes a number of different factors that contribute to mental health (e.g. coping abilities, meaningful employment). The second sentence suggests that the term 'mental health' can be applied to communities as well as to individuals.

1. Using the WHO definition as a starting point make a list of everything you can think of that contributes to mental health. Try to be as specific as possible for example, a healthy diet, exercise and friendship are examples of what helps people cope with the normal stresses of life. Social networking and volunteering are specific examples of community contributions. Spend at least five minutes on this task, jotting down whatever examples come into your head.

2. Once you have completed your list, take a closer look at it. Can its content be organized into groups that represent different types of contributing factor (e.g. individual and community factors)?

As you progress through this chapter you can review and develop your ideas as a framework for mental health is described and elaborated.

1.2 A framework for mental health

Following Wilber (2001), one approach to mapping everything that lies within human experience involves just two key dimensions. The first of these concerns me and you, I and we, mine and theirs. This dimension differentiates between what is you and what is everything else, what is 'self' and what is 'other'. In this chapter, 'community' is substituted for 'other' so that the first dimension runs from 'self' to 'community'. For the second dimension human beings have an interior, subjective sense of themselves but also an exterior objective-self. The former includes thoughts and feelings and the latter the physical body. The subjective-self can be described, even written down, but remains wholly within a person's own experience and is not directly accessible to others. The objective-self can be quantified and measured, and in this sense is accessible to the direct experience of others who may be doing the measuring. It is true also that communities have interior (subjective) and exterior (objective) characteristics. The second dimension therefore runs from 'subjective' to 'objective' and when

crossed with the first dimension from 'self' to 'community' forms a quadrant schema or framework (see Figure 1.1).

Figure 1.1 describes the physical and psychosocial elements that arise within each quadrant. Thus, from the subjective-self quadrant a person formulates their personal intentions while the objective-self exhibits behaviours that can be observed and measured. The subjective-community quadrant is respon-

Figure 1.1 Framework of human experience I (after Wilber 2001)

	Subjective	Objective
Self	Interior individual Intentional (upper-left)	Exterior individual Behavioural (upper-right)
Community	Interior collective Cultural (lower-left)	Exterior collective Social (lower-right)

sible for our sense of culture and in the objective-community quadrant reside social systems and structures. Everything that is within human experience can be mapped onto this framework, which provides an important starting point for understanding the nature of mental health.

 ## 1.3 The nature of mental health

Objective-self

In the upper right or objective-self quadrant reside the physical attributes of an individual. This includes a person's anatomical form and biochemical functioning as well as their physical behaviours. It also includes a person's genes.

Genes

Genetic determinism is a highly contested area though it is now broadly accepted that genes alone are not responsible for most complex traits. Interactions between DNA and signals from other genes as well as from the environment influence the development of a trait. Within such a context it is hard to follow a deterministic line. Genes are not simply the determinants of behaviour but are also the servants of the environment (Dobbs 2007). In essence this means that much can be done by people to promote and maintain good mental health regardless of any genetic risk factors they may have inherited.

Anatomical form

Anatomical form, and in particular the different regions and aspects of the brain, are key factors that influence a person's sense of mental health. Of particular importance are the reptilian brain stem, the limbic system or mammalian brain and the cerebrum, each of which represents a seismic evolutionary leap. The reptilian brain stem drives many of our basic instincts such as the need for food and water. It also stimulates sensorimotor actions essential for self-preservation including reflexes and fight or flight impulses. It is focused in a rather limited way on self, on the preservation of 'me'.

The mammalian brain or limbic system evolved millions of years after the reptilian brain and provides more sophisticated functions including the generation of feelings, desires, emotions, sexual impulses and interpersonal needs. Common to all mammals is their tendency to protect and nurture their young, and to a lesser extent, to experience and communicate empathy. This aspect of the brain introduced a collective sense of 'us' rather than just the limited 'me' of the reptilian brain.

The cerebrum is the rational, analytical brain that evolved only 200,000 years ago. It governs visual processing, sound, speech, calculation and pattern matching. It integrates several functions such as thinking, analysing, conceptualizing and planning. It has allowed humans to develop the written language and to generate ideas and concepts (Plant and Stephenson 2008). It is now recognized that different aspects of a person's brain are associated with different experiences of mental health (or illness). In particular, the older reptilian and mammalian brains generate feelings and emotions, the cerebrum registers those feelings and enables people to express them and to a certain extent control them.

The mammalian brain is also responsible for the physiological functioning of the body's organs. The autonomic nervous system begins in the mammalian brain and spreads throughout the body via two distinct branches: the sympathetic and the parasympathetic nervous systems. The former releases the hormones adrenaline and noradrenaline, which focus a person's attention on threats, increases their heart rate and determines a fight or flight response. The latter releases acetylcholine, which induces relaxation, slows the heart rate and generates calm. This is why humans literally feel their emotions. The sympathetic nervous system creates some of the most unpleasant physical symptoms associated with anxiety and depression including rapid or irregular heartbeats, dry mouth and cold sweats (Plant and Stephenson 2008).

Table 1.1   Neurotransmitters and their general effects (adapted from Plant and Stephenson 2008)

Neurotransmitter	Type of effect
Glutamate	Excitory, agitating
Gamma-aminobutyric acid (GABA)	Inhibitory, calming
Dopamine	Physical arousal
Noradrenaline	Attention
Adrenaline	Fight or flight
Serotonin	Optimism
Endorphins	Pleasure
Acetylcholine	Relaxation

Biochemical functioning

An important biochemical function that mental health nurses should be aware of is the role of neurotransmitters, which control the electrical circuits of the brain and nervous system by allowing messages to transfer between the nerve cells or neurons. If levels of key neurotransmitters become depleted or unbalanced then the electrical circuits will not function properly and mental health is threatened.

Table 1.1 presents an overview of what are considered to be some of the most important neurotransmitters for mental health.

Behaviour

A number of behaviours can support mental health through their direct effect on different parts of the brain and on its chemical messengers. It is possible for example to staunch the flow of anxiety and agitation from the emotional brain by gentle but consistent exercise through which natural endorphins are released (MHF 2005a). It is also possible to help calm the mind by eating a diet rich in the precursors of specific neurotransmitters (McCulloch and Ryrie 2006). There is also evidence for the benefits of behaviours that induce relaxation such as mindfulness exercises, meditation and yoga (NICE 2009; MHF 2010). These promote balance and coherence between the sympathetic and parasympathetic nervous systems, regulating heartbeat and calming the emotional brain.

Subjective-self

In the upper left or subjective-self quadrant reside immediate thoughts, feelings, emotions and sensations all described in first-person terms. This represents a person's interior, subjective world made up of emotions and cognitive processes. There remain difficulties in agreeing a common language and shared definition for this subjective sense of our own mental health. For example, mental health, mental well-being, emotional well-being and quality of life tend to be used more or less interchangeably.

Behind these collective terms lie many more concepts used to describe subjective well-being, which reflect two key dimensions: hedonic (positive feelings, effect, mood) and eudaimonic (positive functioning such as meaningful engagement, fulfilment and social well-being). Keyes (2002) describes the combination of positive feeling and positive functioning as 'flourishing' and proposes six feelings that foster psychological well-being:

- self-acceptance;
- positive relations with others;
- autonomy (or ability to think for yourself);
- environmental mastery (the sense that you can change your circumstances for the better);
- life purpose (having goals and feeling helpful);
- personal growth (being able to learn from the stresses and challenges in life).

Experiencing these positive feelings may be relevant markers for mental health service users on their own recovery journeys.

A form of intelligence that people use to understand and regulate their feelings is known as emotional intelligence (Mayer *et al.* 2000). In objective-self terms it reflects biochemical cooperation between the emotional and cognitive brains. Its subjective-self qualities are characterized by a person's ability to:

- accurately identify their emotional state;
- grasp the natural course of their emotions, what generates them and how they ebb and flow;
- reason about their emotions, being aware of the consequences of different courses of action they could take;
- regulate their emotions, taking charge appropriately (Mayer *et al.* 2000).

We can misinterpret our emotions particularly when faced with constant demands on our time and resources. A frequent misinterpretation is between stress or fatigue and hunger. In a society where food is abundantly available and stress very common, overeating has become quite ordinary. Poor mastery of emotions, fuelled by crude marketing, is one reason for the growing incidence of obesity in society (Servan-Schreiber 2011).

Subjective-community

The community quadrants contain environmental mediators or markers for mental health. The social and physical characteristics of communities and the degree to which they enable and promote healthy behaviours all make a contribution to social inequalities, and mental health is very closely related to many forms of inequality (Marmot 2010). The experience of oppression can gradually dampen the spirit and jeopardize people's mental health.

In the lower left or subjective-community quadrant reside collective thoughts, feelings and world views often referred to as 'culture'. A person's sense of belonging to a friendship, family, community or nation is a key factor that influences mental health, and belonging is also mediated by emotional intelligence, which applies to our relationships with others as well as with ourselves. Thus, emotional intelligence is also characterized by a person's ability to accurately identify, grasp, reason and regulate the emotions of others. This capacity for relating to others makes a significant contribution to mental health and in children is predictive of success in adulthood (Servan-Schreiber 2011).

When people do not belong they feel excluded. The marginalization and exclusion in society of people with mental health problems is a form of social deprivation. 'Stigma' is a related term that refers to the way a society views particular groups of individuals and represents a negative feeling or world view about the group in question. It is pernicious and damaging, not least because of the internalization of those collective messages by the individuals to whom they are aimed. This leads to lower self-esteem and a seemingly self-imposed reluctance to engage in mainstream life and to do the things that a person might really want to do. Furthermore, it stops people seeking help for treatment or sharing their difficulties with others. Stigma is not a tangible commodity therefore, but a subjective quality that resides in the lower left quadrant of the framework.

An antidote to stigma and social deprivation is 'social capital', which describes the invisible 'glue' that binds communities together, giving them a shared sense of identity and enabling them to work together for mutual benefit (Kawachi *et al.* 1997). Research into social capital suggests that community cohesion and efficacy, levels of trust, tolerance, reciprocity and participation are important mediators of mental health (Friedli 2000).

Objective-community

In the lower right or objective-community quadrant are the physical attributes of a community such as its legislature, policy and environment.

Legislation

Legislation has a key role to play, particularly that which promotes tolerance and inclusion. Listed below are two key UK government Acts that support the mental health of the public:

- **The Equality Act 2010** aims to protect disabled people and prevent disability discrimination. In the Act, a person has a disability if they have a physical or mental impairment and the impairment has a substantial and long-term adverse effect on their ability to perform normal day-to-day activities. It provides legal rights for disabled people in the areas of:
  - employment;
  - education;
  - access to goods, services and facilities including larger private clubs and land-based transport services;
  - buying and renting land or property;
  - functions of public bodies, for example the issuing of licences.
- **The Civil Partnership Act 2004** came into operation on 5 December 2005 and enables a same-sex couple to registry as civil partners of each other. Register offices or other approved premises in England and Wales can be used for this purpose, providing a venue and formal procedure for same-sex couples to make a public declaration of their commitment and for families and loved ones to support them in that.

It is worth considering the experiences that some members of society would have if these Acts had not come into force and how this might impact on their mental health.

Policy

Key policy for the mental health field is presented in Chapter 8 of this textbook. However, we draw particular attention to *Healthy Lives, Healthy People*, the UK government's public health White Paper (DH 2010). This seeks to radically shift power to local communities, enabling them to focus on the needs of the local population, improve health across people's lives and reduce inequalities. It recognizes the importance of targeted interventions to develop and strengthen mental health resilience factors at an individual, family and community level.

Environment

Poverty, low wages, unemployment, poor housing, environmental pollution, poor education, limited access to transport and shops, and a lack of recreational facilities all impact on people's mental health. These reflect objective community attributes from the lower-right quadrant of Figure 1.1. They can be referred to collectively as 'material deprivation', which is a corollary to the social deprivation discussed under the subjective-community quadrant.

It is now recognized that the built and natural environments in which we live have marked effects upon our mental health. In a systematic review conducted in the UK, Clark *et al.* (2006) identified relationships between neighbourhood disorder and poor mental health, and between neighbourhood regeneration and improved mental health. It is known also that the availability and regular use of green space can result in:

- improved self-awareness, self-esteem and mood;
- reductions in negative feelings such as anger, anxiety and fear;
- improved psychological health, especially emotional and cognitive function;
- restored capacity for attention and concentration (Maller *et al.* 2002).

The Association of Public Health Observatories (www.apho.org.uk) has developed a range of indicators for public mental health. These echo many of the points raised in discussions of the four quadrants including employment, alcohol and drug use, physical activity, healthy eating, social capital, social networks, neighbourliness, violence and safety. Mental health nurses can use this type of information to better understand the contributions they can make to community and public mental health.

Thinking Space 1.2

Having reviewed the four quadrants in Figure 1.1 and examined those elements in each that contribute to our sense of mental health, consider the following challenge.

- You have been asked to prepare a simple health education campaign to promote and protect people's mental health. The campaign must be brief and take the form of 'top tips' to promote and protect mental health. What would be your 10 top tips?

Figure 1.2 Framework of human experience II (after Wilber 2001)

	Subjective	Objective
Self	I	IT
Community	WE	ITS

1.4 Integral mental health

Integral mental health has four dimensions (the quadrants), each of which provides a vital though partial explanation of human experience. This implies that every moment of awareness contains elements from all four quadrants. This is illustrated by Figure 1.2 which shows the framework introduced previously but now containing the pronouns that major languages use to describe different aspects of human experience. Thus, a person can witness an event from the point of view of 'I' in terms of what I see and feel about the event; or from the point of view of 'we' in terms of how others or 'we' collectively feel about the event; and then again it can be viewed as an 'it' or 'its' in terms of the objective facts of the event (Wilber 2007). All events or phenomena in the manifest world can be interpreted from each of these four dimensions (I, it, we and its), each of which are vital though partial accounts. Integral mental health therefore implies that different treatment approaches, reflecting different quadrants, should have beneficial effects for the same condition. For example, an orthodox or conventional medical practitioner (upper right quadrant) might prescribe anxiolytic medication to calm the limbic and sympathetic nervous systems, both of which are involved in the development of anxiety and depression. However, the integral approach suggests there are other dimensions to the physical phenomena of excited limbic and sympathetic nervous systems, one of which is expressed through a person's thoughts and feelings (upper left quadrant). It should therefore be possible to calm these physiological functions by non-physiological approaches as the integral framework suggests. Research into the mechanisms by which talking therapies, including cognitive behavioural therapy (CBT), have a therapeutic effect confirm this.

Brain scans of individuals who receive CBT for depressive symptoms indicate that the therapy may help the prefrontal cortex (cognitive brain) take better control of the emotional brain (Plant and Stephenson 2008). Thus, there is an integrated system through which brain chemistry alters our emotions and, equally, our emotions alter brain chemistry. This highlights the importance of identifying the wider issues that impact on brain function, in this instance the subjective, integral correlates of an over-stimulated limbic and sympathetic nervous systems. Integral mental health also implies that a deficit or damage experienced in one quadrant is likely to have implications for the other quadrants. In human beings and other mammals, physiological balance (upper right quadrant) is dependent on the love we receive from others (lower left quadrant). This was strikingly demonstrated in a study conducted in the 1960s and published in the *British Medical Journal* (Parkes *et al.* 1969). The team of researchers studied two groups of elderly men of the same age. One group had been widowed while the wives of the other group were still alive. The average survival time of the widowers was significantly less than the married group. Servan-Schreiber (2011) has used this study and others, which demonstrate clear links between emotionally supportive relationships, social networks and health to argue that the physiology of social mammals is not separate from the rest of their being, particularly their mental health. Humans are integral beings and optimum mental and physical functioning depends on relationships with others, especially those that offer close emotional ties. It is of little surprise therefore that when mental health service users are asked about the strategies they find 'most helpful', relationships with others is top of their list (Faulkner and Layzell 2000). Psychiatrists at the University of San Francisco refer to this phenomenon as 'limbic regulation' and argue that a relationship is a physiological process as much as it is a social process, as real and as potent as any pill or surgical procedure (Lewis *et al.* 2000). People can die from broken hearts and Servan-Schreiber (2011) argues that love is quite literally a biological need.

A further implication of integral mental health is that interventions aimed at the group (community) should also have benefits for the individual (self). In this respect Huppert (2005) has developed an argument for shifting the health of the whole population in a positive direction rather than focusing on individuals per se (see Figure 1.3). By reducing the mean

number of psychological symptoms in the population, many more individuals would cross the threshold for flourishing. Similarly, a small shift in the mean number of symptoms or risk factors would result in a decrease in the number of people in both the languishing and mental disorder tail of the distribution. This is an important insight for nurses who have been trained in the care of individuals and who may find it difficult to change focus to communities and populations.

1.5 Implications for nursing

Figure 1.4 presents mental health as a complex phenomenon that arises from the integration of everything that is within human experience and fluctuates as all things relative to that experience change. The figure also represents the art and science of mental health nursing. It contains its subjective and objective orientations, and its interpersonal and evidence-based traditions. Those traditions, which developed principally around the care of people with mental illness, can now be understood in relation to mental health. In this respect there are two overarching themes that have implications for the practice of mental health nursing. The first concerns the delivery of care to promote the mental health of people who experience mental disorders. This is additional to the profession's established tradition of delivering interventions designed to manage the mental disorder itself. The second concerns extension of the profession's role to support the mental health and well-being of communities and the public.

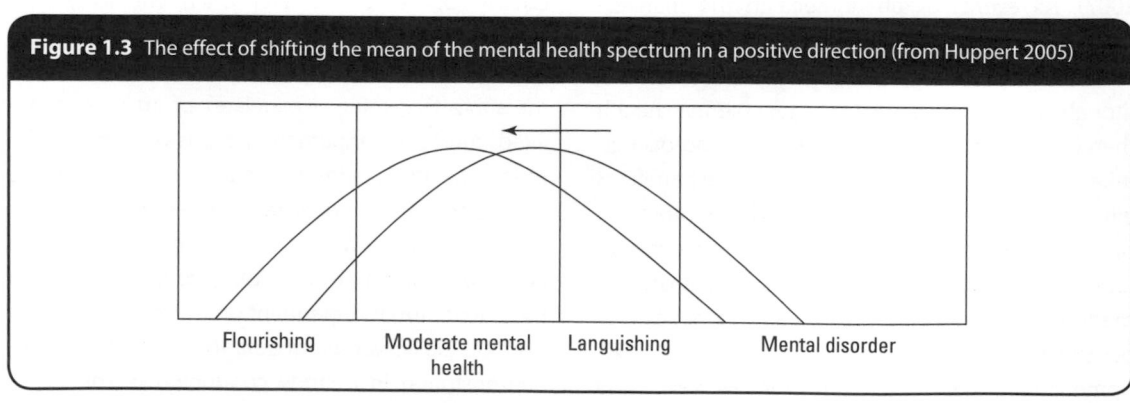

Figure 1.3 The effect of shifting the mean of the mental health spectrum in a positive direction (from Huppert 2005)

Feedback to Thinking Space 1.1

Figure 1.4 provides one possible answer to the two questions posed in the Thinking Space on page 4. The four quadrants represent different types of influence on our mental health (Question 2) and in each quadrant are specific examples of contributing factors (Question 1). We have selected these from other chapters in this volume and from work carried out by NHS Health Scotland (Friedli *et al.* 2007) and the Mental Health Foundation (MHF) (McCulloch and Ryrie 2006). Another possible answer to these two questions is provided in Chapter 4, Figure 4.1.

Feedback to Thinking Space 1.2

The MHF (2009) has produced simple guidance on activities and behaviours that protect and promote people's mental health. They are presented as ten top tips:

- talk about your feelings;
- keep active;
- eat well;
- drink sensibly;
- keep in touch with family and friends;
- ask for help when you need it;
- take a break;
- do something you are good at;
- accept who you are;
- care for others.

Mental health of the individual

While the care and management of mental disorders remains a primary focus for mental health nursing, a complementary focus on mental health provides nurses with opportunities to strengthen their clients' resilience to the debilitating consequences of their condition and to help them forge a meaningful quality of life irrespective of that condition. Opportunities of this type are considered in Chapters 4 and 5, which deal with mental health promotion and recovery respectively. Additionally, we draw attention to the value of intentional activities to promote subjective well-being.

Sheldon and Lyubomirsky (2004) suggest there are three types of intentional activity: overt behaviours, such as taking regular exercise; positive cognitions (e.g. interpreting events in a positive way, appreciating the moment); and motivations towards activities and goals which are perceived as worthwhile. These goals should also be achievable and involve action rather than avoidance (e.g. pursuing the goal of becoming healthy, rather than the goal of giving up fatty foods or smoking). Motivations to participate in social activities and with one's community are also associated with increased life satisfaction.

These activities are not undertaken in the pursuit of pleasure and happiness (hedonic well-being) but fulfilment (eudaimonic well-being). As Huppert (2005) points out, activities of this type produce subjective well-being not because feeling happy is their aim, but because happiness is a by-

Figure 1.4 Integral mental health (After Wilbur 2001)

	Subjective			Objective
Self	Thought			Brain function
	Feelings			Autonomic nervous
	Self-acceptance			System function
	Cognitive style			Physiological balance
	Emotional intelligence			Exercise
	Spirituality			Diet
	Creativity			Alcohol and drug use
	Talking	I	IT	Rest
Community	Relationships	WE	ITS	Legislation
	Belonging			Policy
	Inclusion			Services
	Social support			Employment
	Social capital			Material wealth
	Community			Built environment
	Participation			Nature
	Tolerance			Public health indicators

product of being fully engaged and functioning. An increasing variety of interventions have been tested in trials for their contribution to happiness and well-being. Examples given by Huppert (2005) include:

■ cognitive behaviour therapy, which has been shown to reduce the impact of negative emotions;

■ pleasant activity training, which helps us to identify the activities that make us happy and through practising them enhances our stock of positive emotions;

■ mindfulness meditation, which involves helping people to focus on what is taking place at the moment in their internal and external environment, has been shown to enhance subjective well-being and to reframe their problems positively.

Mental health of the public

Public health or population level interventions are those that are regarded as desirable for everyone. Compulsory wearing of seat belts, fluoridation of drinking water and avoiding smoking are examples of such interventions to prevent physical illness. School-based interventions which teach children life skills, identify positive life goals, value the process of goal attainment rather than the outcome alone, and to find or create social support are the equivalent of these in preventing mental disorder.

The Royal College of Psychiatrists (2010) has reviewed population level interventions for their effectiveness at promoting well-being and strengthening resilience against adversity. Those for which robust evidence exists include:

■ interventions to improve parental health;

■ pre-school and early education interventions;

- school-based mental health promotion and mental illness prevention;
- prevention of violence and abuse;
- early intervention for mental illness;
- alcohol, smoking and substance abuse reduction and prevention;
- promoting healthy lifestyle behaviours;
- promoting healthy workplaces;
- prevention of mental illness and promotion of well-being in older years;
- addressing social inequalities;
- enhancing social cohesion;
- housing interventions;
- reduced stigma and discrimination.

These interventions span the life course and are aimed fundamentally at developing awareness and understanding of mental health among infants, adults and older people whether in relation to their personal lives, work contexts, housing stock and so on. Understanding mental health (and illness) and how to seek mental health information, along with an awareness of risk factors and knowledge of the self-treatments and professional help that are available is collectively referred to as 'mental health literacy' (Chesterson 2009). This has led to the development of mental health first aid (MHFA) training programmes that aim to raise awareness among the general population. A key rationale for such programmes is that many more people in our communities than at present could offer and/or benefit from support, information and access to services, which in turn will enhance positive health-seeking behaviours (Chesterson 2009).

Originally conceived in Australia by Betty Kitchener and her husband, Professor Tony Jorm (Jorm et al. 1997), MHFA was brought to the UK in 2003 when Kitchener visited Scotland to train MHFA instructors. MHFA England was developed later in 2006 by the Department of Health (DH) and involved another visit by Kitchener to train English instructors. MHFA work in the UK is now part of an expanding international movement, currently involving 16 countries (www.mhfaengland.org). Courses run by MHFA England span the equivalent of two full days and teach participants to:

- spot the early signs of a mental health problem;
- feel confident helping someone experiencing a problem;
- provide help on a first aid basis;
- help prevent someone from hurting themselves or others;
- help stop a mental illness from getting worse;
- help someone recover faster;
- guide someone towards the right support;
- reduce the stigma of mental health problems.

Many public level interventions capitalize on mass marketing methods (e.g. anti-bullying, stop smoking and sensible drinking campaigns). Huppert (2004, 2005) has argued that interventions to promote positive well-being should adopt 'social marketing' strategies through which product marketing principles are used to sell ideas, attitudes and behaviours that have social benefits. Box 1.1 provides an example of a population-based information campaign that was designed and delivered by a mental health nurse in partnership with communications experts.

 ## 1.6 Conclusion

In this chapter we have outlined an integral understanding of the human condition and used this to map those elements that have a bearing on the mental health of individuals and communities. This understanding offers potential to develop mental health nursing roles to promote the health and well-being of individuals with whom they currently work and also of the public. Mental health nurses may feel cautious moving from a dedicated focus on the needs and care of the individual to one that is oriented toward the public. However, the integral nature of mental health demonstrates that interventions at the public or community level also have an effect on the experience of individuals. In this respect we have outlined the potential benefits for people suffering from mental disorder of increasing

Box 1.1 Population-based intervention

The MHF's 'Feeding Minds' campaign was designed as a population-based intervention using television, newspapers, magazines and the internet to raise public awareness of the relationship between food and mental health, and to equip people with strategies, ideas and recipes to support their mental health. It was undertaken in partnership with Sustain: the alliance for better food and farming. The key products for this campaign were a report on the relationship between food and mental health (MHF 2005b) and web pages for the public that included mentally healthy recipes, top tips, personal stories, a nutrition table and web guide (www.mentalhealth.org.uk/campaigns/food-and-mental-health). The Foundation's director of research, a mental health nurse, was at the forefront of this campaign in partnership with the chief executive and the director of communications. The project's dissemination strategy used traditional media channels, which on the day of the report's launch included:

- a broadsheet front page story (*Guardian* 16 January 2006);
- 13 national television items featuring campaign staff;
- 16 national radio items featuring campaign staff;
- website to support healthy eating.

Subsequent to its launch the story was reported a further 19 times in national newspapers and 49 times in consumer and trade magazines. The report was downloaded from the Foundation's website 135,000 times in the three months following publication. Following this work the Big Lottery Fund (BLF) sought advice from the Foundation regarding a funding round. A total of £180 million was subsequently allocated by BLF to be spent on projects that addressed mental health, diet and exercise.

the mental health of the population as a whole. We have also provided some pointers for mental health nurses who may wish to move beyond the care of individuals to promote public mental health through interventions to change attitudes and behaviours that create environments in which people's mental health can flourish. In summary, the key points of learning from this chapter are:

- Mental health can be understood using a four quadrant framework that incorporates its objective and subjective elements as well as those that relate to the individual and their communities.

- Individual quadrants include people's physical attributes and their subjective sense of themselves.

- Community quadrants contain environmental mediators of mental health including a community's social and physical characteristics.

- Mental health is a complex phenomenon that arises from the integration of everything that is within human experience (the four quadrants) and fluctuates as all things relative to that experience change.

- The integral nature of mental health means that different treatment approaches, reflecting different quadrants, should have beneficial effects for the same condition, and that a deficit or damage experienced in one quadrant is likely to have implications for other quadrants.

- Integral mental health means also that public-level interventions have benefits for the individual in so far as any reduction in the mean number of population-level psychological symptoms would allow many more individuals to cross the threshold for flourishing.

- This framework understanding provides mental health nurses with the opportunity to develop their role in two respects: to promote the health and well-being of people who experience mental disorders and also of the public at large.

Annotated bibliography

Servan-Schreiber, D. (2011) *Healing Without Freud or Prozac.* **London: Rodale International Ltd.**
This textbook demonstrates how it is possible to support mental health without recourse to traditional or orthodox treatments. It provides an overview of seven highly effective interventions that work through the body to tap into the emotional brain's self-healing process. It combines cutting edge science with alternative medicine and points the way to the mental health practice of the future.

Plant, J. and Stephenson, J. (2008) *Beating Stress, Anxiety and Depression.* **London: Piatkus Books.**
Jane Plant and Janet Stephenson provide a contemporary account of the ways in which we can all support our own mental health and prevent the onset of mental health problems. It provides a rigorous analysis of the physiological correlates of mental health and offers 10 lifestyle and nutritional factors that can decrease the chances of mental illness and dramatically improve mental well-being.

- MHF (www.mentalhealth.org.uk):
  - (2005) *Up and Running: Exercise therapy and the treatment of mild or moderate depression in primary care*
  - (2005) *Feeding Minds: The impact of food on mental health*
  - (2005) *The Impact of Spirituality on Mental Health*
  - (2006) *Cheers? Understanding the relationship between alcohol and mental health*
  - (2010) *Mindfulness report*

These are just five of many publications produced for public consumption by the MHF. They explore a range of factors that contribute to mental health, case study innovative interventions and provide individual guidance to those who wish to care more effectively for their mental health.

References

Chesterson, J. (2009) Mental health promotion and prevention, in P. Barker (ed.) *Psychiatric and Mental Mealth Nursing: The craft of caring,* 2nd edn. London: Edward Arnold.

Clark, C., Candy, B. and Stansfield, S. (2006) *A Systematic Review on the Effect of the Built and physical Environment on Mental Health.* London: MHF.

DH (Department of Health) (2010) *Healthy Lives, Healthy People: our strategy for public health in England.* London: DH.

Dobbs, D. (2007) Eric Kandel: from mind and brain and back again, *Scientific American Mind,* 33: 33–7.

Faulkner, A. and Layzell, S. (2000) *Strategies for Living: A report of user-led research into people's strategies for living with mental distress.* London: MHF.

Friedli, L. (2000) *Mental Health Improvement 'Concepts and Definitions': Briefing paper for the National Advisory Group.* Edinburgh: Scottish Executive.

Friedli, L., Oliver, C., Tidyman, M. and Ward, G. (2007) *Mental Health Improvement: Evidence based messages to promote mental wellbeing.* Edinburgh: NHS Health Scotland.

HM Government (2011) *No Health Without Mental Health: A cross-government mental health outcomes strategy for people of all ages.* DH: London.

Huppert, F.A. (2004) A population approach to positive psychology: the potential for population interventions to promote well-being and prevent disorder, in P.A. Linley and S. Joseph (eds) *Positive Psychology in Practice.* New York: John Wiley & Sons.

Huppert, F. (2005) Positive mental health in individuals and populations, in F. Huppert, N. Bayliss and B. Keverne (eds) *The Science of Well-Being.* Oxford: Oxford University Press.

Jorm, A., Korten, A, Jacomb, P. *et al.* (1997) Mental health literacy: a survey of the public's ability to recognize mental disorder and their beliefs about the effectiveness of treatment, *Medical Journal of Australia,* 166: 182–6.

Kawachi, I., Kennedy, B. and Lochner, K. (1997) Health and social cohesion: why care about income inequality? *British Medical Journal,* 314: 1037–40.

Keyes, C. (2002) The mental health continuum: from languishing to flourishing in life, *Journal of Health and Social Research,* 43: 207–22.

Lewis, T., Amini, F. and Lannon, R. (2000) *A General Theory of Love.* New York: Random House.

Maller, C., Townsend, M., Brown, P. and St. Leger, L. (2002) *Healthy Parks, Healthy People: the health benefits of contact with nature in a park context: a literature review.* Victoria, Australia: Deakin University.

Marmot, M. (2010) *Fair Society, Healthy Lives: Strategic review of health inequalities in England post 2010,* available at: www.marmotreview.org, accessed 15 August 2011.

Mayer, J., Salovey, A. and Capuso, A. (2000) Models of emotional intelligence, in R. Steinberg (ed.) *Handbook of Intelligence.* Cambridge: Cambridge University Press.

McCulloch, A. and Ryrie, I. (2006) The impact of diet on mental health, *The Mental Health Review*, 11: 19–22.

MHF (Mental Health Foundation) (2005a) *Up and Running: Exercise therapy and the treatment of mild or moderate depression in primary care.* London: Mental Health Foundation.

MHF (Mental Health Foundation) (2005b) *Feeding Minds: The impact of food on mental health.* London: MHF.

MHF (Mental Health Foundation) (2009) *How to Look After Your Mental Health*, available at: www.mentalhealth.org.uk/help-information/10-ways-to-look-after-your-mental-health, accessed 12 September 2012.

MHF (Mental Health Foundation) (2010) *Mindfulness Report.* London: MHF.

NICE (National Institute for Health and Clinical Excellence) (2009) *Depression: Treatment and management of depression in adults, including adults with a chronic physical health problem.* (NICE clinical guidelines 90 and 91; update of NICE clinical guidance 23). London: NICE.

Parkes, M., Benjamin, C. and Fitzgerald, R. (1969) Broken heart: a statistical study of increased mortality among widowers, *British Medical Journal*, 646: 740–3.

Plant, J. and Stephenson, J. (2008) *Beating Stress, Anxiety and Depression.* London: Piatkus Books.

Royal College of Psychiatrists (RCP) (2010) *No health without public mental health: The case for action.* London: RCP.

Servan-Schreiber, D. (2011) *Healing without Freud or Prozac.* London: Rodale International Ltd.

Sheldon, K.M. and Lyubomirsky, S. (2004) Achieving sustainable new happiness: prospects, practices and prescriptions, in P.A. Linley and S. Joseph (eds) *Positive Psychology in Practice.* New York: John Wiley & Sons.

Wilber, K. (2001) *A Theory of Everything.* Dublin: Gateway.

WHO (World Health Organization) (2007) *Mental Health: Strengthening mental health promotion, Fact Sheet No. 220*, available at: www.who.int/mediacentre/factsheets/fs220/en, acessed 12 April 2012.

Chapter 2

Mental Disorder

Iain Ryrie and Ian Norman

For me hearing voices is [my] most common [psychotic symptom], they are usually male voices, being very critical of me or telling me to harm/protect myself against others.

PaulD

2.1 Introduction

Chapter 1 described mental health as a state of balance that includes the self and community in both their subjective and objective forms. This chapter uses the same framework to examine mental disorder. The point at which an individual's experience or behaviour might be considered disordered is a highly contested area since different schools of thought have their own explanatory models. We do not draw conclusions in this respect but encourage the reader to consider an integrated explanation of human experience, and thus, of mental disorder. Different models or ways of understanding mental disorder are described both as singular explanations and as building blocks for a more integrated understanding. From this perspective, and as a corollary to mental health, mental disorder is presented as a state of imbalance that includes the self and community in both their

Thinking Space 2.1

Different schools of thought have developed different theories or models to explain mental disorder. Before reading this chapter, take some time to reflect on your own beliefs about the causes of mental disorder.

1. As a starting point, make a list of everything you can think of that might contribute to the development of a mental disorder. Spend at least five minutes on this task, jotting down whatever examples come into your head.

2. Once you have completed your list take a closer look at it. Can its content be organized into groups that represent different types of explanatory factors/models of mental disorder?

To help with this task have a look again at Figures 1.1 and 1.4 in Chapter 1, and use the framework to guide and summarize your thoughts. As you read through the next section of this chapter you can review and develop your ideas as key models for mental disorder are described.

subjective and objective forms. Systems that classify mental disorder are reviewed, and the prevalence and symptoms of key disorders are described.

In summary this chapter covers:

- models of mental disorder;
- the classification of mental disorder;
- key symptoms of mental disorder;
- prevalence and incidence of mental disorders.

2.2   Models of mental disorder

The disease model

A disease is present if it harms the individual, reduces his or her capacity to reproduce and thereby places them at a biological disadvantage (Scadding 1967; Tyrer and Steinberg 2005). This can be understood in terms of a physical disease, such as a cancer, a damaged heart valve or a pathogen that can be transmitted between people. Disease theorists similarly attribute mental disorders, or psychiatric illnesses, to physiological and chemical changes in the individual, particularly in the brain but also in other parts of the body (Tyrer and Steinberg 2005).

Thus we can understand clearly the basis for disorders of perception and cognition among people with dementia or those who have suffered brain injuries. Observable physiological changes in brain structure have correlates in human behaviour. The disease model extends beyond these organic conditions to explain disorders such as depression, which can be attributed to changes in serotonin levels or to some other chemical fluctuation. Similarly, schizophrenia has been attributed to chemical abnormalities and also to physiological differences such as the size of the temporal lobe in the human brain.

The disease model, following traditional medicine, endeavours to identify through scientific objectivity the presence of a stable phenomenon that is called 'mental disorder'. Clinical syndromes become refined into diagnoses, which are essentially codes for heterogeneous, and often unstable, collections of symptoms (Craig 2006). Objectivity in psychiatry is at best quite 'fuzzy' but remains a gold standard. Such a gold standard affords incredible

power to its possessor. Clinical syndromes and diagnoses are codified languages, available only to those who have willingly immersed themselves in that particular paradigm. They can provide an efficient means to communicate complex phenomena, but only to those in the know.

Correspondingly, the treatment armoury of the disease theorist is elitist, being available only to the qualified practitioner. Medicines are prescribed to balance chemical imbalances, electroconvulsive therapy is administered to shunt neural pathways into shape, positron emission tomography may be requested to measure the size of temporal lobes and, in the most extreme of cases, pieces of the brain may be removed.

Diagnostic capability can be enhanced by specific assessment methods. For example, the biochemical correlates of mental disorder in the form of organic compounds can be analysed in urine and blood samples to determine which neurotransmitters are too high or too low. Saliva samples can be analysed to determine levels of cortisol, which provide an indication of the degree of stress an individual is experiencing. Some commentators recommend that these procedures should be included in assessments for mental disorder, particularly before prescribing medications that act on specific neurotransmitters (Plant and Stephenson 2008).

A consistent criticism of the disease model is the possibility that people with mental disorders can become passive recipients of treatment and the nurse or doctor an authority on the person's experience. However, this is not a consequence of the disease model per se, but reflects something of the way in which practitioners apply their knowledge. Passive receipt of care can accompany any model if practitioners fail to speak to people as people, but instead believe they are dealing with symptoms, syndromes or a collection of behavioural problems. There is no reason why the disease model cannot take account of the person behind the symptoms or syndrome, and indeed in our experience this has largely been the case, though not always so.

The psychodynamic model

The psychodynamic model is more accurately described as a style of human interaction and understanding that draws on a broad philosophy, which includes clinical, biological and evolutionary theory as well as religion and the arts (Tyrer and Steinberg 2005). Psychodynamic practice may conjure an image of the psychoanalyst listening to their patient's stream of consciousness as the patient lies on a couch at their side. This may occur, but the psychodynamic model has many branches including some forms of family therapy, group therapies and art therapy (Tyrer and Steinberg 2005).

Common to all psychodynamic approaches is their primary focus on the ideas and feelings behind the words and actions that constitute human behaviour. Psychiatric disorders are not viewed as illnesses with disease-based aetiologies but as conflicts between different levels of mental functioning. Of critical importance are the conscious and unconscious levels. Substantial amounts of mental activity that occur beyond human awareness are believed to determine much of our behaviour. Human development is important in this respect since a person's early experiences can produce a particular *gestalt* or view of the person and their world, which they will take with them into adult life. This *gestalt* will include unconscious mental tricks and mechanisms to protect the person's sense of self. Problems may arise if a person's *gestalt*, that they necessarily cling to, is at odds with the real circumstances they find themselves in as adults. The psychodynamic therapist views psychological distress as the upshoots of unconscious thought (Tyrer and Steinberg 2005). This simple principle is central to most if not all psychodynamic therapies.

The founding father of the psychodynamic school was Sigmund Freud (1856–1939), a biological thinker interested primarily in an organism's attraction to pleasure and repulsion from pain. Application of the pain/pleasure continuum to the human mind and its development led Freud to divide mental life into the *id*, *ego* and *superego*.

The id represents basic primitive instincts, present at birth, which tend toward the pursuit of pleasure or gratification. As gratification is pursued people become aware also of an external reality separate from themselves and this realization necessitates the formulation of a self or ego. Others

in their world have helped shape the external reality in terms of laws, rules and social expectations. This realization leads to the development of the superego, which is more easily understood as a person's conscience. Psychological distress arises from struggles between the id, ego and superego, most of which take place in the unconscious. Freud's contemporaries and his followers have built subsequently upon his work to elaborate the psychodynamic school. Carl Jung (1875–1961) studied the great mythologies of the world, particularly their totems, ancient symbols, images and mythological motifs. He discovered that these primordial images, or *archetypes* as he called them, are common to all people. They do not belong to single individuals but are in fact transindividual or transcendent of the self and reside in the *collective unconscious*. Jungian therapists are therefore interested in people's key dreams and their symbolism with reference to ancient mythology. Knowing what mythological images have meant over time to the human race as a whole enables people to understand what the images may mean in their experience of the *collective unconscious*.

Melanie Klein's (1882–1960) work focused on the first two to three months of a child's life at a time when she believed the ego struggles to differentiate between itself and external reality. Unable to comprehend that good and bad can be present in the same object, the infant assumes the *paranoid position* in which all things are either good or bad but never both. When able to comprehend that these qualities do exist in a single object (e.g. both the mother's love and her chastisement) the infant moves to the *depressive position*. Therefore, in Kleinian terms, the experience and acceptance of depression is considered a maturational step necessary for personal growth (Tyrer and Steinberg 2005).

The influence of these early works on more contemporary psychodynamic therapies such as 'humanistic therapy', 'drama therapy', 'art therapy' and some forms of counselling is without doubt (Tyrer and Steinberg 2005). Equally, the psychodynamic tradition has influenced mental health nursing, particularly through the works of Hildegard Peplau and Annie Altschul (see Chapter 3).

The behavioural model

The behavioural model has a scientific basis in learning theory. Symptoms are considered to be learned habits arising from the interaction between external events or stressors and an individual's personality. Persistent, distressing symptoms are considered maladaptive responses rather than being markers for some underlying disease or illness. For the behaviour therapist the symptoms and their associated behaviours *are* the disorder (Tyrer and Steinberg 2005).

Learning theory posits that two forms of conditioning are responsible for the formation of symptoms: *classical* and *operant*. Classical conditioning refers to a neutral stimulus that becomes associated with an unrelated but established stimulus response sequence. Seminal experimental work in this area was conducted by the Russian physiologist Pavlov (1927) who conditioned dogs to salivate in response to a bell rather than to the established stimulus of food. Initially food was provided to the animals when a bell sounded. After several such trials the animals would salivate at the sound of the bell even when unaccompanied by food.

Operant conditioning results from behaviour rather than as the consequence of a stimulus. Skinner (1972) conducted seminal work in this field with a box in which one or more levers could be pressed. Rats would be placed in the box and through natural curiosity they would eventually press one or all of the levers. When the appropriate lever was pressed food would be deposited in the box. Gradually the rats would learn to continually press the appropriate lever until their appetites were satisfied. Thus it is not a neutral stimulus or the manipulation of an experimenter that conditioned the rats, but their own behaviour.

These theories provide a rationale for the development of some human behavioural problems. Take as a simple example a phobia or fear of spiders in a parent. It is possible that the children in this family will develop a similar fear since they have been subject to the classical conditioning of the parent. They may learn to avoid spiders, which can become self-perpetuating as their fear confirms the danger spiders pose, and their avoidance misses any opportunity to realize that spiders pose no threat.

The behaviour therapist helps people replace maladaptive responses with adaptive behaviour patterns. This is usually done by gradually removing the fear response through such techniques as graded exposure and systematic desensitization. The parent in our example may first be encouraged to imagine spiders, then view pictures of them in a book, followed by seeing them in a jar across the room, then holding the jar and finally holding the spider. Each of these stages will invoke a fear response but these will gradually subside if the person is supported to remain with the present situation.

An important part of behaviour therapy is the collaborative working partnership between client and therapist. The therapist does not view the person as abnormal or ill, but regards them as an equal partner in an unlearning, or new learning, process. This partnership is critical if the individual is to maintain and develop their new adaptive behaviours once therapy has finished. This approach to managing human behaviour has had a major influence on mental health nursing, for example, through the work of Isaac Marks (Marks *et al*. 1978) who, though not a nurse, has championed nurse behaviour therapists. Their contribution to health care has since been evaluated by Gournay *et al*. (2000).

The cognitive model

The cognitive model states that people interpret their thoughts, which in turn are the main determinants of behaviour (Tyrer and Steinberg 2005). This stands in sharp contrast to the behavioural or disease models, which do not include the cognitive mechanisms involved in behaviour and illness. For the cognitive therapist, primacy is given to errors or biases in thinking and it is these dysfunctional thought patterns that create mental disorders.

A key framework used by many cognitive therapists is the ABC model, first described by Ellis (1962): A 'activating event'; B 'beliefs'; C 'consequence'. A person who comes across a spider (activating event) may think it harmless or dangerous (beliefs) and will either continue their usual activity or be unable to do so (consequence). The client is encouraged to explore their thinking patterns and consider more appropriate and adaptive thoughts that fit the evidence. While the behavioural model would focus on the fear response, or consequence in the above example, the crux of the problem according to the cognitive model rests in the beliefs that people hold. Repetitive thoughts (ruminations) can lead to persistent actions (rituals), which can prevent normal functioning. Significant change in a person's mental health necessarily involves significant change in their cognitions (Tyrer and Steinberg 2005).

Though the reverse of the behavioural model, the two are rarely in conflict. Open, collaborative working partnerships are nurtured by respectful therapists and there is a long established discipline of cognitive behavioural therapy (CBT) that combines the two models.

The social model

The social model is concerned with the influence of social forces as the causes or precipitants of mental disorder. While the psychodynamic model is principally concerned with the individual and their personal relations, the social model focuses on the person in the context of their society as a whole (Tyrer and Steinberg 2005). Evidence that social forces are central to the aetiology of mental disorder can be traced to the work of Emile Durkheim (1897) who demonstrated that social factors, particularly isolation and the loss of social bonds, were predictive of suicide. We may be more familiar with associations between poor living circumstances in deprived geographical areas and the incidence of physical health problems. However, this relationship holds also for mental disorders, perhaps because the associated deprivation is usually accompanied by unemployment, loss of social role and a subsequent sense of alienation from mainstream society (Pilgrim and Rogers 2010).

At the heart of this model is the premise that people are prone to mental disturbance when unpleasant events strike them without warning. This led Holmes and Rahe (1967) to develop the Social Readjustment Rating Scale, which attributes a severity score to 42 life events according to the degree of change or adaptation they produce in people. Bereavement, divorce and starting a new job are high on the list. There is an intuitive appeal to the social model since many people are likely to have experienced major upheavals in their lives that may have caused them to feel psychological distress. Anxiety and low mood, for example, may be experienced in the run up to a series of exams or in response to the frustrations associated typically with moving house. The social model provides also a rationale for the origin of other types of psychological distress in which delusions, hallucinations and an apparent loss of contact with reality occur. Unexpected life events are associated with the onset of schizophrenia (Brown and Birley 1968) and the levels of critical 'expressed emotion' experienced by a person with schizophrenia from family members are predictive of the severity of the person's condition and, in particular, the likelihood of relapse (Falloon 1995).

Proponents of the social model do not have fixed ideas about what constitutes a psychiatric illness. The model is concerned that labelling people with a psychiatric illness may create a disorder itself (Tyrer and Steinberg 2005). All symptoms and behaviour have to be understood in the context of the society from which they emanate. There are no independent, objective criteria for mental disorder according to the social model, only a boundary line between normal and abnormal that has been set by society.

Supporters of the social model aim to help people take up an acceptable role in society once more, rather than to correct a chemical imbalance or recondition specific behaviours (Tyrer and Steinberg 2005). This may involve social skills training, some systemic family therapies and more general family interventions involving education on the influence of critical 'expressed emotion' (Gamble and Brennan 2006).

Integrating models of mental disorder

There are key features that differentiate each of the models according to the quadrant framework introduced in Chapter 1. For example, the disease model is concerned with physical, biological and chemical markers of mental disorder. These markers can be observed and measured, and are therefore representative of an *objective* orientation. In contrast, the cognitive model deals with internal thought processes unique to individuals. This orientation is therefore primarily *subjective*.

Additionally, the behavioural model is concerned with *a person's* behaviour, which is orientated to the *self*. In contrast, the social model is concerned not with *self* but with forces beyond a person's control in the society in which they live. This orientation is referred to as *community*. These two dimensions, *subjective–objective* and *self–community*, are used to formulate the quadrant framework (see Figure 2.1) with each of the models positioned in their respective quadrants.

The disease model, which is concerned with a person's biophysiological profile is upper right (*objective–self*). Similarly, the behavioural model, which deals with a person's observable behaviours is also upper right. The cognitive model however, is upper left (*subjective–self*) since its primary focus is on the internal thought processes of the individual.

Freudian psychodynamics are upper left (*subjective–self*), dealing as they do with our inner world and specifically our sense of self. However, Jungian psychodynamics are premised on a transcendent self, borne of intersubjective culture and mythology (community). For this reason they reside in the lower left quadrant (*subjective–community*). The social model is certainly community oriented but straddles both lower quadrants. Unemployment and poverty are quantifiable attributes, and each is associated with mental disorder. This interpretation of the social model reflects the lower right quadrant (*objective–community*). Intersubjective experiences such as kinship and expressed emotion are also associated with mental disorder; an interpretation that reflects the lower left quadrant (*subjective–community*).

Figure 2.1 illustrates the general orientation of different schools of thought in explaining the aetiology of mental disorder and points of comparison and contrast. But things are more complex than appear here, and there is certainly blurring

Figure 2.1 Framework for models of mental disorder

	Subjective	Objective
Self	Cognitive	Disease
	Freudian Psychodynamics	Behavioural
Community	Jungian Psychodynamics	
	Social	Social

across the quadrants. CBT is a good example, since cognitive therapists might argue that although they deal initially with unique internal thought processes, they endeavour to alter these with recourse to external, observable evidence (*objective–self*). Nevertheless, it remains true that they are primarily concerned with, and rooted in, a person's subjective experience. All models have something to contribute to our understanding of mental disorder precisely because human experience is made up of a subjective and objective sense of self and community.

We suggest, therefore, that the models of mental disorder considered here have many more points in common than difference because they each tap into a limited but, nevertheless, vital aspect of the human condition. Human experience arises from all the quadrants and mental health nurses need to draw on them all in their practice rather than discount some but not others on grounds of preference or prejudice.

The stress vulnerability model

An integrated, second-order model developed by Zubin and Spring (1977) to explain the aetiology of schizophrenia is used more widely now to understand the development of mental disorders. Incorporating all other models, it has as its common

Feedback to Thinking Space 2.1

Figure 2.1 provides one possible answer to questions 1 and 2 in the thinking space at the start of this chapter. Each model is briefly elaborated below to provide more detail on the possible causes of mental disorders (Question 1):

- disease model: genetic endowment, physiological/chemical changes and abnormalities;
- psychodynamic model: conflicts between different levels of mental functioning, upshoots of unconscious thought;
- behavioural model: learned habits and maladaptive responses;
- cognitive model: errors or biases in thinking that result in dysfunctional thought patterns;
- social model: influences of social forces and significant life events.

denominator the relationship between stress and vulnerability. Stress is the variable that influences the manifestation of symptoms and a person's vulnerability represents their predisposition to such manifestations.

There are two types of stress. The first is ambient stress and reflects the general concerns and pressures that people face in their everyday lives. Although such stressors are necessary to function and perform, some people experience more ambient stress than others. The second type of stress arises from life events such as those included in Holmes and Rahe's (1967) Social Readjustment Rating Scale. Similarly, there are two types of vulnerability. The first is inborn and will probably include genetic loading and the neurophysiology of the person. The second is acquired and will be specific to an individual's life experiences, but may include perinatal complications, maladaptive learned behaviours or thought patterns, and adolescent peer interactions (Zubin and Spring 1977). Notice that these descriptions include features from the single models previously described and can, therefore, be mapped according to the quadrants in Figure 2.1: for example, vulnerability can be upper left (thought patterns) or upper right (genetic loading) but also lower left (adolescent peer interactions).

Zubin and Spring's central hypothesis is that the interface between an individual's vulnerability and the stress they experience in the course of their lives is the basis for the development or otherwise of schizophrenic symptomatology. There will, of course, be a range of vulnerabilities in any population, with some people being extremely prone to illness even when experiencing relatively mild levels of stress, to those whose vulnerability is so low that they are able to tolerate high levels of stress for significant periods without any trace of psychiatric symptoms.

Since its publication in 1977 this model has had considerable impact in the field of mental health care. It offers hope to those who experience mental disorders because it suggests that coping mechanisms can be acquired to counter the effects of stress and thus reduce the risk of continued illness or relapse. The model is also of value to mental health staff, since it provides a rationale for the use of psychosocial as well as medicinal interventions, and nursing has been able to develop its psychosocial skills base as a result.

2.3 The classification of mental disorder

Systems for classifying mental disorder or 'illness' stem from the medical model, which as Tyrer and Steinberg (2005) point out is not an aetiological model itself but an approach to diagnosing individual disorder. In a general sense all the models apply this process, with the exception perhaps of the social model. For example, the cognitive model uses Ellis's (1962) ABC framework for defining specific cognitive problems that arise between an activating event and the behavioural or cognitive consequence. Problem-oriented statements can be constructed from such an analysis, which represent one approach to classification. For example, 'When I make eye contact with strangers in public (Activating event), I believe they immediately think bad of me (Belief), and therefore I avoid social interaction (Consequence).' This statement classifies a cognitive or behavioural problem depending on your perspective.

Medical diagnosis is another classification system, which represents the dominant frame of reference for most mental health workers internationally. These diagnoses are described in two classification systems – the *International Statistical Classification of Diseases and Related Health Problems* (ICD-10) (WHO 1992) and the *Diagnostic and Statistical Manual for Mental Disorders* (DSM-IV) (APA 1994). At the time of writing both systems are undergoing consultation and development. ICD-11 is scheduled for implementation in 2015 and is being designed in three formats – for primary care, specialist services and research. DSM-V is scheduled for publication in May 2013 with development news and preliminary draft revision available at www.dsm5.org.

ICD-10 diagnostic categories

ICD-10 is the dominant frame of reference in the UK. Table 2.1 presents the main diagnostic groupings together with their key features. The table presents an overview and readers are referred to subsequent chapters for more detailed accounts of many of these conditions.

Psychoses and neuroses

The terms 'psychoses' and 'neuroses' are second-order classifications that group several of the conditions in Table 2.1. The psychoses are disorders in which people's capacity to recognize reality, their thinking processes, judgements and communications are seriously impaired, together with the presence of delusions and hallucinations (Craig 2006). In turn, these are divided into 'organic' and 'functional' psychoses. The former are represented by the group F00–F09 in Table 2.1 in which pathological processes affecting the brain result in psychotic symptoms. The functional psychoses are group F20–F29 and include schizophrenia and delusional disorders but also affective psychoses in which a primary disturbance of mood is accompanied by psychotic symptoms. In keeping with the hierarchical nature of diagnosis, any disorder in the F30–F39 group that incorporates psychotic symptoms will be elevated to a diagnosis within the F20–F29 group.

Individuals who experience neuroses are different from the general population only in the degree of the symptoms they experience. Thus, anxiety and low mood are common to people's experience of life. Indeed anxiety needs to be present to some degree before an important exam in order to enhance performance. However, if this anxiety becomes so great that it debilitates an individual, this may indicate a mental health problem. In contrast to the psychoses, in which a person's grasp of reality is uncertain, the neuroses are characterized by the heightening of normal human experiences but to levels that interfere with a person's ability to function. The neuroses are represented by groups F30–F39 and F40–F48 in Table 2.1.

A group that falls outside of the psychoses/neuroses divide are the personality disorders represented by F60–F69. Personality is a familiar concept and one that people use to describe friends and colleagues. We might say that someone is always cheerful or shy. However, the personality disorders contained in F60–F69 are indicative of habitual behaviours that lead people into conflict with society. These deeply ingrained maladaptive behavioural patterns have been classified into different types of personality disorder including obsessive, avoidant, schizoid, paranoid, borderline, antisocial, dependent, schizotypal, histrionic and narcissistic (WHO 1992).

Table 2.1 ICD-10 classification of mental and behavioural disorders (adapted from WHO 1992 and Tyrer and Steinberg 2005)

Diagnostic groupings	Key features
F00–F09	
Organic mental disorders including dementias and delirium	Brain dysfunction resulting in disturbances of cognition, mood, perception and/or behaviour
F10–F19	
Psychoactive substance use including intoxication, abuse, dependence and withdrawal states	Typically present when substance use interferes with a person's physical, mental or social functioning to the detriment of their well-being
F20–F29	
Schizophrenia, schizotypal, delusional and schizoaffective disorders	Mental states characterized by distortions of thinking, perception and mood, but not due to an organic condition
F30–F39	
Mood (affective) disorders including depression, manic disorder and bipolar disorders	The key symptom is a disturbance in mood though other features will also be present associated with this mood change, for example social isolation accompanying depression
F40–F48	
Neurotic, stress-related and somatoform disorders including phobias, obsessive compulsive disorder and stress reactions	A range of symptoms may be present including tension, anxiety, problems with concentration and ritualistic behaviours
F50–F59	
Behavioural syndromes including eating disorders, sleep disorders and post-partum mental disorders	Symptoms vary according to the condition, for example weight loss with certain eating disorders. However, physiological and hormonal factors appear to play a part in these conditions
F60–F69	
Disorders of adult personality and behaviour including personality disorders, gender identity disorders and impulse disorders	Disorders in which clinically significant behaviour patterns are persistent and reflect the person's lifestyle and way of interacting with others
F70–F79	
Mental retardation of varying degrees from mild to profound	Usually manifest by the impairment of skills associated with intelligence
F80–F89	
Disorders of psychological development including autism, speech disorders, disorders in scholastic skills and developmental disorders of motor functions	Originating in infancy or childhood these disorders delay the development of functions related to maturation of the central nervous system
F90–F98	
Behavioural and emotional disorders of childhood including conduct disorders and hyperkinetic disorders	Only common features are an onset early in life and a fluctuating or unpredictable course

Thinking Space 2.2

Psychiatric diagnoses provide a succinct way of classifying the mental health difficulties that people experience and for organizing services. However, what might be the disadvantages of such an approach particularly for those of us who receive a diagnosis? Take a few minutes to critique the use of psychiatric diagnoses, listing the potential pitfalls you can envisage.

2.4 Key symptoms of mental disorder

The key symptoms of mental disorder are typically classified according to their impact on a person's mood, thought processes, perceptions and behaviour.

Mood
Anxiety
Anxiety is distinguished from general tension by its accompanying physical sensations (autonomic nervous system arousal), including palpitations, sweating and tremor. Anxiety may occur in response to phobic situations or specific thoughts but can also occur independently of any such trigger (free-floating anxiety), or be linked to a sense that something dreadful is about to occur (anxious foreboding) (Craig 2000). Anxiety may also occur abruptly for short periods during which the person experiences marked fearfulness and may feel they are losing control (panic attacks).

Depression
'Sad', 'gloomy' and 'low spirits' are synonymous with depressed mood. More severe forms of this experience encompass additional features including a reduced emotional response to the ups and downs of life (flattened or blunted affect). The individual may also experience disturbed sleep patterns, loss of appetite and a lack of interest in and engagement with life. More extreme forms of this experience can be accompanied by feelings of hopelessness, possibly leading to suicidal thoughts. Other terms associated with this experience include *self-deprecation* (loss of confidence in self and a developing sense of worthlessness) and *pathological guilt* (feeling responsible for actions that may be inconsequential to others).

Elation
Individuals who experience elation in the course of a mental health problem may feel euphoric and excited but also irritable and impatient (Craig 2000). Typically, concentration is impaired, there is over-talkativeness, a reduced need for sleep and reckless acts are not uncommon – for example, excessive spending sprees. Common to these symptoms is an underlying self-esteem that is exaggerated, and grandiose beliefs, such as having special intelligence, are not uncommon.

Thought processes
Obsessional thoughts and compulsions
A person's thoughts are considered obsessional when they become intrusive, unwanted and no longer amenable to self-control (obsessional ruminations). *Obsessional incompleteness* refers to an overriding desire to ensure every aspect of a task has been correctly executed before the individual can consider it complete. Intrusive thoughts of this type may be accompanied by repetitive, *ritualistic behaviour*. An important feature that distinguishes these types of thought is the person's awareness that they are their own.

Delusions
A delusion is a false impression or belief that we can all be subject to from time to time. In the mental health field, additional qualities associated with delusional thought distinguish it as a symptom of mental disorder. The belief is usually held with absolute and compelling conviction, and is typically idiosyncratic and resistant to modification through experience or discussion (Craig 2000). Different types of

delusion have been classified including *delusions of persecution* and *delusions of reference*. The latter often involves people feeling that news items on the TV, radio or in newspapers have a double meaning and make reference specifically to them.

Thought possession

Some people with mental health problems encounter the sensation that the innermost workings of their mind are amenable to outsiders (Craig 2000). Different sorts of experience have been described including *thought broadcasting* (a person believes that their thoughts are heard aloud by those around them), and *thought insertion* (a loss in the ownership of a person's own thoughts, usually accompanied by a delusional explanation for how thoughts are placed in their mind).

Perceptions

Perception among people who experience mental health problems can become diminished, heightened or distorted (Craig 2000). Hallucinations are a key symptom in this respect, which are defined as false perceptions in so far as there is no adequate external stimulus for the experience. Each of the five human senses can be affected by hallucinations. Thus, hallucinations are typically referred to as auditory, visual, olfactory, tactile and gustatory.

Behaviour

The behaviour and appearance of people with mental disorders may appear strange or unusual. A lack of self-care and accompanying self-neglect are not uncommon, but neither are they necessarily an indication of mental disorder. The specific patterns and qualities of a person's speech are more useful indicators of a mental disorder. Symptoms may include *pressure of speech* (a rush of words that is difficult to stop), *flight of ideas* (skipping from topic to topic with no logical association), and *poverty of speech* (speaking freely but in such a vague manner that no meaningful information is communicated).

2.5 Prevalence and incidence of mental disorders

Prevalence, expressed as a percentage, refers to the number of people with a particular disorder within a given population. Incidence, also expressed as a percentage, refers to the number of new cases that arise within a given population in a given time period. Actual estimates of prevalence and incidence of mental disorders vary from one epidemiological study to the next. Different samples will have been studied and there may be real differences between populations. Additionally, different instruments might have been used and their results may have been interpreted in different ways to define a 'case'.

There have been three national surveys of treated and untreated psychiatric disorder in the UK. The first two, in 1993 and 2000, covered England, Scotland and Wales. The most recent provides 2007 prevalence data for the English adult population aged 16 and above (McManus *et al.* 2009). This section draws on the most recent data, which includes comparisons with the two earlier surveys, along with work from the Mental Health Foundation (MHF 2005, 2007) that collates evidence on the prevalence of mental health problems from various sources.

- Approximately 1 in 4 people will experience some kind of mental health problem in the course of a year. Most recent data for England estimate this to be 23 per cent with 7.2 per cent of the population having two or more disorders.

- Common mental disorders (CMDs) include different types of depression and anxiety. Overall, the proportion of people aged 16–64 meeting the criteria for at least one CMD increased between 1993 and 2000, but did not change between 2000 and 2007 (15.5 per cent in 1993, 17.5 per cent in 2000, 17.6 per cent in 2007). In 2007 women were more likely than men to have a CMD (19.7 per cent and 12.5 per cent respectively), and the largest increase in rate of CMD between 1993 and 2007 was observed in women aged 45–64, among whom the rate rose by about a fifth. Somewhere between 1 in 4 and 1 in 6 people will have serious depression at some stage in their lives. Clinical depression is second only to coronary heart disease in terms of international health burden. One in 10 people will have a disabling anxiety disorder at some stage in their lives. This may be a general anxiety mental health problem or a more specific phobia or obsessive compulsive disorder. Most neuroses last under one year, although there is a strong chance of recurrence.

■ Psychoses are less common. In 2007 the overall prevalence of psychotic disorder in the past year was 0.4 per cent (0.3 per cent of men,0.5 per cent of women). In both men and women the highest prevalence was observed in those aged 35 to 44 years (0.7 per cent and 1.1 per cent respectively). There was no change in the overall prevalence of probable psychosis between the 2000 and 2007 surveys: 1 in 100 people will suffer from bipolar illness and 1 in 100 from schizophrenia at some stage in their lives. Between a quarter and a half of people recover completely after a psychosis. Most people have multiple 'acute' episodes but only a minority of these have systematically reduced psychological function between episodes. An estimated 10–15 per cent of people with schizophrenia develop severe long-term disabilities.

■ Eating disorders are often not recognized or reported and studies may underestimate prevalence. In 2007 6.4 per cent of adults screened positive for an eating disorder of which 1.6 per cent also reported that their feelings about food had a significant negative impact on their life. At 9.2 per cent, women were more likely than men (3.5 per cent) to screen positive for an eating disorder and prevalence decreases with age. One woman in 5 (20.3 per cent) age 16–24 screened positive, compared with 1 woman in 100 (0.9 per cent) aged 75 and over.

■ The 2007 survey included antisocial and borderline personality disorders (ASPD, BPD). ASPD was present in 0.3 per cent of adults aged 18 or over (0.6 per cent of men and 0.1 per cent of women). The overall prevalence of BPD was similar to that of ASPD, at 0.4 per cent of adults aged 16 or over. There was no significant difference in ASPD or BPD prevalence between the 2000 and 2007 surveys.

■ About 5,000 people a year in the UK take their own lives, usually as a result of mental ill health especially, of course, clinical depression. In 2007 16.7 per cent of people reported that they had thought about committing suicide, 5.6 per cent had attempted suicide and 4.9 per cent had engaged in self-harm. The proportion of women reporting suicidal thoughts in the previous year had increased between the 2000 and 2007 surveys. An increase was also found in the proportion of people who reported self-harm, particularly among women aged 16–24.

■ Problems with drinking alcohol are common. In 2007 the prevalence of alcohol dependence was 5.9 per cent (8.7 per cent of men, 3.3 per cent of women). The highest levels of dependence were identified in men between the ages of 25 and 34 (16.8 per cent), and in women between the ages of 16 and 24 (9.8 per cent). The prevalence of alcohol dependence was lower for men in 2007 than in 2000 but had remained at a similar level among women.

■ In 2007, the prevalence of drug use in the last year was 9.2 per cent (12.0 per cent of men, 6.7 per cent of women). Most people who had taken drugs in the last year had used cannabis. Drug dependence prevalence was 3.4 per cent (4.5 per cent of men, 2.3 per cent of women). Symptoms of dependence were most commonly reported by adults aged between 16 and 24 (13.3 per cent of men, 7.0 per cent of women in this age group). The prevalence of drug dependence had been higher in 2000 than in 1993 but has not changed significantly since then.

- In 2007 approximately two-thirds (65.9 per cent) of adults spent money on a gambling activity in the previous year. Men were more likely than women to gamble. Among adults, 3.2 per cent met one or more of the criteria for problem gambling.

- Mental health problems in children and young people are also common. Studies have shown that 10 per cent of children and young people require specialist help and 1 in 5 have psychiatric symptoms at any one time. Anxiety, depression, hyperactivity and conduct disorder are the most common mental health problems. Estimates of prevalence vary widely because of different definitions and the high level of hidden morbidity.

- Common mental health problems affect older people but may go unrecognized or untreated. Dementia affects 1 per cent of people aged 60–65, 5 per cent of those over 65 and perhaps as many as 20 per cent of those aged over 80. One in 1,000 people under 65 have Alzheimer's disease (the most common form of dementia).

Mental health problems do not affect all groups of people equally. Different factors are particularly associated with different conditions. However, it must be recognized that association is not the same as causality. Epidemiological studies have found the following associations.

- **Isolation:** people with a neurosis and more markedly people with a psychosis are more likely than the general population to be separated or divorced and/or to live in a one-person family unit.

- **Social class:** people with a probable psychosis are more likely to be defined as being in social classes IV or V.

- **Unemployment:** 39 per cent of people with a neurosis and 70 per cent with a psychosis were found to be economically inactive compared to 28 per cent with no disorder.

- **Social deprivation:** there are clear associations between social deprivation (e.g. poor housing/homelessness, employment and education) and mental illness. The Department of Health's (DH) psychiatric needs index shows a four-fold variation in need between the most affluent local authorities and the most deprived. Many authors argue that the variation in need is even greater for the most severe mental health problems.

- **Physical ill health:** 57 per cent of people with a neurosis and 62 per cent with a psychosis reported having a physical complaint, compared to 38 per cent of those with no mental health problem.

- **Ethnicity:** in 2007 there was little variation between white, black and South Asian men in the rates of any CMD. However, in women all CMDs (except phobias) were more prevalent in the South Asian group. For psychotic disorders these were significantly higher among black men (3.1 per cent) than men from other ethnic groups (0.2 per cent of white men, no cases observed among men in the South Asian or 'other' ethnic group). The prevalence of psychosis among black African and African-Caribbean men is a much contested area of research and practice. Whatever the underlying issues it is clear that black men are considerably over-represented in secure settings and detentions under the Mental Health Act. Many authors have argued that the cause is institutional racism, although this is seldom seen as the only factor and interventions coming too late in the development of problems are also a major concern.

- **Criminal Justice System:** all forms of contact with the police, courts, prison and probation system are associated with high prevalence rates of mental health problems. For example, 56 per cent of sentenced women and 37 per cent of sentenced men are considered to have a psychiatric disorder. The prevalence of mental health problems is higher for remand prisoners.

2.6 Conclusion

Various models of mental disorder have been described, each of which taps into different aspects of the human condition. We have emphasized the importance of mental health nurses embracing an integrated understanding of human experience, through which all models have something to contribute. From this position the profession is better placed to provide holistic, integrated care by either broadening its own perspective, or by working with others who possess complementary specialist knowledge. The profession needs also to develop a theoretical and practical understanding of mental health and well-being (see Chapters 1 and 4). The combined evidence base will enable the profession to fully realize the contributions it can make to the well-being and recovery of people who experience a mental disorder. To conclude, we summarize the main points of this chapter below:

■ Mental disorders represent shades in the spectrum of human experience, which comprise a subjective and objective sense of self and a subjective and objective sense of community.

■ Models of mental disorder describe aetiology and treatment implications in relation to different levels of human functioning: biophysiological organism (disease); the unconscious (psychodynamic); thought processes (cognitive); actions (behavioural); and self in context (social).

■ The models can be mapped against a quadrant framework of human experience (Figure 2.1), demonstrating their partial, though necessary contribution to the treatment and care of people who experience mental disorders.

■ Mental health nurses need to develop an integrated understanding of mental disorders, to be demonstrated in collaborative partnerships with service users and professional colleagues.

■ The profession needs also to integrate considerations for mental health and well-being into its practice in order to promote comprehensive services to the whole person.

Feedback to Thinking Space 2.2

We have grouped a number of problems or disadvantages with the use of psychiatric diagnoses under three headings.

■ **Labelling:** there is a risk that people are understood simply in terms of their diagnoses and the stereotypes associated with those labels (e.g. 'Mr Brown is a schizophrenic'). Where psychiatric diagnoses are used by nursing staff they should be employed as an adjunct to any description of the person (e.g. 'Mr Brown is a 47-year -old man with a diagnosis of schizophrenia'). We believe this to be true of all medical diagnoses (e.g. 'Mrs White was diagnosed with type II diabetes six months ago', rather than 'Mrs White has been a diabetic for six months').

■ **Depersonalization:** closely related to labelling is the risk of depersonalization. If people are reduced to a collection of symptoms and their associated psychiatric diagnoses then this can obscure our understanding of the whole person and limits our potential to help them in ways that are meaningful to the person. This argument has been instrumental in the development of recovery-orientated practice in which the whole person is supported to grow and develop within and beyond the perceived limitations of their condition or diagnosis (see Chapter 5).

■ **The myth of mental illness:** a consistent critique of modern psychiatry over the past 50 years is that the discipline rests on a basic conceptual error – i.e. the systematic misinterpretation of human behaviour into diagnoses of mental illnesses susceptible to pharmacological treatments. A leading proponent of this school of thought, often referred to as 'anti-psychiatry', is Thomas Szasz, who argues that the claim that mental illnesses are diagnosable disorders of the brain is not based on scientific research but is a deception to benefit the standing of psychiatrists and the pharmacological industry (Szasz 2011). For Szasz the use of psychiatric diagnoses means that mental hospitals can be more like prisons, that involuntary hospitalization is a type of imprisonment and that coercive psychiatrists operate more as judges and jailors than as physicians and healers. Szasz considers so-called 'mental patients' as active players in real-life dramas rather than passive victims of psychopathological processes beyond their control, and for this reason does not view their circumstances as being matters for medicine, treatment or science.

Annotated bibliography

Tyrer, P. and Steinberg, D. (2005) *Models for Mental Disorder: Conceptual models in psychiatry*, 4th edn. Chichester: John Wiley & Sons.
Now in its fourth edition, this text provides a detailed yet accessible explanation of the main models of mental disorder in contemporary practice. We have adopted Tyrer and Steinberg's five basic model structure in this chapter but have pursued a different path to integration. However, we recommend also Tyrer and Steinberg's approach, which in this latest edition includes chapters on integration and application of the models in multi-disciplinary teams.

Gamble, C. and Brennan, G. (eds) (2006) *Working With Serious Mental Illness: A manual for clinical practice*, 2nd edn. London: Elsevier.
Though primarily a practice manual as the title suggests, this text devotes a chapter to the stress vulnerability model and a section, comprising eight chapters, to interventions based on a stress vulnerability understanding of serious mental illness. This has been a highly successful text for mental health nurses and is now in its second edition.

MHF (Mental Health Foundation) (2007) *The Fundamental Facts*. London: MHF.
This is an invaluable resource that provides a round-up of information on the prevalence and incidence of mental health problems. It also contains an overview of service provision in the UK and of the costs of mental health problems to the nation.

References

APA (American Psychiatric Association) (1994) *Diagnostic and Statistical Manual for Mental Disorders*, 4th revision. Washington: APA.
Brown, G. and Birley, J. (1968) Crises and life events and the onset of schizophrenia, *Journal of Health and Social Behaviour*, 9: 203–14.
Craig, T. (2006) Severe mental illness: symptoms, signs and diagnosis, in C. Gamble and G. Brennan (eds) *Working with Serious Mental Illness: A manual for clinical practice*, 2nd edn. London: Elsevier.
Durkheim, E. (1897) *Le Suicide*. Paris: Alcan.
Ellis, A. (1962) *Reason and Emotion in Psychotherapy*. New York: Stuart.
Falloon, I. (1995) *Family Management of Schizophrenia*. Baltimore, MD: Johns Hopkins University Press.
Gamble, C. and Brennan, G. (2006) *Working with Serious Mental Illness: A manual for clinical practice*, 2nd edn. London: Elsevier.
Gournay, K., Denford, L., Parr, A.-M. and Newell, R. (2000) British nurses in behavioural psychotherapy: a 25-year follow up, *Journal of Advanced Nursing*, 32: 1–9.
Holmes, T. and Rahe, R. (1967) The Social Readjustment Rating Scale, *Journal of Psychosomatic Research*, 11: 213–18.
Marks, I., Bird, J. and Lindley, P. (1978) Behavioural nurse therapists: developments and implications, *Behavioural Psychotherapy*, 6: 25–6.
McManus, S., Meltzer, H., Brugha, T., Bebbington, P. and Jenkins, R. (2009) *Adult Psychiatric Morbidity in England, 2007: Results of a household survey*, available at: www.ic.nhs.uk/pubs/psychiatricmorbidity07, accessed 12 April 2012.
MHF (Mental Health Foundation) (2005) *Lifetime Impacts*. London: MHF.
MHF (Mental Health Foundation) (2007) *The Fundamental Facts*. London: MHF.
Pavlov, I. (1927) *Conditioned Reeves*. London: Oxford University Press.

Pilgrim, D. and Rogers, A. (2010) *A Sociology of Mental Health and Illness*, 4th edn. Maidenhead: Open University Press.

Plant, J. and Stephenson, J. (2008) *Beating Stress, Anxiety and Depression*. London: Piatkus Books.

Scadding, J. (1967) Diagnosis: the clinician and the computer, *Lancet*, ii: 877–82.

Skinner, B. (1972) *Beyond Freedom and Dignity*. London: Jonathan Cape.

Szasz, T. (2011) The myth of mental illness: 50 years later, *The Psychiatrist*, 35: 179–82.

Tyrer, P. and Steinberg, D. (2005) *Models for Mental Disorder: Conceptual models in psychiatry*, 4th edn. Chichester: John Wiley & Sons.

WHO (World Health Organization) (1992) *International Statistical Classification of Diseases and Related Health Problems*, 10th edn. Geneva: WHO.

Zubin, J. and Spring, B. (1977) Vulnerability – a new view of schizophrenia, *Journal of Abnormal Psychology*, 86: 103–26.

FOUNDATIONS

Mental Health Nursing: an Art and a Science

Ian Norman and Iain Ryrie

I came to realize that it was only because of the nursing input that any of the treatments were effective at all. Pills sent by post will not do any good at all. Physical treatments for mental illness, given where the patient has trust in the doctor and where hope is given, will allay some symptoms, but the help given to re-engage with social life and find some contentment only comes from the nursing contribution.

Felicity Stockwell, retired mental health nurse and tutor, reflecting on her period as
ward sister in an acute psychiatric ward in 1959 (Stockwell 2009).

 ## 3.1 Introduction

This chapter provides a historical perspective on the practice of mental health nursing, upon which nurses and other mental health care workers of the future must build. The first part traces the origins of mental health nursing from the eighteenth century to the present day and outlines recent influences on its development. The second part traces the history of mental health nursing as an academic and practice discipline and the origins of the profession in two traditions; what we refer to as the interpersonal relations tradition (the art of mental health nursing) and the evidenced-based health care tradition (the science). We see today reconciliation between the

artistic and scientific traditions of mental health nursing as the focus of mental health policy turns to promoting core values which support recovery oriented practice.

In summary this chapter covers:

- the origins of mental health nursing;
- the decline of the old mental hospitals and the development of a community-based service;
- UK government reviews of mental health nursing;
- the 'interpersonal relations' and 'evidence-based practice' traditions within mental health nursing;
- fusion of these traditions within contemporary nursing practice.

3.2   Origins

Eighteenth and nineteenth centuries

Throughout the ages people with mental disorder have been the recipients of various forms of care and control. From the twelfth century, the asylum provided a setting for such care, although the importance of the asylum system grew from the late seventeenth century under the influence of the intellectual tradition of the Enlightenment. Notable pioneers were Philippe Pinel in France and the Quaker William Tuke in England who, almost simultaneously, but independently, introduced reforms that unchained the lunatics, and turned the asylums into havens for the insane.

Tuke founded the Retreat at York in 1792 on principles of 'moral treatment'. Tuke believed madness and deranged behaviour to stem from the mode of service provision in eighteenth-century 'madhouses' where 'lunatics' suffered degradation, repression and cruelty. Scull (1981) wrote about care of mentally ill people before the nineteenth century as being a way of solving society's difficulty in knowing how to handle socially disadvantaged groups. Tuke replaced physical constraints with moral constraints based on reason, supported by purposeful work and social and educational activities in a normal domestic environment. The 'moral therapists' challenged medical dominance in the treatment of the insane, arguing that medicine had abused care, and medical treatment was unnecessary in moral therapy because carers were selected for their attitude and personality. The moralists considered the newly industrialized society to be the source of mental instability and that cure could be found in calm, productive, non-competitive communities (Scull 1981). The asylum attendants in the Retreat and other similar communities were the first official care agents, and are often regarded as the predecessors of the mental health nurse.

The moral therapy movement marked the start of changing social attitudes towards the insane, which by the first half of the nineteenth century were influenced by a growing social conscience based on a belief that the community had a responsibility to the weak. This found expression in the Lunatics Act 1845, which was a major achievement of the work of the Earl of Shaftesbury, as was the construction of a number of Victorian asylums. Changing attitudes to the insane had implications for the role of 'lunatic attendants' who, by the mid-nineteenth century, were expected to set a positive example to patients and to offer them guidance rather than simply be custodians. But it was difficult to recruit attendants of the right type. Dr Browne, writing in 1897 of male attendants, described them as 'the unemployable of other professions ... if they possess physical strength and a tolerable reputation for sobriety, it is enough; and the latter is frequently dispensed with' (cited by Connolly 1992: 7). According to Connolly, women attendants of the right type were easier to recruit than men because nursing was widely perceived to be in women's nature.

These recruitment problems are not surprising when one considers working conditions of the time, which were very poor. Records from Springfield Hospital in Tooting, London (then the Surrey Lunatic Asylum) referred to by Connolly, show that in 1842 attendants worked from 6.00 a.m. until 9.00 p.m. and slept in rooms adjacent to the wards. There were nine male and nine female attendants for 350 patients. In a report to Visiting Justices that year, attendants were described as 'the instruments for carrying into effect every remedial measure', the work requiring 'firmness and self control blended with humanity and forbearance' and involving 'many menial offices'. For this, male attendants working in the Surrey Asylum received between £25 and £30 per year. This compared well with the national average salary of male attendants, which was £26 per year. But attendants were among the lowest paid people in the country, and female attendants were paid substantially less than their male counterparts.

Given the developing role of the asylum attendant beyond a purely custodial function, a number of medical superintendents became convinced of the need for some sort of education and training for attendants. The first course of lectures for attendants was probably given by Alexander Morrison, the Surrey Lunatic Asylum's medical superintendent in 1843. This course served as a stimulus for the spread of similar courses of instruction, which culminated in publication of the *Handbook for Instruction of*

Attendants on the Insane by the Royal Medico-Psychological Association (RMPA) – the 'Red Handbook' – which became a standard text. By 1889, 100 hospitals offered programmes of instruction based on the Red Handbook and in 1890 the RMPA established the first register for attendants who had completed successfully a two-year training programme. Thus, mental health nursing as a practice discipline represented by qualification is just over 120 years old.

In spite of these positive developments it would be incorrect to interpret the history of mental health nursing as one of progressive improvement in the conditions for patients and their carers in the asylums. Moral treatment, which had heralded positive changes in social attitudes to the insane and the notion of attendants as therapeutic agents, lasted only 50 years in Great Britain because a growing number of patients gradually outstripped the human resource to provide moral treatment to an adequate standard. By the mid-nineteenth century asylums were being built for thousands at a time to, in effect, warehouse madness. These institutions quickly became overcrowded: for example, by 1909 the number of patients in the Surrey Asylum, built originally for 350, had risen to 1,235. Bureaucratic organization of patients' lives based on rigid doctor, nurse, patient hierarchies became the norm and attendants were once again relied upon for strength and intimidation, rather than friendliness and common sense.

The beginning of the nineteenth century also marked the start of a shifting and often uneasy relationship between mental health and general nursing, which continues to the present day. The British Nursing Association (later the Royal British Nursing Association – RBNA) founded for general nurses in 1887 refused entry to the nursing register to graduates of the RMPA register for attendants. Mrs Bedford-Fenwick, the RBNA president, set out the reasons for this in 1895 when she pointed to the narrow training received by asylum attendants and concerns about the possible effects of admission on nurses' social status:

No person can be considered trained who has only worked in hospitals and asylums for

the insane ... considering the present class of persons known as male attendants, one can hardly believe that their admission will tend to raise the status of the Association.

(Adams 1969: 13, cited by Connolly 1992: 9)

The College of Nursing (eventually to become the Royal College), which was established in 1916, maintained the stance taken by the RBNA by continuing to refuse admission to registered attendants. However, the later established General Nursing Council (GNC) started its own course and examination for attendants, thereby introducing an alternative qualification.

Connolly (1992) points out that the drive for equal status with general nursing was spearheaded by medical superintendents and senior attendants, and was of little concern to rank and file asylum attendants who, through the National Asylum Workers' Union, were concerned to improve conditions of service and pay, but were not concerned with status or professionalism for many years. Moreover, qualifications were not a requirement for a senior position in an asylum and many asylum matrons had general nursing training only and no experience of asylum work.

Twentieth century

The first half of the twentieth century was marked by renewed optimism in psychiatry. In the inter-war period nomenclature changed, asylums became mental hospitals, male and female attendants became nurses, and the management of mental health was incorporated into the National Health Service (NHS), so providing free care as a right of citizenship. However, mental hospitals remained overcrowded, particularly during both world wars when many staff members were enlisted in the forces or redeployed, so that patients had to be redistributed. Thus the main role of the mental nurses during the first half of the twentieth century remained containment and management of large numbers of patients in overcrowded conditions.

During the early twentieth century, allegations of malpractice rose sharply with nurses being the main target for criticism. Such allegations led to calls for a Royal Commission into Lunacy Laws which was established in 1926 and led in turn to the Mental Treatment Act 1930. This Act introduced categories of 'voluntary' and 'temporary' patients, which avoided the pessimistic experience of certification for some patients. The category of 'voluntary patient' was extended and by 1957 this group constituted 75 per cent of admissions. However, admission procedures and rights of patients remained unchanged until the Mental Health Act 1959, which, as Connolly (1992) points out, marked the end of the power of magistrates over the asylum system and a regaining of control by mental health professionals.

During the 1930s many men from depressed areas of the country entered mental health nursing. Ideal entry requirements for nurses from this period into the 1950s were that they should be physically fit, able to take part in organized games or play a musical instrument – criteria that contributed to active sporting and community activities within and between asylums, but did little to improve standards of patient care. While mental nurses were expected to show kindness and forbearance towards patients and set them a good example, asylum regulations in the early twentieth century governing the conduct of staff were strict and gave little opportunity for the exercise of responsibility or common sense – as envisaged by advocates of moral treatment so many years before.

From Connolly's account, mental nurses of the time, with their general nursing counterparts, were much preoccupied by cleanliness and orderliness to the extent that beds would be lined up with pieces of string to ensure regularity. Task allocation was the dominant form of work organization and time periods were set aside for these tasks to be accomplished – such as bed making and mealtimes, when staff and patients would eat together in the wards. Nursing work was varied, with an emphasis on organizing patients' work: in the wards (e.g. cleaning and maintaining the wards, cleaning or feeding other patients), on the farm, in the hospital grounds (e.g. rolling the cricket pitch) or in the laundry or tailor's shop where they would make and maintain clothing and bedding. In spite of the emphasis on constructive activity for patients, little was done to prepare them for return to the world outside hospital.

3.3 Psychiatric hospitals in decline

The community had long been considered a brutalizing environment for people with mental health problems (Wing 1990), but in the 1960s a number of factors combined to make it an increasingly attractive care location for local authorities and the government. These factors included:

- gross overcrowding of hospitals, the population of which had reached 150,000 by the mid-1950s, which was more than the buildings could satisfactorily accommodate;
- crumbling building stock which required expensive repairs and most of which was unsuitably located to serve the major centres of population;
- escalating NHS labour costs, particularly in the 1960s following substantial pay increases for mental health nurses after successful trade union campaigns;
- the majority view that new drugs offered a genuine opportunity for the control of symptoms and, in some cases, cure; and
- the Mental Health Act 1959, which placed a strong emphasis on community involvement in psychiatric care services.

The shift away from the old hospitals to a community-based service was accelerated by other factors, in particular the diminishing power-base of the physician superintendents in the hospitals, which was undermined by new consultant psychiatrists created within the new NHS. The power-base of the consultant psychiatrists was strengthened by the transfer of services such as radiography, pathology and surgery, formerly provided within the mental hospitals, to purpose-built general hospitals. Moreover, the consultants were empowered by new drugs on the market, and were free to select their own treatments independent of the physician superintendents' views. Eventually, in 1960, the post of physician superintendent was declared obsolete.

With the demise of physician superintendents, and the change in the philosophy of psychiatric care away from manual labour and towards therapeutic relationships and environments, the psychiatric hospitals began to change. Wards were unlocked, military-type uniforms (brass buttons, peaked caps) for male nurses were abandoned in favour of white coats, hospital farms which had once provided employment and income were run down and sold off, and ancillary staff were employed to carry out the manual tasks once carried out by nurses and patients.

The influence of the anti-psychiatry movement was, in the 1960s, at its peak. Leading figures in the movement – Laing, Szasz, Sedgewick and Foucault – came from very different philosophical and political positions but were united in their mistrust and scepticism of orthodox psychiatry. Anti-psychiatry saw psychiatry as performing a role of social control and so it could not claim to be a branch of medicine or a respectable science. The anti-psychiatrists were criticized for underestimating the effectiveness of modern psychiatry in diagnosing and treating mental illness and for overestimating its control function. However, their ideas were influential in drawing attention to the coercive aspects of psychiatry in which nurses were perceived to be front-line agents of social control.

Criticism from the anti-psychiatry movement was supported by growing evidence about the effects of institutional life on patients. The structure and organization of traditional hospitals was gradually seen to be pathogenic as the new therapeutic regimes at the Cassel, Claybury and Fulbourne hospitals demonstrated the benefits of an 'open-door policy' and a partnership approach to care between staff and patients.

Goffman's *Asylums* (1961) is a landmark in the history of care of the mentally ill and of the anti-psychiatry movement. His attack on the 'total institution' in the USA, with its emphasis on block treatment, denial of individuality and social distance between staff and patients, caused the USA and the UK to rethink institutional care. Other critics in Britain were also condemning conditions in mental hospitals at the time (e.g. Barton 1959; Townsend 1962). Nurses who ran the hospitals felt powerless to respond because they had no decision-making power (Nolan 1993).

The final blow to the mental hospital system came from a series of psychiatric hospital scandals and public inquiries in the 1960s and 1970s that exposed professional neglect and suffering of mentally ill patients, and that seriously weakened psychiatric nursing. In 1961 Enoch Powell, the then Minister of Health, declared that mental hospitals must close and the development of community care for the mentally ill remained a policy of successive governments. Throughout the 1960s and 1970s only limited progress was made in moving patients from the larger hospitals into community settings, and community care itself lacked conceptual clarity. Although overcrowding and the resident population of large psychiatric hospitals had gradually decreased, by 1975 none had closed.

Nevertheless, the government's White Paper, *Better Services for the Mentally Ill* (DHSS 1975), claimed that the government's policy was working. The development of local services with a shift away from hospital provision and towards community-based social services care was still the target although the White Paper declared also that the hospital would remain the centre for mental health care services for the foreseeable future; that is, until adequate community care facilities were in place to prevent 'revolving door' patients – those who needed supervision of their medication, followed by a rapid return to the community, perhaps precipitating readmission. *Better Services for the Mentally Ill* set the tone for the future community-based care of people with mental illness and continues to provide a useful reference point from which current mental health care services can be judged.

Development of community mental health nursing

Closure of the large mental hospitals and their replacement by smaller units attached to local district hospitals, along with the development of day hospitals and community care facilities, had a marked impact on the practice of mental health nursing from the 1960s. May and Moore (1963) describe the work of two (later four) nurses seconded from Warlingham Park Hospital in 1954 to visit patients discharged from hospital and now living in Croydon. Their role was clinical: investigation and reporting of patients' family and social circumstances was not expected; this was the remit of the psychiatric social worker. Each nurse was responsible for a ward of patients. They attended a weekly ward round, and also outpatient clinics and evening aftercare groups.

McNamee (1993) reports that Moorhaven Hospital established a 'Nursing After-Care' service in 1957. This differed from the Warlingham Park Hospital service in that it involved nurses working both in the wards as well as with patients who had been discharged. Moorhaven Hospital community psychiatric nurses (CPNs) were expected to build relationships with their patients and to use this as a medium for care delivery and for helping patients to cope with the effects of their illness. Thus, the nurse was envisaged as a therapeutic agent, a role that served also to enhance the status of nursing at the time. The CPN role continued to develop. According to Hunter (1974) their functions in the 1960s included:

- giving advice, particularly to patients' families on medication, monitoring its side effects and cooperating with general practitioners (GPs) and psychiatrists to reduce medication;

- providing practical assistance to patients and their families (e.g. help with bathing and shaving patients);

- acting as a link between the ward and community and facilitating admission in the event of relapse;

- ensuring continuity of care for designated groups of patients (including those with schizophrenia, recurrent depression and organic psychosis);

- supervising patients in outpatient clinics;

- assisting in running social clubs and work groups;

- assisting patients to gain employment and accommodation on discharge from hospital.

The CPN role expanded to assume social and rehabilitative functions particularly following the Local Authority Social Services Act 1970, which abolished specialist social workers for people with mental health problems. CPNs began to offer crisis intervention, group work, psychotherapy and behaviour therapy (Hunter 1974). However, in the 1960s and 1970s CPNs worked primarily within hospital treatment teams, received all referrals from hospital consultants and carried out care programmes that were medically oriented.

A change of emphasis away from medical domination towards a more autonomous social model of care followed attachment of CPNs to general practice in Oxford and elsewhere in the 1970s. These CPNs accepted referrals from many sources (open referral system), including each other, and developed into far more independent practitioners responsible for patient assessment, and also planning and implementing an appropriate care package. Later, though, attachment of CPNs to primary care teams was criticized (e.g. White 1990; Gournay and Brooking 1994) for deflecting the attention of nurses towards the so-called 'worried well' and away from the needs of people with serious mental illness who were a government priority for mental health care.

In the early 1970s, and particularly following the White Paper *Better Services for the Mentally Ill* (DHSS 1975), there was a growing lobby for specialist community training for mental health nurses, and in 1974 the Joint Board of Clinical Nursing Studies (JBCNS) published the *Outline Curriculum in Community Psychiatric Nursing for Registered Nurses* (1974). This 36–39-week course was designed to prepare Registered Mental Nurses (RMNs) to work in multi-professional environments and to give both rehabilitative and therapeutic care in the community. CPNs worked from general practice clinics or accepted referrals from other agencies, and developed specialist skills to assist and work with care groups and organizations.

Increased specialization of CPNs and other mental health nurses from the 1970s mirrored and was sometimes forced by increased specialization by their medical colleagues. An important example was the development of training of nurses as behaviour therapists by Isaac Marks at the Maudsley Hospital from 1972, which was the first of a series of post-registration courses to provide community mental health nurses with specialist skills and a specific therapeutic orientation. A more recent example was the Thorn Programme developed and disseminated from the Institute of Psychiatry, King's College London, and the University of Manchester, which trained mental health nurses and other professionals to deliver research-based care and treatment to people suffering from severe and enduring mental illness (Gournay 1997).

> ## Thinking Space 3.1
>
> Compare and contrast the role and responsibilities of mental health nurses today compared with those of their forebears working in mental hospitals in the 1950s and 1960s.

 ## 3.4 UK government reviews of mental health nursing

A major review of psychiatric nursing, *Psychiatric Nursing: Today and Tomorrow*, published in 1968 by the then Ministry of Health (Standing Mental Health and Standing Nursing Advisory Committees 1968), focused particularly on inpatient psychiatric nursing, which was the dominant setting for care in that period. This report highlighted the importance of the personal relationship between the nurse and patient as central to the nurse's role. Among other recommendations it identified the need for psychiatric nurses to develop skills in psychotherapy, a view which resonated with Peplau's (1952) interpersonal relations approach to mental health nursing (of which more later).

A further 26 years were to pass before the next government review of mental health nursing, *Working in Partnership* (Mental Health Nursing Review Team 1994), by which time the context of mental health nursing was much changed. The Thatcher years (1979–90), the NHS and Community Care Act 1990 and the development of the internal market in health care with purchaser and provider

roles had led to a very different care environment. Marked advances in medical science had led to new drugs (for example, Prozac) and a growing confidence in some psychological therapies (e.g. cognitive behavioural therapy – CBT), and patients' expectations for care and treatment had risen. In addition there had been major changes in nurse education, consequent upon Project 2000 (UKCC 1986) which had moved education from hospital-based training schools into higher education, and a gradual acceptance that nursing should be a research-based profession, leading more nurses to question their existing practice and seek clarification of their role. In the light of these changes, by the 1990s it seemed to many that a review of mental health nursing was timely.

The strongest message of *Working in Partnership* was that the relationship between the nurse and service user is at the heart of nursing practice. The report states:

'This review starts from a belief that the work of mental health nurses rests on their relationship with people who use mental health services. This relationship should have value to both parties'.

(Mental Health Nursing Review Team 1994: 9).

Among its recommendations was that nurses should act as key workers, become involved in supervised discharge and take the lead as providers of information to service users. The report urged increased opportunities for patients to become involved in their care in partnership with nurses and for nurses to focus their work on the care of people with serious and enduring mental illness; this recommendation is perhaps the most enduring contribution of the report to mental health nursing policy.

Working in Partnership contained little that was new, and much of it endorsed conventional wisdom of the time. But it was valued by mental health nurses for clarifying their roles at a time of great change in the development of mental health services, and for shoring up the boundaries of the specialty by rejecting generic pre-registration education which would, many feared, dilute mental health nurses' unique identity and contribution to care (Norman 1998). However, it paid too little attention to psychological and other interventions of proven effectiveness delivered by nurses to patients, and the skills required to do this.

Chief Nursing Officers' reviews of mental health nursing

The clearest statements of recovery-oriented practice with regard to mental health nursing are contained in reviews of the profession by the Chief Nursing Officer for England (CNOE 2006) and Scotland (CNOS 2006). The title of the Scottish review, *Rights, Relationships and Recovery*, reflects its key messages, which are: a *rights* based approach to practice; developing *positive relationships* as the starting point for all interventions with service users, carers and families; and *recovery* as the underpinning principle of therapeutic interventions.

The report from the CNOE addressed the question: *How can mental health nursing best contribute to the care of service users in the future?* The review endorsed an approach to contemporary mental health nursing practice based upon broad mental health policies which promote user-centred goals, a recovery approach and evidence-based health care, so bringing together the artistic and scientific traditions in mental health nursing which we discuss in the following section of this chapter.

A national evaluation of progress towards and impact of implementation of the English review's recommendations on mental health trusts and universities (Callaghan et al. 2009) found that implementation of the CNOE's recommendations was limited overall. In universities the review had appeared to help shift the focus of education towards recovery approaches and greater involvement of service users in the education process. However, in trusts, implementation was not widespread and there was little evidence that changes reported were attributable directly to the review. Callaghan's evaluation concludes that implementation was hampered by the lack of an evidence-based implementation plan at both local and national level, competing demands on trusts and

lack of awareness of the review by mental health nurses themselves.

 ## 3.5   Traditions

In this section we trace the origins of two contrasting traditions which have shaped contemporary mental health nursing: the influential ideas of Hilda Peplau and the rise of evidence-based health care.

Nursing in the interpersonal relations tradition: Peplau and her legacy

The interpersonal relations tradition of mental health nursing is as old as mental health nursing itself, and has its origins in Tuke's moral treatment. However, it found its first formal expression in the work of Hildegard (Hilda) Peplau, who exercised a major influence on mental health nursing from the early 1950s until her death in 1999. Peplau coined the term 'nurse–patient relationship' and her book *Interpersonal Relations in Nursing* (1952) became a classic and is still widely read, having been reprinted in 2004.

It was at Chestnut Lodge in Maryland that Peplau came into contact with Harry Stack Sullivan, a psychiatrist, who was developing an interpersonal theory of psychiatric illness (Sullivan 1947). For Sullivan psychiatry was not concerned simply with the study of mentally ill people or group processes, but was a broader enterprise concerned with '*the study of what goes on between two or more people, all but one of whom may be completely illusory*' (Peplau 1987: 202). Peplau's major contribution in *Interpersonal Relations in Nursing* was to apply and so develop Sullivan's theoretical perspective to the interpersonal world of the nurse and patient.

For Peplau, mental health nursing is an important, therapeutic, interpersonal process characterized by three overlapping and interlocking phases in the nurse–patient relationship – orientation, working and termination. Her study of interpersonal relations revealed various roles for the nurse;

as, for example, a resource person, teacher, surrogate parent and leader. Later she was to describe these as 'sub-roles' and the role of counsellor or psychotherapist as the heart of psychiatric nursing. Through the medium of their relationships with patients nurses strive to create conditions that aim to promote health and develop patients' ability to engage with those around them.

Peplau's influence on UK mental health nursing

Peplau's ideas took a long time to influence academic psychiatric nursing in the UK and it was not until the late 1970s and early 1980s that they gained a secure foothold. A number of mental health nurses contributed to the diffusion of Peplau's ideas in the UK, notable among whom were Annie Altschul and Philip (Phil) Barker.

During a study trip to the USA, Altschul was introduced to a nursing curriculum that focused on helping nurses to establish relationships with patients, to use these relationships to move forward patients' recovery and rehabilitation, and to terminate these relationships at an appropriate time. Altschul became convinced that this was the way forward for mental health nursing in the UK. Such relationships she believed evolved over time and were fostered by good mentoring, supervision and support of students, and also by nurses being accountable for their actions. Over the next four decades Altschul was well placed to promote her ideas, first as principal tutor at the Maudsley Hospital in London and then as professor of nursing at the University of Edinburgh until her death in 2001.

Altschul's main contribution to the psychiatric nursing research literature, published in 1972 as *Patient–Nurse Interaction*, is her observation study of how therapeutic relationships between nurses and patients could be established and developed in an inpatient ward. Altschul's study looked for evidence of therapeutic principles underpinning interactions between nurses and patients, but in this she was to be disappointed. She found that nurses in her study did 'not have any identifiable perspective to guide them in their interactions with patients' and the nurses themselves saw mental health nursing as 'just common sense' (Altschul 1972: 192). She concluded that the relationship between the nurse and the patient was 'irrelevant to psychiatric treatment' (1972: 193). In spite of this, most patients described their relationship with the nurses as helpful, although this finding must be considered in the light of patients' reluctance to criticize nurses, particularly when they are hospitalized and feel vulnerable.

Although Peplau's writings were popular in the USA, nurse training in the UK in the 1960s did not emphasize nurse–patient relationships. Thus, Altschul's finding that nurses regarded their practice as just common sense could have been confidently predicted. However, her study proved a great impetus to UK mental health nurse education being oriented towards providing nurses with knowledge and skills to form relationships with patients and use these therapeutically. It also influenced the direction of, in particular, pre-registration nurse education in the UK in the late 1970s and 1980s, which emphasized the acquisition of interpersonal skills (see e.g. ENB and WNB for Nursing, Midwifery and Health Visiting 1982).

An interesting footnote is that towards the end of her life Altschul was to revise her view on the central position of the nurse–patient relationship to nursing practice. Reflecting on her professional life she concluded that while the concept of the therapeutic relationship offered substantial benefits for nurses, it was not so clear that patients benefited (Altschul 1999). Her position in 1999 appears to be that the continuing interaction between the nurse and patient, as occurs in inpatient care, is not conducive to the development and constructive use of therapeutic relationships, since giving attention to a ward of patients is too draining for nurses and relationships with several nurses, simultaneously, is too demanding for inpatients.

The continuing development of the interpersonal relations orientation in UK mental health nursing literature and practice is well illustrated by the work of Phil Barker, currently a psychotherapist

3.6　Capabilities for contemporary practice

Fears that the interpersonal relations tradition of mental health nursing would be eclipsed by the rise and rise of the evidence-based health care tradition have not been realized. Indeed, over the past eight years, since publication of the first edition of this book, we have observed increasing consensus that both traditions are integral to the practice of mental health nursing.

Nurses influenced by both traditions have been reconciled through adherence to a set of recovery-oriented values and objectives that underpin mental health policy, some of the more important of which are:

- supporting service users to overcome social exclusion through work or other productive activity and building and maintaining supportive relationships;
- upholding service users' rights;
- increasing service users' choice of treatment through promoting access to information;
- delivering mental health care without discrimination on grounds of race, gender, sexuality, age or abilities; and
- providing holistic care which addresses the needs of individuals as defined by the individuals themselves.

The CNOE's review of mental health nursing (CNOE 2006b) lists the competencies and capabilities needed by mental health nurses to deliver care based upon these values and principles. These are summarized in Table 3.1.

These competencies and capabilities demonstrate an integration of the artistic and scientific traditions of mental health nursing. Evidence-based health care and interventions are now framed within a recovery-oriented approach which emphasizes the central place of the person with mental health problems and the impact of services upon his or her life journey.

3.7　Conclusion

In our distinction between the interpersonal relations and evidence-based practice traditions in mental health nursing we see a long-running debate between those who emphasize the 'art' of mental health nursing and those who emphasize the 'science'. The debate between artists and scientists is not unique to nursing; it is present in all practice disciplines. It reflects differing research traditions (phenomenological vs scientific) and differing views about what passes as knowledge.

Contemporary mental health nursing practice demonstrates a fusion of these traditions. Evidence-based interventions are being practised in a 'recovery oriented' way that recognizes the importance of reducing the extent to which remaining symptoms interfere with people's efforts to pursue their goals and interests and emphasizes how they can be helped to make the most of their lives. Moreover, in evaluations of mental health care interventions, outcomes oriented towards service users, values such as independence, employment, satisfying relationships and good quality of life (the social dimensions of recovery) have assumed their proper place alongside more traditional outcomes, such as adherence to treatment, relapse or re-hospitalization prevention.

In summary, as the title of this book highlights, mental health nursing is an art and a science. The art of nursing is concerned with therapeutic relationships, with a person's internal world and sense of self (with the left-hand quadrants of the framework we introduced in Chapter 1 – see Figures 1.1 and 1.4). The science of nursing, in contrast, is concerned with a person's biophysiological profile and their observable behaviour (with the right-hand quadrants of our framework). Thus nurses are concerned with change in all four quadrants in response to pharmacological and psychosocial interventions, different forms of care organization or the therapeutic power of caring relationships.

To conclude, the main points of this chapter are:

- The practice discipline of mental health nursing arose under the patronage of the medical profes-

Table 3.1 Best practice competencies and capabilities for pre-registration mental health nurses in England (CNOE 2006b)

1. Putting values into practice
Values Promote a culture that values and respects the diversity of individuals, and enables their recovery.
2. Improving outcomes for service users
Communication Use a range of communication skills to establish, maintain and manage relationships with individuals who have mental health problems, their carers and key people involved in their care. *Physical care* Promote physical health and well-being for people with mental health problems. *Psychosocial care* Promote mental health and well-being, enabling people to recover from debilitating mental health experiences and/or achieve their full potential, supporting them to develop and maintain social networks and relationships. *Risk and risk management* Work with individuals with mental health needs in order to maintain health, safety and well-being.
3. A positive, modern profession
Multi-disciplinary and multi-agency working Work collaboratively with other disciplines and agencies to support individuals to develop and maintain social networks and relationships. *Personal and professional development* Demonstrate a commitment to the need for continuing professional development and personal supervision activities, in order to enhance knowledge, skills, values and attitudes needed for safe and effective nursing practice.

sion and its development has been linked closely with developments in psychiatric medicine.

- The origins of the much discussed therapeutic nurse–patient relationship can be traced to 'moral treatment', which was, however, undermined by asylums becoming dumping grounds for socially disadvantaged people who were difficult to manage.

- The breakdown of the asylum system heralded a period of insecurity but also of opportunity for nursing to grow and develop new ways of working with people with mental health problems in the community.

- UK government reviews of mental health nursing conducted in 1968 and 1994 sought to clarify the identity and remit of mental health nursing at times of great change.

- We identify two traditions which have shaped UK mental health nursing: the interpersonal relations approach (the artistic tradition) and the evidence-based practice approach (the scientific tradition). These traditions are fused within contemporary mental health nursing practice. Evidence-based interventions are practised in a 'recovery oriented' way that recognizes the importance of reducing the extent to which remaining symptoms interfere with people's efforts to pursue their goals and interests.

- The CNO for England's 2006 review of mental health nursing sets out best practice competencies and capabilities for pre-registration education which are required for recovery oriented practice.

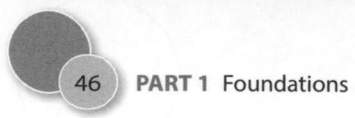

Annotated bibliography

Nolan, P.A. (1993) *A History of Mental Health Nursing.* **London: Chapman & Hall.**
Probably the most authoritative and comprehensive history of UK mental health nursing yet written.

Journal of Psychiatric and Mental Health Nursing, **5(3) and 6(4).**
These issues are devoted to a consideration of the contribution of Hilda Peplau and Annie Altschul to mental health nursing.

Peplau, H. (1952) *Interpersonal Relations in Nursing.* **New York: G.P. Putman.**
To her supporters Peplau presents an empirically precise theory of nursing that can be verified and developed through further research. To her critics Peplau's theory of nursing, based on psychodynamic principles, bears little relation to the work that nurses carry out, contains few operational (empirically testable) definitions and fewer tests of validity. Read Peplau's classic text and judge for yourself.

Barker's ideas on the proper focus of mental health nursing are set out in a series of published papers (two of the more important of which are cited below) and also on his 'Tidal Model' website (www.tidalmodel.co.uk).
Barker, P. (1989) Reflections on the philosophy of caring in mental health, *International Journal of Nursing Studies,* 26(2): 131–41.
Barker, P.J. (2000) Reflections on a caring as a virtue ethic within an evidence-based culture, *International Journal of Nursing Studies,* 37(4): 329–36.
Barker, P.J. and Buchanan-Barker, P. (2011) Myth of mental health nursing and the challenge of recovery, *International Journal of Mental Health Nursing,* 20: 337–44.

Mental Health Special Issue of the *International Journal of Nursing Studies* **(2007), 44(3). This Special Issue includes:**
A critique of the CNO for England's review of mental health nursing by Brooker.
Findings from the national consultation of mental health nurses conducted as part of the review.
Review and discussion papers on: user and carer involvement in training and education of health professionals; interventions delivered by mental health nurses; and physical health problems associated with serious mental illness.

References

Altschul, A.T. (1972) *Patient–Nurse Interaction: A study of interaction patterns in acute psychiatric wards.* Edinburgh: Churchill Livingstone.
Altschul, A.T. (1999) Editorial, *Journal of Psychiatric and Mental Health Nursing,* 6(4): 261–3.
Barton, R. (1959) *Institutional Neurosis.* Bristol: Wright.
Callaghan, P., Repper, J., Lovell, K. *et al.* (2009) *Evaluation of the Chief Nursing Officer's Review of Mental Health Nursing in England.* Nottingham: University of Nottingham, available at: www.nottingham.ac.uk/nursing/cno-review/resources/CNO-Review-Final-Report.pdf, accessed 26 September 2012.
CNOE (Chief Nursing Officer England) (2006) *Review of Mental Health Nursing: from values to action.* London: DH.
CNOE (Chief Nursing Officer England) (2006b) *Best Practice Competencies and Capabilities for Pre-Registration Mental Health Nurses In England.* London: DH.
CNOS (Chief Nursing Officer Scotland) (2006) *Rights, Relationships and Recovery: the report of the National Review of Mental Health Nursing in Scotland.* Edinburgh: Scottish Office.
Connolly, M.J. (1992) History, in J. Brooking, S. Ritter and B. Thomas (eds) *A Textbook of Psychiatric and Mental Health Nursing.* Edinburgh: Churchill Livingstone.
DHSS (Department of Health and Social Security) (1975) *Better Services for the Mentally Ill.* London: HMSO.
ENB and WNB for Nursing, Midwifery and Health Visiting (1982) *Syllabus of Training: Professional Register – Part 3 Registered Mental Nurse.* London: ENB.
Goffman, E. (1961) *Asylums: Essays on the Social Situation of Mental Patients and Other Inmates.* Harmondsworth: Penguin.
Gournay, K. (1997) Responses to: 'What to do with nursing models' – a reply from Gournay, *Journal of Psychiatric and Mental Health Nursing,* 4: 227–31.
Gournay, K. and Brooking, J. (1994) Community psychiatric nurses in primary healthcare, *British Journal of Psychiatry,* 165: 231–8.
Hunter, P. (1974) Community psychiatric nursing: a literature review, *International Journal of Nursing Studies,* 11: 223.
JBCNS (Joint Board of Clinical Nursing Studies) (1974) *Outline Curriculum in Community Psychiatric Nursing for Registered Nurses.* Held by The National Archives, kew.
May, A.R. and Moore, S. (1963) The mental nurse in the community, *Lancet,* 1: 213–14.
McNamee, G. (1993) A changing profession: the role of nursing in home care, in P. Weller and M. Muijen (eds) *Dimensions of Community Mental Health Care.* London: W.B. Saunders & Co.
Mental Health Nursing Review Team (1994) *Working in Partnership: A collaborative approach to care.* London: DH.
Nolan, P. (1993) *A History of Mental Health Nursing.* London: Chapman & Hall.
Norman, I.J. (1998) Priorities for mental health and learning disability nurse education in the UK: a case study, *Journal of Clinical Nursing,* 7: 433–41.
Peplau, H. (1952) *Interpersonal Relations in Nursing.* New York: G.P. Putman.

Peplau, H. (1987) Interpersonal constructs in nursing practice, *Nursing Education Today*, 7: 201–8.

Rogers, C. (1942) *Counseling and Psychotherapy*. Boston, MA: Houghton Mifflin, available at: http://archive.org/details/counselingandpsy029048mbp.

Sackett, D.L., Straus, S.E., Richardson, W.S., Rosenberg, W. and Haynes, R.B. (2000) *Evidence-based Medicine*, 2nd edn. Edinburgh: Churchill Livingstone.

Scull, A. (1981) *Madhouses, Mad-doctors and Madmen*. London: Athlone.

Standing Mental Health and Standing Nursing Advisory Committees (1968) *Psychiatric Nursing Today and Tomorrow*. London: Ministry of Health – Central Health Services Council.

Stockwell, F. (2009) A history of mental health nursing: a personal perspective. In Clarke V, Walsh A *Fundamentals of Mental Health Nursing*. Oxford, Oxford University Press.

Sullivan, H.S. (1947) *Conceptions of Modern Psychiatry*. Washington, DC: William A. White Psychiatric Foundation.

Townsend, P. (1962) *The Last Refuge: a survey of residential institutions and homes for the aged in England and Wales*. London: Routledge & Kegan Paul.

UKCC (United Kingdom Central Council for Nursing, Midwifery and Health Visiting) (1986) *Project 2000: A new preparation for practice*. London: UKCC.

White, E. (1990) *The Third Quinquennial National Survey of Community Psychiatric Nursing*. Manchester: University of Manchester.

Wing, J.K. (1990) The function of asylum, *British Journal of Psychiatry*, 157: 822–7.

Chapter 4

Health Promotion in Mental Health Nursing

Alison I. Machin and Sandra Moran

I've been greatly helped by having access to the gym and physio assistance at my local psychiatric hospital – I attended a ladies only exercise class and the deep stretch and relaxation class is fabulous. I am trying to eat a better diet, although this has not been easy due to a lack of energy and motivation.

Sally

4.1 Introduction

This chapter provides mental health nurses with an overview of the knowledge and skills necessary for promoting people's mental health. Health promotion as a discipline allied to public health is a broad subject that encompasses the health of individuals and of communities. It has implications also for the promotion of mental health among those people who experience mental health problems as well as among people more generally. The chapter begins by examining definitions, strategies and models of health promotion and does this in the broadest sense. It then considers the application of mental health promotion in practice and focuses in this respect on promoting the health of individuals with and without pre-existing mental health problems. The chapter covers:

- definitions of health promotion;
- strategies and policies;
- models and theories of health promotion;
- health promotion application in practice.

4.2 Definitions of health promotion

Mental health is fundamental to the health of people and populations. It influences physical health, educational attainment, employment, criminality and social exclusion (DH 2009). It is suggested that one in four people in England will experience a mental health problem in their lifetime, with mental ill health costing the English economy £105 billion per year (DH 2011a). Mental health is therefore linked to the human, social and economic development of societies (Moodie and Jenkins 2005).

Potentially there is much to be gained from health promotion, which is concerned with actions to improve the health behaviour of individuals and generate healthy public policy to improve the health of populations and groups (Green and Tones 2010). Scriven (2010) suggests that health promotion is about making, supporting, encouraging and placing health higher on the agendas of individuals and policy-makers.

The World Health Organization (WHO) (1986) has defined health promotion as 'the process of enabling people to take control over, and to improve, their health'. Health promotion is a term often used synonymously with 'public health' and the overlap is clear in some definitions. For example, 'Public health is the art and science of preventing disease, prolonging life and promoting health through the organised efforts of Society' (Acheson 1998).

Despite an early tension between the two approaches, under the auspices of the 'new public health' movement, health promotion and public health responsibilities are increasingly merged (Parker 2009). Health promotion is often viewed as a dimension of public health policy and practice which is targeted at addressing the social determinants of ill health and reducing health inequalities (Marmot 2010).

The UK *Public Health Skills and Career Framework* (Skills for Health 2008) suggests eight dimensions of public health practice, four core and four specialized. These are:

- surveillance and assessment;
- assessing the effectiveness of health interventions;
- policy development;
- leadership and collaborative working;
- health improvement and health protection;
- public health intelligence;
- academic public health;
- health and social care quality.

While public health has surveillance, research and managing outbreaks as core functions, health promotion focuses on developing health promotion policies, education for behaviour change and

working with communities. The key challenge highlighted by Naidoo and Wills (2010) is to bring both disciplines together effectively in the overall task of health improvement.

 ## 4.3   Strategies and policies

The potential for health promotion to address key global health issues emerged through the WHO's Alma Ata Declaration in 1978. The principles of the international 'health for all' movement were further enshrined in the *Ottowa Charter for Health Promotion 1986* (WHO 1986), which identified five objectives that formed the basis for improving mental and physical health:

- build healthy public policy;
- create supportive environments;
- strengthen community action;
- develop personal skills;
- reorient health services.

The current UK coalition government has demonstrated its ongoing commitment to the provision of effective services to promote positive mental health in the population. The recent cross-departmental strategy paper *No Health Without Mental Health* (HM Government 2011) acknowledges the economic, social and personal cost of mental ill health and proposes a number of critical measures to improve the mental health of people with existing mental illness, while seeking to prevent mental ill health in the wider population. In line with the recommendations from the Marmot Review (2010) and the public health White Paper (DH 2011a) the strategy proposes taking a life course approach to promoting health and well-being. It recognizes the importance of early identification of risk factors and problems, and targeted timely interventions to develop and strengthen resilience factors at an individual, family and community level to prevent mental ill health. It seeks to address health inequalities and the impact that wider determinants of health such as employment status, poor housing, education and social isolation have upon mental health and well-being. The strategy reinforces the importance of mental health promotion and the capacity of all persons to derive benefit. However, achieving the desired outcomes for individuals, families and communities will only be possible through a whole-systems, joined-up approach between sectors, services and stakeholders.

It has been acknowledged internationally that health inequalities are worsening, despite collective health promotion activity. The WHO's Bangkok Charter (2005) called for urgent action and global commitment to ensure health promotion is: high on the agenda for global development; the shared responsibility of all governments; a key focus for all communities; and core to responsible business practice in the private sector.

 ## 4.4 Models and theories

There are many different approaches to health promotion, all linked to the overarching aims of improving public health and health inequalities. Health promotion activities may be focused on the prevention of ill health, which can be employed at three different levels (Caplan 1964):

- **Primary prevention:** preventing the onset of disease in the general population.
- **Secondary prevention:** preventing the development of disease in individuals in at risk groups.
- **Tertiary prevention:** keeping people with well developed disease as healthy as possible.

Using post-natal depression as an example, primary prevention-level activities might aim to promote healthy behaviours in women that contribute towards a sense of mental well-being and the development of emotional resilience, along with fostering support networks. Secondary prevention activities would include screening pregnant women to monitor for those at risk of post-natal depression and referral to support agencies if necessary. Tertiary prevention activities might target women with pre-existing long-term depression and explore ways of helping them stay as healthy as possible during pregnancy and childbirth, within the con-

straints of their depressive symptoms. Case studies presented later in the chapter explore these levels further and show how they can be applied in nursing practice.

Chesterson (2009) asserts that mental health promotion is concerned with the promotion of emotional and social well-being. In this sense its primary functions are to:

- "protect, support and sustain emotional and social well-being;
- promote mentally healthy lifestyles and living, and support productive and meaningful lives;
- increase a sense of belonging, social awareness and connectedness;
- promote healthy communities, schools, workplaces and social support;
- strengthen personal, family, educational, occupational and economic growth and functioning;
- build community acceptance, tolerance and understanding (personal, social, cultural and spiritual differences/preferences);
- improve coping skills, capacity and adaptation of individuals and communities;
- build resilience – increase/strengthen protective factors, reduce risk factors/behaviours that threaten emotional and social well-being;
- improve mental health literacy."

Naidoo and Wills (2010) emphasize that the primary aim of health promotion practice should be to empower individuals to make positive health choices. This might encompass activities such as information-giving, social marketing, improving self-efficacy and building resilience.

Information-giving

Health education, perhaps the earliest form of health promotion, is most often associated with information-giving. The premise of this approach is that by providing people with information and educating them about the risks associated with unhealthy behaviours, they will be able to make an informed choice about the actions they take. This may take the form of media information campaigns, posters and leaflets, or health messages delivered in school education curricula. The success of this activity is likely to be influenced by the message, the medium of transmission, the credibility of the person delivering the message and the readiness of the person to accept the information given. However, using this approach alone to achieve better health outcomes has increasingly been seen as simplistic. For example, giving written information to someone who is blind or who cannot read or retain information is unlikely to be effective without additional support or advocacy. In addition, literacy levels are lower among groups with the poorest health and in the poorest socioeconomic circumstances (WHO 2007). Using an information-giving approach alone may serve to perpetuate health inequalities, which despite successive targeted public health policies, still exist in the UK and across the world.

Information alone also fails to take into account other social and environmental factors which influence choice and opportunity. Key health education messages are often understood by people, however they continue to make unhealthy choices for other reasons. For example, people might say, 'I know I shouldn't smoke but it helps me relax when I'm stressed' or 'We usually have cheap takeaway food because I don't have the time, money or energy to make healthy meals'.

To begin to address some of the inequalities in the uptake of health education messages, health education has evolved over time. There is now a specific focus on improving health literacy in the population. Health literacy as a term is suggested by Nutbeam (2000) to incorporate: functional literacy (basic reading, writing and skills of everyday functioning); critical literacy (the ability to interpret the information given and make critical value judgements about it); and interactive literacy (the ability to apply the new information in a range of changing life situations).

Improving health literacy at any level is likely to provide individuals with an accelerated opportunity for self-development through improved access to help, support and advice that they may not otherwise have been able to utilize. In keeping with a shift to an asset-based approach to public health development (IDeA 2010), debate has more recently focused on whether health literacy should be framed as a problem to be solved or as an asset to be built upon. A shift to positive thinking is in keeping with the mental health notion of recovery and positive growth (see Chapter 5). While education and information-giving might not necessarily result in attitude and behaviour change it can be useful as a starting point for helping people change.

Social marketing

Social marketing is a relatively recent concept in health promotion which combines providing targeted health messages and engaging people in behaviour change. The theory underpinning it is based largely on exchange theory (Lefebvre and Flora 1988) which involves a voluntary exchange between two parties, not of a commercial product, but of a positive health benefit. It combines health knowledge and expertise with theory from the commercial business sector about how to best 'sell' concepts to particular markets (French 2010). There are several core principles which underpin a social marketing approach, including: consumer orientation; knowledge of the competition; mutual exchange; segmentation of the target population to identify, focus and maximize impact; and marketing mix, which includes consideration of the four 'Ps' – price, product, place and promotion (Kotler and Lee 2008). An example of a successful initiative with a clear mental health promoting benefit using this approach is a project tackling worklessness in Lincolnshire. Details of this and others can be found on the National Social Marketing Website at http://thensmc.com/resources/showcase/worklessness-collaborative-programme. Although social marketing tends to group people together in populations for the purposes of clarity and targeted action, its success rests on individuals choosing to change their behaviour in response to the social marketing message or indeed the process of active engagement. Whether or not they choose to change will be affected by their level of self-efficacy.

Improving self-efficacy

Self-efficacy refers to an individual's perceived level of confidence in and/or ability to make behaviour changes. Becker (1974) suggests that four major psychological processes influence an individual's sense of self-efficacy:

- affective (how they feel about the change and its consequences);
- cognitive (how they understand the change and its potential benefits and costs);
- motivational (what is influencing their desire to change);
- selective (the rationalizing and rehearsing of different courses of action).

In an interactive sense the self-efficacy of the health promotion practitioner is also of influence.

Sturt (1998) studied primary care practitioners' perceptions of the notion of self-efficacy as a framework for health promotion. One of the key determinants of the perceived success of the work was linked to the outcome expectations of practitioners. The degree of confidence that the practitioners had that they would be able to help someone change to healthier behaviours also influenced their ability. Mental health nurses could explore ways of improving the self-efficacy of service users in different situations as a foundation for changing health behaviour (Scriven 2010) (see Chapter 23 which describes motivational approaches for supporting behaviour change).

Thinking Space 4.1

Think about the expectations you might bring to your encounters with service users as well as the environment and the resources that are available to you in practice contexts. What could you do differently to improve service users' self-efficacy? To help you consider this, Greens and Tones (2010) suggest there are three aspects to the health promotion role for improving self-efficacy:

1. Influencing an individual's self-efficacy perceptions directly.
2. Influencing efficacy through the development of the skills and knowledge needed for confidence-building.
3. Influencing any environmental barriers that are inhibiting the development of self-efficacy in the individual.

Influencing self-efficacy directly is likely to involve some assessment of the health beliefs of the individual and their readiness for change (Prochaska and DiClemente 1983). The Health Belief Model suggests that the impact of health promotion activities and the likelihood of change in individuals is dependent on several interrelated factors including: perceived susceptibility to the illness; perceptions of the likely severity of any suffering and its consequences; the perceived benefit of responding to health promotion advice; and the perceptions of the psychological costs to the individual of changing their behaviour (Pender *et al.* 2011). Although used widely in nursing research and practice, the Health Belief Model has also been criticized for its lack of applicability to, for example, children and young families, without adaptation of some of its core concepts (Roden 2004). Despite such criticisms, nurses seeking to help people make healthy lifestyle changes or a reduction in risk taking behaviour will need to carefully analyse the health beliefs of the individual with whom they're working, to better understand and influence individual factors that affect the likely success of their input.

Building resilience

Being able to cope with adversity and not struggle in the face of significant stressors is a key life skill but one that can vary in strength and quality. It is generally recognized that resilience reflects a combination of constitutional and environmental factors and that protective factors can modify an individual's response in 'at risk' contexts, thereby protecting their well-being. Following Chesterson (2009), Box 4.1 presents key risk and resilience factors for mental health.

Chesterson (2009) asserts that the content of Table 4.1 should be routinely incorporated into care practices by nursing staff and their multi-disciplinary colleagues. Some risk factors are identified as part of mental health assessments during early case identification and treatment, but this is rarely true of the protective factors. Incorporating protective factors into routine practice would help promote optimum recovery, coping skills and higher levels of functioning consistent with a recovery and strengths model.

Box 4.1 Risk and resilience factors for mental health

Risk factors

- Poor or interrupted development or maturity
- Unstable or dysfunctional relationships
- Overwhelming adversity, grief and loss
- Absent or poor parenting and role-modelling
- Family discord, domestic violence and abuse
- Parent(s) with serious mental disorder and disability
- Loneliness, lack of friends, peer and social support
- Persistent physical illness, disability or distress
- Drugs or excess alcohol use, poor nutrition and sleep
- Social exclusion, disadvantage, injustice, poverty, stigma

Protective factors

- Nurturing, affectionate, secure family relationships
- Positive/rewarding school and work environments
- Personal and shared opportunities and achievements
- Social connectedness and belonging
- Reliable friendships and social support networks
- Positive temperament, humour, patience, tolerance, hope
- Presence of mind, emotional intelligence, expression
- Self-awareness, esteem, acceptance, courage
- Mentors of personal encouragement
- Healthy lifestyle

4.5 Health promotion in practice

This section provides an overview of where health promotion practice fits within mental health service provision. Two case examples are presented, drawn from practice, of how the different approaches to health promotion can be employed.

Chapter 1 uses the interrelationship of four dimensions (self, community, objective and subjective) to analyse potential influences on mental health. Figure 4.1 applies this framework in a health promotion context. It illustrates where different components of the discussion in this chapter fit together to influence the health of mental health service users, providing examples of opportunities for health promotion activity in mental health nursing.

Figure 4.1 A framework for health promotion

	Subjective	Objective
Self	Health beliefs	Smoking
	Self-efficacy	Obesity
	Motivation	Mental illness
	Experience	Physical illness
	Perceived health status	Physical activity
	Educational attainment	Risk-taking behaviour
	Health literacy	
Community	Culture	Public health policy
	Family support	Mental health policy
	Peer support	Service delivery systems
	Schooling	Service guidelines and protocols
	Participation	Resources
	Collaborative commitment	Community assets
	Communication	Environment
	Employment	Workplace
	Income	Schools
		Housing

Case Study

Amber

Amber is a 30-year-old lady who lives alone. She is employed in the public sector and is responsible for the management of a team of people. She has always felt confident within this role which also includes contact with the general public. She has a good network of friends and family who live nearby and has always had a lively social life and a lot of interests outside her employment. Amber has been under increasing pressure recently because of changing terms and conditions to her employment, with an increased level of responsibility and workload including managing new staff members who are also adjusting to the changes.

Over the last six weeks Amber has felt tearful, irritable and has been having difficulty in sleeping. She has noticed deterioration in her concentration levels and confidence, and often feels anxious. She is avoiding working with other team members and believes they are all making negative comments about her performance. She also doubts her ability to fulfil the requirements of her role, suffering feelings of reduced self-efficacy. Outside work she has started to withdraw from friends and social activities that she would usually have engaged in.

Overwhelmed by the feelings she has been experiencing Amber visited her general practitioner (GP) who referred her to the Increasing Access to Psychological Therapies (IAPT) programme (Department of Health 2011b), which has a team that offers a range of talking and self-help therapies. Amber was assessed and the outcome of the assessment indicated that she was experiencing symptoms of anxiety and mild depression attributed to work-related stress. She subsequently worked with a psychological well-being practitioner (PWP) from the IAPT team who provided low intensity interventions with the aim of helping Amber to be able to understand how her feelings were affecting her behaviour, empowering her to change the behaviour which was affecting her mental health.

The service offered flexible appointments with sessions being delivered face to face, via telephone and email. In addition to this Amber could contact the PWP in between appointments and contact could be maintained via email or telephone. This minimized the need for Amber to take time off work which she was reluctant to do. The interventions delivered were based on cognitive behavioural therapy (CBT) and included computerized CBT to help Amber modify her thinking using programmes such as 'Beat the Blues' and 'Fear Fighter' (NICE 2006). She was also given access to health promotion information in the form of guided self-help workbooks through the 'books on prescription' scheme, learning about sleep hygiene techniques and building up her self-esteem. Throughout the self-help programmes Amber completed questionnaires and the scores from these were used as an indicator of the progress that was being made.

To begin with Amber found the IAPT programme challenging and her progress was slow. Gradually however she did begin to derive benefit and realized this was associated with the amount of effort she put into working through the self-help programmes and workbooks. Each week her PWP encouraged her to undertake specific tasks in the form of homework and although she found this difficult to begin with her PWP's expectations spurred her on. After the first month scores from her completed questionnaires showed a clear if small improvement in self-esteem and anxiety levels, which in turn motivated Amber to progress further through the self-help programmes regardless of other people's expectations.

Towards the end of the second month Amber was experiencing significant improvements in her sense of mental health and her PWP encouraged her to set specific goals to help sustain progress in the future. They revisited the circumstances that led to her initial referral and Amber was clear in her own mind that she needed to renegotiate her workload with her manager. Three months earlier Amber felt that she was failing, whereas now she could see that her employer was being unrealistic and in so doing was letting *her* down. Amber recognized that there were many challenges ahead but felt she now had the confidence to tackle those aspects of her working life that had previously jeopardized her mental health.

Commentary

For those in employment, the workplace is a key factor in mental well-being and this scenario demonstrates the importance of early identification of signs of work-related stress and early intervention to address it. Amber was already experiencing some signs that she was at risk of developing a mental health problem. In health promotion terms, the interventions can therefore be categorized as secondary prevention (Caplan 1964).

Case Study

James

James, aged 28, has experienced symptoms of psychosis since the age of 19. He has been prescribed different antipsychotic medications in the past to treat his symptoms, however in the last few months his psychiatrist has prescribed Clozapine. James believes that this medication has been helpful in alleviating most of his symptoms of psychosis but he has gained a lot of weight and become a lot less active than he used to be. James also smokes.

James now attends the Clozapine clinic weekly to monitor his bloods and medication. During one visit he was introduced to a health trainer who had recently begun outreach work at the clinic. It was a brief encounter in which James joked about his weight and levels of fitness, trying to play down any problem that the health trainer might pick up on. What struck him most after his visit was the way in which the health trainer had accepted his point of view and didn't pressurize him or preach to him. On the one hand this was good but on the other hand James felt a bit cheated. He knew he was unfit and overweight and thought on reflection that he should have been more honest.

It took James a month before he spoke to the health trainer again, even though he was there on each of his visits. When he did speak to him he struggled to explain what was on his mind and the health trainer reflected this back to him in a way that seemed OK. After this second encounter James felt some sense of relief. He was unsure about making any 'healthy' changes to his life but at some level realized that this was normal. He felt he could trust the health trainer and at his next visit plucked up the courage to ask him what his advice would be. The health trainer recommended that they agree a time to sit down together and weigh up the pros and cons of James' lifestyle and then they could work out the best advice together. James wasn't expecting this response and felt a sense of excitement at the opportunity he was being presented.

They actually met on two occasions over successive weeks and James spent most of the time talking about his health fears and anxieties. The health trainer listened carefully and reflected back James' beliefs and feelings in ways that seemed to motivate him to do something. Eventually they drew up a list of James' health concerns and the health trainer encouraged James to select a few to begin with and provided a menu of possible activities that could help him address those concerns.

Three months after initially meeting the health trainer James attended his GP for a physical health check and then began an organized cycling programme. He plans to return to his GP for a physical health check every three months or so to see how he is progressing. He has now attended the cycling programme on four occasions and besides the activity itself really enjoys the company of others. James hasn't stopped smoking or even changed his diet, both of which were on his list of health concerns, but he has made a note that when he next sees the health trainer he must ask him about other group sporting activities that he could get involved in.

Commentary

This scenario highlights the importance of continuing to take opportunities to deliver tertiary health promotion activities when somebody has an existing mental illness, particularly with the increased likelihood of poor physical health. Increased screening, monitoring of physical health and action to improve health for those with mental illness should be part of routine practice. Equally though, we must be realistic about what can be achieved. In James' case the health trainer used brief motivational interventions that allowed him to realize his own reasons for change and to identify gradual, achievable steps towards improved health (see Chapters 22 and 23). As discussed, collaborative working in care delivery is high on the political agenda and this scenario highlights how effective collaborative working can be, in terms of meeting the needs of service users. Such collaborative interprofessional working should put the service user at the centre of decision-making in order to increase their self-efficacy and the likelihood of health behaviour change.

4.6   Conclusion

This chapter has discussed the concept of health promotion to help mental health nurses understand their role in making a contribution to the wider public health agenda. A range of health promotion theories and models have been presented and discussed, although the literature on this topic is extensive and further reading is encouraged. Practice examples have been used to make the links between health promotion theory and mental health nursing practice, identifying a range of factors influencing the process and potential outcomes of collaborative health promotion. In summary, the key points of learning from this chapter are:

- Health promotion to improve public health is high on the global agenda and there is international recognition of the importance of supporting countries to improve the health of their citizens.

- Health promotion is an overarching term to describe activities which aim to enable individuals, groups and communities to take control and improve their own health.

- Improving physical and mental public health is a key feature of contemporary UK policy with priority given to health improvement activities that aim to reduce national health inequalities.

- A range of health promotion theories and models exist providing a foundation for an evidence-based approach to mental health nursing practice.

■ Health promotion to improve both physical and mental health is a core feature of mental health nursing that requires a commitment to work collaboratively to improve the health of service users.

Annotated bibliography

Green, J. and Tones, K. (2010) *Health Promotion: Planning and strategies,* **2nd edn. London: Sage.**
This book provides a thorough overview of theories, concepts and frameworks in health promotion practice. It will be most useful to you for developing a critical understanding of the evidence that underpins the health promotion strategies you use in your practice.

Scriven, A. (2010) *Promoting Health: A practical guide,* **6th edn. London: Elsevier.**
This book is more practical. It gives well formulated ideas and suggestions for implementing health promotion practice in a range of settings. It will help you to reflect on your practice and develop new health promotion skills.

Trenoweth, S., Docherty, T., Franks, J. and Pearce, R. (2011) *Nursing and Mental Health Care: An introduction for all fields of practice.* **Exeter: Learning Matters.**
This is a contemporary text which provides a more specific understanding of mental health promotion in a mental health nursing context. It sets out the Nursing and Midwifery Council (NMC) standards for mental health nursing which include health promotion. It highlights the importance of your role in improving physical health in patients with mental illness. It also considers strategies to prevent mental illness and improve mental health.

References

Acheson, D. (1998) *Independent Inquiry into Inequalities in Health* (the Acheson Report), available at: www.archive.official-documents.co.uk/document/doh/ih/ih.htm, accessed 12 February 2012.

Becker, M.H. (1974) The Health Belief Model and personal health behavior, *Health Education Monographs,* 2: 324–473.

Caplan, G. (1964) *Principles of Preventive Psychiatry.* New York: Basic Books.

Chesterson, J. (2009) Mental health promotion and prevention, in P. Barker (ed.) *Psychiatric and Mental Health Nursing: The craft of caring,* 2nd edn. London: Edward Arnold.

DH (Department of Health) (2009) *New Horizons: A shared vision for mental health.* London: DH, avaible at: www.dh.gov.uk/en/Publicationsandstatistics/Publications/PublicationsPolicyAndGuidance/DH_109705, accessed 10 October 2011.

DH (Department of Health) (2011a) *Healthy Lives, Healthy People: update and way forward.* London: DH, available at: www.dh.gov.uk/en/Publicationsandstatistics/Publications/PublicationsPolicyAndGuidance/DH_128120, accessed 11 October 2011.

DH (Department of Health) (2011b) *Realising the Benefits: IAPT at full roll-out.* London: DH, available at: www.dh.gov.uk/en/Publicationsandstatistics/Publications/PublicationsPolicyAndGuidance/DH_112982, accessed 11 October 2011.

French, J. (2010) *Social Marketing in Public Health: Theory and practice.* New York: Oxford University Press.

Green, J. and Tones, K. (2010) *Health Promotion: Planning and strategies,* 2nd edn. London: Sage.

HM Government (2011) *No Health Without Mental Health: A cross-government mental health outcomes strategy for people of all ages.* London: HM Government, available at: www.dh.gov.uk/en/Publicationsandstatistics/Publications/PublicationsPolicyAndGuidance/DH_123766, accessed 10 October 2011.

IDeA (2010) *A Glass Half Full: How an asset approach can improve community health and wellbeing.* London: IDeA.

Kotler P. and Lee, N. (2008) *Social Marketing: Influencing behaviors for good,* 3rd edn. London: Sage.

Lefebvre and Flora (1988) Social marketing and public health intervention, *Health Education and Behaviour,* 15(3): 299–315.

Marmot, M. (2010) *Fair Society, Healthy Lives: Strategic review of health inequalities in England post 2010,* available at: www.marmotreview.org, accessed 15 August 2011.

Moodie, R. and Jenkins, R. (2005) I'm from the government and you want me to invest in mental health promotion. Well why should I? *Promotion and Education Supplement,* 2: 37.

Naidoo, J. and Wills, J. (2010) *Developing Practice for Public Health and Health Promotion,* 3rd edn. London: Bailliere Tindall.

NICE (National Institute for Health and Clinical Excellence) (2006) *Computerised Cognitive Behaviour Therapy For Depression And Anxiety: Guidance,* available at: www.nice.org.uk/nicemedia/live/11568/33185/33185.pdf, accessed 11 October 2011.

Nutbeam, D. (2000) Health literacy as a public health goal: a challenge for contemporary health education and communication strategies into the 21st century, *Health Promotion International,* 15(3): 259–67.

Parker, E. (2009) Health promotion, in M. Fleming and E. Parker, *Introduction to Public Health.* Sydney: Elsevier.

Pender, N. *et al.* (2011) *Health Promotion in Nursing Practice.* Upper Saddle River, NJ: Pearson.

Prochaska, J.O. and DiClemente, C.C. (1983) Stages and processes of self-change of smoking: toward an integrative model of change, *Journal of Counselling and Clinical Psychology,* 51: 390–5.

Roden, J. (2004) Revisiting the Health Belief Model: nurses applying it to young families and their health promotion needs, *Nursing and Health Sciences*, 6: 1–10.

Scriven, A. (2010) *Promoting Health: A practical guide*, 6th edn. London: Elsevier.

Skills for Health (2008) *The Public Health Skills and Career Framework*, available at: www.sph.nhs.uk/sph-files/PHSkills-CareerFramework_Launchdoc_April08.pdf, accessed 4 October 2011.

Sturt, J. (1998) Implementing theory into primary healthcare practice: an empowering approach, in S. Kendall (ed.) *Health and Empowerment*. London: Arnold.

WHO (World Health Organization) (1978) *Declaration of Alma-Ata*. International Conference on Primary Health Care, Alma-Ata, USSR. Geneva: WHO, available at: www.who.int/hpr/NPH/docs/declaration_almaata.pdf, accessed 18 October 2011.

WHO (World Health Organization) (1986) *The Ottawa Charter for Health Promotion*. First International Conference on Health Promotion, Ottawa, 21 November 1986, available at: www.who.int/hpr/NPH/docs/ottawa_charter_hp.pdf, accessed 18 October 2011.

WHO (World Health Organization) (2005) *Promoting Mental Health Concepts, Emerging Evidence and Practice*. A Report of the World Health Organization, Department of Mental Health and Substance Abuse in collaboration with the Victorian Health Promotion Foundation and The University of Melbourne, available at: www.who.int/mental_health/evidence/MH_Promotion_Book.pdf.

WHO (World Health Organization) (2007) *Interim Statement of the Commission for Social Determinants of Ill Health*, available at: www.who.int/social_determinants/thecommission/interimstatement/en/index.html, accessed 18 October 2011.

Chapter 5

Recovery and Social Inclusion

Rachel Perkins and Julie Repper

[Recovery is] a deeply personal, unique process of changing one's attitudes, values, feelings, goals, skills, and/or roles. It is a way of living a satisfying, hopeful and contributing life even with the limitations caused by illness. Recovery involves the development of new meaning and purpose in one's life as one grows beyond the catastrophic effects of mental illness.

Anthony (1993)

 ## 5.1 Introduction

Everyone who experiences mental health problems faces the challenge of recovery: the challenge of rebuilding, or, where possible, retaining, a valued and satisfying life. There is no way of going back to the way things were before the difficulties started, but they are not the end of life. Many people who have experienced mental health problems have shown us that there is a way forward: that it is possible to recover meaning and purpose in life.

Traditionally, the primary aim of mental health services and practitioners has been 'cure': interventions designed to change the individual so that they 'fit in' by reducing their symptoms and the attendant deficits and dysfunctions. The success of mental health services has been judged in terms of the extent to which they have been able to do this and so discharge people from their care.

For some people, symptoms may continue or recur from time to time but this does not preclude the possibility of them recovering a meaningful and valued life. It is true also that the elimination of symptoms does not guarantee recovery. Prejudice and discrimination extend beyond the presence of symptoms. People may be excluded because of a history of such problems – 'once a schizophrenic always a schizophrenic'. While treatments to reduce distressing and debilitating symptoms are important, they are only a small part of a person's recovery journey. Rebuilding a meaningful and valued life requires more than the treatment of symptoms.

Recovery requires that we move beyond 'cure' to thinking about how we can help people to make the most of their lives. If we are to do this then we must put the individual at centre stage: think not about 'the patient in our services' but instead about 'the person in their life' and the impact – for good or ill – that services have on their journey through this life.

In summary this chapter covers:

■ the meaning of recovery for people with mental health problems;

■ the principles of recovery and social inclusion;

■ the ways in which mental health practitioners can facilitate the individual's recovery journey and promote their inclusion and participation in community life.

5.2 The meaning of recovery for people with mental health problems

Mental health practitioners are accustomed to thinking about the experience of people with mental health problems in terms of their need for different types of interventions and services such as medication, inpatient care, psychosocial interventions and sheltered accommodation. This is not the best place to start. We cannot provide appropriate supports and interventions unless we understand the nature of the challenge that people face and what gives their life meaning and value. Only then is it possible to consider how we might help them in their individual journey of recovery.

Having mental health problems is a devastating and life-changing experience. You have to cope with strange and often frightening events. Perhaps you find yourself unable to think properly. Perhaps those ordinary, everyday things that you always did without thinking seem impossibly difficult. Perhaps you have experiences that no one around you believes or understands. Your confidence and belief in yourself hit rock bottom. You feel very alone and very frightened. Not only about what is happening to you, but also about the prospect of using mental health services.

Thinking Space 5.1

1. List up to 10 features of your life which help you to live to 'a meaningful life'. Now imagine that you become mentally ill and receive a diagnosis of schizophrenia.

2. Rate each of the features, on a scale of 1–10, according to the threat of losing it (where 1 = no threat of losing it and 10 = extremely likely indeed to lose it) as a result of a receiving a psychiatric diagnosis.

3. Compare your list with that of a friend's or colleague's. What are your conclusions about the threat of mental illness to a meaningful life?

All I knew were the stereotypes I had seen on television or in the movies. To me, mental illness meant Dr Jekyll and Mr Hyde, psychopathic serial killers, loony bins, morons, schizos, fruitcakes, nuts, straightjackets, and raving lunatics. They were all I knew about mental illness and what terrified me was that professionals were saying I was one of them.

(Deegan 1993)

You may be surrounded by people who think you will never amount to very much – views that are too often reinforced by the negative attitudes and prognoses of professionals: 'You have a chronic illness', 'You will not be able to work, have children, live independently ...'. Unthinkable things may happen to you – like being picked up by the police, detained against your will, forcibly medicated – all of which reinforce the frightening stereotypes of madness. People start treating you differently: as if you are stupid, or dangerous, or both. They start talking about you, rather than to you: 'Is she all right? Is she taking her tablets?'. They behave towards you as if they are walking on eggshells, fearful lest you dissolve into tears or explode into anger.

To be diagnosed as having serious mental health problems is a bereavement: it involves loss of the privileges of sanity; loss of the life the person had or expected to lead; loss of the person we thought we were or might become.

Out of the blue your job has gone, with it any financial security you may have had. At a stroke, you have no purpose in life, and no contact with other people. You find yourself totally isolated from the rest of the world. No one telephones you. Much less writes. No one seems to care if you're alive or dead.

(cited in Bird 2001)

Too often, when practitioners focus solely on symptoms and cures, such ordinary bereavement responses are seen as pathological – symptoms of the illness itself. Denial becomes the 'lack of insight' supposedly inherent in the disorder. Hopelessness, apathy and withdrawal become the 'negative symptoms' and 'lack of motivation' that are assumed to characterize the 'illness'. Anger becomes a 'symptom' to be treated or the 'acting out' that may be taken to indicate additional 'personality problems'.

In contrast to these traditions, ideas about recovery have emerged from people who themselves have faced the challenge of life with a mental health problem. Deegan (1988) defines recovery as:

the lived or real life experience of people as they accept and overcome the challenge of the disability ... they experience themselves as recovering a new sense of self and of purpose within and beyond the limits of the disability.

In a similar vein Shepherd *et al.* (2008) define recovery as being 'about building a meaningful and satisfying life, as defined by the person themselves, whether or not there are ongoing or recurring symptoms or problems'. Anderson *et al.* (2003) have studied many personal accounts of recovery and conclude that recovery involves four key components:

- finding and maintaining hope;
- re-establishing a positive identity;
- building a meaningful life; and
- taking responsibility and control.

Recovery therefore involves finding new meaning and purpose in life as people live through and beyond the catastrophic effects of a mental illness.

Mental health professionals cannot meaningfully assist people in this process if they are not able to look beyond the 'psychiatric' signs and symptoms to the whole person and their life context with all its hopes, aspirations and frustrations.

Over the past decade, health and social care policy in the UK, such as the *NHS Improvement Plan* (DH 2004), *Our Health, Our Care, Our Say* (DH 2006) and *No Health Without Mental Health* (DH 2011), have emphasized the need to move beyond services that primarily treat illness to recovery-based approaches that:

- positively promote health and well-being;
- maximize people's life chances;
- enable people to take control of their lives and to manage their own self-care; and
- help people to do the things they want to do and to live the lives they aspire to.

Such approaches are now recognized as being important for many groups in our communities in addition to those with mental health problems (e.g. children, older people and people with a learning disability). Some contemporary policy documents for these groups are cited below together with evidence of the recovery approach that is embedded in each.

- *Every Child Matters: Change for Children* (Department for Education and Skills 2003) – *Every Child Matters* and subsequent policy documents that have built upon it over the last decade (e.g. *Healthy Lives, Brighter Futures* and *The Children's Plan*) emphasize the importance of 'enjoying and achieving' and 'making a positive contribution', to enable all children, whether or not they have mental health or behavioural problems, to get the most out of life, develop skills for adulthood and to be involved as valued members of the community.
- *Living Well with Dementia: A National Dementia Strategy* (DH 2009a) – the aim of this ambitious strategy is for all people with dementia and their carers to be supported to live well with the condition. While the dementias are a devastating set of illnesses with

profound negative effects it is also clear that there is a vast amount that can be done to improve and maintain meaning in people's lives. The *National Dementia Strategy* emphasizes that positive input from health and social care services, and from the third sector and carers of people with dementia, can make all the difference between living well with dementia and having a poor quality of life.

- *Valuing People Now: A new three-year strategy for people with learning disabilities* (DH 2009b) – *Valuing People Now* sets out a clear vision that all people with a learning disability are people first, with the right to lead their lives like any

others, with the same opportunities and responsibilities, and should be treated with the same dignity and respect. They and their families and carers are entitled to the same aspirations and life chances as other citizens.

Thinking Space 5.2

Rethink Mental Illness, the mental health charity, distinguishes between two types of recovery: 'clinical recovery' and 'personal recovery'. How would you define these two forms of recovery?

Feedback to Thinking Space 5.2

- **Clinical recovery** has emerged from the expertise of mental health professionals, and involves getting rid of symptoms, restoring social functioning, and in other ways 'getting back to normal'.
- **Personal recovery** has emerged from the expertise of people with lived experiences of mental illness. It focuses on the process of building a meaningful life as defined by the person themselves.

Rethink works to ensure that people are provided with appropriate therapy and support to reduce or take away symptoms of mental illness. However, the focus on recovery directs attention to the importance of *personal recovery* to assist people living a meaningful life, even when experiencing enduring or fluctuating mental health problems.

5.3 Principles of recovery and inclusion

People with mental health problems may benefit from a wide range of support and treatment – the critical question is how these enable (or prevent) the person to pursue their ambitions and make the most of their life. In this context the principles and values of services and the aims of interventions are critically important (see Box 5.1).

Recovery is about people's whole lives not just their symptoms

There are a variety of different ways in which people may gain relief from distressing symptoms: these

include medication, psychological therapy, self-help and self-management to enable the person to manage their difficulties themselves, and a range of complementary therapies. However, people's problems extend well beyond the expertise traditionally found within mental health services. Rarely is it a person's ambition in life merely to get rid of distressing and disabling symptoms – they want to do this in order to do the things they want to do and live the lives they wish to lead. This is what recovery is about: enabling people to have the homes, jobs and friends that give everyone's life meaning and via which we get our sense of value. Enabling people to access accommodation, material resources, employment, education, relationships, social and leisure activities is at least, if not more, important in

---

Box 5.1 Key principles of recovery

- Recovery is about people's whole lives not just their symptoms.
- Recovery is about growth.
- Recovery is not an end product or result but an ongoing journey.
- Recovery is not dependent on professional intervention.
- A recovery vision is not limited to a particular theory about the nature and origins of mental health problems.
- Recovery is not a linear process.
- Recovery is possible for everyone.
- Carers, relatives and friends also face the challenge of recovery.
- Everyone's recovery journey is different and deeply personal.
- Recovery is not specific to mental health problems but is a common human condition.

---

the recovery process as reducing the mental health problems themselves.

Recovery is about growth

It is very easy for people with mental health problems to become nothing other than their illness, ceasing to be Fred and becoming 'a schizophrenic' or 'a manic depressive'. If practitioners focus only on deficits and dysfunctions then the identity of 'mental patient', at the expense of all other facets of personhood, is reinforced. People are always more than their 'illness'. Recovery involves redefining identity in a way which includes these difficulties, but enables people to grow, develop and move beyond them. However, growth is not possible if you are prevented from doing the things you want to do and excluded within the community in which you live. Growth is often limited not by characteristics of the person, but by the barriers imposed by discrimination and exclusion.

> *My recovery was about how to gain other people's confidence in my abilities and potential … in my own experience the toughest part was changing other people's expectations of what I could do.*

> *Combating a disempowering sense of being undervalued …*

(May 1999)

The mental health world has a lot to learn from the physical disability world. When we think about a person with a broken spine or limited hearing, thoughts do not focus on treatment alone. Instead we think about:

- supports that the person might need – like wheelchairs and personal assistants – to enable them to do the things they do;
- adjustments in the environment that facilitate access – like ramps and induction loops;
- changing the attitudes and skills of others in the community in order to remove 'them and us' barriers and enable people to participate as equal citizens.

The challenge for people with mental health problems, and the mental health practitioners who assist them, is to find the psychiatric equivalents of the wheelchair, the induction loop and the disability awareness training. We need to identify the supports and adjustments that the individual might need, and the support and adjustments that others in the community might require if people with mental health problems are to participate fully in community life.

Recovery is not an end product or result but an ongoing journey

Recovery is a process, not an end point or destination. Recovery is an attitude, a way of approaching the day and the challenges I face ... I know I have certain limitations and things I can't do. But rather than letting these limitations be occasions for despair and giving up, I have learned that in knowing what I can't do, I also open up the possibilities of all I can do.

(Deegan 1993)

People cannot be 'fixed' as one might mend a television or refurbish a building. If recovery is a continuing journey, then assistance and adjustments often need to be thought of as a continuing process of supporting people in that journey. And this must involve not only helping the person to move forward, but also helping them to maintain what has already been achieved.

Recovery is not dependent on professional intervention

Recovery is not a professional intervention to which expert professionals hold the key (Anthony 1993). It is an individual journey in which the person's own resources and those available to them outside the mental health system are central. The sources of meaning and satisfaction in most people's lives do not lie within mental health services – they lie in our work, our homes, our relationships, our leisure pursuits, our religion or spiritual beliefs. If people are unable to access the range of ordinary opportunities that other citizens usually take for granted then it is unlikely that they will be able to rebuild lives that they find satisfying and meaningful. The expertise of experience

can also be important. Many people have described the enormous support they have received from others who have faced a similar challenge (May 1999).

the gift that people with disabilities can give each other ... hope, strength and experience as lived through the recovery process ... a person does not have to be 'fully recovered' to serve as a role model. Very often a person who is only a few 'steps' ahead of another person can be more effective than one whose achievements seem overly impressive and distanced.

(Deegan 1988)

This may be achieved via self-help groups and user/survivor organizations or more informal friendships and networks within which people can share experiences and support each other's journeys.

A recovery vision is not limited to a particular theory

Just as professionals have developed a range of different organic, psychological and interpersonal models for understanding mental distress, so people who have experienced these difficulties understand their difficulties in different ways. Based on the narratives of 30 people with serious mental health problems, Jacobson (1993) identified six frameworks that people have used to understand their difficulties: biological; interaction of biology and environment; abuse or trauma; spiritual or philosophical; political; and the dehumanizing impact of long-term contact with mental health services.

As Anthony (1993) points out, a recovery vision does not commit one to a particular understanding of distress and disability. People need ways of understanding what has happened to them ('Why me?', 'What is the point in my life now?') but whether they choose genes, inter- or intrapersonal problems or the action of various deities, recovery – rebuilding a meaningful and satisfying life – is equally important. The critical issue is not the veracity of a model or explanation but the extent to which it:

- Makes sense to the person: any number of randomized controlled trials are unlikely to persuade a deeply religious person that their lives are wholly determined by their biology.
- Enables them to move forward in their life: genetic explanations, for example, may impede growth if characteristics are seen as fixed and immutable; explanations revolving around abuse and trauma preclude the possibility of growth if they are considered to have done irreparable damage. However, both genetic and traumatic explanations can facilitate growth if they are seen as something over which the person can exercise control or influence and as modifiable by social and environmental circumstances.

If mental health practitioners insist that people adopt a single understanding of their difficulties then they are likely to alienate those who prefer alternative explanations.

Recovery is not a linear process

It is also important to accept that recovery will not be a linear process – there will be problems and setbacks along the way. Relapse is not 'failure', but a part of the recovery process – a learning opportunity that can enable a person to move beyond their limitations by identifying the additional support and adjustments that they, or the people around them, may need to successfully pursue their ambitions. However, if a person is not to become dispirited – give up – they need people around them who can 'hold on to hope': believe in them and their possibilities, during those times when they are not able to believe in their own worth and future.

Recovery is possible for everyone

Recovery is not only for those who are more able. It is not contingent on the removal of symptoms or the development of skills. Some people will remain profoundly disabled, but with the right kind of sup-

port they can find sources of value and meaning in order to move forward in their lives. Some people deny their need for services and reject professional help, but they can still achieve the support and encouragement they need to pursue their ambitions outside specialist services: among those friends, family members and agencies that exist to help all citizens.

Carers, relatives and friends also face the challenge of recovery

The critical issue then becomes not whether the individual has appropriate support from mental health practitioners but whether friends, family and community agencies receive the help they need to accommodate the person with mental health difficulties. All too often informal carers find that their own social networks and life opportunities can become diminished as they also experience the negative effects of stigma and social exclusion. It is vital that services facilitate also the recovery of carers and others who are close to the person, helping them to make sense of what has happened and to rebuild their own lives. Importantly it is these reciprocal relationships with friends, family, neighbours and colleagues, rather than one-way relationships with mental health practitioners, that can foster self-worth and provide meaning in people's lives.

Everyone's recovery journey is different and deeply personal

There are no rules of recovery, no formula for success: 'Once recovery becomes systematised, you've got it wrong. Once it is reduced to a set of principles it is wrong. It is a unique and individualised process' (Deegan 1999). It is easy for the destructive, rigid routines and block treatment of the old psychiatric hospitals to spill over into community services. For example:

- There remain community services where a set of rules dictate how people must use them: you cannot have lunch at the day centre unless you attend a group; in order to live in the hostel you have to cook a meal for all residents once a week and attend the community group each day. If a person needs a hot meal it is a waste of their time and scarce resources to insist that they attend a group as well and just how does cooking a meal for eight people train you to cook for yourself at home?

■ The 'ladder' models adopted by some services insist that people start at point A and then move in an orderly fashion to point Z: you must start in the rehabilitation ward, and then show that you can manage in a staffed hostel before you can have a flat of your own. It is entirely possible for someone to move directly from hospital to independent accommodation, or be sustained in their own place during a crisis – is this not what home treatment and assertive outreach services are designed to achieve?

■ The often implicit assumption that there exists a hierarchy of skills in which you can only move on to more 'advanced' endeavours when you have mastered 'basic' ones: you must be able to wash your socks before you can go to work. Yet it is entirely possible for a person to need help in many aspects of daily life and still hold down a responsible job: how many high-flying executives do their own cleaning and cooking?

Such rules inevitably mean that services cannot be tailored to the individual needs and aspirations of the people who use them. Not only is this likely to impede recovery, it is also likely either to de-skill people – prevent them from using their skills/abilities to the full – or alienate them by offering support in a manner that they find unacceptable and infantilizing.

Recovery is not specific to mental health problems but is a common human condition

As indicated, recovery is important for many people in society in addition to those with mental health problems, including children, older people and people with a learning disability. However, it is equally true for all of us as we experience significant changes in our lives such as the loss of a loved one, a pet, a job or the realization that a goal or aspiration we had for ourselves is no longer in reach. At such times we need to re-evaluate and rebuild our lives to regain purpose and meaning. Perhaps the best way of understanding recovery is by considering a difficult event in our own lives.

> ### Thinking Space 5.3
>
> The concept of recovery is not confined to mental health difficulties. Consider an event that has had an impact on your life (such as losing a job, the death of a loved one, serious illness, moving house …) and think about the effect this had on you, ways in which you coped, what helped you and what did not.
>
> Discuss this with another person and note the similarities and differences in your experiences of recovery. How has the experience changed you/your life in the longer term?

5.4   Promoting recovery, facilitating inclusion

Promoting recovery and facilitating inclusion requires not only a major change in the guiding philosophy of services – moving away from a focus on minimizing symptoms and reducing dysfunctions towards a focus on enabling people to do the things they want to do and live the lives they want to lead – but also a change in the approach and skills of mental health practitioners. And we must look to the expertise of personal experience for guidance – what people who are recovering from mental health problems have found helpful in their journey.

There are a number of common features that seem to be critically important in the recovery process: hope; relationships; coping with loss; spirituality, philosophy and understanding; taking back control; finding meaning, purpose and opportunity.

It is also clear that these do not constitute a recipe for, or set of predetermined stages of, recovery. They are intimately interlinked and follow no set sequence.

If mental health practitioners are really to support people in their recovery journey then three interrelated components are central: fostering hope and creating hope-inspiring relationships; facilitating personal adaptation; and promoting access and inclusion (see Figure 5.1).

Maintaining and fostering hope

Hope has been described as the 'anchor stabilizing our lives in the present and giving life meaning, direction and optimism' (Lindsay 1976). It is critical in recovery and central to the lives of most people – without hope there is no reason to carry on.

There is a considerable body of research into the importance of hope in coping with physical illness (e.g. Hickey 1986). In the mental health arena, hope has long been recognized as key to successful psychotherapy (Frank 1968); there is a link between hopelessness and suicide (Beck *et al.* 1990); and the importance of practitioners' hopefulness has been emphasized as central in rehabilitation (Anthony 1993; Kanwal 1997). Hope may be a generalized sense of some future positive development or related to a specific, valued outcome (like getting a job or getting married).

For people with mental health problems, hope lies at the heart of a person's willingness to take on the challenge of recovery and rebuilding: without hope there is no point. In the face of the prejudice and exclusion that many people with mental health problems have experienced it is very easy to lose hope. And if a person can see no possibility of a positive future then it is all too easy for them to give up trying to do anything at all.

But hope does not, and cannot, exist in a vacuum – relationships are central. If everyone around you believes that you have little to offer – that you will never amount to anything very much – then it is difficult (if not impossible) to retain a belief in your own worth. Everyone needs people around who believe in possibilities. Relationships are important

not only as a source of help and support: always to be on the receiving end of support and help from others is a devaluing experience. Giving is as important as receiving and reciprocity in relationships is critical. Relationships in which people can contribute to the well-being of others – help and support them – are an important source of value.

The contribution of people with serious mental health problems often goes unrecognized: family and friends become 'carers' who provide the support and help that people need to survive. Rarely do we recognize the support and help that people with mental health problems offer to those around them – both others with mental health problems and friends, and family outside mental health services. Greenberg *et al.* (1994) have shown that people with a diagnosis of schizophrenia can and do contribute a great deal of practical, social and emotional support to other members of their families. If hope is to be fostered, then we must move beyond ideas about 'carers' and those who are 'cared for' – reciprocal relationships with friends and family in which people support each other are critical to the restoration of hope and self-worth.

Russinova (1999) has described a number of practitioner 'relationship skills' that are important in developing effective, ongoing hope-inspiring relationships that can enable people to gain the confidence and self-belief that are critical if they are to rebuild their lives and access the opportunities they value:

- believing in the person's potential and strength;
- valuing the person as a unique human being;
- accepting the person for who he/she is;
- listening non-judgementally to the person's experiences;
- tolerating the uncertainty about the future developments in the person's life;
- accepting the person's decompensations and failures as part of the recovery process;
- tolerating the person's challenges and defeats;
- trusting the authenticity of the person's experiences;

Figure 5.1 Promoting recovery, facilitating inclusion

Facilitating personal adaptation

" Over the years I've worked hard to become an expert in my own self care... I've learned different ways of helping myself."
(Deegan 1993)

- Offering a range of acceptable and accessible treatments to reduce distressing and disabling symptoms as much as possible
- Helping people to take control of their own problems and the help they receive
- Enabling people to reach an understanding of what has happened that makes sense to them and allows the possibility of moving forward in life
- Fostering self-belief and mobilising personal resources
- Fostering and promoting peer support and relationships with others who have experienced mental health problems

Promoting access and inclusion

" I don't want a CPN, I want a life."
(Rose 2001)

- Facilitating access to material resources (like money, food, housing, transport etc.)
- Helping people to access those roles, activities and resources that other citizens take for granted
- Enabling people to identify and articulate their dreams and aspirations
- Supporting people to maintain valued roles and acitivities that they value and establish new ones that are in line with their ambitions
- Enabling people to access mainstream sources of support and help wherever possible
- Supporting individuals and agencies outside mental health services (like primary care, employers, colleges, housing authorities, churches...) to enable them to accommodate people with mental health problems

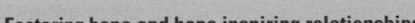

Fostering hope and hope inspiring relationships

" For those of us who have been diagnosed with mental illness and who have lived in sometimes desolate wastelands of mental health programmes, hope is not just a nice sounding euphemism. It is a matter of life and death."
(Deegan 1988)

- Creating hope inspiring relationships with those whom we serve:
  - Valuing people for who they are
  - Believing in the people's worth
  - Having confidence in people's abilities and potential
  - Listening to and heeding what they say
  - Believing in the authenticity of their experiences rather than dismissing them as merely symptoms
  - Accepting and actively exploring their experiences
  - Tolerating uncertainty about the future
  - Seeing problems and set-backs as part of the recovery process

- Fostering and supporting reciprocal relationships with family, friends, peers, partners and others who are important to the person

- expressing a genuine concern for the person's well-being;
- using humour appropriately.

This list may sound simple and self-evident, but we should never underestimate how difficult it is to deliver. Most people do not want to need our services and many are too distressed and/or disturbed when they arrive with us to be grateful. Valuing a person, being non-judgemental and expressing genuine concern for their well-being can be hard if someone is angry and abusive or rejects what you offer them, yet these are the core skills of any mental health worker.

Facilitating personal adaptation and taking back control

Mental health problems are often presented and perceived as uncontrollable – the province of experts. If a person is to take back control over their life they need to both develop ways of understanding and accommodating what has happened to them and ways of taking control over their symptoms and problems, the help they receive and their life and well-being more generally.

As we have already described, the experience of mental health problems constitutes a bereavement: multiple losses that appear to be beyond your control and profoundly change the way you see yourself, your world and your future. In the process of recovery – rebuilding their life and sense of self – people face the task of accommodating what has happened so that they can move on (Repper and Perkins 2002).

- **Grieving that which has been lost.** People need space and time to grieve, to tell their stories – and to tell them over and over again if necessary: new issues, meaning and understanding can emerge with each telling. In reclaiming a sense of identity and value in the present, it is often necessary for a person to talk of identities and valued roles of the past. And expressing at least some of the anger, fear, despair, resentment and shame that they may feel over what has happened. Sometimes anger

and resentment may be directed towards the practitioner and the advantages that they have: we may not feel privileged, but in comparison with many of those with whom we work, we are very fortunate. The process of grieving may be slow. It is difficult to live with mental health problems and there may be little we can do to substantially change the material realities of the person's situation. But we can share the person's burden: understand and accept their distress, and help them to feel less alone.

- **Information.** Many of the popular myths and misconceptions that surround mental health problems are inevitably shared by those who experience them, and are regularly reinforced in the popular media. These make the experience even more frightening. Many of those who deny that they have such difficulties do so in order to reject the images of themselves as dangerous and incompetent. It is important that practitioners make active efforts to dispel such myths and in doing this the personal accounts of people who have succeeded in rebuilding their lives can be powerful. There are a number of anthologies in which these can be found (see e.g. Read and Reynolds 1996; Simpson 2004) and papers in journals such as *Open Mind* and *Schizophrenia Bulletin*. Information about the many successful people – great painters like Van Gogh, scientists like Einstein, writers like James Joyce, politicians like Churchill – who have had mental health problems can also be useful (see e.g. Jamison 1995; Post 1996).

- **Understanding what has happened.** As we have already discussed, people need to find a way of understanding what has happened that makes sense to them and allows them a way forward. The experience of serious mental health problems often prompts people to explore broader spiritual and philosophical issues concerning the meaning of their lives: 'Why me?', 'What did I do to deserve this?', 'What's the point?' Without prescribing particular religious and philosophical frameworks, it is important that practitioners enable people to think about these issues as well.

Specialized treatment from professionals – psychological, pharmacological, systemic – can help to control a person's distressing and disturbing symptoms. But if a person is to rebuild their life then it is important that they are able to take back control over both their problems and well-being:

To me, recovery means I try to stay in the driver's seat of my life. I don't let my illness run me. Over the years I have worked hard to become an expert in my own self-care. For me, being in recovery means I don't just take medications. Just taking medications is a passive stance. Rather I use medications as part of my recovery process. In the same way, I don't just go into hospital. Just 'going into hospital' is a passive stance. Rather, I use the hospital when I need to.

(Deegan 1989)

People who have themselves had experience of dealing with a range of mental health problems have developed a range of different responses (see e.g. the self-management training developed by the Bipolar Organization – formerly the Manic Depression Fellowship – www.bipolaruk.org.uk – and Rethink – formerly the National Schizophrenia Fellowship – www.rethink.org.uk). Many of these initiatives are based on the Wellness and Recovery Action Plan (WRAP) developed by Mary Ellen Copeland (1997). WRAP is not a care plan developed by professionals. It is 'a self-management and recovery system developed by a group of people who had mental health difficulties and who were struggling to incorporate wellness tools and strategies into their lives'. WRAP is designed to:

- decrease and prevent intrusive or troubling feelings and behaviours;
- increase personal empowerment;
- improve quality of life;
- assist people in achieving their own life goals and dreams.

WRAP is a structured system to monitor uncomfortable and distressing symptoms and help you reduce, modify or eliminate those symptoms by using planned responses. This includes plans for how you want others to respond when symptoms have made it impossible for you to continue to make decisions, take care of yourself, or keep yourself safe (see www.mentalhealthrecovery.com). It incorporates:

- a daily management plan describing how you feel when you are well and identifying those things you need to do to stay well.

The identification of:

- triggers: those events and situations that may lead to the onset of uncomfortable symptoms and what you find helpful to do when these occur;
- early warning signs: the often subtle indications that indicate things are beginning to worsen and what to do when you notice these;
- symptoms that occur when things have got worse but not yet reached crisis point, and what you can do if these happen.

Along with:

- a crisis plan that identifies those symptoms that indicate to you that you are no longer able to take make decisions for yourself and keep yourself safe; this tells supporters and health care professionals what you think they should do on your behalf;
- a post-crisis plan describing what you find helpful in working your way out of a crisis and resuming your day-to-day life.

Traditional treatments may be one component of the way in which a person can take control over distressing and disturbing symptoms but this might also include self-help, support from friends and a range of strategies that the person has developed for dealing with particular problems:

stress does play an enormous part in my illness [schizophrenia]. There are enormous pressures that come with any new experience and environment, and any change, positive or negative is extremely difficult. Whatever I can do to decrease or avoid high stress environments is helpful in controlling my symptoms. In general terms all of my coping strategies consist of four steps: (1) recognizing when I am feeling stressed, which is harder than it may sound; (2) identifying the stressor; (3) remembering from past experience what action helped in the same situation or a similar one; and (4) taking that action as quickly as possible after I have identified the source of stress.

(Leete 1989)

People can benefit from the experiences of others who have faced similar difficulties, either individually or within local self-help groups and national networks. People can also access the expertise of others who have experienced similar difficulties via their writings (see above). It is important that mental health practitioners actively foster both direct and indirect peer relationships and maximize opportunities for peer support.

However, if people are to take back control over their own lives, then practitioners must give up that control. It is easy to support people in making choices for themselves when they agree with you: the real challenge arises when the person makes choices that the practitioner considers to be wrong (see Perkins and Repper 1998). There are, of course, occasions when it would be unethical or illegal for the practitioner to accede to the individual's wishes: we may not, for example, help people to kill themselves, obtain illegal drugs or put others at risk, and all of these things are likely to impede the process of rebuilding a valued and satisfying life. However, such instances are few and far between.

More frequently, people make decisions that the practitioner considers unlikely to be successful. Often from the best of motives, practitioners are eager to help people to avoid failure and its potentially destructive consequences. For example, we may discourage a person going to the Job Centre because we think they are not yet ready for employment; or recommend that they live in sheltered accommodation because we do not think they will be able to look after themselves; or suggest that they do not go out clubbing with their friends for fear that they will get drunk or use drugs and make their problems worse.

Making the most of one's life necessarily involves the risk of failure. Entering relationships involves the risk of rejection; trying to get a job involves the risk of being turned down; studying for qualifications involves risking failure of examinations or assessment. Growth and development necessarily involve the risk of failure. And we can learn as much about ourselves, and our possibilities, from our failures as we can from our successes. It is also the case that people with serious mental health problems are often more expert in coping with failure – because of the numerous losses and disappointments they have experienced – than are the practitioners who are helping them.

Instead of attempting to dissuade people from their chosen course of action we need to:

- offer any support and help that we can to maximize their chances of success;
- endeavour to find ways of circumventing the difficulties that might prevent a person from achieving their chosen goal;
- help them to learn from their experiences and try again if they are unsuccessful (and always avoid saying 'I told you so').

Thinking Space 5.4

List the main reasons why mental health difficulties too often lead to and reinforce social exclusion.

Promoting access and inclusion

It is impossible for a person to rebuild a meaningful and satisfying life without the opportunity to do the

Feedback to Thinking Space 5.4

The Social Exclusion Unit (2004) identified five main reasons for social exclusion of people with mental health difficulties:

- *Stigma and discrimination* against people with mental health problems. Fewer than 4 in 10 employers say they would recruit someone with a mental health problem. Many people fear disclosing their condition, even to family and friends.

- *Low expectations by professionals* of what people with mental health problems can achieve. There is limited recognition by health professionals that returning to work and overcoming social isolation is associated with better health outcomes.

- *Limited promotion of vocational and social outcomes* for people with mental health problems.

- *Insufficient ongoing support to enable people with mental health difficulties to work.* People on benefits often do not believe they will end up financially better off if they try to move into work. Many people lose jobs that they might have kept had they received better support.

- *People with mental health difficulties face barriers to engaging in the community.* They can struggle to access basic services such as decent housing and transport. Education, arts, sports and leisure providers often are not aware how their services could benefit people with mental health problems or how to make their services more accessible. Many people do not want to participate in activities alone, but feel there is no one they can ask to go with them.

things they value. But prejudice and discrimination frequently limit the access of people with mental health problems to the opportunities that are available to non-disabled citizens.

In order to facilitate recovery, people with serious mental health problems require access to a range of accommodation possibilities; work/education, leisure and social opportunities; and sources of support. However, Bates (2002) and Repper and Perkins (2002) have outlined things that individual practitioners can do to facilitate a person's access to valued roles and activities. At a general level, these may include:

- **Information.** Providing people with information about the facilities, opportunities and services available in the local area.

- **Bridge-building.** Actively creating links with local facilities to facilitate access. This may involve getting to know key people at the local college, leisure centre, church or job centre;

understanding the demands and expectations of these facilities; and the sort of people who use them.

- **Capacity-building.** Increasing the capacity of community facilities to accommodate people who have experienced mental health problems. This typically involves two elements: breaking down myths and misconceptions about people with mental health problems and providing facilities with the support they feel they need to accommodate people with such difficulties.

At an individual level there are a number of different strategies that practitioners might use to assist a person to access the opportunities and activities that they seek. These include:

- **Planning and target-setting.** Helping people to think about their goals and ambitions, breaking these down into manageable steps and planning the necessary interim goals and targets on the way.

- **Practice.** Helping the person to rehearse what they are going to do and practise it until they feel comfortable doing it.

- **Skills development.** Using a variety of techniques – instruction, prompting, modelling, guided practice, feedback – to help a person develop the skills they need to engage in their chosen activities.

- **Graded exposure/return** to help people overcome fears and anxieties that stop them doing what they want to do or resuming valued activities in which they have previously been involved.

- **Just visiting** a place or activity beforehand as a way of becoming familiar with how to get there and what to expect.

- **Time-limited experience** (like work experience or college 'taster sessions') in order to try something out before deciding whether it is what they want to do.

- **Providing transport** to help the person to get to the activity, or actually going with them to help reduce their anxiety.

- **'Doing with'.** Helping someone to do something by doing it alongside them. This may involve a mental health practitioner, but having your nurse with you in a college class can be stigmatizing. There may be others who are better placed to join the person in the activity and who are less likely to attract negative attention: friends, relatives, volunteers, someone already engaged in the activity, others who experience mental health difficulties.

- **Subsidy.** Helping to meet the costs of the activity by providing money for things like transport, refreshments, course registration fees and/or exploring other sources of subsidy like bus passes or reduced rates of entry for unemployed or disabled people.

- **Special groups within ordinary settings.** For example, special groups or classes to introduce people with mental health problems to the local sports centre, college or library.

- **Staff from different facilities coming into mental health facilities** to introduce them, to familiarize people with the activities involved before going to the community facility.

- **Mentoring.** Arranging for someone who is already involved in the setting/activity to provide information about what will be expected before they go, introduce them to the activity and provide advice and encouragement when they are there.

- **Helping people to make new friends.** Often people lack the friendships and relationships on which most of us rely so heavily. Practitioners can help people to increase their social networks and contacts by, for example, enabling them to access activities where they are likely to meet people who share their interests; accessing internet chat-lines and e-groups (some of which are designed specifically for people with mental health problems like the Yahoo 'uksurvivors' e-group); placing or replying to advertisements in 'lonely hearts'/'contact' columns of local newspapers and listings magazines; befriending; or facilitating contact between service users who share interests/aspirations.

- **Help and support when difficulties arise.** The fluctuating nature of mental health problems often means that it is important to ensure that assistance is readily available when difficulties arise.

- **Working out ways of coping with symptoms/difficulties in the setting.** Leete (1989), for example, offers numerous examples of strategies that she has found useful in coping with the symptoms of her schizophrenia in a work setting.

- **Self-help and support groups** where people with mental health problems who are engaged in similar activities (e.g. working, going to college) can get together and gain encouragement and support from each other.

■ **Negotiating adaptations and adjustments on the part of the provider.** These involve changing the physical or social environment, and/or the expectations on the person, so that they are able to engage in the activity. The UK Disability Discrimination Act 1995 not only outlaws discrimination against people with mental health problems but also requires that employers and providers of education, goods and services make 'reasonable adjustments' to ensure that people with such difficulties can access the opportunities they offer.

■ **Helping people to obtain their rights under the law.** As indicated above, the Disability Discrimination Act 1995 covers people with mental health problems and has been used by people with such difficulties to good effect. Sayce (2002) has suggested that mental health practitioners should:

● Be aware of the rights and protection that the Disability Discrimination Act provides for people with mental health problems and inform people with whom they work of these. Such information can be obtained from the Equality and Human Rights Commission helpline or website.

● Provide information about the assistance available from the Equality and Human Rights Commission helpline and case-work team (see www.equalityhumanrights.com for more information and contact numbers), and helping them to access this.

● Help employers, colleges, and the providers of goods and services to decide what 'reasonable adjustments' a person with mental health problems might need to facilitate access (either on an individual basis or as part of a more general 'capacity building' initiative – see above).

● Provide advocacy in relation to employment, education, leisure and other services.

There are many ways in which practitioners can enable people to access opportunities that they seek, but it is important that any such assistance is tailored to the needs/preferences of the person concerned. In choosing an appropriate approach, practitioners might consider the following (Repper and Perkins 2002):

■ **Individual acceptability.** What sort of help does the person want?

■ **Social acceptability.** What sort of help would draw least negative attention to the person?

■ **Amount and availability.** How much help does the person need and what support might be available?

■ **Existing abilities and resources.** How can the person's abilities, social contacts and other resources be used to best effect?

■ **Issues of control.** How far can the person themselves control the amount, timing and nature of the help they receive?

■ **Evidence of past effectiveness.** What sorts of help have been effective/ineffective in the past?

■ **The research evidence.** For example, skills development and practice are more effective when conducted in the setting in which the skills will be used because things learned in one setting do not always generalize to other situations. Bond *et al.* (2001) have identified a number of factors important to the success of programmes in facilitating access to employment including rapid job-search and minimal pre-vocational training; the availability of time-unlimited workplace support and the integration of clinical treatment with vocational rehabilitation.

 5.5   Conclusion

Recovery originates from service user-led ideas of self-determination and self-management. It emphasizes the importance of hope in sustaining motivation and supporting people's aspirations for a rich and fulfilling life. At its heart is the process of rebuilding meaningful lives despite the continuing presence of mental health problems. We cannot hope to assist in this process unless we understand both the nature of the challenge facing people with mental health problems and the ways in which they are responding to that challenge. In summary, the main points from this chapter are:

■ Recovery is about whole lives, not just symptoms, so services must focus on helping people to do the things they wish to do by adopting a whole-team, multi-agency approach with clear coordination and continuity, and by fostering relationships outside services.

■ Recovery is about growth, so services must focus on a person's strengths and possibilities and change the environment rather than the individual.

■ Recovery is not an end point but an ongoing journey, so services must maintain, as well as optimizing, a person's possibilities, adopting a long-term perspective and continuity of support over time.

■ Recovery is not a professional intervention but an individual's journey towards a meaningful life, so services need to emphasize social integration and maximize opportunities for people with mental health problems to support and learn from each other.

■ Recovery is not limited to any particular theory about mental health, it is based on the perspectives, wishes and aspirations of each individual.

■ Everyone's recovery is different and deeply personal so services need to adopt an individual approach to assessment and support, and respond flexibly to individual needs and wishes.

■ Recovery is possible for everyone; services need to help everyone identify and make the most of their abilities, and identify the types and sources of support that are acceptable to each individual.

If services are to promote and facilitate recovery, then three interrelated components are essential:

■ Facilitating personal adaptation through a range of acceptable and accessible treatments to reduce distressing and disabling symptoms, enabling people to reach an understanding of what has happened to them, and fostering peer support and relationships.

■ Maintaining and fostering hope, and creating hope-inspiring relationships with the individual and those important to them.

■ Promoting access to material resources, roles, relationships, activities and sources of support, and supporting agencies outside the mental health system to accommodate people with mental health problems.

Annotated bibliography

Repper, J. and Perkins, R. (2003) *Social Inclusion and Recovery. A model for mental health practice.* **London: Bailliere Tindall.**
This text provides a more detailed analysis of recovery and inclusion by the authors of this chapter. It draws on service users' experiences of living with mental health problems, and their accounts of recovery, to construct a model for practitioners seeking to promote recovery and inclusion.

Slade, M. (2009) *100 Ways to Support Recovery: a guide for professionals.* **London: Rethink.**
During 2007 Dr Mike Slade spent time away from clinical practice and research programmes to learn about recovery practices across Europe, America and Australia. This report presents his findings and suggestions.

Sayce, L. (2000) *From Psychiatric Patient to Citizen: overcoming discrimination and social exclusion.* **London: Macmillan.**
An in-depth analysis of the discrimination and exclusion experienced by people who have mental health problems with reference to extensive US and UK literature, research and personal contact. Various ways of overcoming this exclusion are debated through practical examples and theoretical debate.

Perkins, R.E. and Repper, J.M. (1996) *Working Alongside People with Long Term Mental Health Problems.* **Cheltenham: Stanley Thornes.**
Again, somewhat dated, but this remains one of very few texts available for direct care workers about the process of rehabilitation – facilitating access to socially valued roles, relationships, opportunities and facilities. It examines a range of different approaches that might be useful, and draws attention to the challenges that (still) remain.

Sainsbury Centre for Mental Health (2009) *Doing What Works: Individual placement and support into employment.*
Briefing Paper 37, available at: www.centreformentalhealth.org.uk/pdfs/briefing37_doing_what_works.pdf, accessed 6 May 2012. This briefing outlines the evidence base for Individual placement and support and provides information on how to 'do what works'.

References

Anthony, W.A. (1993) Recovery from mental illness: the guiding vision of the mental health system in the 1990s, *Innovations and Research*, 2(3): 17–24.

Bates, B. (2002) A–Z of socially inclusive strategies. Unpublished text. First presented at 'Piece of Mind' Conference, New College, Nottingham, January 1999.

Beck, A.T., Brown, G., Berchick, J., Stewart, L.B. and Steer, R.A. (1990) Relationship between hopelessness and suicide: a replication with psychiatric outpatients, *American Journal of Psychiatry*, 147(2): 11–23.

Bird, L. (2001) Poverty, social exclusion and mental health: a survey of people's personal experiences, *A Life in the Day*, 5: 3.

Bond, G.R., Becker, D.R., Drake, R.E. *et al.* (2001) Implementing supported employment as an evidence based practice, *Psychiatric Services*, 52(3): 313–22.

Copeland, M.E. (1997) *Wellness Recovery Action Plan.* Dummerston, VT: Peach Press.

Deegan, P. (1988) Recovery: the lived experience of rehabilitation, *Psychosocial Rehabilitation Journal*, 11(4): 11–19.

Deegan, P. (1989) A letter to my friend who is giving up. Paper presented at the Connecticut Conference on Supported Employment, Connecticut Association of Rehabilitation facilities, Cromwell, CT.

Deegan, P. (1993) Recovering our sense of value after being labeled, *Journal of Psychosocial Nursing*, 31(4): 7–11.

DfES (Department for Education and Skills) (2003) *Every Child Matters: Change for Children.* London: DfES.

DH (Department of Health) (2004) *NHS Improvement Plan 2004: Putting people at the heart of public services.* London: DH.

DH (Department of Health) (2006) *Our Health, Our Care, Our Say: A new direction for community services.* London: DH.

DH (Department of Health) (2009a) *Living Well With Dementia: A national dementia strategy.* London: DH.

DH (Department of Health) (2009b) *Valuing People Now: A new three-year strategy for people with learning disabilities.* London: DH.

DH (Department of Health) (2011) *No Health Without Mental Health: A cross-government mental health outcomes strategy for people of all ages.* London: DH.

Frank, J. (1968) The role of hope in psychotherapy, *International Journal of Psychiatry*, 5: 383–95.

Greenberg, J.S., Greenley, J.R. and Benedict, P. (1994) Contributions of persons with serious mental illness to their families, *Hospital and Community Psychiatry*, 45: 475–80.

Hickey, S.S. (1986) Enabling hope, *Journal of Cancer Nursing*, 9(3): 133–7.

Jacobson, N. (1993) Experiencing recovery: a dimensional analysis of recovery narratives, *Psychiatric Rehabilitation Journal*, 24(3): 248–55.

Jamison, K.R. (1995) Manic depressive illness and creativity, *Scientific American*, February: 46–51.

Kanwal, G.S. (1997) Hope, respect and flexibility in psychotherapy, *Contemporary Psychoanalysis*, 33(1): 133–50.

Leete, E. (1989) How I perceive and manage my illness, *Schizophrenia Bulletin*, 15: 197–200.

Lindsey, H. (1976) *The Terminal Generation.* Old Tappan, NJ: Fleming-Revel.

May, R. (1999) Routes to recovery – the roots of a clinical psychologist. Paper presented at Strangefish Conference 'Recovery: An Alien concept', Chamberlin Hotel, Birmingham.

Perkins, R.E. and Repper, J.M. (1998) *Dilemmas in Community Mental Health Practice: Choice or control.* Oxford: Radcliffe Medical Press.

Post, F. (1996) Verbal creativity, depression and alcoholism: an investigation of one hundred American and British writers, *British Journal of Psychiatry*, 168: 545–55.

Read, J. and Reynolds, J. (1996) *Speaking Our Minds.* London: Macmillan.

Repper, J. and Perkins, R. (2003) *Social Inclusion and Recovery: A model for mental health practice.* London: Bialliere Tindall.

Russinova, Z. (1999) Providers' hope-inspiring competence as a factor optimizing psychiatric rehabilitation outcomes, *Journal of Rehabilitation*, 16(4): 50–7.

Sayce, L. (2002) *Beyond Good Intentions: Making anti-discrimination strategies work.* London: Disability Rights Commission.

Shepherd, Boardman and Slade (2008) available at: www.rethink.org/living_with_mental_illness/what_is_recovery/?shortcut=recovery, accessed 20 April 2012.

Simpson, T. (ed.) (2004) *Doorways in the Night: Stories from the threshold of recovery.* Local Voices: Yorkshire Arts Circus.

Social Exclusion Unit (2004) *Mental Health and Social Exclusion: The Social Exclusion Unit report.* London: Office of the Deputy Prime Minister.

Chapter 6

Improving Mental Health Services

Iain Ryrie and Jean Penny

I am beginning to witness the positive outcomes of my suggestions on placement now, which prior to this module I would not have felt confident in suggesting let alone researching, process mapping, explaining and justifying to others and indeed implementing these improvements.

My previous perception was that the organisation in the NHS was all set by government legislation and NHS management. The truth is that small improvements developed by all workers in the health service can be put in place to change services for the better.

Testimonials from two students who participated in the NHSI improvement in pre-registration education programme

6.1 Introduction

Mental health services in the UK have undergone a period of unprecedented change in recent decades. The expressed wishes of service users, emerging practice evidence, shifts in public policy and economic constraints make for a context in which change is now constant. Mental health nurses need to be flexible and seek opportunities to adapt and enhance the services they provide as part of continuous quality improvement processes. In this chapter

we examine drivers for change in mental health services and introduce the discipline of improvement, its tools and techniques. Application of the improvement discipline is demonstrated through the use of case studies. The chapter covers:

- drivers for change;
- origins of service improvement;
- the discipline of improvement;
- improvement tools and techniques;
- applications in practice.

6.2   Drivers for change

Drivers for change in public services typically arise from policy directives, the expressed wishes of service users and from developments in a practice evidence base. Readers are referred to Chapter 8 for detail on the policy context of mental health care and its implications for change. However, a significant contemporary policy concern is the need for the National Health Service (NHS) to save £20 billion by 2015 and the associated financial challenges that public services in the UK and other European countries face. This dominant policy strand requires that more is achieved for increasingly less, and in such a climate quality and the expressed wishes of service users may receive less attention.

A useful summary of policy aspirations for mental health services was produced by the then Care Services Improvement Partnership (CSIP) in 2006 and remains relevant today. Service users were at the heart of the CSIP working group so that the aspirations reflect their preferences for better quality, safer and more person-centred services. Ten high impact changes proposed by CSIP are summarized in Box 6.1. Key to these aspirations and evi-

dent also in the current UK government's Health and Social Care Bill 2011 is closer partnership working with service users and the public in the design, development and governance of services. How mental health service users and their carers think and feel about the quality and range of services available to them matters a great deal and will reveal important opportunities for improvement.

These opportunities were first collated into the *NHS Improvement Plan* (DH 2004), sponsored by the then Labour government and originally designed to provide ongoing commitment to a 10-year process of NHS reform. The Health and Social Care Bill 2011 builds on this reform process with very specific quality improvement implications for professional disciplines. Embedded in the Bill is the assignment of positive duties to the Secretary of State for Health, the NHS Commissioning Board and the new clinical commissioning groups to secure continuous improvement in the quality of services (DH 2011).

Potentially, front-line staff will have much greater freedom and accountability for finding ways to deliver better and safer care to service users and their families. However, they will also be charged with achieving more for less, given the increasing financial constraints faced by public services. It is

---

Box 6.1 Ten high impact changes for mental health services

1. Treat home-based care and support as the norm for delivery of mental health services.
2. Improve flow of service users and carers across health and social care by improving access to screening and assessment.
3. Manage variation in service user discharge processes.
4. Manage variation in access to all mental health services.
5. Avoid unnecessary contact for service users and provide necessary contact in the right care setting.
6. Increase the reliability of interventions by designing care based on what is known to work and that service users and carers inform and influence.
7. Apply a systematic approach to enable the recovery of people with long-term conditions.
8. Improve service user flow by removing queues.
9. Optimize service user and carer flow through an integrated care pathway approach.
10. Redesign and extend roles in line with efficient service user and carer pathways to attract and retain an effective workforce.

therefore more important than ever for the providers of services to employ grass-roots methods for understanding and collating the preferences of service users for quality improvements and to build these arguments into any case they make for change. Service improvement capability needs to be part of professional development for all NHS staff. The mental health nursing profession must position itself within this vision and provide methods for students, qualified staff and managers to make meaningful contributions to the improvement agenda.

6.3 Origins of service improvement

NHS modernization and service improvement began in earnest in the late 1980s and early 1990s when two industrial, corporate-led and organization-wide change concepts predominated: business process reengineering (BPR) and the all-encompassing total quality management (TQM) (McLeod 2005). BPR aims to achieve massive gains by forcing organizations to fundamentally rethink their basic processes, while TQM puts an emphasis on continuous and incremental improvement (Gadd and Oakland 1996). These two change models have helped shape the development of service improvement in health care today.

The literature of the late 1990s reported problems with implementation and goal achievement from industries using BPR techniques. The largest obstacles were lack of sustained leadership and commitment, unrealistic expectations and resistance to change (Malhotra 1998). BPR therefore evolved over time by integrating incremental process change methods and incorporating various philosophies, concepts, methods and tools, similar to TQM (Malhotra 1998; Blanton 1999). Key to this evolution has been the integration of learning and staff empowerment in a bottom-up approach to change.

The Leicester Royal Infirmary became a national pilot site for this change methodology (McNulty and Ferlie 2002). In an evaluation completed 10 years after the pilot, Thomas *et al.* (2002) reflected on the state of readiness for whole systems change. They concluded that the NHS is unused to the idea of systematic change since it is full of linear structures that inhibit learning across boundaries.

Strategies were needed to support change in people's thinking and behaviour so that the knowledge and skills of health care improvement would become firmly embedded in NHS culture (Fillingham 2004). This was the beginning of the movement to build service improvement capability in the NHS, which recognized that alongside the tools and techniques, there was also a need to understand and influence the attitudes and behaviours necessary for change to happen.

6.4 The discipline of improvement

A seminal paper that helped introduce British audiences to the discipline of improvement was published in 1996 and authored by Dan Berwick, president and CEO of the Institute for Healthcare Improvement. Berwick begins by asserting the central law of improvement: that every system is perfectly designed to achieve the results it achieves. Consequently, it is an understanding of systems that lies at the heart of the improvement discipline.

Berwick views performance as a system characteristic that tends to vary around an average (e.g. waiting times for a service or treatment). It is only when those performance results are used to instigate the creation of a new system that we would expect to see new results. Tinkering with performance alone will not achieve new results since performance is a characteristic of an existing system. The improvement discipline seeks therefore to change health care systems rather than to bring about change within an existing system.

This is a tall order since health care systems are complex, involving multiple actors and pathways that the users of a service might follow. Berwick draws on the work of Langley *et al.* (1992) to present a model for improvement that captures this complexity. Figure 6.1 contains four elements: three

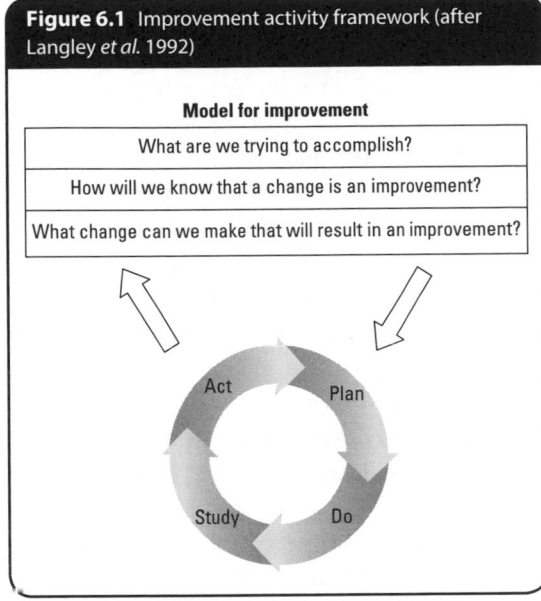

Figure 6.1 Improvement activity framework (after Langley *et al.* 1992)

key considerations and a process for testing new ways of working, which together provide a framework to guide improvement activity.

What are we trying to accomplish?

It is important to establish specific aims for improvement activity and for all involved in the activity to be in agreement with those aims. This can be difficult to achieve in multi-disciplinary environments where different disciplines may have different aspirations or motivations for change. Improvement leaders need to work with all those directly involved in a service as well as wider key stakeholders to forge a consensus on proposed improvement opportunities. Taking a grass-roots approach that identifies and anchors any change ideas in the expressed wishes of service users or clients is an important and powerful principle of the improvement discipline that can cut through interdisciplinary rivalries and resistance to change.

How will we know that a change is an improvement?

Measurement is now commonplace throughout health care, often undertaken for the purpose of governance or performance monitoring. The improvement discipline places considerable emphasis on measurement for the purpose of learning rather than as a means of judging. When an improvement is implemented it is necessary to know what the effects are and whether the improvement should be maintained, adjusted or rejected.

Careful selection of measures may necessitate adjustments to the aims of an improvement project. For example, a project to monitor attendance at an accident & emergency (A&E) department of people with primary mental health problems noted that over two thirds of attendances were made by individuals who had attended the department more than once in the last six months. The project team considered the wider health and social care system and hypothesized that these individuals may feel insufficiently supported by their own community services. Project measures were therefore adjusted to monitor *repeat attendances* and the work was refocused on those users who, if managed more effectively through local mental health teams, would make a significant difference to patient flow in A&E.

What change can we make that will result in an improvement?

When service staff are asked for ideas to achieve an improvement aim, there may be many possible suggestions, including a desire to maintain the status quo. Berwick (1996) therefore stresses the importance of improvement leaders communicating change ideas or concepts clearly and confidently.

Two generic change concepts often cited in the improvement literature are:

- **Waste removal:** stopping work activities that are unnecessary or which help no one (e.g. three separate professionals taking a very similar history from a service user over the course of a day and a half) (note that high impact change number 5 in Box 6.1 refers to the avoidance of unnecessary contact for service users).

- **Continuous flow:** not batching people into waiting lists, or forms and equipment into piles, but instigating less costly and more satisfactory continuous flow processes (note that high impact changes numbers 2, 8 and 9 in Box 6.1 refer to improving the flow for service users and carers).

The 'plan, do, study, act' cycle is a method or technique for testing improvement ideas and is described in detail in the next section of this chapter.

A framework that complements Langley *et al.*'s (1992) model depicts the evidence or information that would be necessary to address each stage in the model (Penny 2002; Penny *et al.* 2004). It organizes this evidence into four domains: understanding user needs and experiences; processes and systems; people and cultures; and initiating and sustaining improvements. Box 6.2 summarizes these domains by way of a series of questions, the answers to which provide staff with the information they need to design and undertake improvement projects.

Thinking Space 6.1

Reflect on your current place of work or a recent placement you have experience of. Work through the four domains in Box 6.2 and answer the questions in relation to your workplace experience. You may not be able to answer all the questions. Jot down your answers and ideas as you go. Once you have completed the four domains consider the evidence you have as a whole and answer the following questions:

1. What improvement ideas have you identified and who would they benefit?

2. What threats or challenges to change have you identified?

3. What strengths or opportunities for change have you identified?

4. How do your ideas relate to the 10 high impact changes in Box 6.1?

Evidence of effectiveness

It is now 16 years since Berwick published his call to service improvement in the *British Medical Journal*. These ideas were taken up originally by a small band of enthusiasts and have since been used by large numbers of providers internationally (Marshall 2009). What evidence is there then for the effectiveness of service improvement methods?

In 2009 Marshall concluded that service and quality improvement approaches have been successful at engaging and enthusing staff and that they often lead to changes in working practices. However, little evidence exists to demonstrate that they have a significant or sustained effect on service user outcomes. Marshall suggests that this is an absence of evidence of effect, rather than evidence that the interventions are ineffective.

More recently Dixon-Woods *et al.* (2012) acknowledged that service improvement projects have encountered similar difficulties to other methods, resulting in patchy and inconsistent results. They review evaluation reports from five improvement programmes sponsored by the Health Foundation to identify the common challenges that improvement projects face. Box 6.3 presents the challenges together with some proposed actions to overcome them.

It is important to note that over-ambitious projects that talk of service transformations can often alienate staff and struggle to deliver change. In reality change is rarely transformational in complex contexts such as health service delivery. More often it is incremental. We need then to have realistic expectations of what quality improvement initiatives can achieve in the short term or we may remain eternally disappointed and miss numerous opportunities to make a difference.

An important principle that informs the improvement discipline is that the smallest changes can make significant differences to the quality of services for clients. Taking a grass-roots approach that begins with clients' and service users' experiences of a system can reveal where simple improvements can bring about appreciable changes. Frontline staff are well placed to work from this perspective and need to be encouraged and equipped to

Box 6.2 Service improvement evidence base

User needs and experiences

- Do you really know what happens to users and their carers as they use your service?
- Do you know what is important to them?
- Do you know what they need to make their experience better?
- Do you know what they would like more of and what they do not want?
- How do you involve them in ideas to improve your service? Do you really listen to them?

People and cultures

- Do you like change yourself? What would encourage you to do things differently? Do your colleagues and leaders like change?
- Are there always lots of ideas and encouragement to do things differently or are people generally reluctant to move from the status quo?
- What is the culture like in your team or organization? Does it embrace change or is it reluctant to do things differently?
- Are there identifiable factors in your team culture that facilitate or inhibit the adoption of change?

Processes and systems

- Have you ever mapped the processes in your service?
- Do you know how users arrive at your service and where they go to when they leave you?
- Do you know where and why users experience frustrations or where their care may be delayed? Do you know how long they have to wait at different stages of their journey?
- Do you understand how your part of the system impacts on others?

Initiating and sustaining

- What do you measure about your service? Are they the things that matter to your users and their carers?
- Do you know how to test your idea before implementing?
- If your improvement idea has been tested and shown to be an improvement, do you know what to do? How does your improvement idea fit with the business plan of your organization?
- What factors influence the sustainability of the improvement and how would you know that a change is actually a sustainable improvement?
- How do your improvement ideas fit with the goals and strategy of your organization? Which corporate leaders will help you and champion your improvement work?

> ## Box 6.3 Improvement challenges and solutions (Dixon-Woods *et al.* 2012)
>
> ### Designing and planning
>
> 1. Convince people that there's a problem – use hard data and service user stories and voices to secure emotional engagement from staff.
> 2. Convince people of the solution – use clear facts and figures with measures of impact that demonstrate the advantages of your solution.
> 3. Data collection and monitoring – this always takes more time and energy than initially thought. Assess local systems and train people.
> 4. Ambitions – over-ambitious goals and too much talk of transformation can alienate staff.
>
> ### Contexts, professions and leadership
>
> 5. Organizational context, culture and capabilities – explain requirements and provide ongoing support. Make sure improvement goals are aligned with the goals of the wider organization.
> 6. Lack of staff engagement – be clear about who owns the problem and solution, agree roles and responsibilities, work to common goals and use a shared language.
> 7. Leadership – use 'quieter' leadership oriented towards inclusion, explanation and gentle persuasion.
> 8. Incentivizing participation – the intrinsic motivations of staff can drive improvement projects especially if incentives are provided (carrots).
>
> ### Sustainability, spread and unintended consequences
>
> 9. Securing sustainability – sustainability can be jeopardized when improvement activities are seen as projects or when they rely on particular individuals.
> 10. Side-effects of change – change in one area may cause problems in another so be vigilant about detecting unwanted consequences and be willing to learn and adapt.

identify and manage small changes. The NHS Institute (NHSI) has had some success in these respects, designing simple service improvement training modules for pre-registration students that use very few improvement tools to enable small-scale change at the local level (NHSI 2008).

6.5 Service improvement tools and techniques

Improvement tools and techniques are many and varied, ranging from statistical methods to simple questions that generate everyday data. They can be used as stand-alone tools or as part of improvement packages.

It is not necessary to be skilled in the use of sophisticated tools to achieve improvements in service provision. The NHSI 'improvement in pre-registration education' programme found that two simple tools were enough to empower students to propose and in some circumstances implement service improvements (NHSI 2008). In this section we describe the two tools along with an improvement package designed for use in the mental health field.

Process mapping

Service improvement begins with a willingness to listen to and understand the issues that face service users and their carers. By first really listening and then looking in detail at how current processes and systems impact on their experiences, safety and outcomes, improvement ideas can be generated. Process mapping is used for these purposes.

Mapping the journeys or processes that service users navigate as they engage with health care systems is a good way to begin to understand their experiences. Process maps have an agreed start and end point such as 'service user is referred for assessment' to 'service user completes a treatment programme'. All the steps and actions the service user encounters between these two points are written down. The areas that cause problems for the service user, their carers or staff, such as delays, duplication of work or lack of communication, are identified and, through discussion, ideas for improvement captured. Figure 6.2 presents a simple process map of an imaginary journey through a mental health service.

Figure 6.2 essentially describes stages in a process, which can be elaborated by incorporating additional information about each stage such as the experience of service users in terms of their feelings, thoughts or reactions. Process mapping systems often include a series of symbols that are used to highlight key features of the process (e.g. black diamonds that signify problems/blockages in a system, golden stars that signify high levels of service user satisfaction with particular stages).

The Cabinet Office (2008) publishes *Customer Journey Mapping*, a methodology that tracks and describes the experiences of customers (or service users) as they encounter a service or set of services, taking into account not only what happens to them, but also their responses to their experiences. Process mapping for service improvement therefore maps a system as well as the experiences of service users who are engaged with the system.

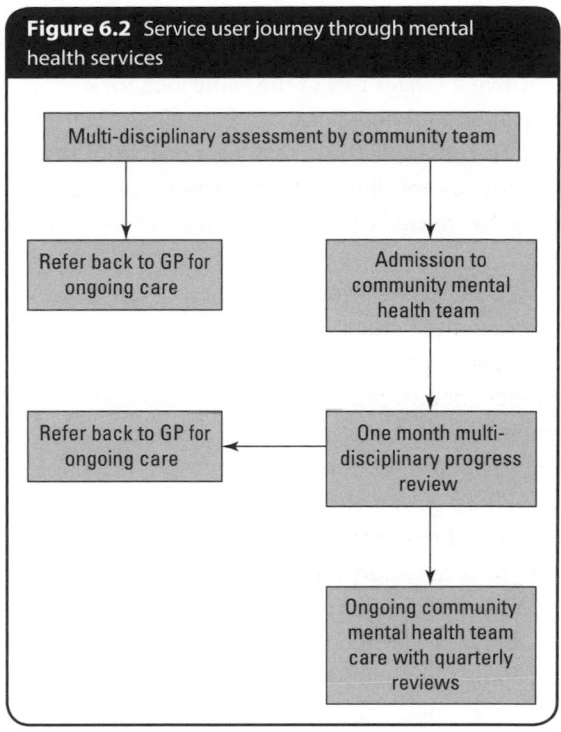

Figure 6.2 Service user journey through mental health services

This type of information reveals important opportunities for improvement that are grounded in the real world experience of service users. As such they can act as a powerful stimulus for change and help ameliorate inter-disciplinary rivalries that might otherwise emphasize competing improvement priorities. Each of the participating pilots in the NHSI programme involved service users either directly in the presentation of improvement ideas or by way of recordings, both visual and audio.

Plan, do, study, act cycle

The plan, do, study, act (PDSA) cycle is an inductive loop that generates learning in respect of any actions that may be taken to test new ideas. A test for each selected idea is planned including where, how and who will test and what the expected effects are in terms of any measures of improvement. Test results are then studied to understand what happened and how it compares with what was expected. Subsequent actions are considered according to this assessment. If the effects were positive a bigger test of the same idea for a longer period would be advisable. If the effects were not as good as expected it may be possible to repeat the test by modifying the improvement idea or it may be necessary to try another improvement idea.

PDSA cycles are repeated until an effective improvement idea has been identified which receives support from all key stakeholders. This model not only promotes a continuous approach to improvement but supports the development of an improvement culture. The method encourages people to get involved, to understand user experiences and the processes and systems they encounter. It tests improvement ideas, measures their effects and captures the learning.

Berwick (1996) emphasizes the importance of regularly testing promising changes on a small scale. It is not necessary to create complex research designs or to engage in months or years of data collection. Often, the smallest changes can make a significant difference to the experience of service users. Berwick asserts also that clever, informative PDSA cycles can often start within days or hours of their original motivation. The power of this method lies in the act of reflection so as to learn from the actions we take.

The productive mental health ward

This is an improvement package produced by the NHSI specifically for inpatient mental health facilities (NHSI 2006). It forms part of the NHSI Productive Ward series and comprises 13 modules for self-directed learning at the ward level.

The improvement package aims to increase the amount of direct care time given to patients in mental health wards as well as improving the effectiveness, safety and reliability of the care. The 13 modules offer a systematic way of making those improvements and include foundation and process modules. The former incorporates ward leaders', project leaders' and executive leaders' guides while the latter covers such topics as admissions and planned discharge, safe and supportive observations, ward round and patient well-being.

The productive mental health ward improvement package includes a number of ready prepared tools in electronic formats for easy use. For example:

- **Activity follow analysis:** prepared as an Excel tool this instrument allows project staff to capture data on intended and actual time spent on key tasks within the ward environment (similar tools are available for other contexts). The tool presents results, including variances in practices, in tabular formats and as simple charts that facilitate the rapid identification of improvement opportunities.
- **Measures template spreadsheet:** this tool divides the productive mental health ward measures into five areas: safety, observations, patient satisfaction, carer satisfaction and other measures. It allows staff to transform the data they collect in respect of any improvement opportunities into cross-sectional and longitudinal charts that enable a comparison of progress across time.

Improvement products of this type have been well received by NHS services with approximately 80 per cent of all NHS trusts signing up to one of the NHSI packages.

 6.6 Applications in practice

Service improvement methods are now commonplace in many NHS trusts and are used more widely in the health field. See, for example, the work of the Health Foundation, which champions service improvement methods in many of its projects (www.health.org.uk). In this section we present some case studies of service improvement projects covering an NHS trust and the experience of student nurses who received service improvement training as part of their professional education.

Case Study

Productive ward

Derbyshire Mental Health Services NHS Trust applied productive mental health ward improvement methods to enhance its care pathways across inpatient and community services (NHSI 2009). A two-year programme of work involved 10 teams including three inpatient wards, the crisis resolution and home treatment team (CRHT) and local community mental health teams (CMHTs). Derbyshire Mental Health Services was the first trust to apply these methods across a whole pathway.

What they did:

- Customized productive mental health ward modules to make them relevant across the entire patient pathway: inpatient to community services.
- Created a red, amber, green traffic light zoning system with agreed criteria for each stage that was used to track patient progress and prepare for discharge.
- Created a series of 'patient status at a glance' boards to map service users across zones as they travelled along the pathway.
- Used the 'Knowing How we are Doing' module to ensure early discharges did not impact on readmission rates.
- Used the activity follow tool to track different people in different roles and thereby understand what really happens during a shift.

What they achieved:

- Increased early discharge of patients by 400 per cent over a five-month period.
- Enhanced patient satisfaction with services and their sense of safe, consistent and comprehensive care as they progressed through hospital and community services.
- Reduced the average number of bed days per patient from 70 to 50.
- Ensured readmission rates did not increase.
- Changed shift patterns in the CRHT team to better match patient needs.
- Achieved a 5 per cent reduction in staff sickness/absence rates.

When invited to reflect on their achievements, key programme staff noted that the modules had provided a framework for teams to understand their own problems and find innovative solutions. They emphasized the importance of a bottom-up approach through which front-line staff were able to lead the changes themselves by reviewing, measuring and adapting the way they delivered services (NHSI 2009).

By working at a systems level, the programme team was able to guard against any negative effects from their work such as increases in readmission rates. Systems thinking also allowed service staff to be more aware of the impact of their work on other parts of the system. Staff reported greater cohesion and better working relationships as a result.

Commentary

Referring back to Box 6.1 it is clear that the Derbyshire Mental Health Services' programme addresses a number of high impact actions, primarily numbers 9 (optimizing patient flow through integrated care pathways) and 3 (managing variation in service user discharge processes).

The size and scope of the Derbyshire improvement programme is impressive as are the outcomes it was able to achieve. However, it is possible to make significant service improvements on a much smaller scale.

Student nurses

The NHSI (2008) improvement in pre-registration education programme worked with universities across the UK to provide nursing and other students with a service improvement learning experience as part of their undergraduate training. The curricula incorporated the four components of the service improvement evidence base (see Box 6.2) into a core day during which students were introduced to the subject, the PDSA cycle, process mapping and Langley et al.'s (1992) model for improvement.

During this core day students were also exposed to the experiences of service users and patients from which opportunities for service improvement could be identified. This was achieved by having service users present in the 'classroom' or using specifically designed case studies based on real scenarios. Some universities developed DVDs with patients that recounted in imaginative ways their experiences with health and social care systems.

Each programme required students to further develop and apply their improvement learning in a clinical or related setting. This was achieved in different ways. Typically the core day was broken down into a number of sessions with students encouraged to apply the learning between each session (e.g. 3 × 2 hour sessions). This provided students with time to reflect on practice, on the service improvement opportunities they had identified and their proposed approaches to address those needs.

Key to this programme was belief in the improvement principle that small changes can make significant differences to the experiences of patients and service users and that the achievement of such changes are in the power of nursing students equipped with simple tools (process mapping and PDSA cycles) and an understanding of the improvement process (Langley et al.'s model for improvement). The case studies that follow provide testament to this belief.

Case Study

Three vignettes:
NHS parking fees

A student on hospital placement in Burton-on-Trent, Staffordshire, initiated a change to NHS car parking fees. She process-mapped patient journeys which often incurred car parking fees at an initial hospital visit and then again at other service sites they needed to attend on the same day. Many of the patients and relatives voiced their concerns about this aspect of their contact with NHS services.

The nurse presented this case to her placement managers and asked if the fees paid on one site could be used on other NHS sites in Burton-on-Trent if there was unspent time on the car parking ticket. Representation was made by the manager to hospital authorities and an NHS car parking ticket in Burton-on-Trent is now transferable between sites.

Medical photography

Two students on placement in a medical photography unit process mapped patients' journeys from having photographs taken to being seen by a consultant. Two separate appointments were required as staff had to mount the photographs before the consultant could see them.

The students proposed that staff print out the photographs immediately so that the consultant could see them that day, hence saving the patient from having to attend two appointments. This simple adjustment to a referral pathway has now been implemented in the department.

Mental health physiotherapy

A student was on placement with a mental health physiotherapy team that had use of a gym. They provided sessions for women with common mental health problems such as anxiety and depression. Some of the women attended spasmodically and some had been attending for many months. When process mapping the women's journey into and through the service it was evident that many were uncertain about the progress they were making and how long they would need to attend. The student identified the need for some objective markers so that a client's progress could be monitored and appropriate adjustments made to their programme.

The student reviewed a number of available indicators and selected a 60-metre walk test and use of the BORG scale. The latter provides a rating of perceived exertion for different activities and pieces of equipment. Completing these simple tests over time would then provide an indication of progress.

The student tested the approach with two women who agreed to participate (PDSA cycle). The tests were unobtrusive, easy to administer and worked well within the gym context. Test results revealed where the women were having difficulty with equipment or activities and where they were ready to progress. It was concluded that this approach ensures exercises are suited to the needs of the individual and provides participants with a measure of their progress across time. It also provides a systematic way for staff to ensure throughput of women over time, thereby freeing spaces for other women who could benefit from this service. The student has written up this work and provided a protocol and pro-forma for ongoing use by the mental health physiotherapy team.

Commentary

Again, with reference to Box 6.1 it can be seen that these student projects have the potential to contribute to a number of high-impact actions, specifically numbers 5, 6, and 8. These vignettes and others captured by the NHSI demonstrate how simple changes can make a significant difference, and how the tools and techniques of improvement can be used effectively by nursing students (NHSI 2008).

6.7 Conclusion

The pace of change in health and social care is set to continue and nurses should expect that their roles and the contexts in which care is delivered will continue to evolve. Mental health nurses need an approach to engage with this agenda as part of their routine contact with users and carers. Improvement and change management skills are no longer the sole responsibility of higher managers and strategy planners. Indeed, at this level the literature is equivocal about the effectiveness of quality improvement methods with over-ambitious projects that herald service transformations often falling short of

the mark. Smaller scale, incremental change at the local level may be a more realistic pursuit for which knowledge of improvement methods is needed by all levels of the workforce. In summary the main points from this chapter are:

- UK government health policy requires that front-line staff find ways to deliver better, safer and more cost effective services. Service improvement and change management are therefore core skills for nurses working at all levels.

- Real improvements arise when systems are changed, not when performance within an existing system is adjusted.

- To successfully bring about change it is necessary to be clear about what you are trying to achieve, how you will know that a change has led to an improvement, and what changes you can make that will result in an improvement.

- By focusing on improvements that arise from patient need and/or their expressed wishes it is possible to galvanize multi-disciplinary support.

- Measurement is best used for the purposes of learning rather than for governing or judging a service.

- The use of process mapping techniques and PDSA cycles is sufficient to make improvements in care.

- These tools and techniques can be applied effectively by staff of varying experience, from novice to expert.

Annotated bibliography

Health Foundation (2012) *Overcoming Challenges to Improving Quality: Lessons from the Health Foundation's improvement programme evaluations and relevant literature*, **available at: www.health.org.uk/publications/ overcoming-challenges-to-improving-quality, accessed 1 May 2012.**
Based on the Health Foundation's NHS service improvement programme this report explores the challenges faced and suggests ways to overcome them.

Ashworth, R., Boyne, G. and Entwistle, T. (2010) *Public Service Improvement: Theories and evidence.* **Oxford: Oxford University Press.**
A more academic text that describes drivers for improvement from private industry and assesses their suitability and impact in public services.

Lloyd, C., King, R., Deane, F. and Gournay, K. (2008) *Clinical Management in Mental Health Services.* **Chichester: Wiley-Blackwell.**
Although the focus of this book is on clinical management it deals with a number of issues relevant to improvement including leadership, change, evidence-based practice, communications and public relations. It offers a practical guide to improve prevention, care and recovery for people who have mental health problems.

References

Berwick, D. (1996) *A Primer on Leading the Improvement of Systems*, available at: www.bmj.com/content/312/7031/619.full, accessed 6 January 2012.
Blanton, G.A. (1999) Total quality management, in J. Juran and A. Blanton Godfrey (eds) *Juran's Quality Handbook*, 5th edn. London: McGraw-Hill.
Cabinet Office (2008) *Customer Journey Mapping: An introduction*, available at: http://interim.cabinetoffice.gov.uk/contact-council/contact-council-resources.aspx#customer-journey, accessed 15 January 2012.
DH (Department of Health) (2004) *The NHS Improvement Plan: Putting people at the heart of public services.* London: The Stationery Office.
DH (Department of Health) (2011) Factsheet C1: *Improving Quality of Care: The Health and Social Care Bill*, available at: http://healthandcare.dh.gov.uk/factsheets, accessed 15 January 2012.
Dixon-Woods, M., McNichol, S. and Martin, G. (2012) Ten challenges in improving quality in healthcare: lessons from the Health Foundation's programme evaluations and relevant literature, *BMJ Quality and Safety*, 10: 1136.
Fillingham, D. (2004) Modernisation Ideas, *Health Service Journal*, 22 January.
Gadd, K. and Oakland, J. (1996) Chimera or culture? Business process reengineering or total quality management? *Quality Management Journal*, 96: 20–38.
Langley, G., Nolan, K. and Nolan, T. (1992) *The Foundation of Improvement.* Silver Spring, MD: API Publishing.
Malhotra, Y. (1998) Business process redesign: an overview, *Engineering Management Review*, 26: 3.
Marshall, M. (2009) Applying quality improvement approaches to health care, *British Medical Journal*, 339: b3411.
McLeod, H. (2005) A review of the evidence on organizational development in healthcare, in E. Peck (ed.) *Organizational Development in Healthcare*. Oxford: Radcliffe.
McNulty, T. and Ferlie, E. (2002) *Reengineering Healthcare: The complexities of organizational transformation.* Oxford: Oxford University Press.

NHSI (2006) The Productive Series, available at: www.institute.nhs.uk/quality_and_value/productivity_series/the_productive_
series.html, accessed 15 January 2012.

NHSI (2008) Evaluation of the improvement in pre-registration education programme: final report. Unpublished paper for the
NHS Institute for Innovation and Improvement.

NHSI (2009) *The Productive Times*, available at: www.institute.nhs.uk/quality_and_value/productive_mental_health_ward/case_
studies.html, accessed 15 January 2012.

Penny, J. (2002) Building the discipline of improvement for health and social care: next steps for NHS improvement, the early
vision and way forward. Unpublished paper, MA Management Board, November.

Penny, J., Bevan, H., Swaby, V. and Wilcock, P. (2004) Building the discipline of improvement in health and social care.
Unpublished paper.

Thomas, P., McDonnell, J., McCulloch, J. and Ferlie, E. (2002) Facilitating learning and innovation in primary care organizations.
Unpublished paper, Imperial College London Business School, Brent NHS PCT.

Chapter 7

Continuing Professional Development and Advanced Practice

Sue Gurney

When I started nursing there was everything to learn from those that went before me. After nearly 20 years in the profession I'm nowhere near achieving that goal and now there's everything to learn from all those that have come after me. CPD has necessarily become part of my professional life.

Anon

 ## 7.1 Introduction

Continuing professional development (CPD) is a professional obligation for all registered nurses. CPD provides a means by which we can keep up to date with changes in policy and practice and develop our knowledge and skills. Advanced practice in nursing is a broad term whereby, following initial registration, nurses have acquired a minimum standard of both wider and in-depth knowledge, skills and experience. The aim of both CPD and advanced practice in nursing is to contribute to more effective patient care.

This chapter covers:

- what is CPD?
- professional registration;
- barriers and pathways to CPD;

- advanced practice;
- CPD and clinical supervision;
- work-related stress in nursing;
- implications for mental health nursing practice.

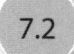 ## 7.2 What is CPD?

The Nursing and Midwifery Council (NMC), as the professional regulator for nurses in the UK, sets standards of conduct, performance and ethics which state that nurses must have the knowledge and skills for safe and effective practice. The NMC stipulates that nurses are required to undertake appropriate learning and professional activities (CPD) that demonstrate the development and sustainability of their practice.

Apart from meeting NMC regulatory standards participating in CPD also plays a part in meeting personal ambitions to improve practice, meet performance and/or work targets, progess career development and promote lifelong learning. Participating in CPD has been shown to increase skills acquisition and job satisfaction, and to reduce burnout (Schweitzer and Krassa 2010). The career progression from novice to expert practitioner (or advancing practice) cannot be met without undertaking CPD. CPD is also a means by which organizations and employers can manage and support workforce capability and capacity. In summary, CPD in nursing is important to the individual practitioner, their employing organization, the professional regulatory body for nursing and the public nurses serve.

7.3 Professional registration requirements and standards

The NMC exists to safeguard the health and well-being of the public. It does this by:

- setting standards of education, training, conduct and performance for nurses;
- ensuring that nurses keep their skills and knowledge up to date and uphold the NMC's professional standards;
- having clear and transparent processes to investigate nurses who fall short of the NMC standards.

The NMC maintains a register of all the people who have fulfilled its registration requirements and who are, therefore, entitled to practise in the UK. If you are not registered with the NMC you cannot be employed to practise as a nurse in the UK.

Requirements for renewal of registration with the NMC

Nurses must maintain their NMC registration by meeting the post-registration education and practice (Prep) standards set by the Council. When nurses renew their registration they must provide a signed notification of practice form declaring that they have complied with the Prep standards. The NMC may request proof of compliance. If the standards have been falsely declared, then the registrant will be subject to fitness to practice proceedings.

The NMC has published a handbook (NMC 2011) to support nurses to meet the Prep standards, which should be read in conjunction with *The Code: Standards of Conduct, Performance and Ethics for Nurses and Midwives* (NMC 2008a). Like many other professional regulators the NMC is continually reviewing and updating its information and standards, so for the current version the reader should visit the NMC website at www.nmc-uk.org.

NMC Prep standards

There are two Prep standards that affect registration: the Prep (practice) standard and the Prep (CPD) standard.

Prep practice standard

To meet this standard nurses must have undertaken a minimum of 450 hours of registered nursing practice (relevant to their nursing qualification) in the previous three years. This time period allows for absence from work (e.g. maternity leave). Alternatively the nurse may have successfully completed an NMC approved return to practice course within the last three years. This practice standard can be met through administrative, supervisory, teaching, research and managerial roles as well as providing direct patient care.

Prep CPD standard

Assuming the Prep practice standard has been met then meeting the CPD standard requires that the nurse:

- undertakes a minimum of 35 hours of learning activity, relevant to their practice area, every three years;
- maintains a personal profile of the learning activity;
- complies with any NMC requests to audit how this standard has been met.

The NMC has additional standards for nurses, in particular roles such as mentors or non-medical prescribers, whereby focused evidence to meet specific outcomes has to be collected (NMC 2008b, 2008c).

Meeting the Prep CPD standard

CPD activity undertaken to meet this standard needs to be relevant to the nurse's area of practice. There are no NMC approved courses or CPD activities. Instead, the NMC adopts a flexible approach and CPD can be met through: formal learning activities such as study days, best practice updates, conferences, workshops, courses and education programmes; or informal learning activities such as reflective practice, staff appraisal-development plans, individual study, action learning sets and directed reading. Whatever the CPD activity, it needs to be documented in a learning profile and in a way which demonstrates what was learned and how new skills and/or theory was applied to develop or reinforce practice. The NMC also advises the routine collection of CPD documentation such as attendance and completion certificates, as evidence to add to the profile. In general, mandatory training is not considered to be CPD activity.

There is no NMC approved format for the learning profile, which can be held in either hard copy or electronic form. The structure and presentation will vary according to personal preference. Box 7.1 provides suggestions about what to include and Box 7.2 illustrates a template suggested by the NMC, to show how the profile might be organized.

 7.4 Barriers and pathways to CPD

The Chief Nursing Officer's (CNO) (England) review of mental health nursing defined CPD as:

> *A systematic and planned approach to the maintenance, enhancement and development of knowledge, skills and expertise that continues throughout a professional's career and is to the mutual benefit of the individual, the employer and the professional body.*
>
> (DH 2006: 61)

The combination of increasing professionalization of nursing, the changing nature of mental health nursing and the move to an all graduate pre-registration programme has highlighted the importance of CPD. CPD is needed to equip mental health nurses with the diverse range of knowledge and skills required to meet their practice, professional and organizational accountability.

Key barriers to participating in CPD for nurses include:

- **Situational barriers:** lack of time because of work responsibilities; child care and home responsibilities; programme costs; fear of losing benefits; difficulty with numeracy and academic reading and writing; and non-supportive relationships.

- **Attitudinal barriers:** negativity arising from unpleasant past learning experiences; low career aspirations; doubts about the value of learning; low self-esteem and lack of confidence in ability; negative peer influence; and failure to take personal responsibility for CPD, expecting it to be the sole responsibility of the employer.

- **Structural barriers:** unavailability of suitable or relevant programmes and/or education institutions; staff shortages which limit opportunities to be released for study; lack of awareness and knowledge about learning opportunities; inflexible work patterns; prohibitive entry requirements; late advertising of CPD opportunities; lack of coherent staff development plans; difficulty in obtaining study leave; and lack of support from managers (Richards and Potgieter 2010; Schweitzer and Krassa 2010).

In response to these findings it is suggested that there should be collective responsibility by the individual, the organization and the education institution to develop flexible approaches to CPD that meet practice and career development (Richards and Potgieter 2010; Schweitzer and Krassa 2010). Staff appraisal and personal development plans are seen as key processes through which to plan and review individual CPD. However, there remains wide variation among employing organizations, resulting in many nurses not receiving regular appraisal and development plans (Scott 2011).

Gass *et al.* (2007) found that both qualified and student mental health nurses valued flexible approaches to CPD such as journal reading, teaching sessions, networking, clinical supervision, short, flexible, clinically focused learning activities and closer links between higher education and practice. Eraut (1994) points out that too often CPD activities focus on new learning with little thought given to refreshing, renewal and consolidation of existing learning. In relation to both new learning and refreshing old learning, CPD activity should be approached through creative and flexible workplace strategies (Deacon 2011).

Role performance and career development

The NHS Knowledge and Skills Framework (KSF) (DH 2004) offers a structure for health care organizations to manage and develop their workforce. Organizations using the KSF are able to demonstrate that staff are either working towards or have appropriate knowledge and skills for their role (measured in the KSF as dimensions). Meeting KSF role dimensions is also closely linked to pay, development and career progression, through the process of annual development reviews and personal development planning. The KSF core dimensions apply to all staff with additional dimensions reflecting the scope of the role. In 2011 a new National Health Service (NHS) Leadership Framework was launched which provides a single overarching framework for the leadership development of staff at any stage in their career. This new framework has clear links to the core dimensions of the KSF (NHS 2011).

As part of the Modernising Nursing Careers Programme (DH 2011) the UK Department of Health (DH) has developed a pathway-based nursing career framework, which demonstrates the breadth of nursing roles across settings and sectors. Indirectly linked to the KSF, this framework provides a point of reference when reviewing and developing nursing roles. It also articulates how nurses can progress both up through a specialty and across specialties by engaging with CPD and personal development. The learning profile provides a way of evidencing role performance and CPD activity in either working towards or meeting these and KSF dimensions.

Accreditation of prior learning

In addition, the learning profile can be used as evidence for accreditation of prior learning, whereby academic credits can potentially be awarded for previous formal learning that has been undertaken (Accreditation of Prior Certified Learning – APCL) or through informal learning (Accreditation of Prior Experiential Learning – APEL). Different educational awarding bodies have different criteria. Local universities often offer further study to support health professionals to develop learning profiles – portfolios and a range of published information and literature is available on the topic.

Box 7.1 What to include in a learning profile (Casey and Egan 2010: 547–8)

- Biographical information
- Educational background
- Employment history with brief description of roles and responsibilities
- Professional qualification certificates
- Training and competency records
- Appraisal and personal development plan records

- Professional development activities with supporting notes outlining the learning from each activity and some reflection on how it has informed and influenced practice
- Activities to support learning and assessment of others including mentoring, preceptoring and teaching activities
- Practice development activities undertaken to support evidence-based practice such as audits, protocols, guidelines and change management projects
- Publications and conference presentations
- Professional body membership and any associated work
- Written reflections on episodes/incidents of care

Box 7.2 Suggested template for organizing the learning profile (after NMC 2011: 9)

Your record could provide:

- A list and description of your workplace or organization and your role for the last three years.
- The nature of the learning activity – what did you do?
- Description of the learning activity – what did it consist of?
- Outcome of the learning activity – how did the learning relate to your work?

You may find it helpful to routinely collect documentation from any learning activity you undertake such as appraisals, attendance or completion certificates.

 ## 7.5 Advanced practice

Nurses have always been extending and expanding their scope of practice, even more so over recent years as practice has become more specialized. The development of advanced nurse practitioner (ANP) roles has occurred internationally although in an ad hoc fashion, resulting in lack of clarity and consistency of titles and roles (Duffield *et al.* 2009).

In the UK, in the 1980s, the nurse practitioner role developed in primary care with titles such as 'advanced practitioner' and 'advanced nurse practitioner' emerging in the 1990s. In 1997 the role of 'nurse consultant' was introduced and in 2001 the role of 'modern matron'. There continues to be lack of consistency and clarity about these titles and roles.

The classification for advanced practice nurses in the UK comprises:

- nurse practitioner (sometimes called 'nurse clinician');
- clinical nurse specialist;
- specialist practitioner (formerly district nurses and health visitors);
- specialist community public health nurse;
- nurse consultant (Duffield *et al.* 2009).

What is advanced practice?

'Advanced practice' is often used as an umbrella term, which is unhelpful because it suggests that it applies to all practice roles above that of initial practice (AANPE 2012).

There has been much debate to reach a consensus on what is advanced practice and this reflects differences in philosophies and political and contextual factors. Elsom *et al.* (2005: 182) summarize the situation as follows:

For some authors, the degree of autonomy enjoyed by the nurse in the form of extended and expanded practice roles defines advanced nursing practice, whereas for others, the scope of clinical practice is less important in defining advanced practice than the level of expertise of the nurse in performing identified nursing tasks.

There has also been debate about whether, on a vertical continuum, specialist practice is at a lower level than advanced practice. AANPE (2012) recommend that the term 'specialist' be considered as one end of a generalist–specialist continuum, rather a vertical development continuum which ranges from novice to expert. Thus, specialist practice is related to a specific nursing context consisting of patient group, skill set and/or organizational context and it would be possible to identify roles that occupy junior-level specialist or senior advanced-generalist levels. Increasingly advanced nursing practice is seen as a level of practice rather than a role or job title (AANPE 2012).

A position statement from the DH (2010a) describes advanced-level nursing as a level of practice, not a specialty or role, which should be evident as being beyond that of first-level registration. This level of practice is viewed as a minimum benchmark and comprises a number of assumptions and 28 elements clustered under the themes of: clinical/direct care practice; leadership and collaborative practice; improving quality and developing practice; and developing self and others.

Regulating advanced practice

Advanced nursing practice in the UK is currently encompassed within, and regulated by, the NMC *Code* (NMC 2008a). In 2010 the Prime Minister's Commission on the Future of Nursing and Midwifery

(DH 2010b) thought this was insufficient, and recommended that the NMC increase its regulatory framework for advanced practice. At the time of writing, this work remains in progress. However, regulation and governance of elements of advanced practice also sit within a wider framework of employment and employee responsibilities.

Thinking Space 7.1

Look at NHS Education for Scotland's Advanced Nursing Practice Toolkit which is designed to enhance nurses' understanding and application of advanced practice. Visit www.advanced practice.scot.nhs.uk/home.aspx.

 ## 7.6 CPD and clinical supervision

Clinical supervision, as a way of using shared experiences and reflective practice, plays an important part in contributing to CPD and lifelong learning. The NMC supports the provision of clinical supervision and together with the NMC's Prep standards this forms an important part of professional assurance and clinical governance. The main objectives of clinical supervision are similar to those of clinical governance: to maintain and improve standards, provide best quality care and continued development of professional practice.

Definitions of clinical supervision vary but primarily refer to a semi-structured process whereby a nurse (the supervisee) meets regularly and confidentially (within agreed parameters) with a more experienced practitioner (the supervisor), to discuss issues of relevance to the supervisee's practice. The supervisor is usually, but not necessarily, from the same profession (Cleary *et al.* 2010).

An often cited definition of clinical supervision from the NHS Management Executive is:

a formal process of professional support and learning which enables individual practitioners to develop knowledge and competence, assume responsibility for their own practice and enhance consumer protection and safety of care in complex situations.

(NMC 2008d)

The NMC proposes that clinical supervision enables registered nurses to:

- identify solutions to problems;
- increase understanding of professional issues;
- improve standards of patient care;
- further develop their skills and knowledge;
- enhance their understanding of their own practice.

The NMC does not advocate any particular model or provide guidance about the nature and scope of clinical supervision for nurses. However it has produced a set of principles which should underpin any system of clinical supervision and these are summarized in Box 7.3.

Approaches to supervision

Clinical supervision has its roots in the helping professions, namely counselling, social work and psychotherapy, and it can take place individually or in groups. Models of nursing clinical supervision, that straddle a spectrum of perspectives, have been reported in the literature since the 1980s. These range from a focus on the psychodynamic relationship between the supervisor and supervisee in facilitating the educational and professional growth of the supervisee, to a more behavioural perspective that analyses issues and problems, identifies goals and develops an action plan for goal attainment (Fowler *et al.* 2007). Whatever approach is used, clinical supervision needs to be clinically meaningful, user-friendly and relevant to the nurse's needs (Cleary *et al.* 2010). Some tips for getting the most from clinical supervision are listed in Box 7.4.

The ability to reflect on practice in clinical supervision is associated with improving knowledge, skills and competence and a continued commitment to professional development (Cleary *et al.* 2010). The purpose of reflection is to question one's practice and learn from the experience. Two frequently cited reflective models by Gibbs (1988) and Borton (1970) show that asking a few simple questions can stimulate learning (see Box 7.5).

The approach to clinical supervision used is influenced by the nature of practice and the different theoretical and conceptual frameworks adopted by

---

Box 7.3 Principles of clinical supervision (after NMC 2008d)

- Clinical supervision supports practice, enabling registered nurses to maintain and improve standards of care.

- Clinical supervision is a practice-focused professional relationship, involving a practitioner reflecting on practice, guided by a skilled supervisor.

- Registered nurses and managers should develop the process of clinical supervision according to local circumstances. Ground rules should enable the supervisor and the registered nurse to be open, confident and aware of what is involved.

- All registered nurses should have access to clinical supervision and the number of practitioners per supervisor should be limited.

- Preparation for supervisors should be flexible and principles of clinical supervision should be covered in education programmes.

- Evaluation of clinical supervision is needed to determine its impact on care and practice standards.

Box 7.4 Some tips for getting the most from clinical supervision

Ways of taking material to supervision

- Spontaneous verbal agenda
- Predetermined agenda
- Case review

Tools that can be used to aid the process

- Reflective writing: log, diary, journal
- Critical incident analysis
- Structured reflection
- Audio/video recording
- Process recording: accounts written following interaction with a patient
- Life chart: provides a diagrammatic summary of key events in a person's life over time
- Genogram: identifies relatives and relationships
- Client/patient formulation

Box 7.5 Models of reflective practice

Gibbs' model (1998)

1. Description – *what happened?*
2. Feelings – *what did I feel about it?*
3. Evaluation – *was it a positive or negative experience?*
4. Analysis – *what sense can I make of the experience, where does it fit within my personal development?*
5. Conclusion – *what else could I have done?*

Borton's model (1970)

1. What – *what happened; what was I doing; what were others doing?*
2. So what – *so what more do I need to know in order to understand the situation; so what could I have done that was different?*
3. Now what – *now what do I need to do to make things better? Now what will I do? Now what might be the consequences of this action?*
4. Action plan – *in a similar situation what would I do?*

the supervisor or their employing organization. Within the same clinical setting, there may be different groups of staff who will require and value different aspects of supervision and so supervision needs to be tailored to ensure that specific needs are met (Cleary *et al.* 2010). Within nursing there are several practices that resemble clinical supervision, such as mentorship and preceptorship.

Clinical supervision in mental health nursing

Clinical supervision in nursing has been widely adopted despite the lack of empirical evidence that it enhances supervisee knowledge and skills and improves patient care (Cleary *et al.* 2010). Research in this area is complex and a recent randomized control trial, although in the main inconclusive, did report improved care quality and patient outcomes in one area of practice (White and Winstanley 2010).

The main debates reported in the literature are: lack of consensus on an operational definition of clinical supervision; the tensions between clinical, managerial, personal and professional understandings, expectations and rationales for clinical supervision; and the variability of approaches used to evaluate clinical supervision. These debates take place against a backdrop of the changing nature and a range of understanding about the role of the mental health nurse (Buus and Gonge 2009; Cleary *et al.* 2010). Additionally, given the emphasis of mental health nursing on interpersonal and psychosocial interventions, clinical supervision in mental health nursing is distinctive from clinical supervision in other nursing specialties and may work differently. Thus, research findings from other nursing specialties may not be directly applicable to mental health nursing (Buus and Gonge 2009).

The key elements of clinical supervision that are reported to occur within mental health nursing include: a key focus on clinical practice patient care; dedicated supervision time; a process that supports to the supervisee's learning; a natural pursuit of topics determined by the supervisee, based on the demands of their practice; time to explore mucky and messy aspects of the work and work-related relationships; the ability to engage in reflective practice, leading to improved knowledge, skills and competence; and an overall long-term commitment to CPD (Rice *et al.* 2007; Cleary *et al.* 2010).

Buus and Gonge's (2009) research review revealed that mental health nurses generally found clinical supervision beneficial and facilitating. However they could also have negative experiences, and that while clinical supervision in mental health nursing is perceived as a good thing, there is limited empirical evidence to support this claim.

Thinking Space 7.2

Ask yourself the following questions about your own clinical supervision:

1. Does my supervisor have the necessary expertise and skills?
2. Can I work well together with him/her? Are both of us clear about our roles and responsibilities?

7.7 Work-related stress in nursing

In addition to enhancing nurses' professional capabilities, clinical supervision may also play a part in helping nurses manage psychological stress. Nurses experience a variety of stressors in their daily lives such as heavy workloads, work conflicts, role ambiguity and experiences of difficult and challenging behaviour from patients. In some cases the experience of psychological stress puts nurses' physical and mental health at risk and may affect their work, family and social relationships.

Psychological stress is a naturally occurring part of life. Different theories of stress generally emphasize the interconnectedness between the stressors, the individual's reaction to them and the coping mechanisms/techniques they use. Lazarus and Folkman (1984) proposed that stress could be thought of as resulting from an inequity between the stressors (internal, external or both) and resources. Stress management as a treatment approach was developed on the premise that the stress is not a direct response to the stressor but reflects the response of the individual to controlling the stress. If this is the case then the response can be influenced and managed.

Sorgaard *et al.* (2010) identify four principal sources of stress in the nursing profession:

1. **Educational sources:** assignments, exams, study, relationships with clinical staff and clinical assessments.

2. **Clinical sources:** excessive work pressures and demands, meeting patient expectations and nursing violent and suicidal patients.

3. **Personal/social sources:** home and work life balance, conflicts in personal values and poor support.

4. **Organizational sources:** conflicts with other professions, lack of resources, organizational change, poor management and insufficient salary.

The nursing literature identifies a range of concepts associated with work or occupational stress, the main ones being burnout, compassion fatigue and vicarious trauma.

Burnout is a construct developed by Maslach and Jackson (1986) which is thought to manifest as psychological stress as a result of long-term difficult work with complex and challenging patients. Burnout is generally characterized by emotional exhaustion and a reduced sense of accomplishment. Interestingly, recent research suggests that burnout may arise as a result of a mismatch between the individual and the job role (Sabo 2011).

Compassion fatigue, as a concept, is generally viewed as a form of burnout characterized by a combination of physical and emotional exhaustion associated with caring for very dependent patients. It is thought to result from the demands of showing compassion and care for patients whose situation may be unremitting and irresolvable. What is uncertain is whether caregivers who display high levels of empathy and empathic response to a patient's situation are potentially more vulnerable to experiencing compassion fatigue (Lombardo and Eyre 2011).

Vicarious trauma, as a concept, is applied to situations where front-line trauma and emergency workers are significantly affected by their work. Over time the repeated exposure to the nature of the work can impact on the way the worker perceives themselves, others and the world, with consequent negative effects on their personal and professional lives (Sabo 2011).

How nurses cope with stress

Studies on coping with stress show that most nurses use helpful, adaptive, informal coping strategies (Gibb *et al.* 2010). Informal strategies include gaining social support by: talking through situations with colleagues, peers, family and friends; using problem-solving approaches and cognitive techniques such as thinking positively; benefiting from close teamwork, handovers and team meetings as opportunities to discuss and resolve difficulties; and thinking creatively (Gibb *et al.* 2010; Ward 2011). The literature also highlights the contribution of access to formal work support structures to improved outcomes if those structures are present and effective. Formal support structures include: clinical supervision, staff appraisals and development plans; line and professional management structures; preceptorship, mentorship and support through occupational health departments.

Unhelpful or maladaptive strategies employed by nurses include: avoidance; distancing, isolation and going it alone; panic; displacing emotions such as anger; and drugs, smoking and alcohol (Timmins *et al.* 2011). Relatively little is known about work-related stress and its impact on nurses' personal lives, and personal life stress and its impact on work life (Lim *et al.* 2010).

> ### Thinking Space 7.3
>
> The annotated bibliography (p. 104) lists some web resources for information on stress, self-assessment tools and ideas and tips on managing stress. *Take a look and have a go.*

Mental health nursing and work-related stress

Mental health nursing work is generally inherently stressful and levels of work stress experienced by mental health nurses can be particularly high (Gibb *et al.* 2010). It has been suggested that this is due to the greater emphasis on interpersonal and psychosocial approaches to care in mental health nursing and the consequential tensions experienced in practicing these (Buus and Gonge 2009). Mental health nursing students report additional stressors related to their study such as assignments, exams, clinical placements, working in other jobs and financial concerns (Timmins *et al.* 2011).

Mental health nurses working in inpatient environments are more susceptible to lower levels of job satisfaction and higher levels of burnout than their community counterparts, possibly because of greater severity of patient illness, the unpredictable and challenging nature of the work, aggression and violence, increased record-keeping and poor managerial support (Ward 2011).

Mental health nurses and students may be powerful role models in supporting the physical and mental health of others, and so it could be argued that they have a responsibility to effectively manage their own health and well-being (Gibb *et al.* 2010).

Coping with psychological stress

The literature indicates that mental health nurses make most use of informal strategies to deal with stress, using, for example, immediate opportunities of discussion with a colleague, or at a handover or team meeting, as opportunities to reflect on problems and reduce resultant stress. While much has been written about sources of stress in mental health nursing, relatively little research has been carried out to evaluate stress-reducing interventions with this population (Timmins *et al.* 2011).

'As nurses begin meeting the needs of others, they often neglect their own needs' (Lombardo and Eyre 2011: 1). Developing and sustaining healthy lifestyles and well-being behaviours is important for mental health nurses in terms of looking after themselves. A commitment to taking care of yourself includes paying attention to physical health (diet, exercise and sleep) and mental health (connect, be active, take notice, keep learning and give). The document *Mental Capital and Wellbeing* (Government Office for Science 2008) is helpful here.

Of all the helpful strategies in managing stress in the workplace it appears that talking with an appropriate person about concerns and developing and maintaining helpful coping strategies are among the most successful (Lombardo and Eyre 2011). Of equal importance is the commitment and investment by employing organizations to creating healthy work environments that promote wellness opportunities and reduce and manage those who are experiencing work-related stress: 'Caring for caregivers, whether on a personal or system level, provides the foundation needed for optimal patient and family care' (Lombardo and Eyre 2011: 1).

7.8 Implications for mental health nursing practice

This section discusses the implications of the material covered in this chapter for mental health nursing practice.

Clarifying the role of the mental health nurse

Meeting NMC professional standards and requirements demonstrates to society that nurses are fit to practice. Machin and Stevenson (1997) offer a three-dimensional framework that incorporates the aspects of role adequacy, role legitimacy and role support. This provides a useful framework for clarifying the dynamics of mental health nurses' roles.

Role adequacy is related to the minimum expected level of knowledge and skills of the practitioner. It can be developed through formal and informal education and experience and so has strong links with CPD. Role legitimacy is concerned with the boundaries of professional practice (both self and others) and fits with the scope of practice and role description of the post the nurse holds. Role support refers to both formal and informal support structures provided by the profession and the organization, such as policy and guidance structures, clinical supervision and informal forms of support.

Machin and Stevenson (1997) propose that when there is clarity within each of the dimensions of the framework there is a balanced equilibrium with resultant role security and implied optimal role function. Imbalance within these dimensions threatens role security with negative consequences for optimal role function and possibly delivery of patient care. Applying this framework to our roles offers nurses an opportunity to reflect on the balance of our role security and role function and develop a plan to address imbalances.

Thinking Space 7.4

Apply Machin and Stevenson's framework to your own nursing role and make some notes in response to the following questions:

1. **Role adequacy** (minimum expected level of knowledge and skills) *Do you have these? If not, what plan can you make to start addressing the deficits?*

2. **Role legitimacy** (the boundaries of professional practice – both self and others) *Are you practising within the boundaries of your professional practice and scope of your role? If not, then why not? Does this raise any ethical, legal and professional issues? Make a plan to address these.*

3. **Role support** (formal and informal support structures that are provided by the profession and the organization) *Map out your formal and informal support structures and networks and decide how effective and helpful they are. What does this tell you? Are there areas that need strengthening? If so are you able to influence these? Are there any other forms of support that you've so far not thought of that you might be able to use? Make a plan to address any deficits.*

4. **Role security and function** *When you look at the above findings, what does this tell you? Is everything in these dimensions clear and balanced? If so do you have role security and are you at 'optimal role function'? If not then the exercise has highlighted imbalances in the dimensions and given some thought to planning how to address them.*

5. **What next?** *If you have found the exercise helpful you may find it useful to repeat it in future as your role changes over time. Finally, consider applying the framework to the clinical team of which you are a part.*

Advanced mental health nursing practice

Confusion surrounds nursing titles and roles associated with concepts of expanded, extended, specialist and advanced practice. This has been exacerbated by radical changes in mental health nursing practice consequent to a shift from institutional to a community-based services. The development required for advanced mental health nursing may be different for individual practitioners. Some may follow a specialist route with a focus on high-level skills and decision-making within a particular client group or clinical context. In contrast, others may acquire knowledge, skills and expertise that reflects high-level assessment, decision-making and autonomous practice across a breadth of practice. Advanced nursing practice requires the development of both a wider range and additional in-depth skills (Gilfedder et al. 2010).

There is concern within the profession that the introduction of the nurse consultant role, with associated high status and salary, has eroded the position of nurses undertaking advanced practice. It can be argued that most mental health nurses at various grades have the same core functions and that these do not differ for nurse consultants. Thus, the best method of distinguishing between practitioners with similar functions may be by measuring patient and organizational outcomes (Duffield et al. 2009).

 7.9 Conclusion

This chapter has provided an overview of CPD and advanced practice.

In summary the main points are:

- CPD is a mandatory requirement for all nurses in maintaining and developing current best knowledge and skills in the delivery of practice.

It is the responsibility of the individual practitioner and their employer.

- Meeting the NMC standards for professional registration is a minimal requirement for professional nursing practice.

- Clinical supervision is regarded as a good thing although the evidence for its benefits for quality of patient care and outcomes is limited.

- Good clinical supervision contributes to CPD and may help nurses manage work stress.

- Mental health nurses appear to value access to informal structures rather than formal structures to help them cope with stress; both types of support are important.

- Mental health nurses are role models for their patients and the public and so should look after their own physical and mental well-being.

- Machin and Stevenson's model offers a framework for reflecting on our roles and planning how to meet development needs.

- There is confusion on clarity and consistency related to advanced and specialist titles and roles.

- It is recommended that specialist practice is considered on a continuum with generalist practice.

Annotated bibliography

Mental Health Foundation, www.mentalhealth.org.uk.
This website has lots of useful information on managing stress and mental health. It also offers an online course on mindfulness, although there is currently a cost attached to this.

NHS Choices, www.nhs.uk.
There are a number of pages on stress and stress management linking to other areas of relevant physical and mental health.

Mind, www.mind.org.uk.
Useful information on stress and stress management linking to other areas of relevant mental health.

Emotional well-being website, http://emotionalwellbeing.southcentral.nhs.uk.
This website has started bringing together a range of information on emotional well-being relevant to users, practitioners, organizations and commissioners.

Lombardo, B. and Eyre, C. (2011) Compassion fatigue: a nurse's primer, *Online Journal of Issues in Nursing,* **16(1).**
This free online paper (just Google for availability) discusses compassion fatigue and illustrates approaches to two case studies. Although the study was based in the USA it raises many points for consideration in a UK setting.

Ritter, S., Norman, I.J., Rentoul, L. and Bodley, D.E. (1996) A model of clinical supervision for nurses undertaking short placements in mental health care settings, *Journal of Clinical Nursing,* **5: 149–58.**
This paper describes the use of the genogram and life chart as clinical supervision tools for knowledge development with nursing students taking brief mental health clinical placements.

A Professional Framework for Mental Health Nursing in England 2011–2016, **www.dh.gov.uk/health/2011/10/cno-introduces-mental-health-nursing-framework.**
This video link shows the CNO (England) presenting a new professional framework for mental health nursing. At the time of writing no other information about the framework appears to be in the public domain but this could be very relevant to the future of nurses' CPD.

References

AANPE (Association of Advanced Nursing Practice Educators) (2012), available at: www.aanpe.org.

Borton, T. (1970) *Reach, Teach and Touch.* London: McGraw-Hill.

Buus, N. and Gonge, P. (2009) Empirical studies of clinical supervision in psychiatric nursing: a systematic literature review and methodological critique, *International Journal of Mental Health Nursing,* 18(4): 250–64.

Casey, D. and Egan, D. (2010) The use of professional portfolios and profiles for career enhancement, *British Journal of Community Nursing,* 15(11): 547–52.

Cleary, M., Horsfall, J. and Happell, B. (2010) Establishing clinical supervision in acute mental health inpatient units: acknowledging the challenges, *Issues in Mental Health Nursing,* 31(8): 525–31.

Deacon, M. (2011) Being creative about continuing professional development, *Mental Health Nursing,* 31(6): 14–17.

DH (Department of Health) (2004) *The NHS Knowledge and Skills Framework (NHS KSF) and the Development Review Process,* available at: www.dh.gov.uk.

DH (Department of Health) (2006) From values to action. The Chief Nursing Officer's review of mental health nursing. London: DH.

DH (Department of Health) (2010a) *Advanced Level Nursing: A Position Statement,* available at: www.dh.gov.uk.

DH (Department of Health) (2010b) *Front Line Care: the future of nursing and midwifery in England. Report of the Prime Minister's Commission on the Future of Nursing and Midwifery in England 2010,* available at: www.dh.gov.uk.

DH (Department of Health) (2011) *Modernising Nursing Careers,* available at: http://webarchive.nationalarchives.gov.uk/+/www.dh.gov.uk/en/Aboutus/chiefprofessionalofficers/chiefnursingofficer/DH_108368.

Duffield, C.D., Gardner, G., Chang, A. and Catling-Paull, C. (2009) Advanced nursing practice: a global perspective, *Collegian,* 16: 55–62.

Elsom, S., Happell, B. and Manias, E. (2005) Mental health nurse practitioner: expanded or advanced? *International Journal of Mental Health Nursing,* 14: 181–6.

Eraut, M. (1994) *Developing Professional Knowledge and Competence.* London: RoutledgeFalmer.

Fowler, J., Fenton, G. and Riley, J. (2007) Using solution-focused techniques in clinical supervision, *Nursing Times,* 103(22): 30–1.

Gass, J., McKie, A., Smith, I., Brown, A. and Addo, M. (2007) An examination of the scope and purpose of education in mental health nursing, *Nurse Education Today,* 27(6): 588–96.

Gibb, J., Cameron, I., Hamilton, R., Murphy, E. and Naji, S. (2010) Mental health nurses' and allied health professionals' perceptions of the role of the occupational health service in the management of work-related stress: how do they self-care? *Journal of Psychiatric and Mental Health Nursing,* 17(9): 838–45.

Gibbs, G. (1988). *Learning by Doing: A Guide.* Birmingham: SCED.

Gilfedder, M., Barron, D. and Docherty, E. (2010) Developing the role of advanced nurse practitioners in mental health, *Nursing Standard,* 24(30): 35–40.

Government Office for Science (2008) *Mental Capital and Wellbeing: Making the most of ourselves in the 21st century – Final Project Report,* available at: http://tinyurl.com/ForesightReportMentalcapital.

Lazarus, R. and Folkman, S. (1984) *Stress, Appraisal and Coping.* New York: Springer.

Lim, J., Bogossian, F. and Ahern, K. (2010) Stress and coping in Australian nurses: a systematic review, *International Nursing Review,* 57: 27–31.

Lombardo, B. and Eyre, C. (2011) Compassion fatigue: a nurse's primer, *Online Journal of Issues in Nursing,* 16(1).

Machin, T. and Stevenson, C. (1997) Towards a framework for clarifying psychiatric nursing roles, *Journal of Psychiatric and Mental Health Nursing,* 4(2): 81–7.

Maslach, C. and Jackson, S. (1986) *Maslach Burnout Inventory Manual,* 2nd edn. Palo Alto, CA: Consulting Psychologists Press.

NHS (National Health Service) (2011) *Leadership Framework,* available at: www.nhsleadershipqualities.nhs.uk.

NMC (Nursing and Midwifery Council) (2008a) *The Code: Standards of conduct, performance and ethics for nurses and midwives,* available at: www.nmc-uk.org.

NMC (Nursing and Midwifery Council) (2008b) *Standards to Support Learning and Assessment in Practice,* available at: www.nmc-uk.org.

NMC (Nursing and Midwifery Council) (2008c) Annexe 1 – NMC circular 10/2008, available at: www.nmc-uk.org.

NMC (Nursing and Midwifery Council) (2008d) www.nmc-uk.org/Nurses-and-midwives/Advice-by-topic/A/Advice/Clinical-supervision-for-registered-nurses.

NMC (Nursing and Midwifery Council) (2011) *The Prep Handbook*, available at: www.nmc-uk.org.

Rice, F., Cullen, P., McKenna, H., Kelly, B., Keeney, S. and Richey, R. (2007) Clinical supervision for mental health nurses in Northern Ireland: formulating best practice guidelines, *Journal of Psychiatric and Mental Health Nursing*, 14(5): 516–21.

Richards, L. and Potgieter, E. (2010) Perceptions of registered nurses in four state health institutions on continuing formal education, *Curationis*, 33(2): 41–50.

Sabo, B. (2011) Reflecting on the concept of compassion fatigue, *Journal of Issues in Nursing*, 16(1).

Schweitzer, D. and Krassa, T. (2010) Deterrents to nurses' participation in continuing professional development: an integrative literature review, *The Journal of Continuing Education in Nursing*, 41(10): 441–7.

Scott, G. (2011) Continuing education must be a priority. *Nursing Standard* 26(3): 1.

Sorgaard, K., Ryan, P. and Dawson, I. (2010) Qualified and Unqualified (N-R C) mental health nursing staff – minor differences in sources of stress and burnout, a European multi-centre study, *BMC Health Services Research*, 10(163): 1–12.

Timmins, F., Corroon, A., Byrne, G. and Mooney, B. (2011) The challenge of contemporary nurse education programmes: perceived stressors of nursing students – mental health and related lifestyle issues, *Journal of Psychiatric and Mental Health Nursing*, 18(9): 758–66.

Ward, L. (2011) Mental health nursing and stress: maintaining balance, *International Journal of Mental Health Nursing*, 20(2): 77–85.

White, E. and Winstanley, J. (2010) Does clinical supervision lead to better patient outcomes in mental health nursing? *Nursing Times*, 106(16): 16–18.

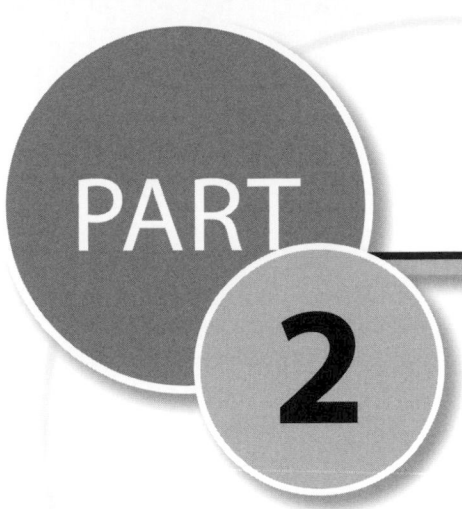

PART

2

Contexts

Chapter 8

The Social Policy Context of Mental Health Care

Paul Calaminus

8.1 Introduction

This chapter considers the social policy context of mental health care in the UK. Rather than focus on specific policy documents it adopts a thematic approach. It outlines a number of key themes and policies that have particular impact on services, and some ways in which such policy has been implemented. In this chapter, social policy is considered to be policy that impacts on the functioning of UK society, with a particular focus on mental health care. This is, deliberately, a broad definition, and the chapter aims to outline the ways in which such policies affect how services are provided. Key elements of social policy considered in this chapter are those that impact on:

- the relationship between statutory providers and the public;
- stigma;
- confidence in health services;
- population change;

- welfare reform;
- public safety;
- information;
- democratic legitimacy;
- methods of implementation.

Each of the above is considered in the context of current UK fiscal policy as it relates to the funding of mental health and social care.

8.2 The relationship between statutory providers and the public

Across the public and private sector, the last 20 to 30 years has seen a sea change in public expectations of service delivery. In many ways, the UK population has become more demanding of service providers in all walks of life, and health care is no exception. Patients have increased expectations of services to provide care that is personalized and customer focused. Users of services have become less willing simply to accept the services on offer, and more inclined to challenge services to provide the care they believe they need. To some extent, this can be characterized as a move away from a paternalistic model of care delivery, towards a model of care that is based on partnership between service users and clinicians.

There are particular complications here for mental health care. To some extent, they go to the heart of what mental health care is. This is because, while service providers often assume that they work in the best interests of patients and their health, this is not the way in which the services can be experienced by those who receive them. This point is strongly made by the service user movement. This movement (exemplified by movements such as the Survivors movement) has always had vocal elements that have argued that mental health services are inherently flawed. Indeed, some argue that services are profoundly abusive towards the human rights of service users, and reject the use of the term 'patients' because they believe that it implies a health care relationship between clinicians and service users that is false. Rather, they argue, mental health services are a form of social control, with health care treatment only a minor part of the range of functions that services fulfil. In support of these arguments they cite not only the historic practice of detaining people within asylums, but also a number of social attitudes towards mental health which may have been perpetuated by services themselves. An example of this is a historic attitude towards parenthood. It was not unusual in the past for the assumption to be made that service users would not be having children. Implications of this included the routine prescribing of risky medication to women of child-bearing age. Indeed, medication per se is often argued to be a form of social control, with side-effects that outweigh the benefits and often cause distress.

Mental health care does remain coercive, however humanely this is done. The fact is that every year several thousand people are forcibly admitted to hospitals and detained there against their will – often with police involvement in the process of sectioning. As at 31 March 2011 there were 20,938 patients detained under sections of the Mental Health Act – a 5 per cent increase on the figure of 31 March 2010 (NHS Information Centre 2011). The impact of this on service users and their families should not be underestimated, and it can continue to affect people and their relationship with services for long periods of time after treatment has been completed.

In this context, the service user movement and general changes in the population's expectation of service providers across health care has provided a major challenge to the culture of mental health care. Overall, these changes have begun a process of working in partnership between service users and organizations that provide care. Thus, it is now normal to find service users involved in the design of services, and in the recruitment of staff. It is also usual to find 'expert patients' who provide advice to service providers. More normal, too, are questionnaires seeking service user experience with a view to taking feedback and using it to improve the service that is provided.

The way in which legal powers are used has also developed to take account of human rights legislation. As the rights conferred by this have become a more fundamental part of English Law, so the way in which mental health legislation is employed has changed. Thus, use of Section 2 of the Act is now much more prevalent (see Chapter 11); the timeliness of tribunal hearings is more tightly monitored; the provision of information to patients is more tightly assessed; and the assessing of capacity has much greater prominence in the statutory *Code of Practice* for the Mental Health Act.

Such changes have led to some specific policy responses. In general, the current coalition government has stated that its National Health Service (NHS) policies are informed by the statement that for every patient it should be true to say that 'there is no decision about me without me'. In mental health services, the shift away from paternalistic models of care has perhaps been best captured in policies on 'recovery' and 'personalization'.

'Recovery' (see Chapter 5) has emerged as a major theme in social policy relating to mental health over the last five years. It emerged from work by Mary Ellen Copeland and her colleagues and represents a significant shifting in the balance of power between providers and those who use services. The impact of this policy is that it provides a framework within which service users define recovery in their own terms as opposed to clinical terms. They also set their own goals on the path to recovery. Frequently these goals are not clinical or about changes in symptomatology; rather, they are about the extent to which people can live and enjoy life as well as the extent to which they feel in control of their care.

Similarly, 'personalization' aims to give control of care provision back to those who are receiving that care. This policy is aimed at social care services, and gives the option of a personal budget to service users, with which they are entitled to buy the care they consider they need from the providers they consider most appropriate. This budget is based on a share of the total overall available budget for mental health social care, and is accessed through an assessment process with social work professionals. This policy has recently been introduced within mental health care but in care groups where it has been policy for a longer period of time it has had a beneficial impact on the lives of service users, and the extent to which they feel in control of their own care (MIND – 'Personalisation in Mental Health' – a review of the evidence, 2010). It is likely that this policy may be introduced to health services more generally, with health personal budgets being piloted in some areas of the country.

Thinking Space 8.1

In the section above we discuss the relationship between statutory providers and the public, but the voluntary sector also makes a major contribution to mental health care.

1. List the voluntary agencies that you are aware of in the mental health field. Then enter a search into Google to find others.
2. What roles do voluntary agencies play?

8.3 Stigma

There can be little doubt that the stigma attached to mental health problems remains a significant social issue. It causes increased distress for those with mental health problems, and can prevent people seeking help for problems as early as they might otherwise do. The stigma attached to mental illness also causes distress for the families of those who are affected, and can lead to discrimination in employment against those who have received treatment for mental health problems. Those who have received treatment or seen family members receiving treatment often describe a sense of shame that was driven largely by the stigma attached to the condition for which they were being treated. In the most extreme cases of stigmatizing behaviour, patients with learning disabilities have been bullied to the point of suicide largely on account of their mental health status. It would appear that this stigma is deeply rooted in UK society (Michael 2007). Topics such as suicide have traditionally been taboo and the provision of asylum care over the last few hundred years arguably reinforced an 'out of sight, out of mind' approach to mental health care.

Over the last 10 years, however, there has been significant social policy focus on equality. This has manifested itself largely in equalities legislation in employment, and duties of equality for all employers. In tandem with this, there have been a number of government-led campaigns aimed at reducing the stigma of mental illness. These have included publicity campaigns, including celebrity disclosures, as well as general health promotion about mental health problems. Mainstream media have also been used to show mental health problems as a 'normal' health problem. These campaigns, along with the general focus on equalities have, to some extent,

begun to change the stigmatized environment in relation to mental health. Recent government policy has also emphasized the importance of mental health across society, and the common nature of the conditions. However, there remains much work to be done before mental health problems can be faced without the additional distress and burden of stigma attached to mental illness.

Thinking Space 8.2

What is social stigma and how would you recognize it?

Feedback

According to the World Health Organization (WHO) (2002: 8), stigma 'results from a process whereby certain individuals and groups are unjustifiably rendered shameful, excluded and discriminated against'. According to Thornicroft (2006) stigma has three key components:

- *Ignorance* (a problem of knowledge) – namely that people are ignorant.
- *Prejudice* (a problem of attitudes) – people hold negative attitudes or preconceived opinions.
- *Discrimination* (a problem of behaviour) – the unjust treatment of people on grounds of sex, race, age or stigmatizing illness.

8.4 Confidence in health services

Over the last few years, confidence in health services generally appears to have been shaken. A number of issues have made a mark in the public consciousness – not least those relating to child paediatric surgery at Bristol Royal Infirmary and standards of care at South Staffordshire Foundation Trust. Mental health services have also had their share of issues – subject to public inquiries – that have raised questions for the general public about the safety and effectiveness of services. Over the last 25 years there have been a number of homicides by people under the care of mental health services which are considered to have damaged public trust in services.

The government's response to these issues of public perception has been to create an explicitly

quality focused regulatory framework to mirror the financial framework that has been in place for a much longer period of time. Currently, this is the responsibility of the Care Quality Commission (CQC) – the regulator of all health care in England. The CQC sets quality standards for the provision of care and carries out unannounced inspections of services across the country.

Service providers have had to register with the CQC since 2010 – the first time that NHS providers have ever had to register as providers of care. By the same token, it is also the first time that it has been possible to de-register health care providers, and prevent them from providing care, or prosecute them for a failure to provide minimum standards. NHS providers are also required to publish quality accounts. These are public documents that describe the performance of the organization against quality standards, as well as priorities for quality improvement. In partnership with the new regulatory arrangements, these are intended to provide a framework within which confidence in the quality of care provided can be maintained. At the same time, policy is also moving towards the creation of fewer, larger, specialist centres where quality of care can be better achieved (there are proven gains in quality and reliability when high enough volumes of certain procedures are carried out) and against the traditional system of district general hospitals providing nearly the full range of services to a local population.

8.5   Population change

Ageing population

A further major issue for social policy is the ageing population of the country, and the health care implications of this. Across the UK, the population is getting older and living longer with chronic disease, not least due to improvements in health care techniques and technology that mean that conditions are now treatable that were not in the past. In part, this is driven by improvements in diet, affluence and living conditions that have led to an increase in general life expectancy. This, in turn, has led to an increase in the long-term care costs for the population (as well as an increased cost of pension provision). The cost of nursing home care, for example, has been a persistent social policy issue over the last 15–20 years, and, as the population ages, the question of how the country can best pay for the cost of this care has become more urgent (DH 2011). This is one area where a real search for cross-party consensus is underway, and ideas have been proposed for some form of universal insurance scheme that will create a means of funding such care at a national level. At present, however, such consensus has not been reached, and such care is means tested, with family assets having to be used to provide funds. Increasingly, this is becoming a political issue, as the number of older voters increases, and it is likely that some form of cross-party consensus will emerge as to how such care should best be paid for. It should be noted that this is one area where there is differ-

ence between Scotland and other areas of the UK as the devolved Scottish administration has a policy that such care be provided free at the point of delivery. However, the shift towards an ageing population has not been universal, and some of the lowest improvements in life expectancy have been for some of the most disadvantaged groups in society.

Using a measure of deprivation such as the Jarman index, which was originally developed to predict demand for primary care in the 1980s and is widely used in the NHS, it is possible to show areas with relatively high levels of social and economic need. These areas usually correlate with localities that have higher levels of health care need and high levels of health risk behaviour (such as smoking and illicit substance misuse). Such areas also often have higher rates of mental illness than areas with lower levels of deprivation. Indeed, as far as mental health is concerned, there does seem to be some correlation between levels of socioeconomic deprivation, high-risk health behaviour and family breakdown, coupled with particular genetic predispositions towards certain mental health problems. Many of these areas are to be found in inner cities across the UK, although this is by no means a hard and fast rule.

Over the past decade, there have been a number of health and social policy responses to this, aiming to address the root causes of ill health as well as to improve the social environment in such areas, including initiatives such as Health Action Zones, which have aimed to bring together a range of agencies (both statutory and voluntary) that work in specific local areas. Substantial sums of money have also been spent on the regeneration of local neighbourhoods – both by the British government and the European Union. This has led to the total regeneration of some inner-city areas and the replacement in part of a generation of high-rise council housing with more modern accommodation.

There have also been specific initiatives that have aimed to ensure that people living in such areas are supported to access services. These have included initiatives such as the Sure Start scheme – a scheme that originally provided services for all children under the age of 4, or the government funding of nursery education for all children aged 3. There have been substantial grants, too, for voluntary sector organizations to try and provide social support and infrastructure that might otherwise not exist in areas of particular deprivation. In general, there has been an emphasis on early intervention where problems are emerging (and, if possible, before problems emerge) to try and prevent more serious issues from developing. This has led to the adoption of more specific schemes, such as the Family Nurse Partnership that works with a defined group of new mothers who are otherwise at risk of not accessing services, and whose children are at risk of being taken into care. In part a more targeted approach is being taken in recognition that some initiatives may have been too general and may, in fact, have simply provided free state support to those who would otherwise have been able to afford to pay for it, rather than be targeted on those most in need.

It has to be said, however, that for all these efforts, the gap between rich and poor in the UK shows limited signs of closing (ONS 2011). There remain areas of deprivation that link with areas of high health need, including high levels of mental illness, and there is some likelihood that the economic situation in the second decade of the twenty-first century will mean that approaches to this problem have to be rethought. Indeed, there is some evidence that such rethinking is already taking place, with greater emphasis on how communities and individuals can help themselves, rather than how the state can help them. This, in turn, builds on policies such as recovery and personalization in mental health services that were discussed earlier.

Immigration

Immigration is also a significant issue in social and public policy. Over the past decade, the UK has, broadly, pursued a policy of multi-culturalism, with great emphasis on ensuring employment and social rights for individuals irrespective of background. The enlargement of the European Union has led to changes in the UK population, particularly in urban areas, and there have been changes in the make-up of populations resulting both from economic migration and from the migration of those from conflict zones. To some extent, this has been a predominantly urban phenomenon, with the majority of non-urban populations remaining almost exclusively white British. Within some urban areas, however, in current school age generations, a majority of children in school are from black or ethnic minority backgrounds (ONS 2010).

This change has created some social policy challenges – in some areas it has led to tensions over employment and housing and some political issues, with a limited rise in more extremist political parties such as the British National Party. To date, this has been very limited, but government social policy has emphasized elements of Britishness and, more explicitly, tried to cap the number of people immigrating to the UK. There is now a citizenship test that people have to undertake before becoming British citizens – a sign of the seriousness with which national government is beginning to treat this area of social policy.

In some ways, immigration has created relatively few issues for mental health care – most services work on the basis that specific services may be required for particular cultural groups and that the organizations providing metal health care will meet their duties under employment and other equalities legislation. However, mental health care has been accused of being institutionally racist – a charge made by the inquiry into the death of Rocky Bennett in 2004 and one that has been repeated since (Heginbotham and Patel 2007).

Racism

Institutional racism is a concept that came to prominence in public life as a result of the MacPherson Inquiry into the death of Stephen Lawrence. This found that in the case of Metropolitan Police, the institution itself had, unwittingly in many cases, enshrined values into its policies and procedures that, taken together, created a system that discriminated on the basis of race. The issue for mental health services is that when one looks at rates of detention under the Mental Health Act (including detention under criminal sections of that Act), there is often a disproportionate number of young black men detained compared with their proportional make-up of the population. The reasons why this is so are not clear. Services have therefore been required to put together action plans to address issues of cultural awareness, and are required to publish a Single Equalities Scheme every year that sets out how they are meeting duties under the legislation, and what work is ongoing to address issues of equality. Annual reports also have to be made to organizational boards on the local workforce and whether or not it is representative of the local population, as well as any work that is ongoing to try and address issues. The issue of over-representation within services does still exist, however, in some areas, and this is likely to remain an area where social policy has an impact on mental health services.

Children, young people and the family

There are also a number of social policy challenges relating to children, young people and the family. These have been brought into stark relief by recent UNICEF reports showing that children in the UK are, relative to children and young people in other European countries, less happy and more affected by poverty than their peers elsewhere (UNICEF 2010). It is easy to be too downbeat about the picture that is presented, but there is at least some sense of crisis among policy-makers about children and young people. The images that dominate the public consciousness are often of 'feral youths' (in a recent study more than 50 per cent of the British public thought that young people in the UK were growing up 'feral' – Barnados 2008) and often family breakdown leading to gang violence. The above is deliberately stereotyped, but it is also a fact that in some (particularly inner-city) areas there are regular acts of youth-on-youth violence (including homicide) and that there are areas that are dominated by gang culture among young people. This is not to say that all young people are engaged in such a culture – that is manifestly untrue – but that there is a signifi-

cant minority who are is also true. The UK also has the highest rates of teenage pregnancy in western Europe (as well as high rates of teenage obesity), and issues with sexual violence and assault among children. Meanwhile, the education system seems stuck in a debate partly about what the best form of school system is (still the debate about grammar schools) and partly about what form of teaching to use to teach basic skills. There are issues relating to academic achievement. Access to university education has been widened, but fees have been introduced, which are to be paid for through a loan – repayable once a graduate reaches a certain salary level on graduation.

At the same time, social policy in respect of children has been influenced by some high profile safeguarding incidents. Perhaps most notable (although by no means the only cases) were the cases of Victoria Climbié and, more recently Baby Peter. Lessons from serious case reviews (carried out into cases where children have been seriously harmed or died) have identified some risk factors common to such cases, including the presence of adults with mental health or substance misuse problems and children aged under 2.

Some politicians and commentators have attributed many of the issues above to the breakdown of families in the UK. Certainly, the UK has higher than average levels of divorce and the absence of parents from family life (possibly through long working hours, for example) has been cited as one reason behind UNICEF findings about childhood in Britain (UNICEF 2010).

Policy responses

The social policy response to the above has been to try and address the root causes of behaviour, to measure the situation and to try and provide support for different forms of family and family life. For example, policies that try and address behaviour include 'restorative justice' in which perpetrators come face to face with victims – with an aim of giving a greater understanding of and empathy for the impact of the crime. In support of families, the government established an Academy of Parenting

Practitioners – training staff across the country in parenting interventions, so that they, in turn, could train parents in how to parent more effectively. A concerted effort has been made to include children in school and limit the level of exclusion, with significant resources going towards special educational needs coordinators (SENCOs) keeping children in mainstream education. Until the impact of the economic downturn in 2010, the Connexions service had been established to try and provide employment opportunities for young people leaving full-time education.

Within the sphere of social care, much greater emphasis has been placed on meeting the needs of children who are looked after, with local authorities formally monitored in their role as corporate parents. The family court system too has attempted to address the needs of children in a more holistic way, making concerted efforts to keep children with their birth families and trying to ensure that the voice of the child is heard throughout legal proceedings. In support of this, a raft of statistics has been gathered about the educational, employment and health status of children and young people.

There have also been structural changes. Every local authority area in England now has a director of children's services responsible for services for children within that area. Generally, they work through partnership arrangements that, although no longer statutory, hold health, social care, police and voluntary sector agencies to account for their work with children, and set local strategic priorities and outcomes for children in their area. Safeguarding boards also exist in every area. These are statutory bodies, chaired by independent people, the remit of which is to hold to account all statutory and voluntary sector agencies in the area that are working with children in respect of their child protection responsibilities. Local, regional and national guidelines have been produced (DH 2006) that set out clearly the responsibilities for child protection. These arrangements have recently been reviewed and a new version of this guidance is expected as a result. At a national level, a childrens' commissioner

has been appointed, with a remit to report to Parliament on any aspect of government policy and practice as it affects children.

All of these have an effect on mental health services. All providers of mental health care will have to comply with the requirements of *Working Together* in respect of child protection. These requirements apply as much to those mental health professionals working with adults and older adults as to those working with children. For those working with adults, their role as parents or potential parents will need to be taken into account. For those working with children, not only will the general social care and educational needs of those children need to be taken into account, their services as a whole will probably be expected to be part of wider social care and multi-agency initiatives that aim to change behaviours as much as treat health conditions. (Examples of this may include how mental health services can help other agencies work with antisocial or highly sexualized behaviour.) It is also clear that policy in this area continues to evolve and does so amidst some unease about the position of children and young people in English society today, and that this evolution will continue to affect mental health services – both for adults and children.

Welfare reform

A major preoccupation of the current UK coalition government is welfare reform. The current welfare benefits bill is some £111.7 billion per annum (PESA 2011). Quite aside from the issues of affordability in the current economic and financial climate, the argument is increasingly being made that the welfare benefits system has become less a safety net for people and more a form of institutionalization in the community. In some areas, there are generations who are welfare dependent, and there is a recognized problem with welfare benefits in the current system that a person coming off benefits and into work can actually be worse off than a person who remains on benefits ('the benefits trap'). Reform is therefore being pursued – both to reduce the overall bill but also based on a belief that the current system is actually disempowering some benefit recipients. Thus, requirements to work are being introduced and all those on Incapacity Benefit are being reassessed for fitness to work. This applies to many mental health service users, many of whom need significant support to undergo what can be an anxiety-provoking experience. This is certainly an area in which mental health practitioners need to support their clients – both to prevent them falling into benefit dependency where possible, but also to prevent the process of reassessment and insistence on work from causing a deterioration in their mental state. Indeed, it is important that mental health practitioners seek ways to support their clients back into work, and a number of vocational and employment schemes exist to support them in doing so.

8.6 Public safety

It is largely true to say that people in the UK today do not feel safe. The UK crime survey reveals this perception (PESA 2011). For obvious reasons, this quickly becomes a political as well as a social policy issue. Crime figures themselves are not always reliable, since they can, by definition, only report recorded crime. What they do reveal, however, is that crime in the UK has fallen consistently. The fear of crime (and violent crime in particular) however has not, and there are few votes for policies that are perceived as being 'soft on crime'.

Since 1997, there have been over 3,600 new criminal laws created in the UK and the prison population has increased to 88,000, while 30 per cent of men aged under 40 in the UK have a criminal record. This has a number of implications for mental health services. First, the number of places in secure hospitals has dramatically increased, with spending in this area increasing to £1.2 billion in 2011 (????). Second, some traditional rules about employing people with criminal records in caring professions have had to be revised – after all, if 30 per cent of the male population under 40 has a criminal record, it is no longer a particularly discriminating employability factor. Third, services have had to engage with a set of risk management

processes known as Multi-Agency Public Protection Arrangements (MAPPA) and Multi-Agency Risk Assessment and Control (MARAC). These are police led, and exist to share risk management information and action plans about known and particularly risky offenders. Mental health expertise is often required for such panels as there can be particular offenders under the care of mental health services, or for whom mental health issues may play a part in their offending behaviour. In such meetings, the role of the mental health professional will be to share such information as is possible and ensure that services are engaged as necessary with this multi-agency planning. Fourth, services have been involved in a general push to address the needs of victims. As an example, there is now a much greater expectation that internal reports into incidents will be shared with the relatives of victims, and that the findings of these reports will be made public in coroners' courts – often with investigators invited to give evidence.

8.7 Information

In terms of information, there have been two major areas of policy development that impact very significantly on the relationship between the citizen and the state, and, in turn, on the relationship between mental health services, their patients and the public as a whole. The first of these is the sharing of information; the second is the Freedom of Information Act. There is now a large amount of information about individuals held on numerous databases throughout the UK. In terms of health and social care, it is now the case that the vast majority of information held about an individual is held in this way. It is also the case that effective risk management is often shown to have been hindered by ineffective information-sharing when untoward incidents are reviewed. This has led to a duty to share information for the purposes of effective risk management – a duty that (in common with child protection duties) overrides any duty of confidentiality towards an individual patient. There is also more generalized information-sharing, with some health systems being used to collect both health and social care data, for example. Mechanisms such as MAPPA and MARAC have already been mentioned – both are examples of the sharing of information for the purposes of effective risk management across agencies. Consent for the sharing of information with other agencies is often requested when a service user first makes contact with services, and should also be requested when any information is to be shared. The ease with which electronic data can be shared, however, can create its own barriers to patients freely sharing data – not being sure how such information might be used. At the same time, when information is effectively amalgamated, it can be used to significantly improve the quality of interventions offered. Virtual wards at home, for example, often rely on sophisticated information-sharing between secondary and primary care, and sophisticated risk stratification software to identify which patients can be effectively supported to live at home, and which need hospital care. It is, however, important that services pay sufficient attention to helping patients understand the reasons for information-sharing, and the extent of it, to avoid jeopardizing the clinician-patient relationship. In some areas this has led to pilots of patient-held electronic information to guide care and to help patients feel in control of the information held and shared about them.

Freedom of Information Act

The Freedom of Information Act has also had a profound impact. This obliges public bodies to share information, unless to do so would cause a disproportionate cost, or where to do so would not be in the public interest. Both these exemptions, however, are tightly applied, with a presumption in favour of the sharing of information. There can be little doubt that this has created a greater culture of openness in the public sector, and certainly a greater awareness in the population of the way in which the public sector operates, and how decisions have been made. This has not always been comfortable, and it is arguable that some of the loss of confidence referred to earlier may have been fed

by the exposure to public scrutiny that the Freedom of Information Act has brought. At the same time, it has engendered greater levels of openness than had previously been the case. The expectation in the NHS, for example, is now that people involved in incidents will follow a 'being open' policy in which details, including those of errors, are shared with relatives of those involved – something that was not routinely part of the culture 10 or 15 years ago. Trust board papers are now routinely published on the internet, with meetings held in public, and both local and national media making use of the Act to inform their reporting.

It is likely that both of these changes will continue to have some significant influence over the coming decades, with greater demands for both information-sharing and, from some patients, greater control over the information that is held about them. At the same time, the demand for access to information is likely to increase and, along with it, the need for organizations to be able to demonstrate open, engaging and accountable decision-making processes.

 ## 8.8   Democratic legitimacy

It has long been a criticism of the NHS that it suffers from a 'democratic deficit' – i.e. that there are no elected representatives in decision-making (or any other) positions (other than ministers). A criticism that can often be made of local NHS decision-making is that it has been driven by a central mandate from Whitehall and that it takes little if any account of the local population's needs or wants for their local NHS services. At the same time, there has, arguably, been something of a decline in the vitality of the democratic process in the UK as a whole. Membership of political parties has declined, and turnout for elections has dropped somewhat (34 per cent in the last European elections and 65 per cent in the last general election). While the idea of a halcyon past when everyone voted at every election is false, this does represent a decline. Given that the core of legitimacy for government in this country is democratic election, the level of voter participation is of great importance. Various proposals have therefore been made to try and increase voter participation in elections and local government generally. These include proposals on party political funding; e-petitions triggering debates in Parliament or councils; neighbourhood forums led by local councillors; compulsory voting and many others. These issues are currently being considered by a commission, charged to propose ways of reinvigorating the democratic process.

For the health service, this is more than an interesting set of observations. Part of the current proposals for change is a greater role for elected council members in NHS decision-making. A general sense of disengagement with local institutions is also, in a more general sense, damaging to the NHS – as stated above, a question that NHS leaders often have to answer is why a change is right for a local area, and how local people have been involved in the decision-making process. As yet, relatively few NHS commissioners have involved the local population (or their elected representatives) in the process of decision-making about the allocation of scarce health resources, let alone in an Oregon-style debate about prioritization in health care, but the need to do so is likely to become more apparent with the challenges posed by current UK fiscal policy. The response to issues of the 'democratic deficit' is likely, then, to be important in shaping the way in which the NHS (and other public sector organizations) engage with their local population.

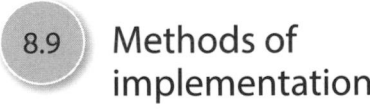

8.9   Methods of implementation

One of the greatest challenges for any government is how to implement social policies effectively. In the last 15 years, much of the approach has been characterized by a target-driven culture. In this culture, targets have been centrally set to determine whether or not policies are being implemented. These have then been centrally reported (usually quarterly) and organizations have been rated (sometimes in league tables) as to whether or not the targets have been met.

In some areas, this approach has been hugely successful. For example, when a target of a 12-hour wait was introduced for accident & emergency (A&E) departments, it was met with considerable scepticism about its achievability. Given the right political priority, however, the target gradually moved to a 4-hour target, and has largely been achieved. The same could be said for targets in mental health services about reducing rates of suicide, which have fostered numerous examples of innovative and effective working across agencies. Indeed, there is evidence that without targets and measurement, improvement is very difficult to achieve. Unless people know the goal they are trying to achieve and how they are performing, it is difficult to know what more needs to be done, or to know when success has been achieved. This is routinely the message reported from service improvement projects. The current Productive Wards and Productive Communities team programme, for example, achieves much of its successes from involving clinical teams and patients in setting goals, measuring achievement and monitoring attainment of targets.

However, the national experience of targets has not been entirely positive. To some extent, this is because many services have experienced target overload and because targets set centrally may often not appear locally or clinically relevant. It is often these two factors that have been behind complaints of too much bureaucracy in the NHS and other public sector bodies.

Another approach has been to follow a more local line, and try and allow local freedom within a national framework. Indeed, the current government has given this approach a statutory framework with its Localism Bill. In health policy, this same government is leaning more in this direction with a requirement to achieve certain outcomes, but less prescription and measurement of the means employed to do so. The dilemma with this approach, however, can be that either policy direction is ignored, or that this very difference in approach leads to accusations of a 'postcode lottery' in service provision, precisely because different approaches have been employed in different areas. For this reason, most administrations steer a path between some national targets (or outcomes), some local decision-making (whether local government, local clinicians or some combination of the two) and, increasingly, some reliance on patients themselves to determine the shape of their care through policies such as personalization.

Competition between providers is also used as a mechanism to drive the implementation of social policy – whether in the health service or other areas of the public sector. This is used, in theory at least, as a way of stimulating the market to deliver both improvements in quality and cost effectiveness. Within local government, there has been a requirement to tender services for a number of years, and in the field of social housing most provision is through housing associations or other independent providers. Within health care too, the market has been opened up to competition – a trend that seems likely to continue. NHS providers, for example, are now required to become NHS foundation trusts (autonomous providers) and are likely to be required to compete with the private sector both on price and quality. In support of this process, a mechanism called Payment by Results (PbR) has been introduced in the acute sector, and will be introduced in adult mental health services in shadow form from April 2012. In community and inpatient services, there are currently private sector providers providing NHS care, and the use of the market seems set to continue as a mechanism for introducing change. Mental health services will not be immune from this, and it is likely that over the next five years many services will be tendered on the market in the search for improvements in quality and cost effectiveness as well, of course, as the effective implementation of government policy (which is usually a condition of any tender). It is worth noting, however, that this is one area where there are substantial differences between the approach in England and the

approach in both Wales and Scotland. In these devolved administrations, a more centralist approach has continued with less emphasis on the market and more on politically-run health care provision. This is often done through health boards, which both commission and provide services.

UK fiscal policy

UK fiscal policy in the second decade of the twenty-first century is likely to have a huge impact on mental health care and the public sector as a whole. The challenging financial environment created by the economic turmoil in 2008–10 will remain for many years to come, and the UK as a whole is very likely to have only limited funds available for any growth in public sector spending. Even if such funds are available, it is by no means certain that they will be spent on a health care system that has, relatively, already been protected from the worst of public sector cutbacks. Even this relative protection means projected savings required from NHS budgets of up to £20 billion just to meet the projections for the increased costs of health care for an ageing population allied to advances in technology. The practical implications of this are likely to be felt both in the salaries and pensions of health care staff, but also in some difficult decisions about the range of health care provision available. Certainly, there is likely to be a continuation of trends towards more care in the community and in primary care, and, at the same time, towards fewer, larger acute centres that can achieve both economies of scale and quality improvements from reducing variability in the application of clinical protocols. At the same time, competition will almost certainly be used to try and drive down the costs to the taxpayer.

A similar process is likely to take place across the public sector as a whole, as central government attempts to reduce spending to an affordable level. The impact of this on the range of policies outlined earlier is hard to quantify, but already there are signs, for example, of moves to water-down equalities legislation in the name of enhancing the competitiveness of small business. At the very least, what will be inevitable is either that these policies are delivered very much cheaper than at present, or to a smaller, more targeted population.

8.10   Conclusion

This chapter has reviewed key areas of UK social policy. The key points of learning are:

- Ensuring public confidence in health services remains a challenge.

- Stigma affects the work of mental health services at a number of levels.

- Population change drives changes in social policy and service provision.

- Welfare reform is a challenge to all political parties and governments.

- Public safety remains an important factor in mental health policy.

- Freedom of information is changing the way public bodies operate.

- The NHS arguably has a democratic deficit which needs to be corrected.

Feedback to Thinking Space 8.1

1. In the UK the most well known voluntary agencies in the mental health field include: Rethink Mental Illness, MIND and the Mental Health Foundation. However, searching Google will have revealed a large number of voluntary organizations at local and community level which are sources of advice and support for people with mental illness and/or their families. No organizational chart could do justice to the complexities of relationships between these many organizations or their diverse sources of funding.

2. From your search of their websites you will see that voluntary agencies play an important function and adopt a variety of roles, which may include:

   - Initiation of pioneering services because of voluntary services' ability to respond more quickly to need than statutory services.

   - Working in partnership with statutory services, so ensuring diversity of service provision.

   - Reaching out to groups with specialist mental health needs (e.g. people with drug or alcohol problems, mentally ill people within closed cultural groups), who may be wary of engaging with statutory services.

   - Ensuring diversity of service provision.

   - Providing a channel and opportunities for people to undertake voluntary work, so fostering social exchange rather than commercial exchange as the basis of human society.

   - Supplementing the work of statutory services through attracting additional resources to mental health care.

   - Offering a critique of statutory provision, and so acting as pressure groups for improved services.

   - Providing information for service users and the public, so combating the social stigma of mental illness.

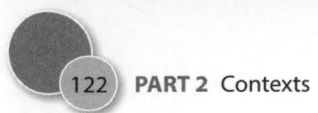

- The way in which social policy is implemented can have a major effect on services and patients.
- UK fiscal policy is likely to most define the social policy context for mental health services.

Annotated bibliography

Shepherd, Boardman and Slade (2008) Making Recovery a Reality.
This is one of the best guides available on the recovery model and movement. It gives an overview of the field and efforts at implementation.

References

Barnados (2008) *Breaking the Cycle.*
DH (Department of Health) (2006)
DH (Department of Health) (2011)
Michael, J. (2008) *Health Care for All: Report of the independent inquiry into access for healthcare for people with learning disabilities.*
NHS Information Centre (2011) annual Mental Health Act data (2011), available at: www.ic.nhs.uk.
Patel, K. and Heginbotham, C. (2007) Institutional racism in psychiatry, *Psychiatric Bulletin*, 31: 397–8.
PESA (2011)
Thornicroft, G. (2006) *Shunned: Discrimination against people with mental illness.* Oxford: Oxford University Press.
WHO (World Health Organization) (2002) *Reducing Stigma and Discrimination Against People With Mental Disorders: A technical consensus statement.* Geneva: WHO.

Chapter 9

The Service Context and Organization of Mental Health Care

Paul Calaminus

9.1 Introduction

This chapter provides an overview of the service context and organization of mental health care. It covers:

- The aims of mental health services.
- The context and systems within which they operate.
- The typical components of mental health services.

Throughout the chapter, the term 'mental health services' is used. As will be described in more detail, this term includes services operated by the National Health Service (NHS), local authorities, private sector providers of health and social care, the voluntary sector and service users themselves.

9.2 Aims of mental health services

Mental health services have a number of aims, all of which affect the ways that they are organized. These include:

- multi-disciplinary treatment of mental health disorders;
- health promotion;
- enhancing the opportunities for recovery for people with chronic conditions;
- addressing the needs of the carers and family members of service users;
- working in a way that is culturally appropriate;
- risk management;
- working within the law;

- ensuring that the physical health needs of mental health service users are met;
- working effectively across service boundaries.

Each of these is considered in turn to demonstrate the effect they have on the way in which mental health care is delivered.

Multi-disciplinary treatment of mental disorders

Effective mental health services deliver evidence-based treatment provided by appropriately trained clinical staff in a way which is compliant and consistent with the best available evidence. Increasingly, this means that the team will be compliant with the standards required by the National Institute for Health and Clinical Excellence (NICE) which sets out both guidelines (for the treatment of conditions) and technical appraisals (for the delivery of specific interventions). They will also provide effective assessment services through staff with well developed assessment skills. Depending on the condition being treated this assessment (as well as the treatment referred to above) may well need to be provided on a multi-disciplinary basis with different members of a clinical team contributing particular skills. This is one reason why most mental health services are provided through multi-disciplinary teams (MDTs). These are seen as the most effective mechanism to ensure that the right range of skills is present in any team to treat the conditions in question. Frequently, this includes more than trained clinical professionals. Many teams include social care staff who bring a range of skills in the assessment of social care needs, and unqualified support workers, whose life experience can, for example, be an important tool in a team's options for engaging with service users.

By focusing on effective assessment and treatment, teams place increasing emphasis on the collection of clinical outcome data. This emphasis on outcomes is an increasing feature of government policy, as across both health and social care funders and commissioners seek to ensure that they are indeed purchasing effective interventions on behalf of clients.

It is, of course, the case that assessing and treating mental health disorders is not a straightforward process – hence the need for a range of skills (and professions) within a team. However, a further reason behind the use of the MDT is to ensure that the range of professional viewpoints about the nature and treatment of mental health problems is adequately represented. The team approach is one way of preventing one professional view or another predominating how patients are assessed and treated. Thus, as well as a range of appropriate skills, MDTs should contain clinicians from those professions that might bring a particular viewpoint to the treatment of any particular disorder. Therefore, in a team focusing on the treatment of early onset psychosis, one might expect psychiatric, psychological, nursing, social work and occupational therapy input as a minimum – each profession bringing its own perspective to the assessment and treatment of each patient as well as each individual in their own right being able to contribute their own skills and experience to the work of the team.

A key requirement of working in a team is that all members need to have an awareness of the treatment plans for all patients seen by the team. As a result, many teams will operate, for example, assessment meetings where the whole team will review the findings of assessment and make decisions about subsequent treatment plans. While this may sometimes seem time-consuming, such communication is essential if all the relevant perspectives in the team are to be brought to bear.

Thinking Space 9.1

What types of multi-disciplinary mental health teams can you identify in your locality and what are their main functions?

Mental health promotion

Mental health services are not, however, just about the assessment and treatment of defined mental health disorders. Services should also aim to provide an element of mental health promotion (see Chapter 4). Traditionally, this has not been seen as the focus of mainstream service delivery, but has an increased profile since the publication of the most recent government strategy for mental health – *No Health Without Mental Health* (DH 2010). This has been reinforced by current government plans to measure and improve the 'happiness' of the population of the UK. Health promotion can include the provision of information and/or training for partner agencies, family members and service users in mental health conditions, how to cope with them and what the protective factors might be. Health promotion also includes a public health perspective by focusing on general mental well-being and assessments at the population level.

Recovery

The concept of 'recovery' for mental health service users is increasingly becoming an expected part of the aims which mental health services are expected to achieve (see Chapter 5). Recovery is not the same concept as effective treatment. Rather, recovery focuses on the achievement of service user-defined goals – not necessarily clinical ones. Increasingly, the expectation on mental health services is that the aim will be not only to provide effective treatment to meet defined needs, but that the services will support service users in achieving their own self-defined goals. Not only is this a significant philosophical change in the way that the aims of mental health services are defined, it also has an impact on the way in which services have to be organized in order to be effective.

The most immediate of these changes is that clinical teams and the organizations they represent increasingly need to find mechanisms that involve service users as co-creators of their care. As a result, it is increasingly common to find clinical services that incorporate service user views into changes in the design and delivery of services. Service user involvement has been formalized under the Expert Patient Programme, which aims to train and support service users to take part in service planning and work with professionals to improve service delivery. It has been successfully implemented across most disease groups in the NHS. The Programme enables service users to provide information to other service users; to act as peer advocates for others using the service and as peer facilitators in the delivery of clinical services; or to be the providers of alternative models of care. These influences are beginning to change the traditional make-up of the clinical teams described earlier in this chapter – with the development of new roles and ways of working that address the requirements of a recovery approach.

Carers and families

The importance of working effectively with carers and families is also increasingly recognized. In some ways, this has been addressed by training members of clinical teams in carrying out carers' assessments and care planning as well as by changes in clinical practice to ensure better recognition of the role of both the family and carers. However, the effective involvement of carers and family members in care planning remains an area of comparative weakness in service delivery. It remains, for example, relatively common that inquiries into failures of mental health services find that either carers or relatives attempted to give important clinical information to the clinical team, but that the information either was not effectively passed into team meetings or was not adequately considered. The aim of a service should be to involve carers in the planning of the care of the service user and that the role of the service user as a family member should be recognized in the work of the clinical team. Thus, many organizations have adapted Care Programme Approach (CPA) policies and procedures to reflect the importance of these groups in care planning.

Thinking Space 9.2

From your professional experience (or otherwise from Google) list the key characteristics of the Care Programme Approach, sometimes referred to as the CPA.

Feedback

The CPA has been part of mental health services in the UK since 1991. It is the statutory framework intended to facilitate joint working across teams and agencies, given that no one team or service can meet the needs of mental health service users with complex needs. Service-level agreements between agencies that commonly work together are an effective way of establishing agreed protocols for joint working, and should include both statutory and voluntary sectors (e.g. primary care, community and inpatient mental health services, voluntary sector housing providers and social services).

If the CPA is working well, mental health professionals will work in partnership with the service user to: assess their needs; jointly draw up a plan to meet them; share responsibility with the service user and their family, carers and other supporters to put the plan into action; and review the plan with the service user and their supporters to see if it is meeting their needs and agree any changes (DH 2008).

Cultural sensitivity

Services need to be culturally sensitive. This means that they must be accessible for and culturally sensitive to the range of users within the local population. Both of these elements are equally important. It is often, for example, the case that some population groups do not access services. This may be because of issues within secondary mental health services, or due to issues with referral patterns. Either way, it is generally recognized as the responsibility of mental health services to design ways in which such discrepancies in access can be addressed. Thus, for example, there may be specific services aimed at outreach to particular age groups (e.g. to older adults who might benefit from cognitive behavioural therapy – CBT), people of certain sexualities, black and minority ethnic (BME) groups (e.g. outreach services aimed at African-Caribbean males) or genders (such as working-age men who may not otherwise access services).

Cultural sensitivity does not just mean improving access to services. It also means providing services that are in tune with the cultural background of the service users being treated. This means being aware of how concepts such as mental health, mental illness, family, caring and social care are perceived within particular communities. Where there are particular issues with the provision of services, it is sometimes necessary to provide specific services for particular groups. However, even if such services are provided, it is still necessary to ensure that staff within clinical teams are trained in culturally appropriate work for their local communities. It is also often both necessary and desirable to ensure that the local community is represented within the workforce of the team.

Risk management

An important part of mental health practice and organization is the effective management of risk. The MDT is considered the most effective mechanism through which to assess and manage risk in mental health services. This is because the range of skills, experience and professional input required to analyse and formulate risk effectively is similar to the range required to provide effective treatment and intervention.

Teams (of whatever type and with whatever care group) will typically use a number of mechanisms to manage risk. The most obvious of these is a risk assessment and management plan. This is often supported by a team method for managing the most risky situations at any point in time. In inpatient units this may include mechanisms such as 'zoning' where a 'red', 'amber' and 'green' categorization is used for the team to structure the management of risk across the unit. Similarly, community teams often structure the working day so that early morning and late afternoon risk meetings are held to ensure that the whole team are aware of particular areas of concern and the planned response to them. Teams also put mechanisms in place to hold team caseloads rather than individual caseloads, so that all members of the team are aware of clients' needs and how they might be met.

Organizations that provide mental health services often put particular emphasis on risk management policies and protocols and their monitoring. These often supplement the CPA – itself introduced as a response to a homicide by a mental health patient, as a means of providing effective coordination of multi-disciplinary care for complex patients. There are requirements placed on teams to ensure that risk assessments are up to date and accurate, and that risk training has been undertaken.

Effective risk management is another reason why there are often limits placed on caseload sizes. It is recognized that there is a limit to the amount of work that any team or individual clinician can undertake safely and effectively. It is also one reason why such importance is placed on ensuring that the electronic patient record is completed in an accurate and timely fashion. This is thought to improve the chances of the effective communication of important information about risk and plans for its management.

Risk management is also an important part of supervision within clinical teams. Typically, supervision will include the discussion of risk management and safeguarding issues and will aim to check that risks have been identified and considered. This is, in cases involving safeguarding for example, usually enhanced by the provision of specific safeguarding leads within the team and the organization as a whole.

It is often the case that there are high levels of risk aversion within teams and organizations providing mental health care. This is, in large part, because both the public and government expectation of mental health services is that they maintain public safety. Thus, significant risk events (such as homicides or suicides) will be followed by not only internal but also external independent inquiries. Whatever the motivations of these (and it is usually to try and learn lessons to prevent the risk event happening again), the existence of this expectation and investigation processes does push organizations and teams towards defensive practice and gives risk management at least as high a profile within mental health care organizations as the provision of effective treatment.

There are also specific teams that are predominantly concerned with risk management – both in inpatient and community services. These forensic services provide treatment and care for people who have been detained under a criminal section of the Mental Health Act. These teams will have specific training in risk assessment and management and also typically provide specific risk management advice to clinical colleagues working in other teams.

Working within the law

Mental health services have to operate within the law and abide by specific legislation (see Chapter 10). In many ways this is self-evident, but it also has a significant impact on the operation and organization of teams and services. Teams have to operate within the Health Act and associated government requirements (e.g. to achieve waiting time targets and to provide care free at the point of delivery). Teams must comply also with registration requirements of the Care Quality Commission (CQC). These are a set of standards that cover the organization and delivery of care across all aspects of health care in England. The standards include the qualifications of staff and the requirement for adequate staffing levels within clinical teams, as well as the effective involvement of service users in their treatment and care. These are legal requirements that all teams have to meet in order to maintain registration and the consequent authorization to provide care at all. Health and safety law also impacts on the organization and delivery of care. In particular it impacts on the levels of training that members of clinical teams should receive (in control and restraint for example) as well as the risk assessment of the environments in which teams operate.

Mental health care is also provided within the context of the Mental Health Act. This sets out a number of specific responsibilities for organizations and practitioners. Thus there are requirements for approved mental health practitioners (AMHPs) (often social workers) and approved clinicians (ACs) (often psychiatrists) to detain people under the Act. There are also requirements on responsible clinicians (RCs) (often psychiatrists) as well as nurses and social workers for the ongoing care of people who are, or who have been, detained under the Act. This, inevitably, means that teams need to include people who are authorized as AMHPs, APs and RCs (see Chapter 11).

Physical health care

Mental health services also need to be aware of the physical health care needs of their service users and to provide a service that enables the mental health needs of those receiving general hospital care to be met. This involves close working and liaison both with general practitioners (GPs) and local acute hospitals, as well as the provision of the right skills and training within the clinical team. In some areas, specialist mental health teams are provided within general hospitals, including accident & emergency (A&E) departments. This is also an important area in the health promotion work of clinical teams. For example, there has been a far smaller reduction in rates of smoking among those with long-term mental health problems than among the general population.

Effective partnership working

Finally, effective mental health services also work across organizational boundaries. Particularly important are the relationships with social services and primary health care. In general, social services staff have

been integrated into clinical teams in adult mental health services (although not everywhere, and not to the same extent in services for children and older adults). Working with primary health care often requires specific input from secondary mental health services. It is particularly important in relation to this work that information is communicated well between the two and that some form of personal relationship is developed between the primary and secondary health care teams. This often takes the form of link workers undertaking regular liaison visits to GP practices to discuss patient care between the team and the practice. Similarly in some areas there are specific primary care mental health teams that aim to bridge this gap, as well as specific arrangements to facilitate communication between GPs and consultant psychiatrists. Arrangements such as these are essential if a working relationship is to be developed. Without a relationship of this sort, it is easy for primary health care and secondary mental health care to feel isolated from each other – to the ultimate detriment of patient care, given that in many cases care will either be shared or passed between them. Effective clinical communication is also essential, and often sub-optimal. It is for this reason that many secondary care organizations insist on regular audit checks of the quality, accuracy and timeliness of communication from secondary to primary care.

 ## 9.3 The context for service delivery

The aims of mental health services are delivered within the context of local health and social care systems, as well as government policy and local population needs. Each of these has an influence on service provision.

National influences

There are a number of organizational principles that are essentially national in character. The first of these is that services are provided in the following care groups:

- children and adolescents;
- adults of working age;
- older adults;
- adults with a learning disability;
- adults with forensic needs;
- adults with behavioural disorders;
- services for people with substance misuse issues.

This categorization runs throughout the NHS (in policy development, commissioning and provision). It is neither a list of conditions nor ages – more a mix of the two. Most of the categories also have sub-categories that are similarly a mix of age groupings and condition-specific groupings.

Perhaps inevitably, on the boundary between each of these groupings, it is not so unusual to find clinical teams disagreeing about approaches to care and there has been much effort to ensure that effective 'transition' takes place from one care group to another. This has included specific transition teams between child and adolescent and adult services, for example. However, it is probably true to say that there remain real differences in approach between care groups and that attention has to be paid to ensure that service users do not suffer fragmentation in their care at points of transition from one care group to another.

Geographical influences

Most services are planned and provided on a geographical basis – often coterminous with local authority (either borough or county council) boundaries. This is similar to most general health community services and means that services are often provided to the funders responsible for that geography. Within organizations, it is common to find all services within a care group in a particular geography grouped together into a service delivery unit such as a directorate. In this way, services in a similar area have the opportunity to develop a shared culture and response to the requirements of working effectively with the local population in that area.

National mental health service strategy ever since the closure of the Victorian asylums has been to prioritize the effective care of service users within the community. This frequently means investment in community services, with an accompanying reduction in inpatient bed capacity, based on the reduction of levels of admissions to inpatient care. The drive behind this strategic direction remains a conviction that inpatient care is best avoided. It can be a distressing and disempowering experience even when provided with high levels of care and skill through a service model based around 'recovery' and empowerment for service users.

Local needs and systems

The NHS in England is organized to try and provide locally sensitive services, consistent with government policy. In practice this means that local clinical commissioning groups take responsibility for the purchasing of health care on behalf of the population of a defined area.

These clinical commissioning groups are made up of GPs, along with some clinicians from secondary care services, and have control of the commissioning budgets for their geographical area. Within the funding available, they are expected to purchase appropriate services from providers that meet the local needs of their population. Usually, they work with local government to achieve this via local health and wellbeing boards.

Clinical commissioning groups are supported to commission health care on behalf of the local population by both the local public health department and specialist commissioners. Local public health departments work across the NHS and local authorities, and have as their remit to improve the health of the population. Every year, the local director of public health provides a detailed report on the health of the local population, making recommendations for areas where improvements are needed and commissioning attention should be directed. Specific analyses (needs assessments) are also carried out at other times as necessary. These often lead to the development of a strategy for service improvement and change. The process of developing such a strategy should be highly inclusive, with opportunities for the involvement of service users, carers, clinicians, local politicians, the general public and any other important local stakeholders. The more inclusive the process is, the more likely it is to lead to successful changes to service delivery and to ensure that services are shaped to meet local need. Such strategies in mental health care have helped to define how many of what types of service should be provided, as well as to set the local aims and objectives for services. Many services that aim to improve cultural sensitivity, for example, have been developed through the process of local needs assessment and the development of services to meet identified need.

Specialist commissioners support the clinicians on clinical commissioning groups to achieve the goals they have set for local health care delivery. They negotiate contracts with health care providers for the delivery of care to the local population, and monitor the delivery of services. Their role is to achieve good value for money for the public (i.e. the best possible service at the lowest possible costs). In practice, commissioners often have the role of demanding that health care providers achieve high standards of care, and higher levels of activity with only modest (if any) increases in funding. Every year, for example, the NHS imposes a 'cost improvement programme' on all health care providers. This means that every year providers are required to reduce costs and provide the same levels of service. Health care providers therefore find themselves in a constant process of trying to reduce costs and, as a result, making constant changes to the way in which services are organized.

Commissioners also use contracts to shape the operation of teams through the application of sanctions and incentives. At present, any provider who is being commissioned by the NHS can be fined up to 10 per cent of the value of the contract (in most cases, several million pounds) if a number of key targets are not met, and given additional funding up to 1.5 per cent of the value of the contract (still over a million pounds in most cases) if other targets are

met. Targets that are sanctioned or incentivized in such a way include:

- whether the home treatment team has seen enough patients;
- whether sufficient levels of clinical outcome scores have been achieved;
- whether key data about patients have been recorded;
- whether or not permission has been sought from commissioners before providing some specialist services;
- whether or not enough patients have been seen by local psychological therapy services;
- whether or not any 'never events' have taken place (nationally defined events that are considered entirely avoidable);
- achievement of national waiting time targets;
- improving transition between different care groups;
- improving patient experience;
- improving the interface between primary and secondary care;
- improving the physical health of mental health service patients.

This approach can have the effect of improving quality. Equally, clinical teams can find themselves required to focus on data collection to prove the achievement of goals as much as on the delivery of care to their patients. Of course, the intention of those negotiating such contracts is usually that they should support providers to work effectively and in the best interests of their patients. However, it is a frequent complaint from clinical teams across the NHS that targets can distort their work – not least because many targets rely on the accurate completion of data systems and have a consequent administrative burden. The requirement however looks likely to remain.

Indeed, current government policy is to move all mental health services onto a contract system called Payment by Results (PbR). In this system, all service users will be allocated to a 'cluster' for which an amount of money will be paid. This amount of money will be based on the average cost of treating a patient in this cluster (weighted for factors such as the cost of living in a given area). This, in turn, will be worked out by agreeing in advance the likely treatment package for patients in that cluster. Treatment packages include not only the types of intervention that will be provided, but also how long (either in time or number of sessions) it is assumed that the intervention will be provided. The aim will be to measure the clinical presentation at the beginning of care in the 'cluster' and to measure in the same way after the treatment package. The tool being used to measure this is based on the Health of the Nation Outcome Scales (HoNOS) – a rating that measures medical, personal, social, risk and employment factors to try and give a holistic picture of a person's presentation to mental health services. The aim, ultimately, is that commissioners should pay a certain amount of money for a certain type of patient to achieve a certain improvement in their mental health status. Whether this system will be effective or not is not yet known. However, its adoption is likely to have implications for the way in which teams and practitioners operate and will require tighter definition (where possible) of the interventions that are being provided; tighter monitoring of the way in which they are being provided; and tighter monitoring of the timescales within which they are being provided. 'Clusters' are also unlikely to be synonymous with teams and team caseloads. This is likely to mean that in order to achieve the improvement in mental health status that is being sought, different teams will need to work together along more formally defined care pathways than is currently the case. For example, the clusters for psychosis include the contribution of a range of different types of team, both in the community and in hospital. In order to establish the packages of care, and the costs that go into each cluster, organizations providing mental health care will have to understand in much greater detail the way in which teams interact together and what the drivers of cost-effective care really are. This will mean teams working

together to define care packages and how they can help each other work in the most cost-effective way possible. To support this, a number of organizations are considering organizing services by care group (e.g. psychosis or affective disorders) rather than by geographical area.

Commissioners' influence on services is, of course, wider than simply contracting. They also have a role coordinating the production of local strategic frameworks, and are responsible for making population-wide decisions about what share of resources is allocated to which client group. The impact of these decisions cannot be underestimated. For most clinical commissioning groups, decisions about 0.5 per cent of the total budget being allocated to one type of health care or another can amount to several million pounds difference in funding levels. Clearly, then, the decision about what percentage of a clinical commissioning group budget should be spent on mental health and what on other areas of health care is a fundamental one and one which significantly shapes the type of service that can be provided in any given area.

Finally, local commissioners will be strongly influenced in their commissioning decisions by central government policy, particularly when this is accompanied by additional grant funding to support its implementation. Even when it is not, commissioners will be strongly influenced by this, not least because they and their organizations will often be judged by the extent to which their commissioning decisions have been implemented in local areas. This judgement can be in the form of formal inspections (as in safeguarding inspections carried out by the CQC for example) but also through the ratings of commissioning groups that are carried out by the Department of Health (DH). There are strong organizational imperatives to achieve good results in such performance ratings, and, so, the pressure to implement government policies will be transmitted from commissioning groups to providers and, thence, into individual clinical teams. This, again, may have a direct impact on operational matters within these teams.

Local authorities

Local authorities are a key part of the local system that impacts on the organization of mental health services. They are the providers and commissioners of social care services in mental health. The services provided by social services usually include AMHP services under the Mental Health Act and general social care services (such as home care, respite care and general social support), accessed through a standard set of thresholds known as Fair Access to Care Services (FACS). If the thresholds for these services are not set in conjunction with NHS thresholds for eligibility for secondary care, there can be significant disconnect between these two different parts of the mental health care system.

One solution to the problem of health and social care not working effectively together has been to integrate health and social care staff within adult mental health teams. In these arrangements, health and social care staff work together as part of the same team, and with a single management structure. This is generally thought to have improved the ability of services to offer a holistic package of care. However, since 2010, there have been challenges to this arrangement, with some local authorities pulling out of such integrated arrangements, often stating that social care staff have become too involved in working to a medical model of care and addressing the preoccupations of the NHS, and not sufficiently addressing the social care agenda within their local authority areas. When coupled with current budget pressures, it may be that less integrated models of care will return. Indeed, in mental health services for older adults and children, formal integration into single teams has been less universal than in services for adults. Rather, in these care groups, the model has been to integrate planning and commissioning of services. In this model, planning for service design and the interaction between different teams across health and social care has been done together, with commissioning responsibility in both the local authority and NHS being shared by a single person or department. In

this way, provision has been integrated and, where appropriate, teams have been developed to meet specific needs.

The influence and importance of local government on the provision of mental health care goes further, however, than simply the commissioning and provision of services. Local authorities continue to have a role in scrutinizing any proposed changes to health services, including mental health services. This function is exercised through a formal scrutiny committee of the council. Made up of councillors, the role of this committee is to scrutinize any proposed changes, to give views on any such changes, to recommend amendments and monitor the impact of service alterations. If a scrutiny committee does not approve of a proposed change it then has the power to refer it to the Secretary of State for review. This is a powerful local process and means of enhancing democratic input to NHS decision-making processes. There are numerous service changes that have been altered as a result of scrutiny committee deliberations, as well as changes that have been stopped – often those relating to proposed closures or the establishment of unpopular local services. Finally, local government plays an important part in the overall context for the provision of services because it is an essential means of engagement with the local population. Councillors, as elected local officials, are an important way of seeking local opinion and input into the operation of teams within their local area, as well as any proposed changes. Thus, for example, local councillors will be visited by their constituents at local constituency surgeries (as will local MPs) and they will therefore have a good perspective on the way in which services are operating and what might be done to improve them. Sometimes, they will raise queries on behalf of these constituents (known as 'members' enquiries') that can both be a useful means of improving care in individual cases, as well as a means of identifying areas where improvements in care delivery need to be made. Most councils also operate 'locality councils' through which the local population and voluntary sector can have an input into local service provision and design. These are important forums for mental health services to use to engage effectively with the local population.

9.4 The organization of care

So far, this chapter has concentrated on the aims of services and how they affect the organization of services, as well as the national and local context and systems in which services operate. This section describes the most common types of service and team for different care groups: adults, older adults, children and adolescents. It also provides feedback to Thinking space 9.1 about clinical teams earlier in this chapter.

Adults

In this care group, the basic element of service delivery is the community mental health team (CMHT). This MDT typically has a core of medical, nursing, social work, occupational therapy and psychology staff. It usually provides services to a defined geographical area, linked with a number of GP practices. Such community teams generally provide secondary mental health care to clients referred by GPs, although they may take self-referrals too. They will typically provide care to anyone with a serious mental health problem. In many areas, the practical operation of the CMHT is supported by medical outpatient clinics. These often act as a means of continued monitoring of and engagement with clients whose mental health is otherwise stable. In some areas, the concept of the CMHT has also been developed to include a primary care mental health team, where care is shared with GPs and a wider range of interventions into primary care is provided than would normally be the case.

Within community services, there should also be a CMHT focused on assertive outreach. The typical make-up will be similar to that of a generic CMHT but the focus of the team will be on outreaching to service users who services otherwise struggle to engage. Part of the remit of the team will

therefore typically be working extended hours, and the team will usually have a smaller than normal caseload size to enable intensive work. Clients who may be assertively outreached include those who have not engaged with generic CMHTs, those who are street homeless and those with particularly chaotic lifestyles.

Early intervention CMHTs are also provided in most areas. These have a typical range of professionals as core members, but with a particular interest and expertise in early intervention psychosis. The aim of these teams is to provide an intensive, time-limited input to those with a first onset psychosis and to enable people and their families and carers to best understand their condition and how to manage it. Such teams will often include the capacity to liaise specifically with GP practices to try and identify those who may be at risk of developing a first onset psychosis. These teams were originally established as a reaction to the long lengths of time between the onset of psychosis and the onset of treatment (known as the duration of untreated psychosis – DUP). An important aim of these services, therefore, is the shortening of this length of time.

Community forensic services are also provided in most areas through a specific forensic CMHT. This team is made up of forensic trained nursing, psychology, occupational therapy, social work and psychiatric staff. The team will work with forensic clients released from secure care (who may well be on some form of restriction order), as well as, on occasion, particularly clients of the local CMHT who are considered to present a risk. Typically this team will provide a particular expertise and focus on risk management.

The next essential element of community mental health services is the locality home treatment team – sometimes known as the crisis resolution team. The core of this team is often medical, nursing and social work staff, with input from psychology staff. The remit of these teams is to offer a community (home) based alternative to hospital admission. They screen all patients who are assessed as needing admission to hospital and see who can be diverted into community-based treatment. They should also be in constant liaison with inpatient wards to identify patients who could be discharged into intensive community care. These teams typically work extended (or 24) hours, 365 days a year.

In support of community services are the inpatient services. In every area, there will be inpatient acute psychiatric wards for those aged over 18 – some provided on general hospital sites, others on stand-alone psychiatric sites. These wards will typically be staffed by predominantly nursing, occupational therapy, psychology and medical staff, often with input from social work staff. Wards should be open 24 hours a day, 365 days a year and will generally accept patients for admission only after a psychiatric assessment, and following screening by the home treatment team. Patients can either be admitted with their consent or without their consent, under a section of the Mental Health Act.

These acute wards are, in turn, supported by psychiatric intensive care units (PICUs). These provide very intensive nursing, medical and psychological interventions to the most acutely disturbed patients. Such wards typically have higher nurse–patient ratios and are often smaller than normal wards. As well as patients detained under civil sections of the Mental Health Act, they may also have patients who have been transferred from prison for assessment under a forensic section of the Act. Like acute wards, PICUs will be operational 24 hours a day, 365 days a year, and will take their referrals almost exclusively from other inpatient environments.

With an even higher level of nurse–patient ratios, and a full MDT, medium secure units provide inpatient care in prison-standard levels of security for those who are detained under criminal sections of the Mental Health Act. These units are often provided on a regional basis, and tend to have many more male beds than female beds, due to the difference in the number of men and women in the prison population, as well as the difference in the number of men and women referred to secure care. The length of stay in such units is typically at least 18 months and, depending on the offence committed, can be much longer. In many cases, discharge and/

or transfer from such units is subject to agreement from the Ministry of Justice. When stepping down from medium secure care, patients are often discharged to low secure care. This is a form of inpatient care that aims to continue the process of inpatient rehabilitation in an environment with slightly lower levels of security than medium. Thus, staffing ratios will be slightly lower than in medium secure units, and the staff mix will be geared more explicitly towards rehabilitation.

Of those service users admitted to general acute wards, those with more chronic conditions may be transferred into inpatient rehabilitation services. These are staffed 24 hours a day, 365 days a year, with a focus on the rehabilitation of services users. Of these services, a particular type is known as a challenging behaviour unit. This will provide inpatient treatment and behavioural interventions for people whose behaviour has been particularly challenging to services. Typically, these inpatient services have lengths of stay of at least 18 months.

In all areas there should also be a range of supported housing available. This is often divided into high support, medium support and low support housing. It is provided to service users who need some support (whether sleeping-in or visiting during the day) to live in the community. These facilities are often provided by housing associations in partnership with clinical service providers.

A range of community-based psychological therapy services will also, typically, be provided. In many areas, these are now known as IAPT services, after the Improving Access to Psychological Therapies initiative. These services are generally provided using a tiered model of service delivery, in which low-intensity (generically trained) workers provide the first line response to presentations of anxiety disorders, while high intensity (clinically trained) workers provide the second line response and the first line response to cases of depression. Typically, such services are provided in general practice and other community settings by single practitioners, the majority of whom will be clinical psychologists. Generally, such services receive referrals from general practice, and also encourage self-referrals. Similarly, in most areas there will be specific services providing psychody-namic psychotherapies – often through a mix of psychotherapists with and without previous clinical training. These services will usually offer both group and individual interventions, and this may, in some areas, include the provision of intensive day treat-ment or therapeutic communities for service users with particular personality disorders. Typically, such services will receive referrals from both primary care and other secondary care services.

Services for eating disorders are usually pro-vided on a regional basis. They will normally include inpatient, day care and community outpa-tient services. Core staffing on these units will usu-ally include nursing (general and mental health), psychiatric, general medical, psychological and social work input. They will generally provide a comprehensive service for clients with an eating disorder, including the capacity to admit to inpa-tient care under a section of the Mental Health Act if required.

Similarly, inpatient services for mothers and babies are provided on a regional basis. These ser-vices provide care for new mothers, often where there are particular safeguarding concerns, and they often have particular expertise in the treat-ment of puerperal psychosis.

A&E liaison services are provided in A&E depart-ments, usually on a 24-hour basis. They provide assessment of all those who attend the department where there appears to be a mental health need. In some cases these services also provide a wider liai-son service for general inpatient wards within the hospital.

Older adults

Services for older adults often have the same structure – based around age-specific CMHTs and acute inpatient beds. In most cases, the core staff-ing will be similar, although the professionals in question will have had specific training in working with older adults. In addition, services now increas-ingly reflect the requirements of the current National Dementia Strategy, with the provision of memory services. These MDTs aim to provide early assessment of memory problems and the timely provision of information and any appropriate treatment.

In addition, older adults services will either provide (or provide in-reach into) continuing care services, as well as in-reach into nursing and, in some cases, residential homes. Some of this con-tinuing care may be provided on an inpatient basis by services themselves (often through intensive nursing care) but it is more usually provided through the in-reach of an MDT (predominantly nursing and medical) into nursing and residential care homes.

Children and adolescents

Services for children and adolescents are generally provided through a tiered model with single (clini-cally trained) practitioners outreaching into com-munity settings such as children's centres, schools and GP practices in Tier 2. In Tier 3, CMHTs provide multi-disciplinary services for children, adolescents and, often, specific services for those children with neurodevelopmental disorders. Some of these ser-vices are provided in partnership with community paediatrics, and the core staffing within the CMHTs is often nursing, psychiatric and psychological ther-apists. In Tier 4, specialist outpatient services are provided as well as acute inpatient services for both children and adolescents. Often, these are provided on a regional basis.

Learning disability services, too, are based around the provision of CMHT services with sup-port from acute inpatient units – staffed by clini-cians with a particular training in working with indi-viduals with learning disabilities. The suitability of general inpatient and community mental health services for clients with a learning disability is assessed through a set of standards known as the Green Light Tool Kit. This was developed as a means of enabling service providers to self-assess the extent to which they provided services that took the needs of patients with learning disabilities into account.

The same can also be said of substance misuse services, where, in effect, a tiered model of service operates – although with a focus as much on the prevention of offending resulting from addiction as on the effective clinical treatment of addictions.

9.5   Conclusion

This chapter has considered the aims of mental health services, and how they affect the way in which mental health care is organized. The context in which services operate has also been described as has the basic organizational structure of mental health care delivery. At the heart of this structure is the MDT, which continues to be considered the means by which community and inpatient services are best delivered. In summary, the main learning points from this chapter are:

- MDTs form the basis of effective mental health care.
- 'Recovery' is increasingly the philosophical framework within which providers operate.
- Services are required to operate within the framework of national policy and the law.
- All providers of services also operate as an integral part of local systems and geographies.
- There are a range of types of services, typically aimed at different age groups and types of patient.

Annotated bibliography

The *Oxford Textbook of Community Mental Health* gives a more detailed overview of themes and provision in community mental health care.

'Components of a modern mental health service' (Thornicroft – BJPsych, 2004, 185.)
This article summarizes available evidence on models of care and their efficacy.

References

DH (Department of Health) (2008) *Making the CPA Work for You*. London: DH.
DH (Department of Health) (2010) *No Health Without Mental Health*. London: DH.

Chapter 10

Mental Health and the Law

Toby Williamson and Simon Lawton-Smith

 ## 10.1 Introduction

Mental ill health and learning disability nursing probably involve more complex legal issues than any other branch of nursing. The vast majority of mentally disordered people consent to their treatment and decisions about their health care, and pose no threat to their own safety or the safety of other people. However, a minority of people with mental disorders cannot or will not accept they are ill and may need treatment because of the risk they pose to themselves or others if left untreated – or do accept they're ill but don't like/want the treatment. Some people are so affected by a mental disorder or impairment that they lack the capacity to make basic decisions about their own care, to consent to treatment or complain when they are victims of abuse. This particularly applies to many people with learning disabilities and those with dementia. It is vital that mental health nurses work both ethically and legally, and understand how ethics and the law apply when working with someone in these situations (see Chapter 11).

This chapter explains the law covering the care and treatment of people with mental disorders (including personality disorders) and decision-making for people with mental illness, learning disability and dementia.

In UK legal terms mental disorder is given special status. This is reflected in the arrangements which exist to detain and treat mentally disordered patients without consent, both under specific mental health legislation and under mental capacity legislation. Although there are no radical differences, different legislative regimes operate within the UK. The Mental Health Act (MHA) 1983 applies to England and Wales, which have traditionally shared mental health legislation. The Mental Capacity Act (MCA) 2005 also applies only to England and Wales although it covers a wider group of people, namely people with an impairment or disturbance of the mind or brain (which includes people with a mental disorder). Northern Ireland has its own separate Mental Health Order (made in 1986, and largely replicating the provisions of the MHA 1983) but no mental capacity legislation at the time of writing (though it plans to introduce a new law in the near future). Scotland has its own Mental Health (Care and Treatment) (Scotland) Act 2003 and an Adults with Incapacity (Scotland) Act 2000. All of these have their own accompanying codes of practice. Wales has recently passed its own Mental Health Measure, creating duties around accessing and providing care and treatment within primary and secondary mental health services (Welsh Assembly Government 2010). Anyone undertaking mental health nursing in Wales should be aware of this legislation, but it does not affect the MHA 1983, other than extending the independent mental health advocate (IMHA) arrangements to patients detained under Section 4 (emergency admission), and Sections 5(2) and 5(4) (doctors' and nurses' powers to detain informal inpatients for a limited time). The MHA 1983 remains the underpinning piece of legislation in Wales concerning the compulsory admission and treatment of people with mental disorders.

In summary this chapter considers English and Welsh legislation around mental disorders and mental capacity with which nurses need to be familiar. It covers:

- the Mental Health Act 1983;
- the Mental Capacity Act 2005;
- related legislation including the Human Rights Act 1998 and the Equality Act 2010;
- children and young people in relation to the Mental Health and Mental Capacity Acts;
- nurses' duty of care and the common law of negligence.

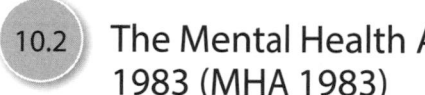

10.2 The Mental Health Act 1983 (MHA 1983)

The MHA is long and complex, and this chapter only deals with those aspects of it that relate most directly to nurses' responsibilities under the Act.

The purpose of the MHA 1983

The purpose of the MHA 1983 is to allow for the detention and compulsory treatment of patients suffering from mental disorder of a sufficiently serious nature or degree to warrant treatment in the interests of their own health or safety or for the protection of others. The Act covers both hospital detention and treatment and treatment in the community under supervised community treatment (SCT).

The Act is the main source of statutory powers and duties for mental health nurses in England and Wales. Among these, they may detain patients who are seeking to leave hospital using the nurse's holding power, or they may use reasonable force to administer treatment.

Over time the original MHA 1983 has been amended, most recently by the MHA 2007, which introduced a broader definition of mental disorder, created new roles for professionals and established new powers of SCT. The 2007 Act also introduced into the MCA 2005 new procedures to authorize deprivation of liberty of mentally incapacitated people. However the MHA 1983 (as amended) remains the fundamental Act of mental health legislation in England and Wales.

Nurses' potential roles under the MHA 1983

Over and above their usual professional nursing duties, nurses are eligible to seek qualification to perform the statutory functions of approved mental health professionals (AMHPs) under the Act. Appropriately qualified nurses are also eligible to become approved clinicians (ACs), and an AC is eligible to become a responsible clinician (RC).

Approved mental health professional (AMHP)

The 2007 amendments to the Act allow for professionals other than social workers, including nurses, to take on the role of AMHP in fulfilling various powers under the Act. This role supersedes the previous role of approved social worker (ASW), although in practice the great majority of AMHPs remain social workers. A first-level nurse whose field of practice is mental health or learning disability may seek to become an AMHP.

The AMHP has a central role, including making an application for detention under the 'civil' (Part 2) procedures of the MHA, either for assessment or for treatment. Similarly, a patient cannot be discharged from hospital under SCT without the approval of an AMHP. The competencies of the AMHP are set out in regulations (the Mental Health (Approved Mental

Health Professionals) (Approval) (England) regulations 2008), and include application of values, skills (working in partnership) and knowledge (both in mental disorder and including the legal and policy framework).

Approved clinician (AC)

Nurses are also eligible to seek approval as ACs. In addition to professional qualification, candidates for approval have to demonstrate competencies in identifying the presence and severity of mental disorder and determining whether the disorder is of a kind or degree warranting compulsory confinement. They will also have to have completed the necessary AC training. The responsibilities of an AC are considerable and it is likely that only experienced senior clinicians will be able to meet the competencies required.

Responsible clinician (RC)

The RC is the AC with overall responsibility for the patient's case. Only an AC may become a RC. The RC has significant powers such as the power to renew detention of a patient detained under Section 3 for treatment and the power to initiate SCT.

Criteria for using the MHA 1983

To be subject to compulsory powers of detention in hospital, the criteria are that:

- the person is suffering from mental disorder of a nature or degree which warrants the detention of the person in hospital for assessment (or for assessment followed by medical treatment for at least a limited period); and
- the person ought to be detained in the interests of their own health or safety or with a view to the protection of other persons.

'Mental disorder' is widely defined in the Act as 'any disorder or disability of the mind' and so is an umbrella term covering mental illness, personality disorder, autistic spectrum disorder and learning disability. It is up to relevant professionals to determine in each case if the individual has such a disorder.

Dependence on alcohol or drugs is not considered to be a disorder or disability of the mind, although of course a person may have a mental disorder which coexists and has an interrelationship with a dependence on alcohol or drugs.

Informal patients

It should be noted that some 60 per cent of patients admitted annually to psychiatric facilities are 'informal' patients – in other words, they are not subject to the MHA 1983. Informal admission is appropriate for patients who consent to admission. In theory informal patients are entitled to leave hospital at any time, but they may be prevented from doing so if staff decide that they need to remain in hospital and invoke the holding power under the MHA 1983, Section 5 (see below).

Powers to admit and treat, and nurses' holding powers

Admission under the MHA 1983 for assessment and treatment generally takes place via the 'civil' (Part 2) sections of the Act, sections 2–5. In 2009/10 some 37,000 people were subject to these powers in England, as described below.

However, people (some 5,000 in 2009/10 in England) may also be detained in hospital under 'criminal' (Part 3) sections that allow mentally disordered offenders to be transferred from courts or prisons to hospital. This is dealt with on pages 298–307 of the *Code of Practice* (DH 2008a) and there is a useful summary of these sections in *The Maze: A Practical Guide to the Mental Health Act 1983* (South London and Maudsley NHS Foundation Trust 2010: 170–85).

Section 2: admission for assessment

A person suffering from mental disorder may be detained under the 1983 Act for assessment for up to 28 days on the application of the patient's nearest relative or an AMHP, supported by two medical recommendations, one of which must be from a doctor approved under Section 12 of the 1983 Act as having special expertise in the diagnosis or treatment of mental disorder. A mentally disordered person does not have to be behaving dangerously to self or others to be compulsorily admitted. They could be detained because it is necessary for their own health, including mental health.

Section 3: admission for treatment

Section 3 provides for compulsory admission for treatment for up to 6 months, renewable for a further 6 months and thereafter at 12-monthly intervals. An application may be made by either the nearest relative or an AMHP and must be supported by medical recommendations given by two medical practitioners. Treatment for mental disorder includes nursing and also psychological intervention and specialist mental health habilitation, rehabilitation and care.

A patient who is detained under Section 3 has the right to apply to a tribunal review for discharge once within the first six months following admission, and once in each period for which the detention is renewed.

Section 4: emergency assessment

There is an emergency procedure under Section 4 of the MHA 1983 for admission for assessment where only one medical recommendation is necessary. The conditions for admission for assessment under Section 2 must be met, and detention may continue for a maximum of 72 hours unless a second medical recommendation is furnished within that time to convert the emergency admission into a full 28-day admission for assessment. Until the second medical recommendation is furnished, the patient may not be given treatment for mental disorder without consent unless he or she lacks capacity to consent and the treatment is immediately necessary in his or her best interests.

Section 5: holding powers

An informal patient who consents to admission but later seeks to leave hospital may be restrained from doing so using the nurse's holding power as set out in Section 5(4). This is a power that may be used by nurses quite often. It enables a registered mental health or learning disability nurse to hold an inpa-tient in a psychiatric ward or hospital for not more than six hours. During that time the doctor or AC in charge of the patient's treatment or his or her deputy should attend to determine whether the managers should be furnished with a report.

The MHA *Code of Practice* (para. 12.25) emphasizes that 'The decision to invoke the power is the personal decision of the nurse who cannot be instructed to exercise this power by anyone else'. The nurse's holding power can only be used where the patient is receiving treatment for mental disorder as an inpatient. The grounds for its use are:

- that the patient is suffering from mental disorder to such a degree that it is necessary for his or her health or safety or for the protection of others that he or she be immediately restrained from leaving hospital; and

- that it is not practicable to secure the immediate attendance of a practitioner (or clinician) for the purpose of furnishing a report.

The MHA *Code* (para. 12.28) sets out a number of factors that should be taken into account, including:

- the patient's expressed intentions;

- the likelihood of the patient harming themselves or others;

- the likelihood of the patient behaving violently;

- any evidence of disordered thinking; and

- any other relevant information from other members of the multi-disciplinary team.

The nurse must record in writing on a statutory form the fact that the statutory criteria are satisfied, and must deliver the completed form to the managers or their appointed officer as soon as possible, but the six-hour detention starts to run from the time when the nurse signed the form. The reasons for invoking the power must be entered in the patient's notes. It is worth emphasizing that this power can be used only where an informal patient is receiving treatment as an inpatient for mental disorder; it cannot, for example, be used on a general hospital ward where the patient is receiving treatment for a physical disorder. A nurse invoking the power is entitled to use the minimum force necessary to prevent the patient from leaving hospital.

The nurse's holding power may only be used to restrain the patient from leaving hospital. The common law allows for reasonable force to be used in self-defence, for the defence of others, or to prevent a breach of the peace. These powers apply regardless of whether the person has capacity. They can only be used to justify detention or restraint within the hospital in so far as it is reasonably necessary. Hence, they would not authorize any restraint or seclusion to continue after the risk had passed. Detaining patients under Section 5 does not confer any powers to treat them without their consent.

Nurses' powers to treat patients without consent

Treatment for mental disorder is defined very widely in the MHA 1983, Section 145(1) providing that 'medical treatment' includes nursing alongside psychological intervention and specialist mental health habilitation, rehabilitation and care. The list in Section 145 is non-exhaustive and treatment for mental disorder also includes such interventions as electro-convulsive therapy (ECT) and the administration of drugs.

Part IV of the MHA 1983 (Consent to Treatment, covered by Sections 56–64) regulates the treatment of people detained in hospital, including those on Section 17 leave, those absent without leave (AWOL) and SCT patients who have been recalled to hospital. Part 4A deals with the treatment of SCT patients in the community.

The administration of medicine

The Care Quality Commission (CQC) in England has issued guidance for nurses on the administration of medication to patients who are detained in hospital under the MHA, and to patients who are subject to SCT in the community and at the point of recall to hospital and revocation of SCT (CQC 2009). This guidance should be read in full by mental health nurses, as the paragraphs below only offer a summary.

Section 63 treatment for mental disorder (first three months)

Section 63 gives the authority to give treatment for mental disorder for the first three months (though see exceptions below), so long as the patient:

- consents to it; or
- does not consent, but the treatment is given by or under the direction of the AC in charge of the treatment. (Nurses should bear in mind that the patient's consent should still be sought wherever practicable.)

The exceptions are where Sections 57 (neurosurgery), 58 (medication after three months) or 58A (ECT) apply. These are treatments subject to special rules, dealt with in Chapter 24 of the *Code*.

Treatment is broadly defined (*Code* para. 23.3) as 'treatment which is for the purpose of alleviating or preventing a worsening of a mental disorder or one or more of its manifestations'. It includes treatment of physical health problems resulting from the mental disorder (e.g. treating wounds self-inflicted as a result of a mental disorder), but cannot otherwise be used to treat a patient's physical health problems.

Section 58 treatment for mental disorder (after three months)

Section 58 also authorizes treatment (medicines for mental disorder) without consent but *only* applies 'once three months have passed from the day on which any form of medication was first administered to the patient during the patient's current period of detention under the Act ('the three month period')' (*Code* para. 24.10).

Medication under Section 58 may be given to patients who are liable to be detained under powers authorizing detention for more than 72 hours, and who are not conditionally discharged restricted patients, or remand patients subject to Section 35. It may *not* be given to some patients (see the list of exceptions at para 23.8 of the *Code*), including patients detained under the nurse's holding powers.

Section 58 treatments require either:

- the patient's consent; or
- a certificate from a second opinion appointed doctor (SOAD) stating that the patient is either (a) incapable of consenting, or (b) capable and refusing, but that the treatment ought to be given.

The SOAD may decide that the patient is capable and consents. In deciding whether drug treatment ought to be given without consent, the SOAD must be satisfied that 'it is appropriate for the treatment to be given'. Before making the decision the SOAD must consult two other people who have been professionally concerned with the patient's medical treatment. One of these must be a nurse, and the other neither a nurse nor a doctor, but someone with knowledge of the patient and the patient's treatment, such as the patient's care coordinator. Neither may be the RC for the patient.

It is the responsibility of the nurse administering the prescribed medication to patients detained under the 1983 Act to ensure that he or she is legally entitled to administer the medication. A copy of the form T2, on which the patient's consent is certified and a description of the treatment is given, or the form T3, on which the SOAD certifies that the treatment outlined on the form should be given, should be kept with the medicine card. The nurse administering the treatment should:

- check the medicine card for date of entry of prescription for the medicine, its dose and route of administration;
- ensure that the route of administration is authorized and that the total dose of the medication is within the limits authorized on the form;
- ensure that where the patient has consented to medication beyond the three-month period, the form T2 is in place and correctly

completed (note that the patient can withdraw their consent at any time);

- ensure that where a second opinion has been obtained the form T3 is in place and correctly completed;
- ensure that the administration of medicine is consistent with Nursing and Midwifery Council (NMC) professional guidance.

Section 62 urgent (emergency) treatment

Section 62 is intended to allow urgent treatment to be given if an SOAD certificate cannot be arranged sufficiently speedily to cope with an emergency (such as to save the patient's life, prevent a serious deterioration in his or her condition, alleviate serious suffering or is the minimum interference necessary to prevent the patient from behaving violently or being a danger to themselves or others), while at the same time protecting patients against hazardous or irreversible treatments. Urgent treatment under these sections can continue only for as long as it remains immediately necessary. If it is no longer immediately necessary, the normal requirements for certificates apply.

Independent mental health advocates (IMHAs)

The MHA 2007 introduced the role of the IMHA. Nurses need to be aware that they may meet IMHAs in the course of their work, and the IMHA's role, which is to help and support patients to understand and exercise their legal rights. IMHAs must be made available to certain 'qualifying patients', namely those:

- detained or liable to be detained under the 1983 Act;
- subject to guardianship under the Act;
- community patients subject to a community treatment order (CTO);
- conditionally discharged;
- being considered for Section 57 or 58A treatments but not otherwise subject to the Act (i.e. an 'informal' patient).

Qualifying patients should be informed that they are eligible for IMHA support as soon as is practicable. An IMHA will meet with a patient on the request of the patient, the nearest relative, the responsible clinician or an AMHP. Where a patient has the capacity to consent and does so, an IMHA may see any hospital or local authority records relating to them. If a patient lacks the capacity to consent, access to such records may still be allowed if it is appropriate and relevant to the help the advocate will provide to the patient. IMHAs have a right to meet patients in private and to visit and interview anyone professionally concerned with the patient's medical treatment, including nurses.

Supervised community treatment (SCT)

A patient who is subject to SCT on discharge from hospital (i.e. is placed under a Community Treatment Order (CTO)) is known as a 'community patient'. The primary purpose of SCT is to ensure that a community patient continues to take his or her medication once they have left hospital, to lessen the risk of relapse and a return to hospital. To be eligible for SCT the patient must be liable to be detained in hospital under Section 3 or, if a Part 3 mentally disordered offender patient, be subject to a hospital order, a hospital direction or a transfer direction *without restrictions*.

To be placed under SCT, the RC must be of the opinion that:

- the patient is suffering from mental disorder (any disorder or disability of mind) of a nature or degree which makes it appropriate for him or her to receive medical treatment;
- it is necessary for his or her health or safety or for the protection of other persons that he or she should receive such treatment;
- subject to his or her being liable to be recalled, such treatment can be provided without his or her continuing to be detained in a hospital;
- it is necessary that the RC should be able to exercise the power to recall the patient to hospital;

- appropriate medical treatment is available for him or her.

It is also necessary for an AMHP to agree that the patient meets the criteria and that SCT is appropriate.

The care plan that every community patient must have should take into account the views of nurses who have been responsible for their care in hospital as well as the multi-disciplinary team that will be responsible for their care in the community, which is likely to involve a nursing member. It is possible for that nurse to be the patient's care coordinator while the patient is under SCT.

In passing, Section 117 of the MHA sets out a duty on health and local authorities to provide aftercare to certain detained patients after they leave hospital (some of whom may also be under SCT). The Section 117 aftercare plan should also take into account the views of nurses involved in caring for the patient in hospital and relevant community mental health nurses.

Treatment of community patients

Part 4A of the Act regulates treatment for community patients. The basic principle is that a patient with capacity may only be given treatment in the form of medicine for mental disorder if they consent and if, beyond the first month of treatment, there is a certificate authorizing the treatment from a SOAD. Accordingly, within one month of being placed on a CTO, a patient should be visited by a SOAD who authorizes the treatment and also specifies what treatment may be given if the patient is recalled to hospital. The requirement of authorization by a SOAD is called 'the certificate requirement'.

Treatment may only be given without consent by recalling the patient to hospital, either as an inpatient or outpatient (see *Code* para. 25.47 *et seq.*).

The *Code of Practice* to the MHA 1983 (England)

We mention at various points above and below the MHA 1983 *Code of Practice* for England (DH 2008a).

The Welsh Assembly Government issued its own *Code of Practice* for Wales in 2008 (Welsh Assembly Government 2008) which should be referred to by nurses practising in Wales.

The English *Code* provides guidance to nurses, doctors, ACs, managers and other staff of hospitals, and AMPHs, on how they should undertake their duties under the MHA 1983, as well as on 'aspects of medical treatment for mental disorder more generally'. Chapter 1 sets out a list of guiding principles that should be considered when making decisions about a course of action under the Act, and nurses should be guided at all times by these principles.

Nurses should be familiar with the whole *Code* but especially with Chapter 23 which details when medical treatment may be given under the Act. This is a central part of nurses' responsibilities in respect of patients detained and treated under the Act, and must be clearly understood and followed. Although the *Code* does not have the same statutory standing as the Act, if a nurse does not follow the *Code* they must be able to give convincing reasons why not.

Treatment plans

The *Code* emphasizes that it is essential for patients being treated under the Act to have a written treatment plan. This should be recorded in their notes, which should form part of a coherent care plan under the Care Programme Approach (CPA), and should be formulated by the multi-disciplinary team in consultation where practicable with the patient. It must include a description of the immediate and long-term goals for the patient and a clear indication of the treatments proposed and the methods of treatment. Where patients cannot (or do not wish to) participate in discussion about their treatment plan, any views they have expressed previously should be taken into consideration.

10.3   The Mental Capacity Act 2005 (MCA 2005)

The MCA 2005 came into force in 2007 (it was passed by Parliament in 2005 but there was a two-year

preparation period before it started). It applies to England and Wales (Scotland has its own legislation, the Adults with Incapacity (Scotland) Act 2000). The MCA replaces previous legal arrangements for dealing with people who lack capacity.

The MCA applies to people aged 16 or over (with some exceptions). It provides a legal framework to empower and protect people who may lack capacity to make some decisions for themselves because of an 'impairment of, or disturbance in, the functioning of the mind or brain'. It therefore applies to people with dementia, learning disabilities, mental health problems, alcohol or substance misuse problems (as well as people with brain injuries and people who are unconscious) who may lack capacity to make certain decisions. This includes people who are unable to make decisions because of the effect of treatment they are receiving. It also provides ways in which people with capacity can plan ahead for a time when they may lack capacity to make decisions.

The MCA makes it clear who can take decisions in which situations and how they should go about this. It covers major decisions about someone's health care treatment, property and affairs, social care and where the person lives, as well as everyday decisions about personal care (such as what someone eats).

The MCA applies to anyone who is caring for someone who may lack capacity, including families and friends, health and social care staff and professionals (whether they are working in the statutory or non-statutory sectors), and others (e.g. police, ambulance staff, solicitors, etc.). However, the degree of involvement and responsibility may vary depending upon the situation and relevant sections of the MCA.

Principles of the MCA

The MCA is underpinned by five key principles set out in Section 1 of the Act:

■ a presumption of capacity – every adult has the right to make his or her own decisions and must be assumed to have capacity to do so unless it is proved otherwise;

- individuals being supported to make their own decisions – a person must be given all practicable help before anyone treats them as not being able to make their own decisions;

- unwise decisions – just because an individual makes what might be seen as an unwise decision, they should not be treated as lacking capacity to make that decision;

- best interests – any decision or action done under the MCA for or on behalf of a person who lacks capacity must be done in their best interests; and

- less restrictive option – anything done for or on behalf of a person who lacks capacity should involve considering options that are less restrictive of their basic rights and freedoms providing they are still in the person's best interests.

The first three principles of the MCA emphasize the importance of people making decisions for themselves. It should never be assumed that just because someone has a mental illness diagnosis or learning disability, for example, they are unable to make a decision. People may need support in making decisions by providing information in a way that is easy to understand, or because of particular communication needs, and this should be provided to help them make the decision for themselves. Again, someone may have a mental illness diagnosis or dementia, for example, and be making a decision that appears to others as being unwise, eccentric or possibly even dangerous but this does not automatically mean they lack capacity. However, a disability or illness that is known to affect mental capacity, together with a decision that seems unwise may be a reason for assessing their capacity to make the decision.

Decisions not covered by the MCA

Certain decisions are not covered by the MCA, even if they involve a person who lacks capacity. These are:

- consent to having sexual relations;
- consent to marriage or civil partnership;

- consent to divorce or dissolution of a civil partnership;
- consent to a child being placed for adoption or to making an adoption order;
- voting;
- decisions concerning the person's compulsory care or treatment authorized under the MHA.

No one can give or refuse consent, or make a decision on behalf of someone who lacks capacity on these issues – this is because they are covered by other laws. However, it is possible that a professional may be asked for their opinion about someone's capacity to make a decision if a situation has arisen involving one of these matters. It also does not prevent action being taken to protect someone from abuse or exploitation.

The MCA and the MHA

If the following conditions apply to an individual who lacks capacity the MHA should be used, *not* the MCA:

- the person meets the criteria for compulsory detention or treatment provided under the MHA;
- the treatment cannot be given under the MCA (e.g. because the person has made a valid and applicable advance decision to refuse the treatment – see section below on 'advance decisions');
- they lack capacity to consent to the detention or treatment and they are showing signs of resisting the detention or treatment (but remember that the MHA does not have a capacity test and can also be used for people who have capacity);
- they may need restraining in a way that is not allowed under the MCA.

If someone is being detained or treated under the MHA, the MCA still applies to *any* mental capacity issue not covered by the MHA — for example, decisions covering personal welfare issues or the person's physical health care needs (unless the physical health problem has been caused by the mental disorder that is being treated under the MHA, e.g. the effects of an eating disorder).

The MCA deals with the assessment of a person's capacity, decisions and actions that could be carried out by any health or social care practitioner including unqualified staff (e.g. nursing assistants, care home staff, etc.), as well as families and friends caring for someone who lacks capacity.

Assessing mental capacity

The MCA sets out a single clear test for assessing whether a person has capacity to take a particular decision at a particular time. It is a 'decision-specific' and 'time specific' test. This means that each decision has to be dealt with separately and no one can be labelled 'incapable' simply as a result of a particular medical condition or diagnosis. Section 2 of the Act makes it clear that a lack of capacity cannot be established merely by reference to a person's age, appearance, or any condition or aspect of a person's behaviour (e.g. simply because they lack 'insight' into their illness, disability, care or treatment needs).

The test only applies to a person who has a mental impairment or disorder that affects their ability to make decisions. If a person is unable to do one or more of the following, regarding a particular decision (e.g. consent to treatment or care) they would be deemed to lack capacity:

- understand the information necessary to make the decision;
- retain the information for long enough to make the decision;
- use or weigh up the information necessary to make the decision;
- communicate their decision (this would usually only apply to someone who is unconscious or in a coma).

Best interests

Section 4 of the MCA explains how an action or decision made for or on behalf of a person who lacks capacity must be in that person's best interests. The MCA provides a checklist of factors that decision-makers must work through in deciding what is in a person's best interests. This includes trying to find out and taking into account the person's wishes and feelings, beliefs and values that are relevant to the decision. A person can put his or her wishes and feelings into a written statement if they so wish, which the person making the best interests decisions must consider. In addition, people involved in caring for the person lacking capacity (either in a paid role or as family member or friend) should be consulted concerning a person's best interests wherever it is practical to do so. A person making a best interests decision should not do it on the basis of what they would want if they were in the same situation. It must also not merely be based upon a person's age, appearance, or any condition or aspect of a person's behaviour. In certain situations an independent mental capacity advocate (IMCA) must be appointed to assist with best interests decisions (see below).

Making decisions about a person's capacity and best interests

Deciding if a person lacks capacity and making best interest decisions are based upon 'reasonable belief' (as opposed to the other legal test of 'beyond all reasonable doubt') – i.e. on the balance of probabilities it appears that the person has or lacks capacity, or that the decision and course of action is in the person's best interests. However, it is very important to be able to provide the reasons for deciding about a person's capacity or best interests. Consideration should also be given to other factors such as:

- delaying the assessment or best interests decision until a time when the person is most likely to have capacity;
- the time and place in which the assessment or best interests decision takes place to optimize the person's capacity;
- involving the person as much as possible, even in a best interests decision – they may be able to indicate preferences about aspects of the decisions even if they are unable to actually make the decision itself;

- involving others who know the person (e.g. family members);

- involving someone who has specialist skills (e.g. a psychiatrist, psychologist, interpreter, speech and language therapist, etc.) that might be necessary to assist with the assessment or best interests decision;

- anything about the person's life that is relevant to the decision involved (e.g. cultural or religious factors).

Apart from the capacity test and best interests checklist described above the MCA does not set out any other formal procedures or requirements about record-keeping to be followed when undertaking these tasks. It also does not specify who can or cannot assess capacity or make a best interests decision. Family carers, paid staff (both in the statutory and non-statutory sectors), professionals and others (including attorneys and deputies – see below), can all do a capacity assessment or make a best interests decision if they need a person who may lack capacity to make a particular decision. For simple, everyday decisions it may be easy to assess capacity or make a best interests decision. However, for more complex decisions it may be advisable to involve a professional with specialist mental capacity skills and assessing capacity or making a best interests decision for some decisions (e.g. a doctor requiring consent to treatment) can only be carried out by the professional involved.

Where paid staff and professionals are carrying out mental capacity assessments or best interests decisions a record should be kept in the person's notes but for more routine, everyday matters (e.g. decisions about daily personal care, food, etc.) record-keeping should be kept as simple as possible to avoid it becoming too time consuming.

Mental capacity assessments and best interests decisions should be a routine part of everyday nursing practice involving people who may lack capacity. Care reviews, CPA meetings, case conferences, ward rounds, multi-disciplinary team meetings, adult safeguarding meetings, etc. are all settings where mental capacity issues can be considered.

Decisions and actions in connection with care or treatment

Section 5 of the MCA offers legal protection from liability where a person makes a decision or is doing something in connection with the care or treatment of someone who lacks capacity. This could cover actions that might otherwise attract criminal prosecution or civil liability if a nurse, for example, has to carry out an invasive intervention to a person's body or their property in the course of providing care or treatment.

Restraint

However there are limits to decisions and actions in connection with a person's care or treatment which Section 6 of the Act sets out. It defines restraint as the use or threat of force where a person who lacks capacity resists, and any restriction of liberty or movement whether or not the person resists. Restraint is only permitted if the person using it reasonably believes it is necessary to prevent harm to the person who lacks capacity, and if the restraint used is a proportionate response to the likelihood and seriousness of the harm. Restraint can therefore be used under the MCA to provide care or treatment providing it meets these strict criteria.

If care or treatment needs to be provided that requires going beyond these criteria then it will almost certainly be a deprivation of liberty which Article 5 of the Human Rights Act (the right to liberty) only permits if there are particular legal safeguards. These safeguards are contained in the MHA but in some situations people may need to be deprived of their liberty to provide care that is in their best interests but they do not meet the criteria for the MHA. The safeguards in the MCA for these situations are known as the Deprivation of Liberty Safeguards.

Deprivation of Liberty Safeguards (DOLS)

In 2009 a further legal framework was added to the MCA to provide legal safeguards for people who needed to be kept in hospital, registered care homes or nursing homes to provide care in their best interests because they lacked capacity to give their consent to this. These are known as the Deprivation of Liberty Safeguards (DOLS) and came about as a result of a legal ruling by the European Court of Human Rights.

An additional *Code of Practice* for DOLS explains when and how they apply (DH 2008b). They are most relevant to the care of people with dementia or learning disabilities but may on occasions also apply to people with a mental illness. A deprivation of liberty is not defined in the MCA but could involve physical restraint, very close supervision, preventing someone from leaving, and possibly even use of medication if it is only used to sedate someone with no clinical or therapeutic benefit, where any of these actions need to go beyond the definition of restraint in Section 6 of the MCA. If staff in a care home or hospital (known as the 'managing authority') believe that someone is being deprived of their liberty an application needs to be made to a local authority (known as the 'supervisory body') to do an assessment which may result in a DOLS authorization being granted. This can be a complex process and the safeguards include representation for the person, a clear plan of care, and rights to review and appeal.

Difficulties may arise in deciding whether the MHA, Sections 5 and 6 of the MCA, or DOLS should be used for people in hospital who have a mental disorder. It is very important to remember that DOLS do not authorize actual treatment. Therefore, according to the DOLS *Code of Practice* if a person meets the criteria for the MHA (i.e. requires treatment to which they do not or cannot give their consent) then the MHA should be used rather than DOLS.

Lasting Powers of Attorney

The MCA allows a person to appoint someone such as a close family member (known as an 'attorney') to make decisions and act on their behalf should they lose capacity in the future. This involves a legal document called a Lasting Power of Attorney (LPA). An LPA can cover decisions about health and personal welfare (including decisions regarding social care) and decisions about a person's property and finan-

cial affairs, or both. Before it can be used it must be signed by someone to verify that the person had capacity when they made it and an LPA must be registered with the Office of the Public Guardian (OPG) (see below). An LPA covering property and financial affairs can be used even when a person still has capacity to make the decision specified in the document but a health and personal welfare LPA can only be used when the person lacks capacity to make the decision specified in the document.

An action or decision authorized by an LPA must be done in the person's best interests if they lack capacity. This means that an attorney who is a family member or friend could refuse consent to a decision involving health or social care even if professionals disagree. However, LPAs cannot apply to decisions covered by the MHA if the person lacks capacity and is under a section of the MHA (with the exception of decisions involving ECT and people on SCT who have not been recalled to hospital). However, LPAs can still be used to make other decisions not covered by the MHA while someone is being treated under the MHA, providing the LPA authorizes these (including ECT and people on SCT). There are additional safeguards where an LPA covers decisions involving life-sustaining treatment. LPAs replace the previous legal arrangements known as Enduring Power of Attorney (EPA) which only applied to decisions about property and financial affairs, although the EPAs created before October 2007 are still valid.

Advance decisions to refuse treatment

The MCA enables people who have capacity to make a decision in advance to refuse treatment if they should lack capacity in the future when the treatment might be provided. An advance decision to refuse treatment (ADRT) is a legally binding document that professionals must respect providing it is 'valid' (i.e. the person had capacity when they made it) and 'applicable' (i.e. it is specific to the particular situation and treatment that has arisen), even if the refusal of treatment it specifies is not considered to be in the person's best interests. An ADRT does not need to be written down except where it concerns a refusal involving life-sustaining treatment. In these situations the decision must be in writing, signed and witnessed. In addition, there must be an express statement that the decision stands 'even if life is at risk' which must also be in writing, signed and witnessed. Like LPAs, ADRTs do not apply to treatment decisions covered by the MHA if the person lacks capacity and is under a section of the MHA (with the exception of decisions involving ECT and people on SCTs who have not been recalled to hospital). However, it is still legally binding for other decisions that it specifies, not covered by the MHA, while someone is being treated under the MHA (e.g. treatment for a physical illness as well as ECT and people on SCTs).

Mental health practitioners need to be confident of the validity of an ADRT held by someone who has mental health problems, especially if it involves refusal of psychiatric treatment. It would be important to know that the person was not mentally unwell when they made the ADRT. However, one should not treat a person with an ADRT who has mental health problems in a discriminatory way and failing to adhere to the first principle of the MCA by assuming they did not have capacity when they made it.

The Court of Protection

The Court of Protection (COP) has jurisdiction relating to the whole of MCA and is particularly important in resolving complex or disputed cases – for example, whether someone lacks capacity or what is in their best interests. It deals with decisions concerning property and financial affairs, as well as health and welfare decisions. The COP has its own procedures, nominated judges and several locations in England and Wales (though it can deal with cases on paper as well as full hearings). It can make declarations, decisions and orders affecting people who lack capacity and appoint 'deputies' to make decisions on behalf of people lacking capacity. Deputies can be appointed to make decisions on health care and personal welfare issues as well as property and financial matters. However, they cannot make decisions involving care or treatment covered by the MHA although they can still make other decisions if they are authorized to do so while the person is being treated under the MHA.

The Public Guardian

The Public Guardian has several duties under the MCA and is supported in carrying these out by the OPG. The Public Guardian is the registering authority for LPAs and deputies. It supervises deputies appointed by the court and provides information to help the court make decisions. Where necessary the OPG works together with other agencies, such as the police and social services, to respond to any concerns raised about the way in which an attorney or deputy is operating.

Independent mental capacity advocate (IMCA)

An IMCA is someone instructed to support a person who lacks capacity and has no one appropriate or able to consult with about their best interests, such as family or friends (though an IMCA must not be used simply because staff disagree with the views of family or friends). An IMCA must be involved where decisions are being made about serious medical treatment (except where it is being given under the MHA) or a change in the person's accommodation involving hospital or a care home, where it is provided, or arranged, by the NHS or a local authority. An IMCA may also be involved in care reviews and cases involving abuse where the person lacking capacity is either the perpetrator or victim (even if there are family or friends who can be consulted), but these are discretionary. It is the responsibility of the decision-maker to refer a case to the local IMCA service (usually provided by a voluntary sector organization).

The IMCA finds out as much as possible about the person's wishes, feelings, beliefs and values in relation to the decision in question and brings to the attention of the decision-maker all factors that are relevant to the decision. IMCAs are entitled to see the medical records and other notes about the person lacking capacity and can challenge the decision-maker on behalf of the person lacking capacity if necessary (e.g. if they have evidence that the person has capacity to make the decision). IMCAs can provide important information to assist with a best interests decision but their role does not involve making the actual decision.

A criminal offence

The MCA includes a criminal offence of ill treatment or wilful neglect of a person who lacks capacity (irrespective of their age). A person found guilty of such an offence may be liable to imprisonment for a term of up to five years. There have already been hundreds of prosecutions involving this offence.

Research safeguards

Research involving, or in relation to, a person lacking capacity may be lawfully carried out if an 'appropriate body' (normally a research ethics committee) agrees that the research is safe, relates to the person's condition and cannot be done as effectively using people who have capacity. The best interests checklist does not apply when deciding if someone who lacks capacity should participate in a research project. The decision is based upon whether the research should produce a benefit to the person that outweighs any risk or burden, but if it is to derive new scientific knowledge it must be of minimal risk to the person and be carried out with minimal intrusion or interference with their rights.

Family carers or nominated third parties must be consulted and agree that the person would want to participate in a research project if they had capacity. If the person shows any signs of resistance or indicates in any way that they do not wish to take part, the person must be withdrawn from the research.

MCA and safeguarding in general

The MCA can link in and support other adult safeguarding policies and procedures that an NHS trust or other organization may have in place. However, the purpose of the MCA is not just about safeguarding, because the principles emphasize the right of individuals to make decisions for themselves wherever possible, the right to make unwise decisions,

and the importance of supported decision-making. The MCA should not therefore be used to justify decisions about safeguarding because of staff concerns about risk or because of disagreements with families – the principles and processes of the MCA must be applied first, before a safeguarding decision is made.

Code of Practice

There is a statutory *Code of Practice* to accompany the MCA (Department for Constitutional Affairs 2007) and an additional code for DOLS (DH 2008b). The codes provide guidance about all aspects of the MCA and DOLS to anyone working with and/or caring for adults who may lack capacity, including family members, paid staff and professionals. Anyone who has a paid role in caring for people who may lack capacity, as well as attorneys and deputies, must 'have regard' to the *Code*. This means that they should normally follow it, but if for any reason they do not follow it they must have good reasons for doing this which they are able to explain.

 ## 10.4 The Human Rights Act 1998 (HRA 1998)

The Human Rights Act (HRA) came into force in 2000 and sets out the fundamental rights and freedoms that individuals in the UK have access to. These include:

- right to life;
- freedom from torture and inhuman or degrading treatment;
- right to liberty and security;
- respect for your private and family life;
- freedom of thought, belief and religion.

As well as the HRA, nurses should also be aware of the United Nations (UN) Convention on the Rights of the Persons with Disabilities (CRPD). It covers people with mental health problems, learning disabilities and dementia and has applied in the UK since 2009. The aim of the CRPD is to ensure that the HRA is meaningful for people with disabilities and includes the freedom to make one's own choices, respect for diversity and the rights of people with disabilities to fully participate in society. It also emphasizes the rights of people with disabilities to have the same access to health, education and employment as people without disabilities.

Nursing practice should positively promote the HRA and CRPD and use of the MHA and MCA must be 'compliant' with them, meaning that they must not be used in a way that contravenes one or more of the HRA or CRPD's rights and freedoms.

However, some of these freedoms are not absolute and can be overridden in certain circumstances where necessary and proportionate, because of limited resources, and if supported by other laws. For example, detention, care and treatment under the MHA or MCA are deemed to be legal under the HRA providing the laws are applied correctly even if it means, for example, interfering in someone's private or family life. Similarly, because of limited resources, health services are not required to provide life-saving treatment in all circumstances. However, under no circumstances can anyone be subject to torture, inhuman or degrading treatment.

10.5 The Equality Act 2010

The Equality Act merges together several laws to simplify anti-discrimination legislation and covers the whole of the UK. Under the Act people are not allowed to discriminate, harass or victimize another person because they have any of what the Act calls 'protected characteristics'. Protected characteristics are:

- age;
- disability (mental and/or physical);
- gender reassignment;
- marriage and civil partnership;
- pregnancy and maternity;
- race;
- religion and belief;

- sex;
- sexual orientation.

The Act defines unlawful discrimination as less favourable treatment (in the broadest sense) because of a protected characteristic (direct discrimination) and applying rules, policies etc. that has a greater negative impact on a people who have a protected characteristic in a way that cannot be justified, (indirect discrimination). For the first time, treating someone less favourably because of something connected with a disability is unlawful (e.g. not providing information about treatment for a mental disorder to a person with a learning disability that is provided to others because the person communicates using picture boards).

The Act applies to all public sector organizations and other service providers including non-statutory sector organizations. Providing different health and social care services (as well as other services) to people simply because of their age is also banned.

The Equality Act does not override the MHA or MCA but it would apply where someone subject to the MHA or MCA is treated less favourably under either of those laws because they have a protected characteristic. For example, giving someone of Caribbean origin who is detained under the MHA more invasive treatment than a white person who is detained under the MHA who has the same presentation and behaviour without a clinical justification would almost certainly contravene the Equality Act.

The Equality & Human Rights Commission provides more information about the Equality Act, Human Rights Act and CRPD: www.equality-humanrights.com.

10.6 Children and young people under the MHA 1983 and MCA 2005

The Children Act 1989 defines a child as a person under the age of 18, and each year there are a small number of children detained under the MHA 1983 either through the civil (Part 2) or criminal (Part 3) process. The MHA broadly applies to children in the same way as it applies to adults, but there are other pieces of legislation affecting children that need to be taken into account. As the *Code of Practice* (para. 36.3) puts it, this includes 'the Children Acts 1989 and 2004, the Mental Capacity Act 2005 (MCA), Family Law Reform Act 1969, Human Rights Act 1998 and the United Nations Convention on the Rights of the Child, as well as relevant case law, common law principles and relevant codes of practice'.

Nurses should become familiar with Chapter 36 of the MHA 1983 *Code of Practice* and Chapter 12 of the MCA *Code of Practice* which cover children and young people under the age of 18. In addition, there are useful summaries produced by the South London and Maudsley NHS Foundation Trust (2010: 186–93) and the Department of Health (DH) (2009).

 ## 10.7 The nurse's duty of care and the common law of negligence

Common law is the law developed through case-by-case precedent by judges. Nurses owe a common duty of care to their patients, to avoid causing them injury by wrongful acts or omissions. The standard of care expected of a nurse is that of responsible practitioners skilled in the specialty. In order for a nurse to be liable for negligence, the patient or other person suing them must establish three basic elements:

- that the nurse owed them a duty of care;
- that the nurse breached that duty;
- that the breach of duty caused them injury.

Nurses owe a duty of care to people who they should reasonably foresee as being likely to be injured by their acts or failure to act. This means that patients and clients are owed a duty of care, as are work colleagues. So the nurse in charge owes a duty of care to a vulnerable elderly mentally ill client who lacks mental capacity and who is seeking to leave the ward late at night in freezing temperatures. Equally, a nurse who is told by a patient that he or she intends to assault another member of staff would owe a duty of care to that colleague to take reasonable steps to avoid that risk coming to pass.

The second issue in a negligence action is whether the nurse broke the duty, that is, fell short of the standard of care to be expected of a nurse. This means that expert witnesses are called to state what they would have considered to be acceptable nursing practice. In the hypothetical example of the frail elderly person with mental illness seeking to leave the ward in freezing temperatures, it would be hard to imagine any responsible body of nursing opinion coming forward to support allowing him or her to leave.

The third issue in a negligence claim is whether the claimant has suffered injury as a result of the breach of duty. This means that the claimant must establish that his or her injury resulted from the negligence of the nurse and was not attributable to some other cause. Moreover, the injury must be of a kind recognized by the law, which allows claims for recognized psychiatric illness or injury resulting from negligence, as well as for physical injury. The injury suffered must also be of a reasonably foreseeable kind. A whole vista of dire consequences would be reasonably foreseeable in the case of the frail elderly woman allowed to leave the ward late on a freezing cold night. If the woman died as a result of hypothermia, or falling into a river, the nurse could be sued for negligence. The employing hospital would be liable to meet the damages claim under the doctrine of vicarious liability whereby an employer is liable for the acts or omissions of his or her employee in the course of employment duties. In addition to suing for negligence, the relatives could ask the health service commissioner (the health ombudsman) to investigate and report, and they could complain to the NMC that the nurse was guilty of professional misconduct.

10.8 Conclusion

To conclude, the main points made in this chapter are summarized below:

- Mental health and learning disability nursing probably pose more acute legal issues than any other branch of medicine, especially around people's capacity to make decisions about their care, and when people's decisions can be overruled.

- In the UK there are different legal regimes for mental health and mental capacity issues between England, Wales, Scotland and Northern Ireland.

- In England and Wales the main source of statutory powers and duties for mental health nurses is the MHA 1983, which governs the care and treatment of people suffering from mental disorder, but consideration must also be given to the MCA 2005 and the circumstances where treatment and admission may take place under that Act.

- Nurses play a key role in caring for, and treating, patients subject to the MHA 1983, both in hospital and in the community. In particular they need to be clear about the legal basis of any treatment they give to patients without consent. Under the MHA 1983 they may also seek to take on additional responsibilities, such as that of an AMHP.

- Irrespective of whether someone is subject to the MHA nurses must adhere to the principles and procedures of the MCA when they are caring for or treating someone with a mental illness, learning disability or dementia in hospital, residential care or in the community, except for care and treatment authorized by the MHA. Wherever possible they must respect and support a person to make decisions independently but also understand how and when they can make a decision on behalf of someone who lacks mental capacity to make a decision for themselves.

- Nurses need to be clear about the legal status of patients they are responsible for who are detained in hospital or residential care, particularly as regards the differences between the MHA and DOLS.

- All those who exercise statutory functions under mental health and mental capacity legislation, including nurses, must be aware of the legal context in which they operate; that they are aware of the circumstances where other legislation (e.g. HRA, Equality Act), common law rights, statutory rights and ethical principles may be engaged, and of how to ensure that their decision-making achieves a fair balance between protecting those rights and the need to detain and treat mentally disordered people.

Annotated bibliography

Bowen, P. (2007) *The Mental Health Act 2007.* **Oxford: Oxford University Press.**
A full account of the MHA 1983 as amended by the MHA 2007 and the MCA 2005.

Fennell, P. (2007) *Mental Health: law and practice.* **Bristol: Jordans.**
A full account of the MHA 1983 as amended by the MHA 2007.

Jones, R.M. (2008) *Mental Health Act Manual,* **12th edn. London: Sweet & Maxwell.**
The MHA 1983 as amended by the 2007 Act and the accompanying rules, regulations and *Code of Practice.*

Maden, A. and Spencer-Lane, T. (2010) *Essential Mental Health Law.* **London: Hammersmith Press.**
A brief guide to the MHA 1983 as amended by the MHA 2007 and the MCA 2005.

South London and Maudsley NHS Foundation Trust (2010) *The Maze: A practical guide to the Mental Health Act 1983.*
    London: South London and Maudsley NHS Foundation Trust (amended 2007).

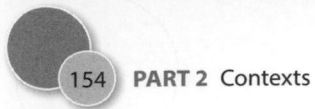

Statutes

Adults with Incapacity (Scotland) Act 2000

Children Act 1989

Equality Act 2010

Family Law Reform Act 1968

Human Rights Act 1998

Mental Capacity Act 2005

Mental Health (Care and Treatment) (Scotland) Act 2003

Mental Health Act 1983 (as amended by the Mental Health Act 2007)

The Mental Health (Approved Mental Health Professionals) (Approval) (England) Regulations 2008 SI 2008 No 1206

Mental Health (Nurses) (England) Order 2008 SI 2008 No 1207

Mental Health (Northern Ireland) Order 1986

References

Care Quality Commission (CQC) (2009) Nurses, the administration of medicine for mental disorder and the Mental Health Act 1983. London, CQC.
Department for Constitutional Affairs (now the Ministry of Justice) (2007) *Mental Capacity Act 2005 Code of Practice*, available at: www.dca.gov.uk.
DH (Department of Health) (2008a) *Mental Health Act 1983 Code of Practice*, available at: www.dh.gov.uk.
DH (Department of Health) (2008b) *Mental Capacity Act 2005: Deprivation of Liberty Safeguards Code of Practice*, available at: www.dh.gov.uk.
DH (Department of Health) (2009) *The Legal Aspects of the Care and Treatment of Children and Young People with Mental Disorder: A guide for professionals*, available at: http://its-services.org.uk/silo/files/publication-cyp-legal-guide-jan-2009.pdf.
South London and Maudsley NHS Foundation Trust (2010) *The Maze: A practical guide to the Mental Health Act 1983*. London: South London and Maudsley NHS Foundation Trust (amended 2007).
Welsh Assembly Government (2008) *Mental Health Act 1983: Code of Practice for Wales*, available at: www.wales.nhs.uk/sites3/Documents/816/Mental%20Health%20Act%201983%20Code%20of%20Practice%20for%20Wales.pdf.
Welsh Assembly Government (2010) *Mental Health (Wales) Measure 2010*, available at: www.legislation.gov.uk/mwa/2010/7/contents/enacted?view=plain.

Acknowledgements

The authors would like to thank Paul Gantley OBE, Ian Hulatt and Dr Tony Zigmond for their helpful comments on earlier drafts of this chapter.

Chapter 11

The Ethics of Mental Health Nursing

Ann Gallagher

 ## 11.1 Introduction

An older person on a dementia unit asks a nurse if he can go home. The nurse says, 'No, you can't go home today Frank. It's Sunday and there are no buses.' Stephanie is a young woman with an eating disorder who is on continuous observation. She asks the nurse if she can have some privacy to use the toilet. The nurse says she has to observe Stephanie at all times. These are just two of the many examples of practices that introduce challenging ethical issues. Did the nurse do the right thing in each of these situations? What should he or she have done? And why? These questions get to the crux of mental health ethics. In the course of this chapter readers will have the opportunity to engage with ethical questions relating to mental health practice. The chapter covers:

- distinctions in ethics – normative and empirical ethics;
- ethical principles and virtues;
- dignity in care – implications for mental health practice;

- application of a deliberative framework to practice examples.

 ## 11.2 Ethics: normative and empirical

When asked to suggest a definition of ethics, respondents often cite words such as 'right', 'wrong', 'good' and 'bad'. This is a good beginning as ethics can be said to relate to right conduct and good character. It relates to what we ought to do and how we ought to be and live. Ethics is not an optional extra but rather a fundamental part of everyday mental health practice – what nurses do and omit to do and how they are, in terms of the moral dispositions they enact, are fundamental elements of ethical practice.

There are different branches of ethics. In addition to an increasing range of normative or theoretical perspectives offering guidance on the 'oughts' of practice, there is a growing body of work in empirical ethics (Widdershoven *et al.* 2008). Normative ethics, also referred to as theoretical, prescriptive or philosophical ethics, requires an understanding of ethical theories, principles, virtues and values and their application to practice situations. Empirical ethics relates to what people do, think and believe regarding ethical issues and involves research relating to, for example, service users' views of dignity in care; nurses' experience of moral distress; the moral or ethical climate of organizations; or staff views on lying in dementia care.

There is a wide range of theoretical possibilities for considering normative ethics in relation to mental health nursing practice. These include: the four principles approach (Beauchamp and Childress 2009); virtue ethics (Banks and Gallagher 2009), ethics of care (ter Meulen 2011), narrative ethics, relational ethics and hermeneutic ethics (Ashcroft *et al.* 2005). Traditional frameworks of ethics derived from moral philosophy include: deontology or duty-based ethics (questions for the nurse include 'What are my duties or obligations?'); utilitarianism or consequence-based ethics (questions include 'What is going to bring about the most good or happiness for the most people?'); and rights-based theory ('What are the service user's rights, and what are my rights?').

The focus of discussion in this chapter is on the four principles approach, virtues-based ethics and the concept of dignity (contextualized within a human rights perspective). Reference is made to other ethical frameworks (e.g. the Nuffield Council on Bioethics work on ethics and dementia) and a deliberative framework will be introduced and applied to four practice situations.

11.3 Mental health nursing: ethical principles and virtues for practice

It has been said that ethics is concerned with what people do and don't do (their conduct) and also with moral dispositions or virtues (their character). Such a view of ethics, I suggest, requires an understanding of ethical principles and also of virtues. One of the most common ethical perspectives on

health care ethics is the 'four principles approach'. The four principles are:

1. Respect for autonomy.
2. Non-maleficence.
3. Beneficence.
4. Justice.

Respect for autonomy

The word 'autonomy' comes from two Greek words *autos* and *nomos* meaning self-rule or self-government. This then relates to mental health service users' rights to make decisions for and about themselves. Autonomy is a key principle underpinning UK health policy. The policy document *Equity and Excellence: Liberating the NHS* (DH 2010), for example, refers to 'no decision about me without me'. In considering the principle of autonomy it needs to be asked, first, if the person is autonomous. There are different views of autonomy and some of these require a high level of cognitive functioning. Beauchamp and Childress (2009) focus on 'normal choosers who act: intentionality; with understanding; and without controlling influences that determine their action' (2009: 110). Autonomous actions are, therefore, on a continuum and there needs only to be 'a substantial degree of understanding and freedom from constraint' (2009: 101).

The two conditions necessary for autonomy are: agency (internal condition) and liberty (external condition). Agency is defined as the 'capacity for intentional action' and liberty as 'independence from controlling influences' (Beauchamp and Childress 2009: 100). There is much potential for both conditions to be compromised in mental health practice. The mental distress experienced by service users may compromise their agency, for example, should they experience psychosis or dementia. Detention under the Mental Health Act (see Chapter 13) will compromise their liberty, that is, when various restrictions and sanctions are imposed. The principle of respect for autonomy directs professionals to acknowledge the service user's 'right to hold views, to make choices, and to take actions based on their personal values and beliefs' (Beauchamp and Childress 2009: 103). It supports rules or obligations to tell the truth, respect privacy, maintain confidentiality, obtain consent and help others to make decisions. The principle of respect for autonomy, therefore, supports some of the most fundamental rules in mental health practice, and most particularly informed consent, truth-telling and confidentiality.

Non-maleficence

This means that mental health professionals should not inflict harm on others. The phrase *primum non nocere* (above all do no harm) has a long tradition in health care going back to the Hippocratic oath. There is much potential in mental health practice for different kinds of harm – physical (e.g. from the side-effects of treatment or other interventions) and psychological, emotional or social harm (e.g. from disrespectful, disempowering or abusive practices). Non-maleficence is generally considered in relation to beneficence. The principles to do good and to avoid harm go hand in hand. The rule 'one ought not to inflict evil or harm' is derived from the principle of non-maleficence (Beauchamp and Childress 2009: 151).

Beneficence

This also has a long tradition in health care. This principle supports rules such as the prevention of harm or evil, the removal of harm or evil, and the obligation to promote and do good. The principles of non-maleficence and beneficence, therefore, require a weighing up of what it means to do good as opposed to what will bring about harm or do wrong. In relation to any mental health intervention, therefore, the professional needs to consider the harms and benefits that will ensue for the service user and others. At times, it may be necessary to have a short-term harm (e.g. involuntary detention) for a longer-term benefit.

Justice

This is one of the most complex principles to grasp and apply to mental health practice. It is described as comprising several principles rather than one. The concept of 'justice' is defined as referring to 'fairness, desert (what is deserved) and entitlement' (Beauchamp and Childress 2009: 241). In health care ethics, justice is generally applied when there are challenges regarding resource allocation. Distributive justice refers to a range of principles that suggest what fair or justice distribution might mean – for example, the allocation of resources on the basis of need, effort, merit, contribution or to give everyone an equal share (Beauchamp and Childress 2009: 243). When mental health care resources are scarce, difficult decisions have to be made to ensure that the criteria for distribution are ethical and people are not discriminated against without good reason. Beauchamp and Childress (2009: 241) state that:

> Standards of justice are needed whenever persons are due benefits or burdens because of their particular properties or circumstances, such as being productive or having been harmed by another person's acts. A holder of a valid claim based on justice has a right, and therefore is due something. An injustice involves a wrongful act or omission that denies people resources or protections to which they have a right.

The four principles approach has limitations but is also very helpful as a deliberative framework to structure thinking in the analysis of ethical problems. The framework also helps with the ethical decision-making that underpins mental health practice. More is required, however, if mental health practitioners are to respond appropriately to the complexities, subtleties and challenges of contemporary mental health practice. They need virtues or moral and intellectual dispositions to engage adequately with the ethical dimensions of practice.

A theoretical approach that focuses on the character and ethical qualities or dispositions of the health care professional is virtue ethics. There is a growing literature relating to virtues and health care (see e.g. Banks and Gallagher 2009) and discussion continues as to which are the most relevant virtues for health care professionals. There are many possibilities and these virtues may change over time – that is, some virtues considered appropriate in one historical era for a profession may now be considered inappropriate.

Professional wisdom

The intellectual virtue of professional or practical wisdom, prudence or phronesis relates to decision-making directed towards a good. Comte-Sponville (2002: 32) describes prudence as follows:

> *Prudence [practical wisdom] does not reign over the other virtues (justice and love each have more merit); it governs them. And indeed, what would a kingdom be without government? Merely loving justice does not make us just, nor does loving peace make us peaceable by itself: deliberation, decision, and action are also required. Prudence determines which of them are apt, as courage provides for them being carried out.*

Professional wisdom is the wisdom required for everyday professional practice and, it has been argued, has the following elements:

- an ability to distinguish between different views of practice that are more technical-rational (involving rules, diagnosis, evidence, training, technical competence, etc.) or more in keeping with professional artistry (emphasizing patterns, interpretation, creativity, uncertainty and ambiguity, and professional judgement); an ability to appreciate salient features of practice situations and to perceive the ethical aspects of mental health practice;
- the ability to exercise the moral imagination – to put oneself, for example, in the shoes of others and to think about people's situations in different ways;
- reflective and deliberative skills that enable practitioners to make decisions and to act.

Courage

Courage is associated with responses to fear-inducing situations and with concepts such as endurance and fortitude. In mental health practice there are many situations that require courage – for example, in responding to extreme mental distress or aggression, in breaking bad news to a service user or relative or in challenging a colleague who engages in unethical practice. A helpful way to think about courage and other moral virtues is in relation to what is called 'the doctrine of the mean'. This has a long philosophical tradition. The Greek philosopher, Aristotle (1976: 1115a, 6–29), described courage as 'the right attitude towards feelings of fear and confidence' and 'as a mean state in relation to feelings of fear and confidence'. The idea is that getting things right in terms of courage requires directing our attention towards the right object, in the right amount, in the right situation and at the right time. We can go wrong in at least two ways in relation to courage – an excess would mean that a person is rash or foolhardy and a deficiency would mean that a person is cowardly. It is not difficult to imagine a mental health nurse who intervenes too early and inappropriately in a situation whereby a service user becomes aggressive, nor to imagine a nurse who is too frightened to speak out about unethical practice. Fear is a prerequisite for courage and different types of courage are called for; not all may be moral. We can, for example, think of people who engage in dangerous sports – this may not involve any moral or ethical purpose. The type of courage required for mental health practice is primarily moral in that it is related to the overall goals and purpose of the profession.

Integrity

This has been described as an 'overarching disposition or capacity that enables the moral agent to hold together and balance the other virtues – characteristic of the good professional Banks and Gallagher (2009:195). The idea of the 'integrated self' suggests that parts of a person are integrated or combined into a harmonious whole. The person orders or ranks values, commitments and desires so there are no conflicts and he or she is 'whole-hearted' about this prioritization. As Banks and Gallagher (2009: 200) point out, this view is not necessarily ethical as a person could be wholehearted in pursuing selfish goals. Integrity is also related to identity whereby people act 'from motives, interests and commitments that are most deeply their own' (Banks and Gallagher 2009: 200). A distinction is made in relation to the integrated self and identity views between personal integrity (relating to consistency) and moral integrity (which has a normative or ethical content). A person could then have personal integrity (e.g. a dictator) and lack moral integrity.

Integrity is also related to conduct or behaviour that is in accord with standards or norms that are socially accepted. Such a view does not include taking into account individuals' motives, commitment or ability to critically reflect on their values. Social integrity goes further and involves a consideration of individuals' roles in a community. Here 'Integrity is a matter of having proper regard for one's role in a community process of deliberation over what is valuable and worth doing' (Banks and Gallagher 2009: 202). Standing up for what one believes in and having regard for what is worth doing is part of social integrity. There are different ways of thinking about integrity in relation to professional life: as personal integrity and as professional integrity. The former (personal integrity in professional life) emphasizes the:

> unity of the personal and professional – seeing either no separation between the two (one simply acts with everyday honesty, reliability and so on in one's work role) or a strong continuity and connection (one has chosen the job as a vocation and actively strives to live up to one's personal values and projects through the job).

(Banks and Gallagher 2009: 205)

It is, of course, not always possible to have harmony between personal and professional life. There may be conflicts and practitioners may feel that their personal values are challenged by organizational constraints in the workplace. In such situations workers may experience moral distress whereby they feel they know the right thing to do but feel unable to do it.

Professional integrity is closely aligned with views of professionalism, which involves adhering to the values of the profession as set out in a professional code; the values accepted by members of the professional community. Professional integrity is also related to 'ideal professional integrity' involving 'holding on to a more timeless service ideal of what the profession should be at its best' (Banks and Gallagher 2009: 207). The elements or features of integrity in professional life include:

- **A commitment to a set of values:** for our purposes here, this involves a consideration of what it means to be a good mental health nurse or professional. The range of values can be said to include, minimally, respect for autonomy, beneficence (do good), non-maleficence (do not harm) and justice.

- **An awareness that the values are interrelated and form a coherent whole:** this interrelationship makes up the purpose or goals of the profession and requires professional wisdom to get it right.

- **A capacity to make sense of professional values:** this requires reflection on the relationship between personal and professional values. Again, there is a role for professional wisdom to enable professionals to reason and reflect.

- **The ability to give a coherent account of beliefs and actions:** in addition to the ability to articulate the nature and value of mental health practice, this is important in relation to professional accountability – to be able to justify actions and omissions in the context of virtue ethics.

- **Dispositions to think, feel and act in accordance with the core values:** the virtue of integrity then involves reflecting on and enacting principles and virtues in mental health practice and through education.

- **Strength of purpose and the ability to implement these values:** integrity requires more than the ability to reflect and assert values but rather involves the ability to act based on a coherent set of ethical values directed towards the purpose or ideals of the profession. At times this will require courage and resilience.

Respectfulness

There are many everyday references to respect and it is a concept that is rarely interrogated. A view of respect that is derived from the work of Joseph Raz (2001) suggests different stages of respect: as an acknowledgement of value and as preservation and non-destruction. The former relates to the appropriateness of our responses in relation to the value of the object or person in question. It could refer to making eye contact and polite greetings and demonstrating good manners in our interactions with others. We need to be wary of assuming that politeness is sufficient for respectfulness as it is possible to be polite and to treat people unethically. The stage of preservation and non-destruction goes further as it involves acknowledging achievement and striving towards preserving, promoting and flourishing rather than diminishing or destroying. A parallel with beneficence (do good) and non-maleficence (do no harm) can be made here. Banks and Gallagher (2009) argue that engagement, which goes beyond the respect stages of Raz, is an important stage in terms of respectfulness in relation to professional practice. Thurgood's (2004: 650) view of engagement in relation to mental health nursing is pertinent here:

> *Establishing and maintaining relationships with clients that are experienced as helpful is fundamental to engagement. To do this requires nurses to learn about their clients' unique perspectives and to respect them as valid and meaningful. Respect for the client's viewpoint provides the basis for collaborative working and open negotiation around informed choices for care and treatment.*

11.4 Dignity in care

At the time of writing a number of media headlines and reports highlight failings in care resulting in service users, often the most vulnerable, being neglected, feeling undignified and not receiving the standard of care they should receive. The following true case study is an example in point.

Case Study

Mr L

The Health Service Ombudsman report *Care and Compassion?* (2011) detailed the experience of 72 year-old Mr L who had a diagnosis of Parkinson's disease. His wife described him as a 'brilliant architect' and as someone who had liked to keep fit throughout his life. As a result of hallucinations and aggressive behaviour he was taken to the Accident & Emergency (A&E) department at the local hospital. He was then transferred to an assessment unit in a mental health trust. Despite being described as being 'in a calm and pleasant mood' he was given 10mg olanzapine, an antipsychotic drug, with devastating results. Mr L's wife described how he was transformed into 'a zombie, a ragdoll' which, the family said, 'robbed him of his dignity' (Health Service Ombudsman 2011: 33). He became unable to walk, had to be fed and could not talk coherently. He then developed pneumonia and died two weeks later.

The family complained to the Ombudsman that Mr L was given antipsychotic medication unnecessarily, contributing to his death. His wife said that the failings had 'fast-tracked her husband to his death' and the trust had 'taken away every last ounce of dignity my husband had left' (p. 34). Following an investigation, the Ombudsman concluded that although it was not inappropriate to prescribe olanzapine, the dose was 'incautious and too high for an elderly man with his symptoms'. The prescription had been changed to a lower dose but this was not written up on Mr L's drug chart so the nurses continued to give the higher dose on a regular basis, 'even though he did not meet the criteria for its administration' (p. 34). There were also shortcomings in Mr L's care more generally with no evidence of an individualized care plan or attention to fluid intake although it was recorded that Mr L had passed very concentrated urine. There did not appear to be regular nursing observation although this had been requested by doctors. The family's complaint was upheld by the Ombudsman. The trust apologised to Mrs L for their failings and agreed to 'pay her £1000 compensation for the distress and anxiety caused to the family' (p. 35). The trust was also asked to prepare plans so that lessons could be learned and other service users and families would not have to endure such distress.

Sadly, Mr L's case is not untypical in the National Health Service (NHS) and care home sectors. Previous reports have detailed practices that have compromised the dignity and well-being of service users and have contributed to a dignity in care agenda with initiatives from the Department of Health (DH) (2009) and the Royal College of Nursing (RCN) (2008). If dignity in care is to be taken seriously in mental health services there needs to be an understanding of what it means, what undermines it and what promotes it. Definitions of 'dignity' relate to worth, value, pride, respect and honour. A definition from the RCN report *Defending Dignity* (RCN 2008: 8) defines dignity as follows:

> *Dignity is concerned with how people feel, think and behave in relation to the worth and value of themselves and others. To treat someone with dignity is to treat them as being of worth, in a way that is respectful of them as individuals.*

Other definitions of dignity discussed in the literature include: 'Dignity is when one can feel important and valuable in relation to others, being able to communicate this to others as well as being treated as such by others in threatening situations' (Haddock 1996) and 'We lack dignity when we find ourselves in inappropriate circumstances, when we are in situations where we feel foolish, incompetent, inadequate or unusually vulnerable' (Shotten

and Seedhouse 1998). Dignity is defined as a core value within international rights' declarations. The Preamble to the Universal Declaration of Human Rights (UDHR 1948 - http://www.un.org/en/documents/udhr/), for example, states that:

> *whereas recognition of the inherent dignity and of the equal and inalienable rights of all members of the human family is the foundation of freedom, justice and peace in the world.*

Article of the UDHR (1948) states that:

> *All human beings are born free and equal in dignity and rights. They are endowed with reason and conscience and should act towards one another in a spirit of brotherhood.*

There is a wide range of philosophical views regarding the meaning of dignity. The Scandinavian philosopher Lennart Nordenfelt (2004), identified four types of dignity as follows:

- **The dignity of *Menschenwürde*:** *Menschenwürde* is a German word referring to a kind of dignity everyone has to the same degree just because they are humans.
- **Dignity as merit:** this relates to the kind of dignity people have on the basis of their achievements in certain roles and due to their actions. They have special rights as a result of this.

- **The dignity of moral stature:** this kind of dignity is based on the moral stature that emerges from people's actions and omissions and from the kind of people they are. A person who could be considered to have dignity of moral stature might be Nelson Mandela. There are degrees of this type of dignity as it is dependent on people's actions, so it may come and go.

- **The dignity of personal identity:** this kind of dignity is related to self-respect and to one's identity as a person. It is related to concepts such as integrity, autonomy and inclusion. This kind of dignity can be taken away from people when, for example, they are humiliated, insulted or treated as objects.

While all four varieties of dignity can be applied to mental health practice, it is dignity of personal identity and *Menschenwürde* that are most pertinent (Wainwright and Gallagher 2008).

Common themes in the literature suggest that dignity can be diminished or promoted in relation to three main areas:

- **People:** the attitudes and behaviour of staff and others makes a significant contribution to service users and families feeling respected, included and empowered.

- **Place (physical environment and organizational culture):** if the physical environment enables service users to have privacy and same-sex accommodation then this is likely to enhance their dignity. The organizational culture is also a factor in people feeling valued.

- **Processes:** some interventions result in people being more vulnerable to indignity, for example, if there is continuous observation, restraint or seclusion (RCN 2008).

Stacey and Stockley (2011: 181) identify the areas 'where dignity is central to providing recovery-oriented care' in mental health practice. These include: challenging stigma and discrimination; promoting social inclusion; respecting diversity; facilitating shared decision-making; promoting awareness of physical health needs; and promoting safe mental health care environments.

 ## 11.5 A framework for ethical deliberation

The ETHICS framework (Gallagher 2008) is but one approach to ethical deliberation (see also Clinical Ethics Network 2011). The stages are as follows:

- **E**nquire about the facts of the situation/case – what are the clinical or medical facts? What evidence applies to the situation? Is there a diagnosis? What interventions have been implemented? What information do the key stakeholders have access to?

- **T**hink/**T**alk through the options available to those involved – what are the practice options or potential interventions that could be tried in this situation?

- **H**ear the views of those involved – who are the key stakeholders in this situation? Who has already been involved and what are their views? Who else should be involved and how might their views best be ascertained?

- **I**dentify relevant principles and other values – how do the four principles (respect for autonomy, beneficence, non-maleficence and justice) apply to the situation? What virtues do practitioners require to respond ethically in this situation? How does dignity apply to the situation?

- **C**larify the meaning and implications of key values – consider the meaning of the principles, virtues and value of dignity in relation to the situation.

- **S**elect a course of action and present ethical arguments to support this – a key element of ethical deliberation relates to professional accountability. Ethics provides arguments to justify actions and omissions, to enable practitioners to reflect, to learn from their practice

Thinking Space 11.1

Apply the ETHICS framework to each of the practice situations in Box 11.1. If possible, work through the situations with a fellow student or practice colleague.

Box 11.1 Practice situations

1. *'You can't go home today' – truth-telling and dementia care*
   An older person on a dementia care unit asks a nurse if he can go home. The nurse says, 'No, you can't go home today. Frank. It's Sunday and there are no buses.' Frank frequently makes his way to the front door of the unit attempting to leave. On one occasion, the door was left open and Frank wandered out onto the main road. He became frightened and bewildered and was returned to the unit by the police. When he is told that there are no buses he appears to become calmer and wanders off in another direction.

2. *Ethical aspects of continuous observation*
   A young woman, Stephanie, has an eating disorder and is on continuous observation. She asks the nurse if she would turn her back when she is in the bathroom. The nurse refuses. Stephanie has been an inpatient for three months and her weight remains dangerously low. She was discovered water-loading and had hidden weights in her underwear so that her weight would appear to have increased. Staff and Stephanie's family are very concerned for her welfare.

3. *Raising concerns or turning a blind eye?*
   A student nurse (Eshan) on placement in an acute unit observes a registered nurse interacting with a service user. He overhears the nurse saying, 'If you don't take your medication we may have to section you.' Eshan feels uneasy but as the nurse is a senior colleague and his mentor he decides not to say or do anything. Eshan has overheard other colleagues on the unit express concern about her mentor. They speculated that he may have personal problems.

4. *'You'll be sorry' – risk and the limits of service user autonomy*
   Davina has a long history of mental distress and arrives at the A&E department on a Friday afternoon saying she feels 'desperate' and wants to kill herself. She is seen by a mental health nurse who, after consulting with the team, tells Davina that admission is not possible. As she leaves she says to the nurse, 'You'll be sorry when I kill myself.'

Feedback to Thinking Space 11.1

Each of these practice situations presents challenges for mental health practitioners and their responses have the potential to enhance or diminish the well-being and dignity of the service users. The ETHICS framework can help you to think through the factual and ethical aspects of the practice situations. You may also have found it helpful to discuss the situations with a colleague.

Enquire about the facts of the situation/case – it is helpful to have background information regarding the service user's experience and journey through mental health services. You might also ask about diagnosis, treatment and care strategies. In Frank's case, for example, you know he is in a dementia care unit. It is important to learn more about dementia and about Frank's capabilities as well as his deficits. Finding out about his home circumstances will help you to decide on the range of interventions that might be offered. Whereas chemical or physical restraint is not conducive to the development of a therapeutic relationship, involving Frank and his family in discussing options such as opportunities for exercise (e.g. walking in the garden) and perhaps technological restraint such as tagging. The nurse's response regarding the availability of buses should be interrogated further – is this an ethical strategy? What happens when this approach is taken? Similarly, in relation to Stephanie, you would need to find out more about her medical and psychosocial history and strategies she has adopted to cope with her situation. Eshan is a student who has observed what may be coercive practice. You might consider what else she needs to know that will guide her in responding appropriately in this situation. What action is already being taken to respond to the nurse's behaviour? How would the nurse explain his approach to the patient? Is there a need to raise concerns and how? The fourth situation, involving Davina, is a very challenging one and involves weighing risks and benefits (short- and long-term) against the service user's wishes. Is it the case that what Davina wants would not be in her best interests in the longer term? Again, finding out more about her background and history will help nurses to make an informed decision and risk-calculation.

Think/Talk through the options available to those involved – In relation to Frank, the intervention adopted involves deception. What other strategies are possible? For example, taking Frank for a regular walk may be very effective. Regarding Stephanie, it would be appropriate to ask whether an attempt has been made to discuss alternative responses when Stephanie is taken to the toilet. Might it be possible to have bathroom privacy as part of her plan or contract of care? Eshan, the student, has opted not to do anything regarding the conduct. She may feel intimidated as the nurse in question is a senior colleague and her mentor. She does have the option to discuss the situation with a trusted practice colleague who can advise her on the approach that is ethical and in accordance with the NMC guidelines. If the nurse's personal problems are intruding his work life, then this is likely to be a matter for his line manager and possibly occupational health. Turning a blind eye when service users are not receiving the care they should, if this is the case here, is not an option for Eshan. The options regarding Davina seem straightforward, that is, to offer or decline admission. The team refused admission and the nurse is confronted with the possibility that Davina may harm herself. The team may consider other alternatives, for example, intensive community support.

Hear the views of those involved – one of the challenges confronting professionals in mental health practice relates to the involvement of families and friends in decision-making regarding service users. In the case of each of the service users featured in the scenarios, family members and friends are likely to have views regarding the most appropriate intervention. They may be motivated by love and concern but this cannot be assumed. It also cannot be assumed that service users are happy to have information shared with family members. It is important that, on first contact and throughout the service user journey, that this is checked out so that information is shared appropriately. In extreme circumstances it may be necessary to share confidential information with others - for example, should there be a risk of significant harm. Within the team, it is helpful to see the views of colleagues who have had most contact with the service user. Should the service user lack capacity, and family and friends not prove to offer a consistent or reliable indication of previous wishes, then it may be helpful to approach the service user's general practitioner (GP).

Identify relevant principles and key virtues – the four practice situations can be analysed using the principles and virtues described in earlier sections of this chapter. Regarding the principle of autonomy, it needs to be asked if each of the service users are in a position to exercise autonomy and what will follow from this. Should the professional respect the autonomy of each service user? For Frank, this could mean permitting him to leave the care home. Stephanie would have privacy to go to the bathroom without continuous observation. Eshan would have to consider whether the service user on the receiving end of his mentor's comments has received information to make an informed choice and if there is any reason why a decision to refuse medication should not be respected. The case of Davina is likely to be complicated by her wish for admission and, perhaps, she may take desperate measures to force professionals to respond to her wishes. In all of the situations, it is necessary to weigh short-term and longer-term harms (non-maleficence) and benefits (beneficence). The principle of justice urges professionals to ask if their practice is fair and non-discriminatory – for example, is the service user being treated this way because they are older, because they have a challenging mental health problem (perhaps being labelled 'personality disorder' or 'PD'?) or on the basis of need? Virtues have a role to play in each of the situations. Without professional wisdom, professionals and students will be insensitive to the ethical aspects of the situation and unable to deliberate and respond rationally and respectfully. If they lack courage they will be unable to take a stand, to speak up and advocate for service users. Or, as in the case of Davina, sometimes decide not to respect the wishes of service users with a view to a longer-term benefit. Respectfulness is a virtue required in everyday mental health practice toward service users, families and colleagues. Similarly, the virtues of trustworthiness and integrity are necessary for the development of therapeutic relationships and to inspire confidence in families and colleagues.

Clarify the meaning and implications of key values – regarding each of the principles and virtues referred to in relation to the practice situations, it is important that professionals and students share a common understanding of the concept and can specify what it means and what it implies for mental health practice. Readers are advised to re-read earlier sections of the chapter and to undertake additional reading in this area. Regarding the situation of Frank, it should be noted that a different interpretation of autonomy is suggested in the Nuffield Council of Bioethics Report (2009) in relation to dementia.

Select a course of action and present ethical arguments to support this – for good reason, much of the discussion in this textbook is on evidence- or research-based practice. This enables professionals and students to give reasons for interventions. However, the evidence base is not available for many interventions and, if it is, it may be that service users, families and professionals have ethical objections. Much of mental health practice revolves around values – those of service users, family members, professionals and the organizational and societal context – and this is an area that requires serious attention. Ethics provides the language and arguments to support professional accountability, enabling professionals to justify why they pursued one course of action rather than another.

experiences and to continue to develop their practice.

11.6 Conclusion

This chapter has provided readers with the opportunity to consider four challenging practice situations and to apply a framework that can assist with ethical deliberation. In addition to understanding the meaning and implications of ethical concepts, it is necessary to adopt an attitude of aspiration and non-complacency. Humans, including mental health professionals, are fallible and may have blind spots regarding ethics. They may work with people they find difficult and not always feel inclined to be respectful and just. It is important that mental health organizations demonstrate a commitment to ethical practice and have mechanisms in place to support professional values. This could involve setting up a clinical ethics committee with a brief to analyse challenging practice situations, offer ethics education and provide opinion on the ethical aspects of mental health policies.

In summary the main learning points of this chapter are:

- Ethics in mental health practice is concerned with prescribing what people do and don't do (their actions) and with their dispositions or virtues (their character) (philosophical ethics), and with describing ethical aspects of practice (empirical ethics).

- Ethical principles (autonomy, do good, avoid harm and justice) and deliberative frameworks guide mental health practitioners, enabling

them to reflect on their everyday practice and to justify their actions and omissions.

- An aspiration to professional virtues such as integrity, courage, respectfulness, justice and wisdom enables practitioners to respond ethically to the complexity and subtleties of mental health practice.

- Unethical practices in mental health services result in service users feeling devalued, humiliated and diminished, thus violating their human rights.

- The promotion of ethical mental health practice is the responsibility of every mental health practitioner. Each has an obligation to enact, role-model and advocate for practice that enables service users and families to flourish.

Annotated bibliography

Barker, P. (ed.) (2011) *Mental Health Ethics: The human context*. Oxford: Routledge.
This book provides a comprehensive and scholarly overview of ethical, legal and ideological aspects of mental health practice. The editor and authors have, among them, a depth and breadth of expertise and experience in mental health practice, research and education. The text provides: opportunities to engage with the perspectives of a range of mental health care professionals; reflection on ethical dilemmas that arise in practices such as restraint and the administration of medication; discussion of ethical and legal issues that arise for service users with different problems and in different care contexts.

Gallagher, A. and Hodge, S. (2012) *Ethics, Law and Professional Issues in Healthcare: A practice-based approach*. Basingstoke: Palgrave Macmillan.
This textbook invites readers to consider key concepts in ethics and law and within professional codes through a consideration of practice examples. The vignettes or practice examples are drawn from the experiences of nurses, paramedics, midwives and operating department practitioners. While not all examples are directly concerned with mental health practice, all of the key concepts (consent, confidentiality, truth-telling, justice and ethical practice) are. Each practice example facilitates reflection on practice.

Nordenfelt, L. (ed.) (2009) *Dignity in Care for Older People*. Chichester: Wiley-Blackwell. And

Matiti, M.R. and Baillie, L. (eds) (2011) *Dignity in Healthcare: a practical approach for nurses and midwives*. London: Radcliffe Publishing.
Both these books offer the reader excellent coverage of the philosophical and practical aspects of dignity in care. The Nordenfelt text engages in more depth with the philosophical analysis of dignity and focuses on the experiences of older people in a European context. The Matiti and Baillie text is more UK- and practice-focused. Chapters are devoted to different care settings and service user groups. In addition to dignity for children, older people and people with learning disabilities, there is a chapter by Gemma Stacey and Theodore Stickley regarding dignity in mental health services. These two texts are complementary and are to be recommended as required reading to inform the development and sustainability of dignity in mental health services.

Williamson, T. and Daw, R. (2012) *Laws, Values and Practice in Mental Health Nursing: A Handbook*. Maidenhead: Open University Press.
This handbook is designed to explain the ins and outs of mental health law and how it intersects with values based practice in a range of mental health settings. The book is practical and designed to give mental health nurses practical guidance on dealing with often complex and daunting scenarios. The book looks at the Human Rights Act, the Mental Capacity Act 2005, the Deprivation of Liberty Safeguards and the Revised Mental Health Act. Each chapter includes case studies.

***Nursing Ethics* journal.**
This is an international peer-reviewed journal that engages with a wide range of ethical issues in health care. There is a good deal of scholarship and research that relates to mental health practice and it is recommended that readers use the search facility to find the topic area they are interested in (see http://nej.sagepub.com).

Clinical Ethics Network.
The network website contains very helpful ethics-related resources that will be of interest to mental health practitioners and will help them with ethical decision-making. There are, for example, articles on competence and decision-making in relation to service users with anorexia nervosa and dementia (see www.ethox.org.uk/research/genetics/uk-clinical-ethics-network-project).

References

Aristotle (1976) *Nicomachean Ethics*. London: Penguin.

Ashcroft, R., Lucassen, A., Parker, M., Verkerk, M. and Widdershoven, G. (2005) *Case Analysis in Clinical Ethics*. Cambridge: Cambridge University Press.

Banks, S. and Gallagher, A. (2009) *Ethics in Professional Life: Virtues for health and social care*. Basingstoke: Palgrave Macmillan.

Barker, P. (2011) *Mental Health Ethics: The human context*. Abingdon: Routledge.

Beauchamp, T.L. and Childress, J.F. (2009) *Principles of Biomedical Ethics*, 6th edn. Oxford: Oxford University Press.

CQC (Care Quality Commission) (2011) *Dignity and Nutrition Inspection Report: A national overview*. London: CQC.

Clinical Ethics Network (2011) www.ethics-network.org.uk, accessed 30 November 2011.

Comte-Sponville (2002) *A Short Treatise on the Great Virtues: The uses of philosophy in everyday Life*. London: Heinemann.

DH (Department of Health) (2009) *Final Report of the Department of Health Dignity in Care Campaign*. London: DH, available at: www.dignityincare.org.uk/_library/Opinion_Leader_Final_Report_to_DH.doc.pdf.

DH (Department of Health) (2010) *Equity and Excellence: Liberating the NHS*. London: DH.

Edwards, S.D. (2009) *Nursing Ethics: A Principle-Based Approach*, 2nd edn. Basingstoke: Palgrave Macmillan.

Fowler, M. (2009) Nursing's ethics, in A. Davis, M. Fowler and M. Aroskar (eds) *Ethical Dilemmas and Nursing Practice*, 5th edn. Massachusetts: Appleton & Lange.

Gallagher, A. (2009) ETHICS framework: Open University A181, *Ethics in Real Life*. Milton Keynes: The Open University.

Gillon, R. (1986) *Philosophical Medical Ethics*. London: Wiley Medical Publications.

Health Service Ombudsman (2011) *Care and Compassion? Report of the Health Service Ombudsman on ten investigations into NHS care of older people*, available at: www.ombudsman.org.uk/care-and-compassion, accessed 31 January 2012.

Mandelstam, M. (2011) *How We Treat the Sick: Neglect and abuse in our health services*. London: Jessica Kingsley.

McMillan and Hope (Widdershoven *et al* 2008 p.19)

Nordenfelt, L. (2004) The varieties of dignity, *Health Care Analysis*, 12: 69–81.

Nordenfelt, L. (ed.) (2009) *Dignity in Care for Older People*. Oxford: Wiley-Blackwell.

Nuffield Council on Bioethics (2009) *Dementia: ethical issues*. London: Nuffield Council on Bioethics.

NMC (Nursing and Midwifery Council) (2010) *Raising and escalating concerns*. London: NMC.

Raz, J. (2001) *Value, Respect and Attachment*. Cambridge: Cambridge University Press.

RCN (Royal College of Nursing) (2008) *Defending Dignity: Challenges and opportunities for nursing*, available at: www.rcn.org. uk/__data/assets/pdf_file/0011/166655/003257.pdf.

Stacey, G. and Stockley, T. (2011) Dignity in mental health: listening to the flying saint, in M.R. Matiti and L. Baillie (eds) (2011) *Dignity in Healthcare: a practical approach for nurses and midwives*. London: Radcliffe Publishing.

ter Meulen, R. (2011) Ethics of Care, in R. Chadwick, H. ten Have and E.M. Meslin (eds) *The Sage Handbook of Health Care Ethics*. London: Sage.

Thurgood, M. (2004) Engaging clients in their care and treatment, in I. Norman I and I. Ryrie (eds) *The Art and Science of Mental Health Nursing*. Maidenhead: Open University Press.

Wainwright, P. and Gallagher, A. (2008) On different types of dignity in nursing care: a critique of Nordenfelt, *Nursing Philosophy*, 9: 46–54.

Widdershoven, G., McMillan, J., Hope, T. and Van der Scheer, L. (2008) *Empirical Ethics in Psychiatry*. Oxford: Oxford University Press.

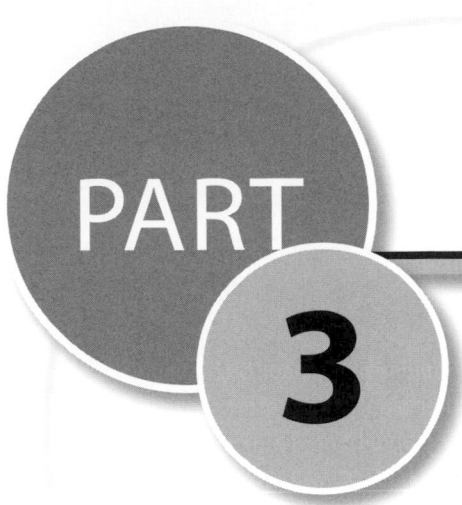

Core Procedures

Chapter 12

The Therapeutic Relationship: Engaging Clients in their Care and Treatment

Megan Ellis and Crispin Day

12.1 Introduction

This chapter examines the key elements that underpin therapeutic relationships and effective client engagement. The chapter covers:

- the different ways that the therapeutic relationship has been conceived historically, and the impact that engagement has on recovery throughout care and treatment;
- three key elements that underpin nurses' therapeutic relationships and effective client engagement: the type of relationships that nurses seek to build; nurses' interpersonal qualities and their communication skills; the tasks of the care and the treatment process.

Much of the content of this chapter draws on our development and experience of the Family Partnership Model (Davis and Day 2010). The model was originally developed to assist practitioners in their work with parents whose children had complex developmental needs. It has since been adopted across many areas of practice including community nursing, child mental health, adult mental health and social care in the UK and internationally.

12.2 What is a therapeutic relationship?

The provision of health care by a practitioner and its receipt by a client inevitably involves an enormous number of interactions. These interactions are affected by the ways in which the client and practitioner relate and respond to each other. Over time, and sometimes very quickly, these interactions can develop into a consistent and continuing relationship, which, if seen as beneficial and restorative to the tasks of care and treatment, are experienced by the client as therapeutic.

By care and treatment, we mean the process that begins with initial referral and assessment, and moves on to the planning and provision of tasks and actions that underpin supportive and structured nursing approaches such as the Care Programme Approach (CPA), as well as the provision of specific pharmacological, psychological and social interventions. Care and treatment ends with client discharge (see Chapter 16).

Without the development and maintenance of an effective therapeutic relationship the client is much less likely to access and make effective use of care and services available. The absence of a therapeutic relationship hampers the planning and provision of the care and treatment that will enable and enhance recovery and may lead to non-attendance or discharge. Its presence ensures that clients can make full and effective use of the expertise, knowledge, skills and human contact offered by nurses.

The therapeutic relationship has been of consistent interest throughout modern health care, though the way that it has been conceived has changed over time. In the early days of psychoanalytic psychotherapies, the therapeutic relationship was seen as a reflection of the client's inner difficulties and the therapist as a treatment vehicle through which the client worked through their own unconscious conflicts. The expertise of the therapist enabled her or him to interpret these conflicts and offer insights to the client that would lead to resolution of their difficulties.

In the middle of the last century, Carl Rogers and other humanistic theorists emphasized the role of the therapeutic relationship as a bedrock, upon which the therapist could create a constructive, respectful, non-judgemental environment. Demonstrations of therapist genuineness, empathy and unconditional positive regard toward the client were considered to be the facilitating conditions that would enable clients to find their own solutions to the difficulties they faced.

More recently, cognitive behavioural approaches have emphasized a collaborative therapeutic relationship between therapist and client as a vehicle through which clients are inducted and engaged in treatment, with the adoption and use of specific cognitive behavioural treatment techniques being seen as primarily responsible for change. Mental health nursing innovator Hildegard Peplau, along with Annie Altschul and latterly Eileen Skellern (Winship et al. 2009) have drawn upon these various conceptualizations to establish the concept of the therapeutic relationship as a cornerstone of mental health nursing practice. Over 50 years ago, for example, Peplau (1952: 16) defined nursing as:

> a significant, therapeutic, interpersonal process. It functions co-operatively with other human processes that make health possible for individuals in communities . . . Nursing is an educative instrument, a maturing force, that aims to promote forward movement of personality in the direction of creative, constructive, productive, personal and community living.

In broad terms, the therapeutic relationship has been conceptualized as both the cause of change as well as the vehicle for change, and the active engagement of clients in their care and treatment is seen as central to achieving successful outcomes and recovery.

Box 12.1 describes the characteristics of therapeutic relationships that effectively engage and

Box 12.1 Characteristics of effective therapeutic relationships

Supportive – emotionally and practically supportive of the client.

Connected – closely connected to the feelings and experiences of the client.

Facilitative – the nurse is able to make things happen on behalf of the client.

Influential – the nurse is capable of helping the client make positive changes to their life.

Purposeful – the nurse and the client are clear about the focus and intention of the relationship.

help clients successfully use their care and treatment.

12.3 What is engagement and why is it important?

The term engagement is used to describe the active and emotional involvement of a client in their care and treatment. It can be contrasted with other forms of participation and even non-participation such as the passive or submissive acceptance of treatment by a client, or the refusal or rejection of treatment. Engagement is often closely associated with the initial stages of therapy, however, we see engagement as not simply confined to the initial phase of care and treatment but an important and consistent feature throughout care and treatment. In the remainder of this chapter some of the key features that underpin the conditions that nurses need to create to facilitate and increase the likelihood of successfully engaging clients positively in care and treatment are discussed.

12.4 The type of therapeutic relationship

In this section we briefly examine six particular types of relationship. The nature and characteristics of the relationship the nurse builds can vary enormously. These manifest in different ways and have different consequences for initial and continuing engagement. They are not mutually exclusive – the therapeutic relationship may have elements of one or more relationship type.

The expert relationship

One of the most common types of relationship that nurses form with their clients is the expert relationship. By this we mean that the nurse is considered by him or herself and/or the client as possessing superior knowledge and insight into the client's experiences, symptoms and life difficulties as well as better understanding and expertise of the care, treatment goals and interventions that should be adopted. In contrast, the client is assumed to have less and/or inferior knowledge, is dependent upon the expertise of the nurse and is assumed to readily accept and be able to put into action whatever course of care and treatment that the nurse offers and recommends. This type of relationship can be viewed as emphasizing the purposeful and influential components of the therapeutic relationship but without the supportive, connected and facilitative components.

> **Thinking Space 12.1**
>
> Considering the following case study, what are the advantages and disadvantages of this type of relationship?

Case Study

Jane

Jane is 34 years old and has had recurring bouts of depression throughout her adult life. Martha has been her community psychiatric nurse (CPN) for a month. Martha looked for and found literature that supports her belief that exercise improves mood. She has also recently discharged a client to whom she had recommended zumba (a dance fitness programme) and who had reported back to Martha that it had been the key to her recovery.

Martha has made a careful and full care plan with her multi-disciplinary team for Jane to follow. Included in the plan is attending zumba classes. Martha has been able to access subsidized session vouchers and has given these to Jane, suggesting she go to the Sunday morning class because it is quieter. Martha is convinced that if Jane follows the plan, her mood will improve and she will be able to discharge her. Martha's manager has agreed to this plan in supervision and is keen for her to make room in her caseload to take on new referrals.

A month after presenting this plan to Jane, Martha is frustrated that Jane hasn't been to zumba and always seems to have an excuse. Jane hasn't come up with an alternative and Martha wonders if Jane doesn't want to get better, and whether she should discharge Jane as she is non-compliant.

Jane felt excited when Martha first visited because she was energetic and seemed determined to help Jane get back on her feet. Now she dreads Martha coming because she still hasn't been to zumba, she can't bear the thought of it and has always detested exercise class type activity. She can't tell Martha. She feels like a failure.

Feedback to Thinking Space 12.1

Martha experiences an increased sense of satisfaction and confidence in her own abilities and expertise in reducing the client's distress and expects this to be helpful for Jane. When passively rejected or when the plan is ineffective, Martha assumes that this is because Jane has failed to act on her advice properly. As a consequence of the pressures of this expert relationship, Martha is considering withdrawing from it, attempting to relieve her frustration and potentially avoid exhaustion. Jane feels disappointed in Martha and more significantly in herself. She wants Martha to give her more appropriate advice. We can see that initially Jane felt comforted and hopeful that Martha was available with a greater knowledge than herself. However, Jane's autonomy is undermined and she has a diminished sense of her own agency, waiting for the omnipotent presence of Martha to be the expert and get it right for her. As a result, Jane has become more passive and is not able to make decisions for herself in relation to her recovery, looking to Martha for guidance as the expert. The likelihood of Martha remaining engaged with Jane is significantly threatened, and in fact Jane is also contemplating withdrawal. Initially providing an expert solution appeared to engage Jane but has not been a sustaining factor.

The friendship

Friendships are another type of relationship that may form between a nurse and a client. This type of relationship may be more likely to develop in settings such as inpatient units where nurses are with clients for extended periods in which there is both formal and informal time spent together, making boundaries difficult to establish and maintain. Close personal bonds may develop where there is a blurring of roles and purpose, informality and mutuality, where the relationship is perceived as meaning the same to each other. This may result in nurses inappropriately sharing personal information and opinions, emotional interdependence and the avoidance of difficult or challenging issues. This type of relationship can be viewed as emphasizing the supportive and connected components of the therapeutic relationship but lacks balance with the facilitative, influential and purposeful characteristics.

Being connected and supportive are required to engage distressed and disorganized clients in their care and treatment, however when this crosses the boundary into a perceived friendship it can be both detrimental to the client and the nurse involved as well as the multi-disciplinary care the client receives.

The dependent relationship

This is a relationship in which the nurse takes on excessive responsibility for achieving the client's outcomes. In doing so, a nurse may assume that her actions are essential for the client's recovery, act on behalf of the client, sometimes without agreement, and offer help and advice that may interfere with the client's personal choices and responsibility. Looking at the components of the therapeutic relationship outlined above in Box 12.1 we can see that there is an emphasis on the facilitative and influential aspects, making things happen for the client without the client's authentic involvement, also an over-involvement.

Thinking Space 12.2

Considering the following case study about Peter, what are the advantages and disadvantages of this type of relationship?

The adversarial relationship

This type of relationship is characterized by antagonism and hostility between the nurse and client. There may be either open or covert disagreement

or an inability to reconcile differences. Each person may blame the other for the difficulties they experience and each may wish to assert their own needs and fail to acknowledge those of the other person. The influential component of the therapeutic relationship may be evident in this type of relationship, an unfortunate distortion of the intent to bring about change and participation that is particularly coercive. Adversarial relationships can result in nurses believing they can exercise unconditional control and authority, and that harsh or punitive actions towards a client are justified.

The avoidant relationship

Avoidant relationships are characterized by the nurse becoming emotionally and intellectually uninvolved, detached and remote from their client. The emotional distance present in avoidant relationships may suit the client and the nurse for different reasons. For example, there may be a struggle between the nurse and client to find a common connection. The avoidance may reflect a desire of

Case Study

Peter

Peter is living in the community and suffers from bipolar disorder. Both Peter and Tracy, his CPN, agreed to set a goal for Peter to enter into paid employment. Tracy helped him to get a job labouring for two days a week for a construction company. Tracy found the advertisement on the internet, prepared Peter's application and took Peter to the interview. They were both very pleased Peter got the job. Tracy decided she would do whatever it took to make it a success. Peter said he would not be able to get to work, he struggled with motivation in the morning and thought he would miss the train. Tracy said she would ring him in the morning and then come past his flat and walk him to the station, it was on her way to work so it made sense to her and Peter said he wouldn't be able to do it without her.

Time has passed, Peter has been working for a month, two days a week. On one occasion Tracy was unable to pick Peter up, due to a change in her own childcare arrangements. Peter didn't go to work that day, he was pleased to have the day off. Peter has now been asked to work three days including Saturday. He thinks he would like to do this and that Tracy should be able to get him up. Peter has started waking at 4 a.m. and has plans for the company but hasn't shared these with Tracy yet. Tracy is feeling a little over-committed to Peter and wants to stop waking him up, as she believes he should be able to do this independently now.

the nurse, client or both not to address difficult or important issues as a result of which the client is perceived as non-compliant and not worth any further effort. Often an avoidant relationship may be prompted by disappointment with and dislike of the client, the nurse's efforts may feel unreciprocated and a subsequent loss of motivation may precede avoidance. The purposeful aspect of a therapeutic relationship is underemphasized or taken at face value, leading to the nurse becoming, on a surface level, task focused.

The partnership relationship

A partnership relationship has several key characteristics that increase effectiveness in achieving

Feedback to Thinking Space 12.3

Jason doesn't want to have any more contact than is absolutely necessary. He knows the staff think he's smelly, and he doesn't want to have to endure the wrinkled noses and looks of disgust. Jamilla feels that she is doing the task asked of her and therefore her job. For Jason, there is a consistent reinforcement that he is not worthy of human contact and he learns to mask his other more disabling paranoid symptoms and continues to manage these with alcohol on discharge. This lack of engagement may be compromising Jason's safety and health, as Jamilla neither knows what Jason's plans are nor is able to investigate Jason's perspective. Additionally there is no possible investigation of Jason's malodorous presentation – for example the urinary incontinence may be associated with an underlying health problem such as prostate cancer. For Jamilla, this superficial nursing practice will not lead to a development of nursing skills in which she may be helpful to a client from a marginalized group. Any further deterioration in Jason's mental state is likely to be missed, ironically while he is under surveillance. Both Jason and Jamilla are engaged in tasks that are related to monitoring and discharge planning without having either engaged with each other or with care and treatment.

engagement in care and treatment (Davis and Day 2010). Partnership relationships give both the nurse and the client the opportunity to openly discuss and mutually agree aims and purpose, as well as identify, negotiate and explicitly resolve differences and conflicts. The shared processes that are at the heart of partnership relationships provide a means by which the complimentary roles, expertise and knowledge of the client and the nurse can be acknowledged and used to fully contribute to achieving the goals and aims of care and treatment. This requires the nurse and client to recognize and accept their shared rights and responsibilities within the therapeutic relationship as well as agree how they will work together in a coordinated and mutually acceptable way. The emphasis throughout is on mutual trust and respect, and the way in which the nurse openly raises and discusses these aspects of the partnership with the client as well as encourages and is influenced by the views and priorities of the client. Partnership relationships require the active and ongoing commitment of both nurses and clients.

Collaborating with clients is more demanding since there is a constant call on the nurse to con-sciously demonstrate a range of qualities and skills (see below) that facilitate this process, and the relationship does not develop automatically.

Some relationship types are more enabling to the client's recovery than others. We believe that partnership is a more sustainable relationship and is more consistent with recovery as a set of principles than the other types of relationship outlined above. A partnership will prove most successful in initial efforts to engage clients and in sustaining that engagement throughout the process of care and treatment.

 ## 12.5 Personal qualities and interpersonal communication skills

Evidence from research and effective practice consistently demonstrates that key interpersonal qualities and communication skills are positively associated with a client's active engagement in care and treatment. The nurse will need to develop these as fully as possible to promote a partnership relationship and subsequently apply them in the context of engaging with and sustaining a client's care and treatment. The qualities listed below are internal to the nurse and underpin her stance towards the client. They are not directly observable but have a major influence on the nurse's behaviour. We have focused on a specific set of key qualities both for simplicity and to provide the nurse with a manageable list to start with and continue to develop over the course of their career. All the qualities in the list are highly interrelated:

- respecting clients;
- being genuine;
- having humility;
- being empathic;
- showing quiet enthusiasm;
- processing personal integrity;
- processing knowledge, experience and technical expertise;
- maintaining intellectual and emotional attunement;
- being constructive and sensitive.

12.6 Tasks of care and treatment

In the preceding sections we have outlined different types of relationships that nurses can build with clients and the effective qualities required of them. These elements provide the bedrock of the relational and interpersonal characteristics required for effectively engaging the client in their care and treatment. Successful engagement requires the nurse to understand how these relational and interpersonal characteristics are used to guide the nurse and their client through the key tasks of care and treatment. One way of conceptualizing the tasks involved in care and treatment that draws on the work of Gerard Egan is the Family Partnership Model (Davis and Day

2010) which is summarized in Figure 12.1 and explained below.

The tasks of the helping process usually begin with the nurse and client building the early basis of their relationship, preferably, in our view, a partnership. This provides the platform for the subsequent engagement of the client in the other tasks of the helping process. The helping process itself is dynamic. For example, the way in which the task of exploration is undertaken will affect the nature and depth of the emerging partnership between the nurse and the client as well as influence the quality and type of shared understanding that subsequently develops between them. This, in turn, will influence the selection of care and treatment goals, the choice of treatment strategies and the methods of implementation and subsequent tasks of the helping process.

While the helping process is generally sequential, the tasks are neither fixed nor is it necessary for each task to be fully completed before moving on to the next. Sometimes, particularly in urgent situations, for example, it is necessary to move rapidly into planning and implementing strategies to address risk and harm. Similarly, it is unrealistic

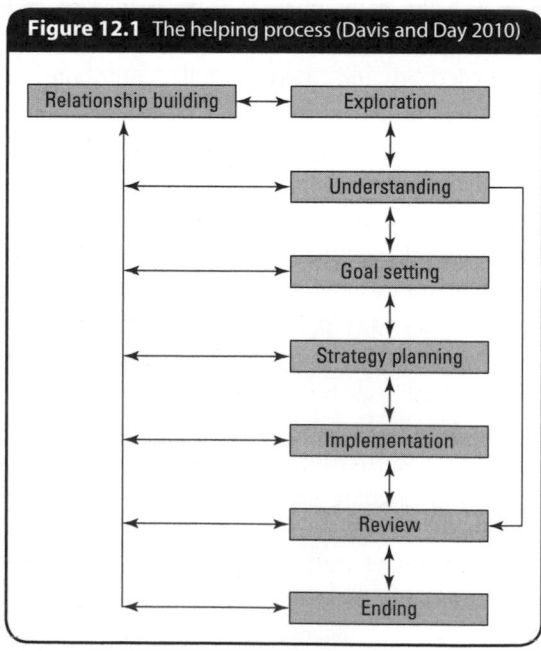

Figure 12.1 The helping process (Davis and Day 2010)

Relationship building ↔ Exploration
Understanding
Goal setting
Strategy planning
Implementation
Review
Ending

Case Study

Thea

Thea is a 54-year-old woman with scizo-affective disorder. She has been using services for over 30 years. She worked with Cathy, a CPN, for 15 years and they shared similar interests in knitting and crafts. Thea particularly loves bright colours, she doesn't like black and when she is unwell she has a particular aversion to it, considering anyone wearing black to be a member of the dark arts. She has chronic asthma during the winter when she has significant bouts of bronchitis and is on high doses of steroids. At this time her fear of black increases and her mental health deteriorates significantly. She becomes isolated and has poor self-care. It has never been established but it is hypothesized that Thea believes she is being poisoned at these times and is very suspicious, particularly about what she eats. Cathy has recently retired and Donna is now Thea's CPN.

Donna met Thea in a psychiatric emergency clinic approximately a year ago when Thea was escorted by the police to services; she had been threatening to 'burn the witches in the house next door'. Thea had been abusive towards Donna and had thought that she was a witch due to the black clothing she was wearing.

Donna was nervous picking up this case as her first meeting the year before had been a disaster. She knew that Thea and Cathy had a very good relationship and Thea adored Cathy. She and Cathy were very different types of people and nurses; Cathy was a motherly soul who wore bright colours and knitted clothes and she connected with Thea around the crafts. Donna on the other hand had a wardrobe full of black and couldn't bear crafts but wanted to build a connected and supportive relationship with Thea that was purposeful. She had discussed with the team her concerns about Thea's significant annual deterioration and admission and had in her mind that she wanted to facilitate both a medication review and develop a relapse prevention plan with Thea to avoid the trauma of winter admission.

On her first meeting, Donna acknowledged the close relationship Thea had with Cathy. She tentatively voiced her concerns that Cathy and her were very different people and suggested they discuss how she and Thea could work together. Donna was relieved when Thea agreed that she was 'Certainly very different in her dark drab clothes and could never replace Cathy.' Donna tentatively expressed empathy towards Thea, saying that she must be sad that Cathy had retired and that she herself would miss Cathy's bright and optimistic personality in the team. Thea got a tear in her eye, softened and told Donna that they 'would be able to work something out'. At the end of this initial meeting Thea said that she really didn't like going to hospital every winter, the food was terrible and she wanted to be able to stay in her cosy flat. Donna said she had been concerned about this too and they agreed they would initially focus on this.

At the next visit Donna wore black trousers and boots but decided to wear a green T-shirt and a paisley scarf. She hoped she would be able to establish some baseline information about Thea's mental state while she appeared well, as this would potentially be helpful in the future. She took a pad of flip-chart paper, a set of multi-coloured post-it notes and a set of 24 brightly coloured markers. She asked Thea if they could explore the 'winter admissions' together and map out and draw the conversation. Thea was very enthusiastic about the materials and doing this. They filled two flipchart pages in this session and came to an understanding that the asthma medication severely altered what Thea thought about colour, food and the people around her. She also told Donna that while she didn't like the black trousers and boots she had on, she did think she looked smart and the green and black looked good together. They decided to draw a picture of Donna on the map with these comments beside it.

Thea said she would like to avoid an emergency admission this winter and identify and plan for an alternative. Together Thea and Donna developed a plan, including a medication review, exploring respite options and a clear set of early warning signs and what to do. Thea asked that Donna come to the medication review and thought that she would probably cover the picture of Donna in black if she was becoming suspicious of Donna. They agreed that should this happen Donna would increase the duties of the support worker, Billy, who Thea always maintained contact with when unwell. Thea wrote down that Billy could get her groceries at this time, and also that Thea's general practitioner (GP) would phone Donna should she need to go on steroids.

A medication review was undertaken and the plan was put in place. In the winter when Thea's physical health started to deteriorate the GP phoned Donna. Donna then discussed the case with the psychiatrist who titrated Thea's anti-psychotic medication. Visits from the support worker were increased and Thea avoided admission. When Donna visited to review the 'winter' action plan, Thea was able to tolerate Donna wearing black items of clothing. She had a twitch of a smile and said to Donna, 'You are looking like a witch, come in but don't make the tea.'

to expect that all clients are fully open about their personal circumstances, needs and life experiences. It can take time for clients to trust nurses, so we should be realistic about what we are told, what we learn and what clients are prepared to tell us.

We can use this framework as a basis for moving forward through the tasks of the helping process, while knowing that as we do so we will subsequently learn more that will prompt further exploration, lead to a better understanding, the formulation of more helpful care and treatment goals and so forth. The purpose of the helping process is to act as a guide and framework. It is not a recipe with specific quantities of each task and exact timings to achieve the right outcome. The key is that nurses have a firm understanding of the tasks involved in the process and use this knowledge to guide them and their clients through care and treatment (see Chapter 15 for more detail).

Relationship-building

Thea's case study is now drawn on to illustrate how the therapeutic relationship and the tasks of helping

interrelate and promote sustained engagement in care and treatment.

The relationship

A 'connection' or rapport may quickly develop during the first contact between the nurse and the client. With Thea and Donna we see that connecting over the loss of Cathy appears to lead to Thea feeling more hopeful and less distressed. Thea feels less alone and even begins to feel clearer about what may be the best way forward for her. This experience for Thea and the reciprocal effects on Donna contribute to building the relationship and strengthen Thea's engagement. With this experience, the potential of Donna as a source of practical and emotional support becomes clearer to Thea. The potential of this relationship will be made real, deepened and strengthened as Thea and Donna negotiate and successfully fulfil the tasks of the helping process together.

On the other hand, the risks associated with initiating another type of relationship, say expert or avoidant, based on Donna's concerns and anxieties, may have been less successful. This could occur at any point in care and treatment and can lead to the practical or emotional withdrawal of the nurse, the client or both from the relationship. This may increase the likelihood of the development of some of the less optimal relationships described above, which may result in disengagement through refusing care and treatment, passive compliance or intermittent attendance, accompanied by little investment or commitment to the relationship or tasks of the helping process. The nurse, in turn, may have little emotional enthusiasm for their work with the client, avoid contact with them, become over-demanding and be unreasonable in their expectations, or blame the client for being resistant or non-compliant.

Exploration/assessment and clear understanding/formulation

Assessment, in our view, describes the structured information-gathering that nurses use to enable them to reach a diagnosis or a formulation about a client's presenting difficulties and strengths. Traditionally, assessment is led by the needs and requirements of the nurse and can focus narrowly on what is important to the nurse and their team rather than what is important to the client. Clients often report that the process of having an assessment 'done to them' feels repetitive and rather disconnected from their experience. Nurses report a separating of relationship-building and assessment, thus not utilizing the tasks of care and treatment to deliberately and consciously engage clients. In contrast, exploration is a joint and interactive task, led by the client and facilitated by the nurse. It involves encouraging a client to tell their story from their own perspective.

However, exploration and assessment are not mutually exclusive. In fact the two tasks can be, and often are, undertaken at the same time. In the case study, Thea is leading the process and talking about the issue that Donna wants to focus on. Had Donna led, this would have had a different effect on both the engagement and the care and treatment.

Goal-setting, planning, implementation

Goals are specific objectives that the nurse and client jointly agree are to be achieved in care and treat-

ment and these result from the exploration and formulation stages. Planning involves clients and nurses jointly looking at the range of actions available to enable clients to reach their agreed goals (see Chapter 15). Nurses need to use their knowledge and expertise in collaboration with the client, not in place of the client's own knowledge and expertise. With Thea we see her understanding her own life, desires and capabilities intimately, and using this information to develop a plan of action. Donna learns what Thea hopes to achieve and helps her to decide her priorities. These prorities are aligned with Donna's own purpose. If this had not been the case, then Donna would have needed to gently challenge Thea to ensure that her goals were relevant, realistic, feasible and clear. Goal-setting may require negotiation, the nurse having some options to offer as choices but the selection should be made based on both agreement and viability. This collaborative, partnership approach to the relationship is fundamental to maximizing any client's commitment and engagement throughout their care and treatment.

Implementation involves Donna encouraging and supporting Thea to put her plans into action. This requires the continued commitment, engagement and involvement of both Donna and Thea.

Review and ending

Finally, reviewing facilitates explicit learning about how a client is progressing in relation to their recovery journey and what is helpful and less helpful in the collaboratively developed care plan, and why. Often review is perceived as a task at the end of treatment, however we suggest that review is an ongoing necessity in the sustained engagement of a client. This ongoing and regular review helps to identify barriers or issues not only in relation to the care plan but in terms of the therapeutic relationship that is the vehicle through which the care plan is being administered. Nurse reflection is one aspect of reviewing that may help to highlight any barriers to engagement and assess the success of a care plan or treatment pathway. Thea is demonstrating an increased sense of her own agency and achievement, strengthening her resilience and increasing her self-esteem in her comment to Donna on a review visit. This also indicates that Thea has remained engaged in her care and treatment throughout.

An equally important function of review is to make explicit the characteristics of the relationship, the successes and barriers (including how they have been overcome), so that the client is empowered with the knowledge of the processes they have been participating in. Common barriers fall into four broad categories: stressors and obstacles, a poor relationship, a perception that treatment isn't relevant or helpful and a perception that treatment is too demanding. By being open and honest about progress the nurse is seeking to accept responsibility for improving care.

 12.7 Conclusion

Peplau (1952) argued that the nurse was the agent of change rather than the mechanism of the therapy. She emphasized that the nurse's self-awareness and self-reflection needed to happen as vigilantly as the tasks and content involved in the assessment of a client's mental health needs.

This chapter has explored how the nurse needs to be consciously aware of the type of relationships that they build, develop and maintain. They need to be equipped with and able to communicate a set of personal qualities and skills and have to have a clear sense of the tasks involved in care and treatment.

In summary, the key learning points from this chapter are:

■ Nurses should be constantly aware of and review the nature and quality of each of the therapeutic relationships in which they are involved.

■ Nurses should consciously identify and consider the way in which they use their interpersonal qualities and skills to maximize their effectiveness.

■ Relationship-building and engagement is not a process that is unique to the beginning of a therapeutic relationship; it is a process that involves initiating, maintaining and sustaining engagement in a therapeutic partnership between the client and the nurse throughout the stages of the helping process.

■ Each stage of the helping process is interrelated with relationship-building. The more the characteristics of the relationship reflect partnership at each stage of the helping process, the more likely engagement will be sustained. Engagement depends on how the task is undertaken.

■ All clients are unique individuals and by working in partnership nurses and clients can identify clients' needs, strengths and priorities in the context of their mental state, enhancing and promoting engagement.

Annotated bibliography

Davis, H. and Day, C. (2010) *Working in Partnership with Parents: The Family Partnership Model,* **2nd edn. London: Pearson.**
This is a clear and easy to read book about the Family Partnership Model and its components. It provides further detailed explanation of the development and maintenance of the partnership relationship in the context of the Family Partnership Model. It extends the ideas about the therapeutic relationship, it's interrelationship with the tasks involved in helping, and provides examples that position the theory in practice.

Rapp, C.A. (1998) *The Strengths Model: Case management with people suffering from severe and persistent mental illness.* **New York: Oxford University Press.**
A unique text that offers detailed theory, values and principles about the Strengths Model, which is used to guide the mental health professional to focus on the individual rather than pathology. It is user friendly, offering the reader theory and techniques to enable engagement of clients in their care and treatment, underpinned by a strengths approach.

Edwards, E. and Elwyn, G. (2009) *Shared Decision-making in Health Care: Achieving evidence based patient choice,* **2nd edn. Oxford: Oxford University Press.**
A theoretical and practical book that provides the evidence, criteria and tools to assist the mental health professional in the complex work of collaborative decision-making and the challenges that may present. Chapter 38 focuses on mental health; however other chapters have easily adapted tools with relevance. The chapters are short and the book is well structured and easily read in bite-sized chunks.

Deveson, A. (2003) *Resilience.* **South Australia: Griffin Press.**
This is a heartfelt book exploring resilience and the business of being human and living life. It is interwoven with heartache, adversity and resilience drawn from the author's life, from her mother growing up in the harsh outback of Australia to familiar and important global figures like Nelson Mandela. Her son and her partner both feature in the book, as does their resilience and her own when facing the anguish and heartbreak of her son's experience of serious mental distress and her partner's illness and eventually both their deaths. This is not a technical book but is a book that touches the reader; it is inspiring and thought provoking.

References

Davis, H. and Day, C. (2010) *Working in Partnership with Parents: The Family Partnership Model*, 2nd edn. London: Pearson.
Peplau, H.E. (1952) *Interpersonal Relations in Nursing*. New York: GP Putnam & Sons.
Winship, G. *et al.* (2009) Collective biography and the legacy of Hildegard Peplau, Annie Altschul and Eileen Skellern: the origins of mental health nursing and its relevance to the current crisis in psychiatry, *Journal of Research in Nursing*, 14(6): 505–17.

Chapter 13

Creating a Therapeutic Environment in Inpatient Care and Beyond

Anne Aiyegbusi and Kingsley Norton

 13.1 Introduction

Staff working on inpatient psychiatric wards report that it is hard to provide both safe custody as well as excellence in clinical care (Haigh 2002), and patients voice their dissatisfaction about the treatment received therein (Beadsmore *et al.* 1998; Ford *et al.* 1998). In one survey of ex-inpatients, over half had found their hospital admission to be untherapeutic, with 45 per cent claiming that it was detrimental to their mental health, and 30 per cent experiencing it as unsafe (Baker 2000). Indeed, in a damning indictment of the UK services they commissioned, the Department of Health (England) (DH) acknowledged that there was 'incontrovertible and compelling evidence' that mental health service users found hospital care to be 'neither safe nor therapeutic' (DH 2002: 8).

Problems with delivering a high standard of care and treatment to mentally ill patients in hospital settings are not new. Over the years, many potential solutions have been conceived. The late eighteenth century, for example, saw a sea change in attitudes to mentally ill patients who were incarcerated, resulting in the so-called 'moral treatments'. This innovative and humane approach (developed by Tuke and others) was based on a concept of 'shared responsibility for the physical maintenance of the shared living space, participation and democratic decision-making in the governance of the project' (Whiteley 2004). Following on from this, although there have been many important pharmacological and psychotherapeutic developments in treatment for mentally ill patients, the latter have not resulted simply in modern inpatient settings – 'milieus' – being therapeutic, as the surveys referred to above attest. It is therefore timely to consider what lessons might be learned from the past.

In this chapter we illustrate the problems associated with providing a therapeutic environment for inpatients and summarize some of the relevant therapeutic milieu literature, with the aim of offering a practical guide to staff, particularly nursing staff. We put the latter centre stage and discuss a range of issues around the theme of what contributes to making an inpatient environment therapeutic.

In summary this chapter covers:

- challenges of creating a therapeutic inpatient environment;
- aspects that can undermine therapeutic endeavour;
- the central role of nursing within inpatient care settings;
- the application of therapeutic milieu principles to working effectively in outpatient and community care settings.

13.2   Therapeutic milieus

The 1960s and 1970s saw an upsurge of academic interest and clinical experimentation in inpatient settings, including the rekindling of interest in some of the ideologies of previous generations of mental health care reformers and psychiatric clinicians. The term 'therapeutic milieu' was coined to refer to 'a method of providing specific treatments in an effective manner' (Abroms 1969: 560). The main aims of the therapeutic milieu were:

- to control or set limits on pathological behaviour (such as destructiveness, disorganization, deviancy, dysphoria and dependency); and
- to promote psychosocial skills (such as orientation, assertion, occupation and recreation).

Achieving these aims required the construction of a 'stable, coherent social organisation, which provides an integrated, extensive treatment context' (Abroms 1969: 560). However, creating such an organization is problematic. In part this is because of the upsetting, anxiety-inducing and disturbing effects of psychiatric disorders, not only for patients but also for those around them, especially those who are emotionally close or attached to them. It is

difficult to produce the necessary degree of organization and integration, relying as it ultimately does on the capacity of staff and patients to work together sufficiently. Delivering a 'therapeutic' outcome, within a given ward, is further complicated because what an individual patient might require, at a specific point in time, can differ markedly from what is appropriate for another patient at the same time, in the same ward. Yet, a single ward environment is required to cater, more or less equally, for all the patients who inhabit it – for the collective, as well as for the individual patient's needs.

To address these challenges it is helpful to consider the therapeutic functions that might need to be undertaken by an inpatient ward, to maximize the chances of it being therapeutically effective. Five functions were defined by Gunderson (1978): containment, support, structure, involvement and validation. These would be enacted according to the prevailing needs of the 'ward as a whole' (see also Badia 1989). At times, the emphasis is on the requirement for the first aim – control – but, at other times, there is scope to promote patients' recovery via the provision of opportunities to acquire pertinent skills. With the high turnover of patients in many modern wards, and the associated short duration of many admissions, some of the functions concerned with the second aim of the therapeutic milieu – promoting psychosocial skills – are increasingly delivered in outpatient and community settings. Nonetheless, a consideration of the whole range of functions helps steer the nurse in the direction of providing an integrated and coordinated treatment package, which remains patient-centred, across different settings – from inpatient unit to wider community.

13.3   Why inpatient settings are not simply therapeutic

Thinking Space 13.1

Read the following case study. What are the challenges of providing Cecelia with therapeutic inpatient care?

Case Study

Cecelia

Cecelia is a 25-year-old woman who has a primary (Axis I) diagnosis of bipolar disorder and a secondary (Axis II) diagnosis of borderline personality disorder. She has a long history of contact with mental health services, presenting as a 'revolving door' patient. She typically spends a few weeks in hospital followed by a short period of time in the community which precedes a further hospital stay. When in hospital, Cecelia poses mental health services with a number of challenging behaviours. She exhibits a range of self-harming behaviours, has engaged in violence as an inpatient and is extremely verbally abusive to staff, launching hurtful personal attacks on professionals. As an inpatient, Cecelia also regularly complains of physical health problems, which when investigated are found to have no organic basis.

Between hospital admissions, Cecelia takes occasional overdoses and consequently attends the local accident & emergency (A&E) department. While there, she tends to be uncooperative and abusive to the medical and nursing staff. They feel confused and annoyed, failing to understand why Cecelia should self-harm rather than ask for help from a health service, and cannot understand why she behaves as though they have attacked her in some way, criticizing them and abusing them personally. Sometimes, Cecelia places herself in dangerous situations, such as threatening to throw herself from a motorway bridge while intoxicated, which require the intervention of the police. When the latter arrive on the scene, Cecelia is similarly abusive towards them, fighting with them and accusing them of manhandling her as they try to restrain her to safety.

When Cecelia is admitted to hospital, her challenging behaviours are dealt with as they occur and are experienced by the clinical team as something to be endured. To ensure her safety, Cecelia is placed on 'increased observations' and receives medication, against her will, as a response to her violent behaviour. She begins to settle and her challenging behaviour gradually lessens and finally stops. There is seldom reflection about what might be mediating her behavioural presentation. Rather, there is concern about the poor use she makes of the follow-up care on offer. Cecelia takes her medication erratically with low compliance with the monitoring blood tests, which form part of the pharmacological management of her bipolar illness. She is discharged back to her flat where she lives alone in social isolation. Inevitably, the cycle continues, with Cecelia bringing herself to the attention of emergency services by putting herself at risk, being taken compulsorily into hospital and then abusing the help on offer there. Worryingly, Cecelia's risk-taking behaviour appears to be increasing. Staff fear that she could kill herself, probably without really intending to do so.

Feedback to Thinking Space 13.1

'Cecelia' is a composite case, based on many actual examples of inpatients known to us, male as well as female. This case serves to paint a picture of a commonplace clinical situation, where a patient has more than one diagnosis and so-called 'complex needs'. Cecelia's case also illustrates the fact that such patients in acute psychiatric wards are not simply helped by their experience therein. This patient's diagnosis of borderline personality disorder suggests a pattern of unstable mood and associated impulsive behaviours, related to profound fears of abandonment, in the face of threatened or actual loss or separation. This forms the backdrop to and complicates the management of her serious mental illness, bipolar disorder. This is especially so as her discharge date nears – the threat of separation. In her case, some symptoms are controllable with medication. However, Cecelia's erratic compliance with the relevant medications, as with other aspects of her care plan, means that it has not been clearly established how much she could be helped by it. Her isolation and lack of social support, between hospital admissions, represent other factors that impact negatively on her capacity for recovery. The clinical management of Cecelia is far from simple.

From the nursing staff's perspective, it feels as if they have no time to think or plan their patient's care. They find themselves 'fire-fighting' – i.e., responding to the next acute and dramatic episode of Cecelia's dangerous or worrying behaviour. In doing so, they are adopting (and accepting) a stance which is essentially reactive. However, not all staff feel the same way about Cecelia and her care. Some feel defeated, despairing and frustrated, believing that she is beyond help and others that she does not merit it. Some believe that the system is failing their patient and that Cecelia might be helped if only others (within the health care, social or penal systems) worked differently or harder. Staff find themselves, at times, arguing strongly against or blaming one another. It is also very tempting for them to become critical of colleagues from other agencies who share Cecelia's case. Failures by the health care system to communicate effectively and work together, consistently and systematically, sometimes do result in their patient being admitted to hospital. Hospital admission may relieve those staff initiating it of some anxiety associated with Cecelia's self-injurious behaviour. The ward-based staff on the receiving end, however, often feel they have little or nothing to offer. Once Cecelia is in hospital, a familiar pattern becomes enacted, as if inevitably, even though none consciously wishes it to be so.

13.4 Controlling maladaptive behaviour and promoting psychosocial skills

Ideally, the inpatient ward provides patients like Cecelia with an interpersonal environment that provides not only a safe place but also avoids reinforcing maladaptive coping strategies, so that some learning of new coping strategies and skills might take place. This state of affairs has been aptly described as, 'preventing "bad" things from happening and allowing "good" things to occur' (Gunderson 1978: 332). However, it is much simpler to describe than to deliver as Cecelia's case testifies. Modern wards may be better at achieving Abroms' first aim – controlling maladaptive behaviour – than his second – promoting psychosocial skills (Abroms 1969). We now outline therapeutic functions and processes of a therapeutic milieu, which represents a brief summary of Gunderson's pertinent concepts. He reasons that to provide a therapeutic setting, inpatient ward staff need to understand the wide range of functions that they may be called upon to deliver. This is so they can select and deploy relevant aspects of care and treatment, based on the changing needs of their patients, according to their mental state, risk status, the stage in their disorder and the phase of their recovery.

Containment

According to Gunderson (1978), the function of 'containment' is to sustain the physical well-being of patients and removes from them the burdens of self-control or feelings of omnipotence. It is effected through the provision of food, shelter and at least temporary removal from the stressors of the outside world. The aim of containment is to prevent assaults and to minimize physical deterioration and dangerousness in those who lack judgement, as was almost always the case with Cecelia's inpatient admissions. The effect of admission is to reinforce, at least temporarily, the patient's internal controls and to reality-test their omnipotent beliefs concerning their destructiveness. Effective containment thus demonstrates to the patient that their violence can be stopped – i.e. they are *not* all powerful.

There is a risk that inpatient wards can overemphasize containment, thereby suppressing the patients' own initiative, reinforcing their feelings of isolation and increasing their sense of hopelessness and despair. Cecelia appeared to suffer from an increase of such feelings, especially once a discharge date for her had been set. The staff caring for her also felt increasingly hopeless and despairing, as readmission relentlessly followed admission. Even though she was not fit to benefit from other functions, outlined below, Cecelia did at least experience some containment. Her physical well-being was sustained. Indeed, her life was almost certainly prolonged by the treatment she received.

Support

'Support' refers to deliberate efforts, effected through the social network of the inpatient environment, to help patients feel better about themselves (Gunderson 1979). There is an acceptance that patients have certain needs, which staff can fulfil, and also that they have limitations which staff need to make accommodation for. Relevant supportive activities include the provision of escorts and other behavioural provisions (such as advice and education) aimed at preserving and reinforcing the patient's existing ego functions. This may also include assisting patients to do things which they protest are impossible but under circumstances where success is almost certainly guaranteed. Those milieus that emphasize support are recognizable as retreats that provide nurturance and permit, encourage and direct patients to venture into other, more specific, therapies such as psychotherapy, rehabilitation or family therapy.

With the costs of health care being intensively scrutinized and carefully controlled, one consequence of shorter acute psychiatric admissions is that there is less time available for forming and strengthening a therapeutic alliance between patient and staff. A weaker alliance means that it is harder to form a secure platform, post-discharge from hospital, upon which to develop further therapeutic interventions that can promote the patient's fuller recovery. Certainly, the suddenness and speed with which Cecelia is usually discharged means that there is little or no time to reflect on what has transpired or to engage actively and meaningfully in her care plan. Cecelia therefore is not in a position to benefit from the functions specified below, which previously were more often part of an inpatient stay, at least in some psychiatric inpatient settings.

Structure

'Structure' represents all aspects of an inpatient milieu that provide for a predictable organization in terms of time, place and person. It acts to make the environment less amorphous and to support the patient's reality-testing, via making the ward's treatment programme intelligible to patients (Gunderson 1979). Structure facilitates the safe attachment of patients to their environment (Haigh 1999). Ideally, the latter feel neither invaded nor detached and alone. Structure promotes changes in patients' symptoms and action patterns, especially where these are considered to be socially maladaptive, for example, as with forensic patients. It can contribute to this outcome through helping them to consider the consequences of their behaviour for both themselves and others. This can gradually help them deal differently with their emotions and impulses, delaying them acting upon depressive feelings or destructive impulses. The beneficial effect of structur is mediated by, among others: hierarchical privilege systems and the use of treatment contracts (see Miller 1989). These draw on the patients' healthy capacities.

In practice, staff in many inpatient environments are predominantly reacting to the prevailing crisis – part of the routine of fire-fighting, as in the case of Cecelia, and not concentrating on making the environment intelligible to patients. This detracts from the setting's capacity to function predictably, with the result that the patient's sense of reality orientation may be even further impoverished, as inpatient surveys have shown (Baker 2000). With little or no negotiation or joint planning (given the short time available between the acute situation being managed and Cecelia's discharge from the ward), the potential for promoting more adaptive behaviour, on the basis of her greater insight, is seldom realized.

Involvement

'Involvement' refers to those processes that cause patients to attend actively to their social environment and to interact with it. The purpose of involvement is to use and strengthen a patient's ego and to modify aversive or destructive interpersonal patterns. In particular, it confronts patients' passivity – i.e. their wishes to have others do things to or for them. Means of facilitating involvement include 'open doors', patient-led groups, negotiation of therapeutic goals, mandatory participation in milieu groups and collective activities. Placing a high emphasis on the interpersonal meaning of symptomatic behaviours (such as deliberate self-harm) conveys to patients the belief that such aspects are within their control and thus their responsibility. Therefore, patients who talk about their 'needs' not being met may find these being re-framed (by staff or fellow patients) as unrealistic or inappropriate 'wants' (Gunderson 1978). The treatment aims to reinforce ego strengths by encouraging social skills and developing feelings of competence. Along with this, patients are expected to relinquish or subordinate private, antisocial or unrealistic wishes. Wards that emphasize involvement will have a distribution of power and decision-making, some blurring of traditional roles and an emphasis on the group processes of cooperation, compromise, confrontation and conformity.

Cecelia's behaviour on the acute inpatient ward reveals that she does little that is constructive and staff have little time to confront, constructively, her lack of engagement. Her challenging behaviour elicits a predictable 'containing' response, which appears only to reinforce more such behaviour. For reasons that are not understood, her destructive behaviour ceases and discharge follows imminently. Cecelia does not appear to have a sense of herself as an effective 'agent', except in relation to her destructive and dangerous behaviour and the impulsive taking of her own discharge.

Validation

'Validation' refers to the processes and activities that occur in the hospital ward setting that affirm a patient's individuality. Patients are validated through the staff's attention to a range of aspects of individualized treatment programming: respect for a patient's right to some privacy, to be alone; frequent exploratory one-to-one talks; an emphasis on issues concerning separation and loss; and encouraging individuals to operate at the limits of their known capacities, including 'opportunities to fail'. This requires the staff's acceptance and understanding of patients' incompetence, regressions or symptoms as meaningful personal expressions. They need to know that such aspects should not be ignored but nor do they necessarily have to be eradicated. Validation, which takes many forms, might include encouraging patients to talk about their hallucinations and to consider them as expressive of some unclear but important aspect of themselves. The patient who self-harms might be asked to recall a recent episode of the behaviour and explain why it had made sense to act in that way (Gunderson 1978). Unfortunately, this ideal is not achieved in respect of Cecelia. It appears to be only her negative self-image that is 'validated' by the vicious circle of readmission.

13.5 Practical application of Gunderson's five principles: tips for ward managers

In terms of practical application, the five principles of the therapeutic milieu are overlapping rather than mutually exclusive constructs. Key aspects of each principle however, are listed below.

Containment

This principle refers to external controls required to assure physical safety and security. Continual risk assessment and management of the physical environment is required with judgements and decisions made about whether doors are locked or open, whether windows are secure and whether furniture and fittings require to be fixed or free-standing. The availability of sharp objects, for example, is another area for continual risk assessment and management. The balance between maintaining physical safety and security and producing a culture of non-thinking and institutional practices which are potentially anti-therapeutic, is an important containment task required of ward managers.

Support

This principle refers to clinical interventions which reduce anxiety while increasing self-esteem. Practical application requires nurse–patient allocation on each shift. Allocated nurses would work alongside patients, rather than, say, waiting for incidents or distress to be manifest before intervening. The allocated nurse who is working alongside supports the patient through their day-to-day activities, providing praise when the patient is coping well, while discussing and problem-solving with the patient when they experience struggles. Organizing communal activites whereby nurses and patients work side by side on a project is a helpful form of support. Providing support in this way takes the focus away from the nurse providing reactive interventions and militates against the institutional risk of the patient engaging in destructive behaviours as a means of gaining input from nurses.

Structure

This principle refers to the provision of a predictable routine and environment, ordering the patient's day. A clear ward programme is required. Also, predictability with regard to staff responses to expressions of

distress and related problematic behaviours is required. With regard to ordering the day, a half hour morning 'plan of the day' is a helpful structure to include on the ward. Patients and staff come together for half and hour and plan individual programmes and ward group activities for the day. An 'end of the day' meeting is an effective way of patients and staff coming together to reflect on the day, provide individual feedback on progress and plan to resolve any outstanding issues. On an individual basis, effective therapeutic structure is offered by the range of available tools for working proactively towards wellness and recovery by identifying triggers, early warning signs and effective interventions, thereby avoiding relapse, encouraging control and greater self-management by patients.

Involvement

This principle refers to including patients in the interpersonal environment to promote strengths and develop coping strategies. The central forum in the therapeutic environment facilitating the practical application of this principle is the ward community meeting which may offer a space for patients and staff to work together to address domestic issues on the ward but also may be used to examine and problem-solve interpersonal dynamics within the ward environment. It is important that the community meeting is attended by all members of the multi-disciplinary team and not just nurses and patients. The community meeting may be a forum for facilitating patient involvement by viewing feedback on patient experience which may be collected by a tool such as the Patient Experience Tracker or from a ward suggestion box. This process would enable patients and staff to develop action plans together for improving patient experience of the ward.

Validation

This principle refers to providing attention to individual needs with respect to feelings and rights. Understanding how problematic or risk behaviours may be better framed as expressions of distress by a person, who for one reason or another cannot verbally express such feelings, is a first step towards providing a validating therapeutic environment. The nurse's task is to be sufficiently attuned to their patient's experiences to be able to work with them to resolve distress. Providing time is essential to enabling the person to resume thinking and to talk about what is worrying them. Understanding the impact of hospitalization on the person and their worries about the future are also basic and essential to providing a validating environment. Key though, is communicating to the patients that they are entitled to feel as they do although it may also be important to work together to identify better ways to express their feelings.

 ## 13.6 Unconscious impediments to effective health care delivery

In the context of an inpatient setting, by definition involving a number of patients and staff, the need to cater for the differing needs of individual patients is potentially problematic. In effect, giving to one can mean taking from another and, due to the priority that crises demand, time that might be spent in conversation with patients is easily eroded. However, even where time is available and patients are motivated, the latter may not be able to confide, for a variety of reasons, including high emotional arousal, fear of stigma, shame, humiliation and feelings of vulnerability. Many patients, such as Cecelia, are unable to speak openly about themselves. Instead, they present themselves as if as a puzzle for the professional to solve, without their own active participation.

Staff may experience this passivity, and lack of engagement, as exasperating. However, patients often have no concept of a shared enterprise of any kind. Their previous experience of the world and of other people has not exposed them to any such mutually respectful encounters. This situation may go unrecognized, with the staff member assuming a level of engagement which is actually missing. It may be only once the 'therapeutic' relationship has become seriously derailed or undermined (e.g. with some violation of the usual professional relationship boundary) that the professional discovers that something is, and has been, amiss. Often relevant training and supervision of complex cases and problematic encounters is not available to those in most need of it. Knowing something of Cecelia's early life history can shed some light on her presentation.

> ### Thinking Space 13.2
>
> Read the case study on Cecelia's early life. What insights does knowledge of this give to her current behaviour on the ward?

Case Study

Cecelia's early life history

Cecelia is the eldest of nine children. Her mother also suffered from bipolar disorder and was frequently hospitalized during Cecelia's childhood. During those times, her father and the other siblings expected Cecelia to stand in for her mother. This involved her doing the bulk of the housework and shopping, with the result that her attendance at school was patchy and her academic achievement poor. However, she undertook the maternal role with energy and not without some success, albeit she was authoritarian, strict and occasionally violent to those in her charge. Partly on account of this, and deterioration in her behaviour at school, Cecelia was placed in care. While there she was subjected to physical, sexual and emotional abuse on various occasions and in various placements.

When her mother was home from hospital, Cecelia was returned to the family setting, which was inevitably chaotic, with all the children (unsettled and insecure after yet another period of upheaval and on occasions, trauma) vying for their mother's attention. The mother was never able to meet the children's needs. Nevertheless, the only periods when Cecelia felt hopeful were when she was awaiting to return home to her family having been in care. Once returned, however, she soon experienced the familiar feelings of insecurity, derived from being part of such a dysfunctional family.

Feedback to Thinking Space 13.2

The effects of Cecelia's past abuse and neglect have left her scarred emotionally (as well as physically) and with an extremely limited behavioural and psychological repertoire to deploy in relation to other people. Her style of asking for help is confusing and misleading. Her mode of interacting with authority figures, including ward staff and police, is unconsciously designed to keep them at bay–at a safe emotional distance. In doing so, Cecelia's inner self is kept private and hence potentially safer. However, this does not permit her any access to emotional closeness, which she both longs for but fears.

13.7 Establishing and maintaining therapeutic alliances in the ward setting

Case Study

John

John was admitted to a medium secure mental health service in his 30s. He was suffering from severe depression and had been drinking heavily for a number of years. He was in and out of prison, on account of offences involving petty theft and acts of minor violence. During the course of his imprisonment, the quality of relationship with his long-term female partner deteriorated, as John became convinced that she was being unfaithful to him. After a particularly large alcohol binge, shortly after having been released from prison, John carried out a frenzied knife attack on her, leaving her paralysed. He had no recollection of the assault.

In the medium secure ward setting, John was difficult to engage. He preferred a solitary existence. On the surface, he appeared to function well, being self-sufficient and having good personal care skills. However, he did not talk about how he felt. With his primary nurse, he spent most of the sessions looking down at the floor and did not make eye contact. He did not provide anything the nurse felt she could work with. She found the individual sessions with John excruciating and persecutory. The whole team treating John felt immense sympathy for his ex-partner, who was also languishing in a long-term hospital bed, and a sense of grievance on her behalf, for the injury their (perpetrator) 'patient' had caused. John evoked little or no sympathy from them. Most believed that he should have been serving a prison sentence. All felt stuck, with treatment achieving nothing.

It was difficult for staff to make any empathic connection with John. However, they had not considered whether, unwittingly, they were playing a part in the therapeutic stalemate. It was only after a presentation of John's case, by a new and relatively junior member of the nursing staff, who had undertaken a particularly thorough summary of his copious case files, that the team began to think more deeply about what was going on, between him and them, and were able to take a step back.

The nurse's presentation revealed that John's mother had suffered from alcohol problems for many years before and after John was born. When he was young, his mother was unable to put his needs before her own need to drink. She managed to cut herself off from John's vulnerability and dependence on her, experiencing his cries for care as deliberately persecutory on his part. This instilled in him an inappropriate degree of 'independence' (actually, withdrawal from authentic emotional contact) from early on. John's father was kindly towards him but the father's priority was to try to pacify and placate his wife. When older, John would find himself drawn into this dynamic and believing his mother's version of events, that he was a nuisance and the cause of her 'bad moods' and hence her need to escape by intoxicating herself. John's fundamental sense of himself was as a person who was evil.

Privately, John believed that he would inevitably damage anybody with whom he tried to get close. Except when under the influence of alcohol, he was solitary and uncommunicative. This pattern was repeated while in hospital. Despite the fact of his lonely, loveless life being documented in his case notes, John was not seen as a person who needed or merited care. This replicated his experience with his mother, who was not able to acknowledge the needs he had. It is possible that John's emotional inaccessibility was too much for the ward nurses to bear, especially his primary nurse. Rather than trying to understand what John's introversion and isolation might represent, it was as if John's nursing team set about confirming the belief that there was nothing wrong with him. Worse, their negative attitudes and avoidant behaviour confirmed his belief that he was too much trouble for others to bother with, reinforcing his existing impoverished self-image.

Thinking Space 13.3

Have you worked with any patients with whom there appeared to be a therapeutic stalemate? What were the reasons for this?

13.8 Recognizing and dealing with destructive processes

Developed in the context of psychoanalysis, 'therapeutic alliance' is a concept that recognizes that the quality of the professional–patient relationship should not be taken for granted (Greenson 1967). The concept refers to a more healthy, 'rational relationship' between patient and therapist (alongside a more 'neurotic', unhealthy one), which makes it possible for the patient to work purposefully in therapy. Within a psychiatric inpatient ward, this more rational relationship, between staff and patient, is often more of an aspiration than an expectation. However, enabling patients to perform their role as patient 'rationally' is a relevant task. It can include information-sharing, for example, so that patients understand what is expected of them, so they get the help they need, which can foster the patient's active involvement in their treatment. However, many factors can interfere with the achievement of this apparently modest goal.

Identifying negative aspects and processes may not be easy because they derive not only from the deliberate, conscious behaviour of people in the inpatient situation but also from factors that come from the unconscious part of their minds. The following destructive processes and phenomena have been described: the destructiveness of the isolated individual; destructive group phenomena; the contribution of staff to destructiveness; and destructive structural manifestations (Roberts 1980).

A patient may carry out actual acts of destruction, aimed at the fabric of the building or their own body, and rarely towards another member of the inpatient ward. Often this behaviour is considered to reflect alienation, which the patient experiences anew within the treatment setting. Certain patients may be especially at risk of isolation: the new patient, the scapegoat (perhaps a patient from a minority ethnic group), the psychotic patient, those with schizoid personality features, the borderline patient, those who repeatedly act out early rejection experiences, and those dependent on alcohol and drugs (Roberts 1980). Cecelia and John both fall into a number of these categories. However, according to Roberts, their behaviour and that of their respective ward staff should not be construed as being solely due to their conscious motivation but to unconscious factors.

Unconscious factors derive, in part, from the operation of defence mechanisms which are deployed involuntarily to or minimize anxiety that would otherwise threaten the psychological integrity of the individual. The effect of the unconscious defensive operation is to distort the 'reality' of the situation, at least by degree. Certain defences, such as 'splitting', 'projection' and 'denial' exert a far-reaching and distorting effect (Kernberg 1984). Often this serves to simplify perceptions. Denial, for example, can remove the anxiety associated with dealing with a painful dilemma, such as being expected to be sympathetic to John, who had been so violent. Defence mechanisms often function in concert. Denial, splitting and projection together therefore could account for staff viewing John as being 'all bad', the perpetrator, and his ex-partner as essentially 'all good', the victim. These perceptions

are clearly oversimplifications or distortions of the true state of affairs.

In the multi-disciplinary staff team, the phenomenon of splitting can result in simple polarizations, often painful and marked by extreme animosity, around a particular contentious issue. Allies to the opposing factions may collect and lead to a paralysis of usual, more cohesive, team functioning. According to Roberts (1980), other manifestations may follow in the wake of splitting, such as 'sub-culturing', 'idealization' and 'splits in leadership'. The last can be particularly destructive in its effect. The leaders' capacity for thinking, which might be directed at solving the difficulties within their team, is otherwise expended in a futile battle between themselves. As above, other staff may be drawn into the battle or elect to retreat as excited or helpless onlookers.

Roberts also considers the role of 'idealization', another important unconscious defence mechanism, the effect of which may be especially hard to recognize for people working in the caring professions. Its operation can cause staff to try to live up to unrealistic expectations placed on them by patients. They may believe that they have the authority or skills to achieve them. Consequently, they can overwork, becoming stressed and eventually even become mentally ill themselves. All of this can foster the development of further destructive splitting processes and so contribute to the breakdown of cooperative working among different members of the team, leading to an inconsistent delivery of the overall treatment programme for a patient, hence a poorer prognosis.

Roberts considers structural manifestations of destructive processes, identifying three main conditions: 'autolysis', 'crystallization' and 'encapsulation'. Autolysis represents the breaking down of internal structures, such as the dissolution of time boundaries for the treatment programme or a lack of clarity between the respective roles of staff and patients. Crystallization reflects an internal organization that has become so rigid and entangled that change is impossible. Flexible functioning suffers; for example, the ward is unable to adapt itself to move swiftly to containment mode in the face of an emergency. Encapsulation is the situation where the institution has stopped interacting effectively with its environment. All of these states can appear within a given part of an organization, for example a hospital ward. In the case of specialist or autonomous units, closure may ensue. In other situations, where closure is not so readily conceivable, the consequence is likely to be an increase in serious untoward incidents. The latter may be the first recognizable signs that destructive processes are operating at an unacceptable level (for a fuller account of relevant aspects please see Campling *et al.* 2004).

 ## 13.9 Unconscious roots of untherapeutic practice

Like Roberts, others have argued that the problematic functioning of health care staff often results from 'unconscious processes' (see Hinshelwood 2002). Therefore, if meaningful behavioural change for the better is to be achieved, health care organizations must address these processes (Obholzer 1994). Obholzer advocates a psychoanalytic approach to understand the difficulties experienced by health care workers in their interpersonal interactions with patients. As the group whose work takes place predominantly in the 'public' areas of the ward environment, nursing is the profession that has been the subject of (mainly psychoanalytic) observational studies (Singanoglou 1987; Donati 1989; Chiesa 1993).

Nurses in mental health services have been found to experience difficulty sustaining interpersonal engagement with patients. In a seminal study, Menzies-Lyth developed the application of a psychoanalytic approach to the evaluation of a general nursing service within a large hospital. She described how many practices were not determined by the needs of patients but were unconsciously applied by nurses to defend them against the emotional effects of close interpersonal proximity to human suffering and death (Menzies-Lyth 1988). She found that the practices, which were unconsciously developed to

defend against relevant anxiety actually impeded the delivery of effective nursing care.

Chiesa (1993) conducted a series of psychoanalytic observations in an acute mental health admission ward and found that nurses tended to neutralize any potentially meaningful human interactions between themselves and the patients. He observed that nurses employed continual motor activity as a 'manic' defence against anxiety provoked by their proximity to the psychological distress patients experienced. Sinanoglou (1987), studying nurses' attitudes in a mental health unit, also concluded that excessive motor activity was employed by nurses to defend against anxieties provoked by making emotional and interpersonal contact with psychological distress associated with patients' psychotic states. Other observational studies have drawn on the perspective of unconscious processes of anxiety and defence to understand the phenomena of nurses' impoverished interpersonal interactions with patients. Donati's observations within a 'chronic psychiatric ward' concluded that nurses made 'high use of inappropriate, defensive maneuvers' (Donati 1989: 42), in response to anxiety associated with their therapeutic impotence in the face of patients' enduring conditions). Other defensive nursing practices were the maintaining of superficial, ritualized interpersonal contacts with patients and ensuring that all feelings of failure and poor self-image remained located in the patients, to raise the nurses' own self-image.

A number of researchers have observed that nurses are less likely to engage interpersonally with patients who present with certain types of behaviours: poor compliance with clinical programmes (Rosenthal *et al.* 1980); demandingness and complaining (Sarosi 1968; Stockwell 1972; Armitage 1980); over-dependence on nurses (Rosenthal *et al.* 1980); and rule-breaking (Spitzer and Sobel 1962; Armitage 1980). Both Cecelia's and John's behaviour would certainly fit into the first category – poor compliance. Altschul's (1972) investigation of nurse–patient relationships by observing interactions between patients and nurses in an acute mental health service found that the patients who nurses engaged most with were more likely to enjoy a good treatment outcome. However, this study also noted that nurses lacked a theoretical framework for organizing, understanding and interpreting their relationships with patients and that they tended to have more contacts and to spend more time with non-neurotic patients (Altschul 1972). Interestingly, it has been shown that an increase in the quality of interpersonal care provided by nurses is associated with higher rates of recovery from illness (Stockwell 1972).

Overall, the (limited) literature paints a picture of impoverished interpersonal communications and interactions between patients and mental health nurses. This has been construed as reflecting unconscious defensive manoeuvres against anxiety, which enable professional survival in the nursing role and the maintenance of self-esteem. The anxiety stems from a combination of the patients' disturbing presentations and the nurses' own (individual and collective) impotence. There is no reason to suppose that any other professional group exposed to the ward environment for such prolonged periods would fare better or operate differently than those in the nursing profession. However it might be that the training, support and supervision of other professional groups allow them greater access to useful theoretical frameworks with which to 'organize' their relationships with their patients.

Thinking Space 13.4

Consider with colleagues the extent to which the ward in which you work, or to which you are connected, embodies the principles and practice of a therapeutic milieu. The following checklist might be helpful:

- Do staff and patients in the ward know what the enterprise is trying to achieve?
- Do patients know how the ward is organized and what ingredients or treatment sessions they might encounter in any given week?
- Are staff clear and explicit with patients about the rules that apply, what is expected of them and what supports are available to help them flourish?
- To what extent do staff from the same and different disciplines work collaboratively with each other and with patients?
- Does the ward regime empower patients and provide them with sufficient opportunities to voice their concerns?
- Is there an explicit statement about the values of the inpatient setting, such as abhorrence of racism and sexism?
- Do staff have regular reflective practice or supervision sessions whereby the unconscious processes at work in the milieu are clarified?

If nursing (and other) staff are to be facilitated to improve the quality of their demanding work within the pressurized and stressful environment of the inpatient ward, they require appropriate training, support and supervision (see also Kurtz 2005). This will vary according to the nature and function of the particular ward. However, without such input, it is hard to imagine that staff could be in a state of mind to develop new perspectives on their work – to have new ways of 'organizing' their interactions with patients. They need this if they are to incorporate an understanding of the role of unconscious processes which influence the process of health care, and translate the new concepts into practical changes in their individual behaviour and the functioning of the teams of which they are members.

> ### Thinking Space 13.5
>
> What practical steps might be taken to increase the therapeutic potential of the inpatient environment? In collaboration with others, draw up an action plan for implementation.

13.10 Application of therapeutic milieu priniciples to outpatient/community settings

With the closure of many inpatient beds – acute, long-stay and rehabilitation – a much greater proportion of psychiatric patients is treated in outpatient or community settings. While outpatients whose needs are relatively straightforward probably get these met satisfactorily (and increasingly via primary care-based services), those with more complex needs fare less well. Among such patient populations are those with dual diagnosis, severe personality disorder, drug addiction, serious eating disorders and learning disability. The list is a long one and, for these groups at least, there is a need to attempt to provide in a dispersed form something in the community that was previously available within the therapeutic milieu.

Managing therapeutic resources outside a hospital requires much planning; probably more than to achieve the same aim within hospital. This is because an integrated package of care, involving a range of professionals and often a range of modalities is needed but with a team which is virtual – i.e. it does meet together on a regular basis. Indeed, the 'team' may not know or agree on its own membership! For most psychiatric patients with complex needs there

is reason to believe that successful treatments (NIMHE 2003) have the following characteristics:

- set out clear aims;
- specify the treatment methods to achieve these aims;
- are consistent during phases of transition from one (part of) a service to another;
- use skilled and motivated professionals;
- have good inter-communication among all those involved;
- are supported educationally and managerially; and
- pay particular attention to the termination phase of treatment.

In practice, however, it is hard to achieve the above, given the geographical dispersal of human resources and the need for all those involved to collaborate, respecting and valuing one another's contributions to the shared therapeutic venture. Patients, such as Cecelia, who might have been catered for previously as inpatients, sometimes over extended periods (months or years), now find themselves seeing a variety of professionals, often in a range of different settings and locations. Like Cecelia and John, many patients are unable to articulate their needs, presenting themselves as a problem to be solved by professionals. Their oppositional or passive presentations may alienate them from professionals who are more comfortable with an insightful and compliant patient. Professionals working outside of the hospital will also face their share of frustrations. Like their inpatient staff counterparts, they may not have ways of 'organizing' their transactions with their patients, so as to avoid some of the pitfalls associated with falling prey to the operation of defence mechanisms (e.g. splitting), which complicate management of the case and can also impair necessary collaborative working. A crucial clinical task therefore is to identify when and how the clinical transaction with a given patient is going wrong – deviating from the straightforward path that was originally envisaged (Norton and McGauley 1999).

Case Study

Cecelia's care in the community

Cecelia's 'local' inpatient team found themselves at loggerheads with the 'crisis team', which functioned as a gateway (or, as the local team viewed it, a barrier) to inpatient wards. This was because the inpatient team also operated within the community but could not directly admit its patients to its ward! The latter had to be referred for an assessment by the crisis team. All proceeded smoothly, when the crisis team agreed with the local team's assessment – i.e. the need for Cecelia to be admitted. But at other times, it worked out differently and there were more of the latter outcomes, when Cecelia was not admitted.

There had been sufficient of the 'disagreeable' outcomes between the two teams to produce a barely concealed hostility, which Cecelia almost certainly noticed. She told her community psychiatric nurse (CPN) she was unsure who was looking after her at any given time while out of hospital, and that she did not know to whom to turn when she felt herself to be in a crisis. Wittingly or unwittingly (i.e. unconsciously), Cecelia added fuel to the fire of division that existed between the local and crisis teams. She would praise the staff member she was speaking to but be scathing of the efforts of staff who were not present to contradict or otherwise defend their reputations. In her case, when it came to the point of giving a date for discharge from hospital, there was often disagreement about which team was better placed to deliver this. The plan to give a date would be thus postponed and Cecelia, as was her norm, took her own discharge, without agreement about the details of follow-up. On one occasion, in this state of limbo, in the community, Cecelia took a substantial overdose, necessitating admission to a general hospital. She spent a number of weeks there, having almost died.

The senior clinicians involved with Cecelia's case felt guilty about the overdose. They thought, not altogether unreasonably, that their indecision and divisions could have exerted a negative influence on their mutual patient's mental state, increasing her suicidality. A psychotherapist was asked to provide a 'second opinion'. She interviewed the patient to provide a psychodynamic assessment that might inform the combined approach of the two teams. Discussion followed, as the formulation was more or less accepted as capturing the main elements. These included, in particular, how staff felt misled, manipulated and rendered ineffectual by the patient and how Cecelia was feeling rejected, confused and abandoned, believing that neither team had her interests at heart.

Commentary

Further meetings enabled the different 'sides' to see things from the other's perspective. At least for a period, Cecelia was more settled in the community and there was a greater sense of working together for the professionals involved. The revised care plan, with her involvement, also included referral to a creative therapy group to help her focus on some of her strengths ('validation') and also to be exposed to forming some more healthy social contacts ('involvement').

Thinking Space 13.6

Think about the challenges you have experienced or observed in forging collaborative working relationships across teams, professions and services.

With patients such as Cecelia, there is a need to create and maintain a network of all the relevant individuals who are involved. This requires the patient's knowledge and permission and should include key players in the patient's own family or social network. In this instance Cecelia had no significant people living locally and her family had only been in intermittent contact. She had kept her condition and circumstances from them, a pattern of secrecy that had started in her childhood.

Information-sharing and clinical networking

Engagement

In the community as in the inpatient therapeutic milieu, staff need to secure the patient's active engagement in their treatment – involvement. This is achieved through education, discussion and negotiation, when the patient is not highly anxious and the professional has adequate time and are not anxious nor too frustrated or angry with the patient. Education, part of Gunderson's 'structure', refers to information being imparted to enable the patient to understand their *responsibilities* – what they should and should not do and also their *rights*, especially in terms of what they can and cannot expect of professionals.

An effective treatment contract can form part of the 'structure' of treatment. It is usually characterized by the following (after Miller 1990):

- being mutually agreed by all parties, including patient and/or carer(s);
- having clear specified responsibilities for all parties;
- bearing a minimum of detail so that it can be readily recalled, when needed;

- providing for alternative strategies for the client to manage intolerable feelings;
- providing positive reinforcement for the client's adaptive change;
- is strictly enforced, but allowing for reasonable negotiated modification;
- fosters a therapeutic alliance.

A contract can fail for many reasons, including it being unduly restrictive of the patient, becoming a substitute for therapeutic activity, and being used by the professional as a punishment, even unwittingly. But a contract can serve as a useful reminder if the actions of one or both parties depart from what was previously agreed.

Information

How relevant information is collected and disseminated varies according to the circumstances of the case but general principles remain the same (see Norton and Vince 2002). In each case the responsible senior professionals need to ensure there is an adequate network, with rules governing the frequency of contact and what should be communicated to whom, if an emergency arises, which could be predicted. Such a network is ideally in place as soon as it is apparent that the case is complex. Otherwise it is likely that it will have to be hastily put together in the face of an unanticipated crisis. The latter is more difficult, as was the case with Cecelia. It also needs to be recognized that collaborative working can be undermined by a range of factors and influences, including the negative effects of unconscious defensive mechanisms.

Information about treatment and the importance of a therapeutic alliance should be imparted with regard to the patient's intellectual, psychological and social circumstances, as well as the overall complexity of the clinical task and treatment package. Going over with a patient what had previously been agreed in a team meeting, and providing a written summary of decisions, can be important to ensure clarity and reinforce commitment.

Information might usefully include facts about the patient's condition as well as what has been agreed about their treatment. Ideally, it conveys the logic of the latter, given the former. The patient's ambivalence to treatment and their difficulty with forming a trusting relationship (possibly on the basis of low self-esteem, fear of stigma and the rekindling of feelings of insecurity) might also be acknowledged, where this is considered to be helpful. The patient should be made aware of the limits of confidentiality – i.e. the conditions under which it will be broken, in what way, and to whom. This should happen at an early stage, before the necessity to do so has been encountered. The relationship network should be monitored to ascertain, as far as possible, the authenticity of the patient's engagement, which should not be seen as 'all or nothing' or 'once and for all'. The client should be informed there will be regular reviews of his or her care, possibly in addition to any statutory requirements. Professionals need to form a shared opinion about the quality of the engagement of their shared client. This usually requires at least some face-to-face meetings of the key personnel.

Regular communication

Regular communication among the relevant professionals, in addition to the monitoring of the therapeutic alliance, is needed to judge if treatment goals are being achieved. This may not be easy. First, the client may provide differing accounts to different 'points' in the network. Second, even if the same account is given to each part of the network, professionals may differ in how they construe it – progress, regress, status quo! Third, sometimes it appears, in relation to the client's gross behaviour, that the patient is not changing. However, seemingly subtle signs, such as the quality of the therapeutic alliance, reflected by the level of the patient's disclosure or emotional candour, can be decisive.

Realizing that 'splits' can develop among those providing treatment in complex cases can also reveal the patient's internal world, and such splits should not therefore be construed as simply negative (Gabbard 1988). Apparently disparate views can sometimes be imaginatively integrated when both 'sides' can be held, with neither party battling

to establish supremacy over the other. Such a mature state of affairs, however, is difficult to achieve, especially where there is high anxiety over a patient's violent potential or over the prospect of blame being apportioned to the professional in the event of an untoward incident (see Davies 1995). Mutually respectful relationships between professionals can have a containing effect on the patient, who may be unused to having people working concertedly with their interests at heart. This became the situation with John and the two staff 'sides' and also with Cecelia, as the 'local' and 'crisis' parties began to appreciate the partial views that they had held.

Terminating treatment

Endings of treatment are often difficult with complex cases, as with Cecelia and John, where many professionals have been involved or where the treatment process has been lengthy. Such situations require substantial attention to effective communication. Meetings between the professionals involved might need to be *increased* in frequency and it should be expected that some patients will regress, with a return of earlier symptoms. There might be disappointment expressed by the patient (or their carers or significant others) that they are 'back at square one'. However, in cases of a relatively sustained and identifiable therapeutic process, rather than abrupt or magical changes for the better, and where there is no particular adverse recent circumstance to account for apparent deterioration, the professionals should not simply agree/collude with the patient's apparently negative evaluation. Regression is a phenomenon that is frequently observed at the latter stages of lengthy treatments, particularly with non-psychotic patients. It may arise solely out of increasing anxiety about the uncertainty of the future, beyond therapy. It is important therefore that the patient is helped to sift the relevant evidence and helped to arrive at a balanced judgement about what they have achieved and what problem areas remain, which might require further work in the future or be endured.

> *Thinking Space 13.7*
>
> Are there one or more patients on your ward who might be alienated from care and treatment? If so, consider with colleagues whether the patient(s) developmental history might make their social behaviour more understandable so that they might feel more socially included.

13.11   Conclusion

Inpatient wards form only one part of the whole mental health care system. As the whole evolves and develops, for instance, in response to policy directives and resource reallocation, so the parts are required to change and realign. The process is dynamic and ongoing. A review of mental health nursing by the Chief Nursing Officer (CNO) for England identified the need for nurses to promote the empowerment of patients and their social inclusion through the development of positive therapeutic relationships. The report *From Values to Action* (DH 2006) describes the set of values and principles that underpin the so-called 'recovery model' (see Chapter 5). Recovery is not so much viewed as necessarily a return to life as it was before illness but to a life experienced as worthwhile which might depend upon the development of new expectations, skills and ways of living. To assist in this process, nurses and other professionals have to approach their roles with hope and optimism regarding patients' capacities to make progress.

At present, in the UK (though the system differs in different locations), overall bed numbers within the inpatient system are fewer than previously. This is one consequence of developing more community-based services, with the corresponding transfer of financial and other resources to enable assertive outreach, crisis and home treatment, and early intervention in psychosis services. The resulting increase in the proportion of ward patients compulsorily detained, with little scope to disperse and rehouse them in wards that might represent a potentially therapeutic mix, means that it is difficult for staff to retain their therapeutic optimism. Staff are more taxed than formerly to provide a therapeutic, as well as a custodial, environment. There is often tension between 'therapists' who visit the ward (or are visited by patients from the ward in pursuit of their therapy) and those staff (mostly nurses and care assistants) who must remain anchored to the inpatient environment. The latter groups of staff are destined to spend the duration of their shift, at least potentially, in close proximity to very disabled, disturbed and socially deteriorated patients. Their personal and interpersonal coping strategies can be tested to the limit and their psychological functioning and mental health can be impaired in the process.

According to some researchers, unconscious processes account for at least some of the failure of concerted and therapeutic action of staff within inpatient settings. Some studies have found that nursing staff defend themselves against contact with their patients by a range of means, which are not usually deliberate, for example keeping on the move, blaming patients and falling out with colleagues. There is no reason to believe that nurses are different from other health care professionals or that their responses are anything but natural human defences deployed in the face of overwhelming emotional difficulty. The fictitious case studies presented in this chapter illustrate the relative failure of many inpatient milieus to do more than contain their patients, with an inability to provide higher functions.

Positive change in ward environments requires training, support and supervision to enable ward staff to understand the processes that operate when extremely disturbed and disordered patients are housed with staff who are not necessarily appropriately trained or experienced (Kurtz 2005) and when their role responsibilities are not clear or clearly understood in relation to those of colleagues (Burns 2000). The consequences of this mismatch, of patient requirement and staff resource, can be damaging to all parties. This situation can be improved if staff, individually and collectively, are aided to reflect on their work. To effect this, protected time and space are required, so that staff's anxiety levels are low enough to enable learning to take place. Training is also needed to facilitate staff to embed new skills, through the provision of supervision, to change overall ward functioning. In this way, some of the 'higher functions' might be able to be reintroduced to wards and integrated during patients' inpatient stay.

By providing a safe transfer from the ward environment to the community, higher functions, required to support patients to 'recover' can be deployed. However, even within the community, coordinated functioning between different health care disciplines and agencies is hard to achieve. Just like ward-based staff, community-based workers also fall prey to the stress of working with patients, such as Cecelia and John, whose needs are complex and behaviours challenging to staff. Sources of anxiety may differ; for example, the lone professional may believe they could be blamed more readily for a 'critical untoward incident', since their own role and influence is more clearly identifiable than for inpatient staff. Splitting is prevalent. Staff training, support and supervision is needed so that its destructive effect on 'team' functioning is recognized and dealt with creatively. Otherwise, the Cecelias and Johns of the psychiatric world will continue to find that they are little helped by the services offered to them and the staff working with them will have low job satisfaction and may even find their own mental health deteriorating.

In summary the main points of this chapter are:

- It is challenging to provide both safe custody and therapeutic care in mental health inpa-

tient wards because of the acuity of patients' mental health related problems and the need to provide for the collective as well as individual needs.

- Ideally the inpatient ward provides patients with long-standing complex needs with an interpersonal environment which is both safe and does not reinforce maladaptive coping strategies; however, such an environment is not easy to achieve.

- Consideration of Gunderson's five functions of mental health care (containment, support, structure, involvement and validation) enacted according to the prevailing needs of the ward as a whole can help nurses to provide an integrated, coordinated, patient centred treatment package across different care settings.

- We provide tips for ward managers which may help them enact Gunderson's five functions in their busy wards.

- Identifying processes which disrupt therapeutic alliances between nurses and patients is not easy because they derive not only from the deliberate and conscious behaviour of people in inpatient wards, but also from processes of which they are unaware.

- With the move to a community-based mental health service there is a need to provide in a dispersed form something that was previously available in inpatient settings for patients with complex needs. Characteristics of successful treatment programmes for this patient group have been identified.

Annotated bibliography

Campling, P., Davies, S. and Farquarson, G. (2004) *From Toxic Institutions to Therapeutic Environments*. London: Gaskell.
A very useful text which describes the processes that support the development of effective therapeutic milieus and those which underpin anti-therapeutic inpatient services.

Hinshelwood, R.D. (2002) Abusive help – helping abuse: the psychodynamic impact of severe personality disorder on caring institutions, *Criminal Behaviour and Mental Health*, 12: 20–30.
A paper which lucidly describes the interpersonal processes that lead to people becoming alienated from mental health care.

Kurtz, A. (2005) The needs of staff who care for people with a diagnosis of personality disorder who are considered to be a risk to others, *Journal of Forensic Psychiatry and Psychology,* **16(2): 399–422.**
A detailed, thorough account of what services require to have in place for staff, including nurses, if they are to work effectively with people who have a diagnosis of personality disorder and who present a risk to others.

Pflaffin, F. and Adshead, G. (2003) *A Matter of Security: The application of attachment theory to forensic psychiatry and psychotherapy.* **London: JKP.**
A book of edited papers applying attachment theory to the forensic context. This is a very useful book and makes a lot of reference to the institutional setting.

References

Abroms, G.M. (1969) Defining milieu therapy, *Archives of General Psychiatry*, 21: 553–5.

Altschul, A. (1972) *Patient Nurse Interaction.* Edinburgh: Churchill Livingstone.

Anthony, W.A. (1993) Recovery from mental illness : the guiding vision of the mental health service system in the 1990s, *Psychosocial Rehabilitation Journal*, 16: 11–23.

Armitage, S. (1980) Non compliant recipients of health care, *Nursing Times*, 76: 1–3.

Badia, E.D. (1989) Group-as-a-whole concepts and the therapeutic milieu on the inpatient psychiatric unit, *GROUP*, 13(3 & 4).

Baker, S. (2000) *Environmentally Friendly?: Patients' views of conditions on psychiatric wards.* London: MIND.

Beadsmore, A., Moore, C., Muijen, M. et al. (1998) *Acute Problems: A survey of the quality of care in acute psychiatric wards.* London: Sainsbury Centre Mental Health Publications.

Burns, T. (2000) The legacy of the therapeutic community practice in modern community health services, *Therapeutic Communities* 21(3): 165–74.

Campling, P., Davies, S. and Farquarson, G. (2004) *From Toxic Institutions to Therapeutic Environments.* London: Gaskell.

Chiesa, M. (2000) At a crossroad between institutional and community psychiatry: an acute admission ward, in R.D. Hinshelwood and W. Skogstad (eds) *Observing Organisations: Anxiety, defence and culture in health care.* London: Routledge.

Davies, R. (1995) The inter-disciplinary network and the internal world of the offender, in C. Cordess and M. Cox (eds) *Forensic Psychotherapy.* London: Jessica Kingsley.

DH (Department of Health) (2002) *Mental Health Policy Implementation Guide: Adult acute inpatient care provision.* London: DH.

DH (Department of Health) (2006) *From Values to Action: The chief nursing officer's review of mental health nursing.* London: DH.

Donati, F. (1989) A psychodynamic observer in a chronic psychiatric ward, *British Journal of Psychotherapy*, 5: 317–29.

Ford, R., Durcan, G., Warner, L., Hardy, P. and Muijen, M. (1998) One day survey by the Mental Health Act Commission of acute adult psychiatric inpatient wards in England and Wales, *British Medical Journal*, 317: 1279–83.

Gabbard, G. (1986) The treatment of the 'special' patient in a psychoanalysis hospital, *International Review of Psychoanalysis*, 13: 33–347.

Greenson, R. (1967) *The Technique and Practice of Psychoanalysis*, Vol. 1. New York: International Universities Press.

Gunderson, J.G. (1978) Defining thetheraputic processes in psychiatric milieus, *Psychiatry*, 41: 327–35.

Haigh, R. (1999) The quintessence of a therapeutic environment: five universal qualities, in P. Campling and R. Haigh (eds) *Therapeutic Communities Past, Present and Future*, Vol. 2. London: Jessica Kingsley.

Haigh, R. (2002) Acute wards: problems and solutions, modern milieux: therapeutic community solutions to acute ward problems, *Psychiatric Bulletin*, 26(12): 380–2.

Hinshelwood, R.D. (2002) Abusive help – helping abuse: the psychodynamic impact of severe personality disorder on caring institutions, *Criminal Behaviour and Mental Health*, 12: 20–30.

Holmes, J. (2002) Acute wards: problems and solutions: creating a psychotherapeutic culture in acute psychiatric wards, *Psychiatric Bulletin*, 26(12): 383–5.

Kernberg, O.F. (1984) *Severe Personality Disorders: Psychotherapeutic Strategies.* New York: Vail-Ballon Press.

Kurtz, A. (2005) The needs of staff who care for people with a diagnosis of personality disorder who are considered to be a risk to others, *Journal of Forensic Psychiatry and Psychology*, 16(2): 399–422.

Macilwaine, H. (1983) The communication patterns of female neurotic patients with nursing staff in psychiatric units of general hospitals, in ?? Wilson-Barnett (ed.) *Nursing Research: Ten Studies in Patient Care.* Chichester: Wiley.

Menzies-Lyth, I. (1988) The functioning of social systems as a defence against anxiety: a report on a study of the nursing service of a general hospital, in *Containing Anxiety in Institutions. Selected Essays*, Vol. 1. London: Free Association Books.

Miller, L.J. (1990) The formal treatment contract in the inpatient management of borderline personality disorder, *Hospital and Community Psychiatry*, 41(9): 985–7.

MIND (2000) *Environmentally Friendly: Patients' views of conditions on psychiatric wards.* London: MIND.

NIMHE (2003) *Personality disorder: no longer a diagnosis of exclusion. Policy implementation guidance for the development of services for people with personality disorder.*

Norton, K. (1997) In the prison of severe personality disorder, *The Journal of Forensic Psychiatry*, 8(2): 285–98.

Norton, K. and Vince, J. (2002) Out-patient psychotherapy and mentally disordered offenders, in A. Buchanan (ed.) *Care of the Mentally Disordered Offender in the Community.* Oxford: Oxford Medical Publications.

Norton, K.R.W. and McGauley, G. (1998) *Counselling Difficult Clients.* London: Sage.

Obholzer, A. (1994) Managing social anxieties in public sector organizations, in A. Obholzer and V.Z. Roberts (eds) *The Unconscious at Work: Individual and organizational stress in the human services.* London: Routledge.

Pflaffin, F. and Adshead, G. (2003) *A Matter of Security: The application of attachment theory to forensic psychiatry and psychotherapy*. London: JKP.

Roberts, J.P. (1980) Destructive processes in a therapeutic community, *International Journal of Therapeutic Communities*, 1: 159–70.

Rosenthal, C.J. *et al.* (1980) *Nurses, Patients and Families*. London: Croom Helm.

Sarosi, G.M. (1968) A critical theory: the nurse as a fully human being, *Nursing Forum*, 7: 349–64.

Sinanoglou, I. (1987) Basic anxieties affecting psychiatric staff and their attitudes to psychotic patients, *Psychoanalytic Psychotherapy*, 3: 27–37.

Spitzer, S. and Sobel, R. (1962) Preferences for patients and patient behaviour, *Nursing Research*, 11: 233–5.

Stockwell, F. (1972) *The Unpopular Patient*, Royal College of Nursing Research Project, Series 1, No 2. London: RCN.

Whiteley, J.S. (2004) The evolution of the therapeutic community, *Psychiatric Quarterly*, 75(3): 233–48.

Acknowledgements

We are grateful to Mark Jenkinson, service manager, St Bernard's Hospital, Middlesex, for his thoughtful comments on an early draft of this chapter.

Chapter 14

Assessment

Iain Ryrie and Ian Norman

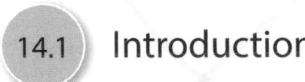

14.1 Introduction

Assessment is a cornerstone of mental health nursing and permeates all aspects of professional work. It can be difficult to comprehend the breadth of activity that represents assessment, and even harder to disentangle different approaches and their associated methods. We draw on the work of Barker (2004) to provide a 'map' of assessment that allows all its 'bits and pieces' to be understood collectively. Each is accorded its legitimate place in the framework, allowing each to be judged for its utility in relation to the person being assessed. The first part of the chapter deals in general with the principles and practice of assessment, from which the framework is developed. The latter part provides specific examples of selected assessment strategies. Further detail on the assessment of people with specific mental health problems can be found in Part 5 of this book. We also draw readers' attention to Part 4 of the book in which specific assessment strategies from the psychological therapies are presented (e.g. Chapters 21, 22 and 23).

This chapter covers:

- defining assessment;
- the purpose of assessment;
- the scope of assessment;
- methods of assessment;
- assessing the whole person.

14.2 Defining assessment

In its broadest sense assessment permeates all aspects of nursing care. It is not just a discrete activity that initiates the 'nursing process' or 'problem-solving cycle', leading to a plan of care, which is implemented and evaluated. The preferences people have for different health care options (planning) necessitate assessment, as do their abilities to engage meaningfully with the intervention itself (implementation), and evaluation requires still further assessment activity. Even then, it would be incorrect to suggest that assessment occurs only at these key points in the nursing process. It is an ongoing cycle of activity that all nurses perform in all nursing situations. Assessment may be implicit or explicit, informal or formal. It may involve simply noting a person's appearance and behaviour during a home visit or observing someone who is deemed to be at risk over extended periods. It can involve structured instruments that specify the type or severity of problem that someone experiences, or it may take the form of a seemingly casual conversation.

Common to all types of assessment is the collection of information.

The information we collect as nurses must be meaningful and necessary. Assessment data traditionally describe a person's appearance and behaviour, or their presentation and performance, or again, the form and function of their thoughts and feelings. Barker (2004) emphasizes the importance of these two viewpoints and their use by nurses to better understand a person. However, Barker cautions also against simply collecting data on the form and function of a person's thoughts and feelings, which can contribute to the formation of a medical diagnosis but will tell us little else about the person in the broader context of their life. Diagnosis is therefore one 'bit' of assessment, which focuses typically on problems, deficits and abnormalities. More broadly, assessment information encompasses a person's overall sense of self and their position in life, including not only problems and diagnoses but also their assets and strengths (Barker 2004).

The collection of information is only one part of the assessment process. Savage (1991) and Barker (2004) point to the inferences nurses draw from the available data, and the decisions they make regarding a person's need for care. Assessment is therefore a two-stage process. It is not enough to only gather information; we must be able to do something useful with it, and that use is nursing's purpose. Hence, assessment is central to all nursing activity. Barker has defined mental health nursing assessment as 'the decision-making process, based upon the collection of relevant information, using a formal set of ethical criteria, which contributes to an overall evaluation of a person and his circumstances' (Barker 2004: 7). This definition is useful since it implies the ongoing nature of assessment by referring to 'the decision-making process', which we take to be continuous and ever-present in the activities of a nurse. Barker highlights also the importance of a 'formal set of ethical criteria', referring to such issues as confidentiality, note-keeping, our style of interaction, how we ask questions, what we ask and why.

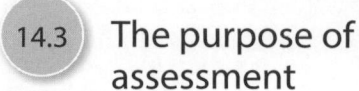

14.3 The purpose of assessment

We have emphasized two assessment stages, the collection of information and the use of that information to infer the need for nursing or other health care interventions. Though medical diagnosis is an important part of assessment, and one we fully acknowledge, mental health nursing is interested not in medical diagnoses per se, but in the way a person functions as a result of their condition. We need to comprehend their life problems (and strengths), and to understand the context within which these problems arise. Nursing diagnoses have been advocated for this purpose, which describe the nature of a person's problem and the effect it has on their functioning (Ward 1992). For example, 'I feel under threat and am angry with everyone I encounter.' This nursing diagnosis could be present in several medical diagnoses however, including paranoid schizophrenia or generalized anxiety disorder. Better then to deal with the nature of the problem and its implications, than with overlapping categories.

Neither of us have been strong advocates of the term 'nursing diagnosis', preferring to use other, non-medical, terms to describe nurses' activity. But we agree fully with Ward (1992) and Barker (2004) that the exploration of relationships between a person's thoughts, feelings and behaviour is a diagnostic process, and one that nurses perform. Whether this procedure is referred to as nursing diagnosis, problem identification or functional analysis may be less important to the person in care.

Barker (2004) identifies four assessment objectives (summarized in Table 14.1), the products of which provide the basis for nursing diagnoses. The information in the table provides an assessment overview; it tells us something about the quality, content and context of a person's health concern, its relationship to contributing factors and its effect on the person's and others' functioning. These data allow us to make judgements about why a problem exists and the factors that seem to be associated

Table 14.1   Assessment objectives and outcome (After Barker 2004)

Objectives	Outcome
Measurement	Key questions such as how often a person experiences a problem or exhibits a behaviour provide information on the scale or size of the problem
Clarification	Key questions such as where, with whom and under what circumstances problems arise provide information on the context or conditions associated with the problem
Explanation	Key questions such as the effects of a person's behaviour, their own and others' interpretation of its meaning provide evidence for the possible purpose or function of the problem
Variation	Key questions such as how the person's problem varies over time and in different situations provide evidence for its seriousness and the degree to which it dominates their life

with it. In turn we are able to identify areas of need and so plan interventions. As a simple example, consider the following problem statement: 'Arguments with my parents mean I don't like to be at home, so I spend my time alone in public parks where I smoke cannabis to make the day more interesting.' We can make several judgements about this person's need for care. The relationship between family tensions and personal isolation represents one possible area of need, and the lack of meaningful daily activity another. We might consider an opportunity to reflect on the positive and negative consequences of cannabis smoking to be a further need.

 ## 14.4   The scope of assessment

Increasing emphasis is placed on assessment of the 'whole person', by which different authors may mean different things. We have suggested that mental health nursing assessments are concerned with how people function in relation to health problems as well as in relation to the broader context of their lives. This focus on functioning provides one way of understanding the whole person and thereby the potential scope of assessment.

Barker (2004) draws out a number of different levels on which people function or live simultaneously, including their physiological self, biological self, behavioural self, social self and spiritual self. Actions as well as thoughts and feelings are included

in Barker's 'behavioural self'. These levels reflect the quadrant framework we introduced in Chapters 1 and 2 to provide explanations of mental health and disorder respectively. By so doing we proposed that human experience is made up of a *subjective* and *objective* sense of *self* and a *subjective* and *objective* sense of *community*. We employ these dimensions again to represent the whole person, and reproduce the framework in Figure 14.1, which presents an overview of the scope of assessment.

Consideration of each of the quadrants is necessary to understand and assess the whole person. The upper left quadrant (*subjective-self*) reflects a person's inner thoughts and feelings. It is concerned with the subjective meaning a person attributes to their life and/or their problems. We would position Barker's (2004) spiritual self and the thought and feeling components of his behavioural self in this quadrant. The upper right quadrant (*objective-self*) reflects a person's quantifiable, observable, external attributes. We would include the action component of Barker's behavioural self in this quadrant, along with the physiological and biological self. Similarly, we would place psychiatric diagnoses in this quadrant for their attempt to categorize people according to external, normative criteria.

The lower left quadrant (*subjective-community*) captures a person's collective sense of self. Their relations with family members and significant others are important here, as are their cultural roots and identity. But there is another side to our sense

Figure 14.1 The scope of mental health assessment

	Subjective	Objective
Self	Thought	Brain function
	Feelings	Autonomic nervous system function
	Self-acceptance	
	Cognitive style	Physiological balance
	Emotional intelligence	Exercise
	Spirituality	Diet
	Creativity	Alcohol and drug use
	Talking	Rest
	I	IT
	WE	ITS
Community	Relationships	Legislation
	Belonging	Policy
	Inclusion	Services
	Social support	Employment
	Social capital	Material wealth
	Community participation	Built environment
	Tolerance	Nature
		Public health indicators

of self in community and this is reflected by the lower right quadrant (*objective–community*). As well as the inter-subjective experiences of culture and kinship there are inter-objective social phenomena in the form of health and social care systems, legislation, financial and other community resources that impact on our sense of self and thus on our sense of health or illness.

We would place nursing diagnoses or problem statements that deal with a person's thoughts, feelings or beliefs (written in the first person and using their words) in the upper left (*subjective–self*) quadrant. Those that deal with external, observable behaviour or actions are upper right (*objective–self*). In reality, problem statements can straddle both quadrants (or all quadrants) dealing with thoughts and behaviours in relation to self and community.

This is to be expected since human experience is made up of all four quadrants. To repeat our earlier example, 'Arguments with my parents mean I don't like to be at home, so I spend my time alone in public parks where I smoke cannabis to make the day more interesting.' Figure 14.1 therefore represents our framework for assessment of the whole person upon which all assessment approaches and methods can be mapped. However, we must also consider in general terms the focus of any assessment in each of the quadrants, which might focus on indicators of health or illness.

Health and illness

Mental health and mental illness are inseparable, relational terms, and the reality they describe is human experience. This is not to say that we only feel ill because *previously* we have felt healthy, but rather that we feel ill against a background sense of health, we feel the two *simultaneously*. We can say we are ill because we experience limitations in our health, but it would be incorrect to say that we are ill because we have no health. Assessment therefore encompasses 'health' and 'illness', or 'mental health' and 'mental illness'. With some notable exceptions that we will come to, mental health nursing has focused largely on 'illness' in assessment practice. By this we mean deficits, problems, abnormalities, negative risks and so on. Their correlates (strengths,

solutions, commonalities, positive risks) have received far less attention.

Health remains a poorly understood concept and is frequently used as a euphemism for illness. For conceptual ease we equate illness with diagnoses, dysfunctions, problems and abnormalities at both the individual and community level. Correspondingly we equate health with strengths, solutions, assets and skills at both the individual and community level. The following case study of Tom emphasizes the importance of health for an individual with a debilitating illness.

Case Study

Tom

Tom is an 80-year-old man with dementia whose mobility is limited, but who insists on a twice-daily walk. His insistence is borne of an inner belief that his ability to walk connects him with life as he has always known it, despite the fact that his mind seems to be deserting him quite literally. His morning walk connects him with the local newsagent where he buys a daily paper, which connects him with the wider world. Throughout his working years as a commuter he attempted to complete the crossword in this daily paper and he feels it is more important than ever to maintain that activity. His walks also expose him to society in general. He comes across people and does what he has always done, says hello, comments on the weather, strokes a dog or simply talks nonsense at the supermarket checkout. He has always been like this, outgoing and happy. He is also very proud of these abilities, these markers of himself, particularly as he knows something is terribly wrong.

In fact, Tom is fast progressing in his dementia. His short-term memory has been virtually destroyed and he can no longer comprehend complex tasks. He has severe arterial restriction in his lower limbs and on two occasions he was found lying by the side of the road that leads from his home into town. Someone saw him fall once and commented that they thought he was drunk as he staggered up the road. At the time this hurt Tom deeply, he began to panic and refused any help.

Now it is true that Tom is facing a progressively debilitating disease but what is far more apparent is his sense of health, those things that he can still do in spite of his illness. He may have lost his short-term memory to a ravaging, organic, pathological process, but Tom is still very much alive in his habits, his long-established routines and fundamental interactions with the world. Tom's community psychiatric nurse (CPN), while acknowledging the disease and its associated problems, set about assessing Tom's health with a view to preserving what was important to him.

Tom now leaves the house with an urban version of a traditional shooting stick which allows him to rest when necessary. The nurse also asked one of Tom's children to write a message for him, which the nurse had laminated, and which now hangs on the back door next to his shooting stick. It simply asks dad to remember to take his stick, and to enjoy his walks. Both his children's names are printed at the bottom of the message. On occasion Tom can now be found on the road leading back to his house, sitting on his stick and bothering anyone who passes with stories about his useless legs.

Although Tom's nurse was aware of his problems/illness (limited mobility and dementia) she was aware also of his strengths/health (outgoing and social). More importantly, in the second stage of assessment she used this information to promote Tom's independence, and sense of self, irrespective of his illness. Tom might have been discouraged from leaving the house alone and offered transport to attend a day hospital where he could mix with others. In this case the information gathered from the assessment would have been used with his limitations (illness) very much in mind.

We can relate Tom's case study to Figure 14.1 to clarify the quadrants. His 'inner belief that his ability to walk connects him with life as he has always known it' is an example of upper left, *subjective–self* information. His diagnosis of dementia and his limited mobility due to arterial restriction are upper right, *objective–self* data. The value Tom places on his social connections reflects the lower left quadrant, or *subjective–community*. Finally, the nurse's knowledge of Tom's family structure and the production of a laminated message by his family is evidence of lower right or *objective–community* awareness.

When considering what to assess we need then to take account of the context, the person's background sense of health, within which an experience of illness is felt. As well as gathering information on a person's problems and deficits we need to know something of their strengths and personal ideals. We need, in short, to develop an understanding of the whole person.

 ## 14.5 Methods of assessment

This section gives an overview of the main methods by which assessment information can be gathered. Selected assessment strategies for each of the quadrants are presented in the final section of the chapter. Information-gathering for assessment can be more or less formal and explicit. Whether a formal or less formal approach is preferred depends on the circumstances. Take for example a person who is talkative and eager to communicate their experience. An informal approach that allows the person free expression would be recommended, particularly in the early stages of their contact with services. On the other hand, a withdrawn individual who finds it difficult to communicate may benefit from a more structured, formal approach. In both cases the information provided (or the information that is sought) is documented and arranged in a systematic way that tells us something about the person, the problems they encounter in relation to their condition and life in general, and the strengths or attributes they may possess. Taking our cue from the person to be assessed, and the reason for assessment, methods are usually selected to increase specificity as the assessment procedure progresses. Thus, a broad overview of an individual leads to the collection of information regarding the nature and implications of a specific problem. We outline three main data collection methods for mental health nursing assessments: interviews; questionnaires, rating scales and structured pro forma; and observations.

Interviews

The interview is a means of eliciting information by questioning people. Typically this will involve the person in care but may also include others who know the person well including their relatives, friends and other health care professionals. There is little benefit in asking questions if we are unable to listen properly to the answers that are provided. A good interviewer requires good listening skills.

Barker (2004) states that a good listener is someone who helps a person to elaborate and qualify what they have to say, and who is able to curb any desire to offer premature interjections or summaries. Active or reflective listening is an important skill in this respect. Reflective listening can involve repeating key words used by the interviewee, perhaps with an inflection in tone, which invites them to elaborate their point. It may be more appropriate to simply ask if someone could elaborate on a topic, or ask them to explain the meaning an issue has for them. Open questions that invite elaboration rather than closed questions, which need only a single categorical answer, are crucial for reflective

Table 14.2 Interview goals and aims (after Barker 2004)

Goal		Aim
Descriptive	Collecting information to form a broad overview or picture of the person and to develop a therapeutic, trusting relationship	Relationship-building
		Trust-building
Diagnostic	Investigation of a problem area in which relationships between a person's thoughts, feelings and behaviour are explored, and from which nursing or medical diagnoses can be formed	Professional collaboration
		Problem identification
Therapeutic	Ongoing face-to-face meetings to help the person through the process of care by clarifying problems, identifying solutions and reflecting with the person on their progress/response	Problem resolution

listening. Summarizing at discrete points during an interview to check for understanding is another example of reflective listening.

Each of these techniques communicates accurate empathy in so far as they convey an interest in, and an understanding of, the person's experience. Research demonstrates that therapeutic change, and the necessary relationship between therapist and client for this to occur, is dependent on the manifestation of accurate empathy by the therapist (Rollnick *et al.* 2008). This is a fundamental tenet of the therapeutic alliance.

Reflective listening is only beneficial if it is accompanied by appropriate non-verbal behaviour. It is no good asking someone to elaborate while we fumble to read a text, or sit with our arms crossed admiring the view from a window, or position ourself in a room with constant interruptions. Interest can be conveyed as much through our non-verbal behaviour and the environment in which we choose to interview someone, as it can by what we say or don't say (see Chapter 20).

Interviews may be more or less structured depending on their purpose and the type of information to be collected. Following Barker (2004), Table 14.2 represents a summary of the possible goals and aims of the interview, with the aims reflecting interpersonal functions between the nurse and the person receiving care.

Questionnaires, rating scales and structured pro formas

Questionnaires and rating scales generate quantifiable measures of human experience. They stem from the objective right-hand quadrants in Figure 14.1 and therefore complement, but cannot replace, the subjective left-hand quadrants. Instruments of this type may invite simple categorical responses (e.g. yes or no) to a question or statement. Many also invite the rating of a statement according to a series of possible responses that reflect different degrees of agreement with the statement. It is also possible to rate or scale the experiences or problems that people encounter on a 10-point scale (e.g. 'how would you rate the intensity of those feelings if 1 represented very low intensity and 10 represented very high intensity?').

These approaches can generate quantified summaries of the person in care. We may say that Tom's dementia is severe following administration of a questionnaire on which he scored poorly. We could reduce this further by saying he scored 2 out of a possible 20, thereby indicating severe dementia. Such an approach can be advantageous. Questionnaires and rating scales are usually developed through extensive research during which the instruments are refined to enhance the accuracy (validity) and consistency (reliability) with which they measure a concept of interest. However, to say that Tom's dementia questionnaire score was 2 tells us very little about the person behind this numeric.

We include various pro formas in this section, such as logbooks and diaries, which allow people to document specific experiences in a structured way (Barker 2004). A simple example is the 'antecedent', 'behaviour', 'consequence' framework, against which the context of a behavioural problem can be mapped. By substituting 'behaviour' for 'belief' in this framework we can map the context of a cognitive problem. Barker (2004) offers a further example using the headings 'action', 'emotion', 'thought', while Fox and Conroy (2000) advocate the acronym 'FIND' (frequency, intensity, number and duration of a problem). The ABC framework is particularly useful when trying to understand the triggers (antecedents) to a behaviour or belief and can generate important information for formulating plans of care that minimize the triggering of a client's problem.

Observations

Observation is a continuous form of data collection within the context of nursing care. It may be relatively informal, such as an overall assessment of a person's appearance and behaviour or the assessment of interactions within a ward environment. Structured observation methods include the prospective use of pro formas such as those described in the previous section. These can be completed by the person receiving care or by nursing staff. Observation schedules can yield important information but can also present a challenge to those who complete them. They require more or less continuous attention or good recollection in order to capture a representative set of data. This can be difficult for a person with a mental health problem and for their nurse who may not be available during periods when a problem is present.

Mental health care involves another type of observation that is concerned with documenting biochemical and physiological indices. Barker (2004) acknowledges this aspect of assessment but does not pursue it as a legitimate activity for the mental health nurse. On the other hand, Plant and Stephenson (2008) emphasize the importance of physiological indices in the assessment of mental

health problems. For example, deficiencies in zinc, magnesium, iron, omega-3 fatty acids and the B vitamins are not uncommon following childbirth and these deficiencies are implicated in depression. Therefore the assessment of postnatal depression in women should always include physiological screening for these deficiencies. Other examples, as indicated in Chapter 1, are the levels of key neurotransmitters which have a role to play in the experience of mental health problems. Although not widely used in the UK at present, methods are available to analyse urine or blood samples to determine whether specific neurotransmitters are too high or too low. Plant and Stephenson (2008) argue that these should be routine observations undertaken in the course of a mental health assessment, especially if there is an intention to prescribe medication that affects neurotransmitter levels.

14.6 Assessing the whole person

In this section we provide some examples of assessment strategies for each of the quadrants in Figure 14.1. We begin with an exploration of the breadth of personal and social information that needs to be collected when people first enter a health care system. Those who are already known to services may have extensive past medical or nursing notes. Though the information contained within these notes may be useful they are not a substitute for the collection of contemporary data regarding a person's presenting problem, or for the opportunity to elicit someone's personal history in their own words.

Presenting problem and personal history

Gamble and Brennan (2006) identify four core elements of the information-gathering process that describes a person's presenting problem and history (see Table 14.3). The core elements in Table 14.3 reflect predominantly the right-hand quadrants of Figure 14.1 (*objective–self* and *objective–community*). They are concerned with external, quantifiable attributes and phenomena, with the exception of

Table 14.3 Core elements of the information-gathering process (after Gamble and Brennan 2006)

Core element	Examples
History of psychiatric disorder and past physical history	■ Family and social background ■ Past treatments, contacts with services and risk levels ■ Current medication and any side-effects
Current financial, social functioning and environmental factors	■ Personal relationships ■ Employment
Psychiatric diagnosis and current symptoms	■ To include effects of symptoms on behaviour
Personal insights	■ Evidence of the person's awareness and understanding of their difficulties

Table 14.4 Admission profile (after Barker 2004)

Component	Examples
Name, age, sex, marital state	
Family	■ Whether any dependants and who they live with ■ Siblings ■ Whether part of an active extended family
Domestic	■ Living alone or with significant others
Occupation	■ Employment status ■ Nature of employment
Socialization	■ Close friends and other acquaintances ■ Membership of clubs or organizations including church
Financial status	■ Access to hard cash or other funds ■ Record of outstanding bills or debt
Medical cover	■ Name and contact details of any physician/social worker ■ Current medication

'personal insights'. This is not to say that Gamble and Brennan are uninterested in a person's subjective feelings, as their work testifies. However, their main approach, in terms of identifying health-related need, tends towards objective assessment. Barker (2004) provides a more integrated approach that begins with the generation of an admission profile and description of the presenting problem. By admission profile Barker refers to any point of entry into health or social care services, whether these be residential or community based. Tables 14.4 and 14.5 contain the key components of an admission profile and a presenting problem inventory.

It is evident that Barker's (2004) initial assessment draws on all four quadrants, incorporating both subjective and objective data of self and community. However, these data are firmly oriented toward problems, which Barker acknowledges. He believes it may be inappropriate to consider a person's strengths or assets at this stage, particularly as it may indicate a fear on behalf of the nurse to deal with a person's problems. We agree, but with one exception: evidence of exceptions to the presenting problem. We have found it useful to ask people early in an assessment process whether there are ever any exceptions to the presenting problems

Table 14.5 Inventory for presenting problem (after Barker 2004)

Component	Examples
Functioning	■ Changes in bodily functions including limbs, speech and memory
Behaviour	■ Changes in behaviour including behaviours that might be upsetting the person or others
Affect	■ Specific feelings associated with problems
Cognition	■ Specific thoughts about the problems, including ruminations and recurring thoughts
Beliefs	■ The meaning the problems have for the person
Physical	■ Physical problems associated with the difficulty, for example pain, loss of appetite, listlessness
Relationships	■ Any changes in usual relations and whether associated with the problem
Expectations	■ What the person thinks will happen to them now they are in touch with services

they describe. If so, we would encourage exploration of those exceptions since this often uncovers potential solutions to the problem (see Chapter 22).

Having elicited an admission profile and inventory of the presenting problem Barker (2004) then recommends the development of a thumbnail sketch. Specific topic headings are provided, which expand the available information to include past history, present circumstances and the way a problem interferes with the person's life experience (see Table 14.6).

During this stage of the assessment process Barker places much greater emphasis on a person's strengths, assets and preferences while maintaining an interest in all four quadrants of human experience, as evidenced in Table 14.6. Barker also draws attention to exploring a person's hopes for the future having examined their past in some detail. Questions pertaining to their aspirations, their expectations and hopes, and their future plans are important in this respect. Through these enquiries a more holistic picture of the person begins to emerge, from which it is possible to identify areas where further investigation may be needed. This investigation may follow any one of the specific strategies we describe in the following sections.

Subjective–self

The upper left quadrant of Figure 14.1 represents a person's inner world, their thoughts, feelings and beliefs. The psychodynamic model and its therapeutic approach (see Chapter 2) tap into this quadrant with their interest in assessing the ideas and feelings behind the words and actions that constitute human behaviour. Though some mental health nurses specialize in this tradition, the profession as a whole does not practise according to psychodynamic principles. Nevertheless, assessment of the *subjective-self* is a necessary component of holistic nursing practice.

Barker (2004) refers to this as 'learning from the person', which necessitates listening to a person's life story or personal narrative. It is true that a personal narrative may allude to behaviours or social structures which are external, observable attributes that belong elsewhere in Figure 14.1. But we can still ask for the meaning they hold for the person. This orientation lies at the heart of *subjective-self* assessments. It focuses on a person's thoughts, feelings, personal values and beliefs, which describe their sense of self and the meaning they attribute to their life experience.

Subjective-self assessments require the use of open-ended questions and reflective listening skills to elaborate a person's description of their experience. We might ask:

■ What are your feelings about that experience?

■ What thoughts did you have at the time?

■ Could you say a little more about what that means for you?

Table 14.6 Developing the history (after Barker 2004)

Topic	Example
Education	■ Description of schooling at basic and advanced level
	■ Attitudes towards schooling and adult learning
Occupation	■ Past and present occupations
	■ Feelings towards present job
	■ Any work aspirations
	■ Degree to which present problems interfere with work
Social network	■ Does the person enjoy going out?
	■ Do they have an extended social network?
	■ What kind of social life would they prefer?
	■ Impact of problem on these social networks
Recreation	■ Way in which free time is used
	■ Hobbies and preferred activities
	■ What changes might be desirable?
General health	■ States of health throughout the person's lifetime
	■ Maintenance of health through diet, exercise, etc.
Drugs	■ Use of drugs whether prescribed, over-the-counter or illicit
	■ How does the person feel about drug-taking?
	■ Amount, route of administration, frequency and duration of any drug use
	■ Is present problem and use of any drugs connected?
Past treatment	■ Any past treatments for presenting problem
	■ Effects of any treatments and preferences/feelings toward them
Coping	■ Coping strategies employed to deal with life's problems
	■ Successful strategies that have been employed previously
Outstanding	■ Problems that the person perceives to be beyond help
Problems	■ Feelings towards them and likely reactions, including anger/attempting suicide

It follows that the information we receive needs to be recorded in the person's own words, otherwise we are documenting our interpretations of what they say and are missing an opportunity to understand fully the person's *subjective-self*. Interpretations and judgements about their need for care will still be made, but in the case of the upper left quadrant

these should be predicated on an individual's verbatim account of their inner world.

Subjective–community

The lower left quadrant of Figure 14.1 represents the meaning, values and beliefs that a person holds regarding their sense of self in community. These include cultural identity and world views. Allied to these are negative correlates including racism, social exclusion and stigma. In Chapter 1 we demonstrated how stigma and social exclusion have a bearing on people's mental health. For example, the experiences of African-Caribbean communities in the UK, which include poorer housing, higher levels of unemployment and lower average incomes than the indigenous population are sufficient to engender mental health problems (Modood *et al.* 1998). In this particular quadrant it is not the quantifiable attributes themselves but the meaning they have for people that contributes to the formation of mental health problems. As with the *subjective–self* (upper left) we can only comprehend the personal meaning of these aspects of a person by asking them directly through open-ended questions and reflective listening. For example, someone may appear socially isolated or excluded but we cannot fully comprehend such observations without understanding the meaning they hold for the person.

Of contemporary interest in this quadrant is the emergence of the recovery approach and the meaning it holds for service users (see Chapter 5). The Chief Nursing Officer's (CNO) review of mental health nursing (DH 2006) recommends that the profession incorporates the broad principles of the recovery approach into every aspect of its practice, including assessment. This means understanding the goals that are important for service users, being positive about change and promoting social inclusion.

Objective–self

The upper right quadrant of Figure 14.1 represents external, measurable, quantifiable attributes of the person. This includes their physiological and biological self, and associated indices, as well as measurements of their functioning or mental state through the use of questionnaires and rating scales. 'Functioning' is a broad term that incorporates thoughts, feelings and behaviours associated with self as well as those associated with self in community. The latter is often referred to as social functioning, which is examined in the next section (*objective–community*). A number of instruments incor-

porate both self and community measures of functioning, particularly global assessments of need such as the Health of the Nation Outcome Scales (HoNOS) (Wing *et al.* 1995) and the Camberwell Assessment of Need (CAN) (Phelan *et al.* 1995). Each taps into personal attributes such as physical health and symptom severity as well as measures of social functioning such as interpersonal behaviours and social engagement.

Gamble and Brennan (2006) provide a detailed account of questionnaires and rating scales that are designed to capture in quantifiable terms the experience of illness. Less evident are instruments that tap into the experience of health, although some are cited in Barker's (2004) work. We draw on this literature to present a selected overview (in Table 14.7) of questionnaires and rating scales that are available for *objective–self* assessments. Readers may wish to review subsequent chapters for assessment instruments relevant to the specific problems/conditions that people experience.

Objective–community

The lower right quadrant of Figure 14.1 represents external, measurable, quantifiable attributes of the self in community. In the earlier section that described presenting problems and personal histories, the collection of information pertaining to these attributes was recommended. For example, in Table 14.6 Barker (2004) emphasizes the importance of enquiring about a person's occupation and social structures. These are examples of self in community data. In the *objective–community* quadrant these attributes are quantified according to questionnaires, rating scales and other objective data. However, we can also seek to understand a person's subjective experience of these phenomena (*subjective–community*).

For objective measurement, instruments that tap into a person's social functioning and to a lesser extent their quality of life are important. We include the latter, which often straddle both the *objective–self* and *objective–community* quadrants of Figure 14.1, but which typically measure an individual's quality of life in its broadest sense, and are, there-

Table 14.7 Instruments to assess illness and health in the individual

Instrument	Commentary
Brief Psychiatric Rating Scale (BPRS) (Overall and Gorham 1962)	One of the oldest and most commonly used instruments for assessing the presence of various forms of mental illness including anxiety, depression and thought disturbance. All items are rated on a 7-point scale from 'not present' to 'extremely severe'. Administered through direct questioning but relies also on observations made at the time of administration.
Beck Depression Inventory (BDI) (Beck *et al.* 1961)	Another much used instrument designed to measure the severity of depressive states. Containing 21 items, each is rated on a 4-point scale and can be completed by the person in care directly or through interview technique.
Positive and Negative Syndrome Scale (PANSS) (Kay *et al.* 1987)	Designed to assess key symptom types associated with schizophrenia. The instrument contains 30 items, a proportion of which are completed through interview and the remainder through observation. Each is rated on a 7-point scale.
Beliefs About Voices Questionnaire (BAVQ) (Chadwick and Birchwood 1995)	Designed to elicit the feelings a person has about hallucinatory voices. The questionnaire contains 30 items, all of which are answered with simple yes or no responses.
Self-Esteem Scale (Rosenberg 1965)	This brief 10-item instrument taps into a key component of health or well-being. It is easy to administer with each item rated on a 4-point scale.
Self-Efficacy Scale (Sherer *et al.* 1982)	A further instrument to gauge aspects of a person's health. Of the 30 items the majority tap into general self-efficacy and the remainder examine social self-efficacy (lower right quadrant). Each is rated on a 5-point scale.

fore, grounded in the self in community. Measures of social functioning are often concerned with problem areas and deficits while quality of life measures are more broadly focused and accommodate measurement of a person's sense of health. We would include also in this quadrant the objective views of carers and significant others involved in a person's care. Table 14.8 presents a selected overview of instruments that are available for *objective–community* assessments.

 ## 14.7 Conclusion

We have presented assessment as an ongoing continuous process, which in its many forms underpins all nursing activity. Its purpose incorporates both the collection of information and the use of that information to make judgements about a person's need for health care. Traditionally these judgements are based on a person's problems, deficits and abnor-

malities though we encourage a broader perspective that accommodates strengths, assets and skills.

We advocate the principle of holistic assessment and have presented a framework for that purpose, which takes account of a person's *subjective* and *objective* sense of *self* and their *subjective* and *objective* sense of *community*. In each respect consideration needs to be given to a person's problems (illness) and their strengths (health).

This holistic framework does not require mental health nurses to be skilled in all areas of assessment, but does require acknowledgement of its scope and thus the need to collaborate with others who have complementary assessment skills.

In summary, the main points of this chapter are:

- Assessment is an ongoing cycle of activity that all nurses perform in all nursing situations.
- Assessments can be more or less explicit and formal depending upon the person being assessed and their reason for assessment.

Table 14.8 Instruments to assess illness and health of self in community

Instrument	Commentary
Social Functioning Scale (SFS) (Birchwood *et al.* 1990)	This instrument covers seven main areas of social functioning including independence in living skills and social engagement. All areas reflect aspects of day-to-day social functioning that can be adversely affected by mental health problems. The authors designed this instrument specifically for use in family intervention programmes.
Instrumental and Expressive Functions of Social Support (IEFSS) (Ensel and Woelfel 1986)	This instrument is designed to assess the function and emotional content of a person's social relationships. A 5-point scale is used to rate 28 problem areas, which cover demands, money, companionship, marital conflict and communication.
Quality of Life Scale (QLS) (Heinrichs *et al.* 1984)	This instrument has 21 items, each of which is rated on a 7-point scale. They cover three key areas deemed to be representative of a person's quality of life: interpersonal relations; occupational role; and richness of personal experience. The scale specifically taps into a person's capability to manage social roles and with this emphasis on capability is oriented towards health rather than illness.
Manchester Short Assessment of Quality of Life (MANSA) (Priebe *et al.* 2002)	In addition to gathering sociodemographic data this instrument asks 16 questions pertaining to employment, finance, friendships, leisure, accommodation, family, safety and health. Each is rated on a 7-point scale. As with the QLS the emphasis is upon health rather than illness.
Carers' Assessment of Managing Index (CAMI) (Nolan *et al.* 1995)	Designed to assess coping style and management of stress in the carers of people with mental health problems. Examples of coping strategies are given, which respondents report their use of and the degree to which they are effective.

- The process of assessment involves decision-making, which requires the collection and interpretation of information to make judgements about a person's need for care.

- Holistic assessment requires information on a person's *subjective* and *objective* sense of *self* and their *subjective* and *objective* sense of *community* and, in each area, indicators of both health and illness should be explored.

- Mental health nurses need to develop an integrated understanding of the scope of assessment to be demonstrated in collaborative partnerships with service users and professional colleagues.

Annotated bibliography

Barker, P. (2004) *Assessment in Psychiatric and Mental Health Nursing: In Search of the Whole Person*, **2nd edn. Cheltenham: Stanley Thornes.**
This text provides a detailed contemporary account of theoretical principles, methodologies and instruments for conducting mental health nursing assessments. Practical examples of how to assess a range of disorders are provided, including anxiety states, psychotic experiences and human relations. The text includes an examination of the moral and ethical issues surrounding assessment, and provides a selected bibliography of assessment instruments.

Gamble, C. and Brennan, G. (2006) Assessments: a rationale and glossary of tools, in C. Gamble and G. Brennan (eds) *Working with Serious Mental Illness: A manual for clinical practice*, **2nd edn. London: Elsevier.**
A valuable chapter in which the authors provide a rationale for systematic assessments, describe the core elements of information to be collected and provide an extensive glossary of standardized assessment tools. The chapter provides also some practical strategies to aid the interpretation and effective implementation of assessment data.

Bowling, A. (2004) *Measuring Health: A review of quality of life measurement scales,* **3rd edn. Maidenhead: Open University Press.**
This text provides a comprehensive collection of quality of life measurement scales that have been selected for inclusion either because they have been well tested for reliability and validity or because considerable interest has been expressed in their content area. The author provides a useful discussion of the conceptualization of functioning, health and quality of life. The text includes instruments and methods to measure functional ability, health status, psychological well-being, social networks and support, and life satisfaction and morale.

Bowling, A. (2001) *Measuring Disease: A review of disease-specific quality of life measurement scales,* **2nd edn. Buckingham: Open University Press.**
Though not specific to mental health this book complements Bowling's 2004 text. The strengths, weaknesses and coverage of a range of instruments designed to measure aspects of disease are reviewed.

References

Barker, P. (2004) *Assessment in Psychiatric and Mental Health Nursing: In search of the whole person,* 2nd edn. Cheltenham: Nelson Thornes Ltd.

Beck, A., Ward, C., Mendelson, M. *et al.* (1961) An inventory for measuring depression. *Archives of General Psychiatry,* 4: 561–71.

Birchwood, M., Smith, J. and Cochrane, R. (1990) The Social Functioning Scale: the development and validation of a new scale of social adjustment in use in family interventions programmes with schizophrenic patients, *British Journal of Psychiatry,* 157: 853–9.

Chadwick, P. and Birchwood, M. (1995) The omnipotence of voices II: the Beliefs About Voices Questionnaire, *British Journal of Psychiatry,* 166: 11–19.

DH (Department of Health) (2006) *From Values to Action: The Chief Nursing Officer's review of mental health nursing – summary.* London: DH.

Ensel, W. and Woelfel, J. (1986) Measuring the Instrumental and Expressive Functions of Social Support, in N. Lin, A. Dean and W. Ensel (eds) *Social Support, Life Events and Depression.* New York: Academic Press.

Fox, J. and Conroy, P. (2000) Assessing clients' needs: the semi-structured interview, in C. Gamble and G. Brennan (eds) *Working with Serious Mental Illness: A Manual for clinical practice.* London: Baillière Tindall.

Gamble, C. and Brennan, G. (2006) Assessments: a rationale and glossary of tools, in C. Gamble and G. Brennan (eds) *Working with Serious Mental Illness: A manual for clinical practice,* 2nd edn. London: Elsevier.

Heinrichs, D., Hanlon, T. and Carpenter, W. (1984) The Quality of Life Scale: an instrument for rating the schizophrenic deficit syndrome, *Schizophrenia Bulletin,* 10: 388–98.

Kay, S., Fiszebein, A. and Opler, L. (1987) Positive and Negative Syndrome Scale, *Schizophrenia Bulletin,* 13: 261–76.

Modood, T., Berthoud, R., Lakey, J. *et al.* (1998) *Ethnic Minorities in Britain: Diversity and disadvantage. the fourth national survey of ethnic minorities.* London: Policy Studies Institute.

Nolan, M., Keady, J. and Grant, G. (1995) CAMI: a basis for assessment and support with family carers, *British Journal of Nursing Quarterly,* 4: 822–6.

Overall, J. and Gorham, D. (1962) Brief Psychiatric Rating Scale, *Psychological Reports,* 10: 799–812.

Phelan, M., Slade, M., Thornicroft, G. *et al.* (1995) The Camberwell Assessment of Need: the validity and reliability of an instrument to assess the needs of people with severe mental illness, *British Journal of Psychiatry,* 167: 589–95.

Plant, J. and Stephenson, J. (2008) *Beating Stress, Anxiety and Depression.* London: Piatkus Books.

Priebe, S., Huxley, P., Knight, S. and Evans, S. (2002) *Manchester Short Assessment of Quality of Life.* Manchester: The University of Manchester.

Rollnick, S., Miller, W. and Butler, C. (2008) *Motivational Interviewing in Healthcare: Helping patients change behaviour.* New York: Guilford Press.

Rosenberg, M. (1965) *The Measurement of Self-esteem.* Princeton, NJ: Princeton University Press.

Savage, P. (1991) Patient assessment in psychiatric nursing, *Journal of Advanced Nursing,* 16: 311–16.

Sherer, M., Maddux, J., Mercandante, B. *et al.* (1982) The Self-efficacy Scale: construction and validation, *Psychological Reports,* 51: 663–71.

Ward, M. (1992) *The Nursing Process in Psychiatry,* 2nd edn. Edinburgh: Churchill Livingstone.

Wing, J., Curtis, R. and Beevor, A. (1995) *Measurement of Mental Health: Health of the Nation Outcome Scales.* London: Royal College of Psychiatrists Research Unit.

Chapter 15

Care Planning

Jane Padmore and Charlotte Roberts

15.1 Introduction

This chapter addresses collaborative care planning by focusing on the role of the mental health nurse at key transition points in a service user's journey through a mental health service. It covers:

- engagement;
- assessment;
- developing a care plan;
- implementation;
- review;
- discharge.

Admission and discharge planning are considered in more detail in Chapter 16.

15.2 Care plans

What is a care plan?

A care plan is the blueprint of treatment drawn up in partnership with a service user that can be used to communicate the type of treatment they are receiving and to review progress. A care plan can either be a nursing care plan or a multi-disciplinary care plan. A service user may have more than one care plan as each plan should address only one difficulty in detail.

Why are care plans used?

Care plans have many purposes and can be useful for the service user, the care team, other agencies and clinical governance. They are used to set goals, to demonstrate the patient's journey within a service or across different services and can provide life-saving information for use in an emergency. Specific activities are allocated and their tasks detailed.

The service user should be involved throughout the care planning process to develop a shared understanding of the difficulties, set goals, plan tasks, implement the care plan and review it. This is important because the success of many nursing interventions is influenced substantially by whether or not the service user considers the intervention appropriate and is willing to give it a try. Clinical experience suggests that it may be helpful to generate a series of alternative interventions together and for the service user to be invited to consider which one is the most appropriate for them. A collaborative approach to care planning will also foster engagement and help to ensure the sustainability of interventions over time.

In some instances the service user may not wish to engage in planning their care or may not even be available – for example, if they have absconded from the ward. It would still be important to have a care plan in place, with the reasons for the service user not participating in the development of the plan and any views of the service user detailed. At the earliest opportunity the care plan should be reviewed with the service user and adapted to include their views.

If, after further discussion, a mutual understanding of the difficulties or tasks cannot be reached, the service user's opinions should still feature in the care plan. Using their words the nurse can ensure the service user feels heard and valued. The care plan can be a valuable tool in the service user–nurse relationship and can ensure that service users participate and their views are represented in their care.

Communication with the service user, carers, other members of the multi-disciplinary team, the general practitioner (GP) and other agencies is of utmost importance in the care and treatment of people experiencing mental health difficulties. Care plans offer a means of communication in a clear and succinct way that can be easily found within medical records, copied to others as well as held by the service user. They promote continuity of care and ensure everyone is working towards the same goals.

Care plans can demonstrate that the service user's care complies with national and local policies and procedures. They not only provide a way to monitor the service user's progress but also to monitor that the care needed is given. They can also be used as quality indicators for the Commission for Quality and Innovation (CQUIN) payment framework.

Types of care plan

Care plans come in many shapes and forms with a variety of foci. They can be documented on a tem-

plate, written within a letter or in a format negotiated with the service user. The Care Programme Approach (CPA) uses multi-disciplinary care plans as an integral part of the process. The CPA describes the framework for supporting and coordinating effective mental health care for people with severe mental health problems in secondary mental health services. Prior to 2008, the CPA applied to all people under the care of mental health services, using an 'enhanced' approach for those with complex needs and a 'standard' approach for others. Revised guidance (DH 2008) means that the CPA only applies to those with more complex needs.

Types of care plan include:

- treatment care plan;
- risk plan;
- physical health care plan;
- contingency plan;
- nursing care plan;
- multi-disciplinary care plan;
- relapse prevention plan.

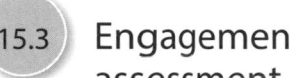 ## 15.3 Engagement and assessment

The importance of engagement and working in partnership is consistent throughout the entirety of a service user's journey. The partnership between the nurse and the service user is a dynamic relationship that changes over time and begins even before the initial meeting. This is explored in Chapter 13.

Initial meeting and care planning

The first meeting with a service user can make the difference between the service user deciding whether or not to engage in the future.

Case Study

Noah

A man in his early twenties, Noah, was referred to a community mental health service as he had started to withdraw from his peer group and not attend university. He had previously been referred a number of times to the service but had not attended. The family were from Eritrea and the mother did not speak English.

In view of previous appointments having been missed a new appointment letter was preceded by a telephone call to Noah to negotiate the assessment care plan. Noah requested a home visit at a specific time. He agreed to an interpreter being present, to ensure communication with his mother.

In Noah's case an urgent home visit was arranged. A discussion took place with the interpreter before entering the home to decide how the nurse and interpreter would work together. Important cultural matters were also considered, such as how to greet the family appropriately in their language.

On arrival Noah's mother was extremely hospitable and had made sweet cakes and poured traditional drinks. Being in the family home enabled the nurse to see that there were no concerns about Noah's physical environment and put Noah and his mother at ease. It came to light that they had not attended the clinic as Noah had been too paranoid to leave the house and his mother was too afraid to contradict Noah as he had become violent.

Once the refreshments were finished, Noah's mother naturally began to tell the nurse her concerns and Noah joined in to contradict or expand as she went along. With an interpreter this took a considerable length of time and the nurse did not need to say much. It was clear that Noah was not very well and needed an urgent admission to hospital but he was very paranoid and his mother was scared of him.

Even though Noah was very unwell, an initial care plan was negotiated. This involved an emergency care plan to use if Noah deteriorated, which was clearly written down by the interpreter. The nurse arranged for a colleague to come and see Noah the following day to further assess the situation. Noah requested that the nurse be present at that meeting so that was put into the care plan. Despite the refreshments and acute situation the session only lasted an hour. There was enough time to develop a relationship and get the key information needed to develop an initial care plan.

Commentary

Noah's case illustrates how important the first contact, both directly and indirectly, with the service user and carer is. This contact gives the service user an opportunity to test out any preconceived ideas they may have. The importance of preparation should not be underestimated. Most teams have protocols in place for managing referrals, how they are administered, allocated and how people are offered appointments. Some teams make contact by telephone, others wait until they have an available appointment to see the new patient and then contact them. This could be a few weeks later, potentially leaving the service user feeling uncertain and anxious. Whatever the local protocol, a care plan can be put in place, negotiated with the service user, to manage the period prior to being seen for the first time.

Noah's first experience of care planning was the care plan that was agreed verbally, over the phone, and documented in his clinical records. He was also involved in the care plan that was developed with his mother at the end of the assessment. Following a session, where sensitive information has been shared, a service user and their carer can feel vulnerable and anxious about what will happen next, even whether they will see a professional again. The collaboratively developed care plan provided clarity to both Noah and his mother about what the nurse was going to implement to ensure Noah received the appropriate care. It also detailed what Noah and his mother would do if the situation deteriorated. This was written down for them and included contact numbers for services both in and out of office hours.

In day-to-day practice, particularly when faced with someone who is acutely unwell, it is tempting for the nurse to move straight into a problem-solving mode, without taking sufficient time to build a relationship with the new patient and their family, to understand the patient's perspective. For the service user the situation is new and can be bewildering. By ensuring that relationship-building is attended to, the service user is more likely to be at ease, feel respected and keep their next appointment. In addition, any risks presented by the patient are more likely to be contained if the family are engaged as partners in care.

Assessment

Assessment is discussed in Chapter 14. In this chapter, assessment directly related to identifying the difficulties to be addressed in a care plan will be considered. Time needs to be spent exploring difficulties as well as strengths, listening and empathizing, and at the same time asking questions to gain a fuller understanding. The exploration of these issues can bring to light many different strands of difficulties and identify those which are a priority to the service user.

It may be tempting to curtail assessment and move quickly on to solve problems. This is particularly so in a service environment concerned with meeting performance indicators, moving patients along a pathway of care and delivering evidence-based interventions. But a clear model of the problem, developed by the service user and the nurse in partnership, is essential to identify the service user's difficulties and strengths while also providing a clear mutual understanding of treatment priorities.

The difficulties and strengths of service users are many and varied. They can manifest in any or every part of the context within which the service user exists. Also, what is presented as the primary problem, or the diagnosis, is often not a stand-alone issue, nor

the highest priority for the service user. Many factors are at play and both strengths and difficulties contribute to the situation the service user finds themselves in. In addition, there is the question of whether or not the service user wants help, is able to access help, or knows what help is available.

Broadly, the difficulties and strengths could be categorized using a biopsychosocial model as defined by Engel (1977) which, although conceptualized a considerable time ago, remains relevant. A complementary framework is demonstrated in the diagrams that follow.

Figure 15.1 illustrates how the service user is at the centre of the presentation to services and at the centre of the work being done. However, other things (e.g. people, organizations, environment, government) have an influence on the person to a greater or lesser extent. Strengths and difficulties can occur in any or all of these areas. Those in the diagram do not represent an exhaustive list, rather they are examples of the kind of influences there may be and the service user can develop their own unique representation of their situation.

Once the service user has developed their personal representation of their strengths and difficulties at the current time, they can then be

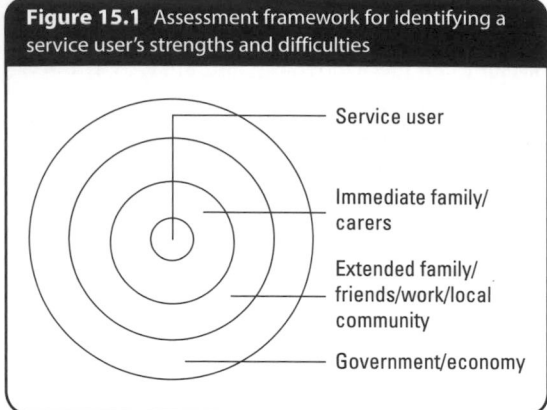

Figure 15.1 Assessment framework for identifying a service user's strengths and difficulties

- Service user
- Immediate family/carers
- Extended family/friends/work/local community
- Government/economy

explored over time. Figure 15.2 gives an example of how these areas may impact on the person through the progression of time. The presentation to services offers just one cross-section in time. This map shows the fluidness of strengths and difficulties and the constant interplay between the different areas. The impact one area has on another can have repercussions on the other areas and the nearer to the service user it is the more of an impact it is likely to have. The service user can adapt the diagram, adding arrows and additional rings, so that they have generated a model that is meaningful to them and assists them in identifying where the priorities for their care plan are.

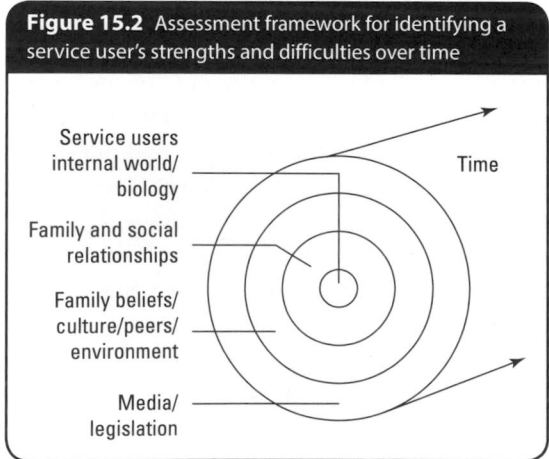

Figure 15.2 Assessment framework for identifying a service user's strengths and difficulties over time

- Service users internal world/biology
- Family and social relationships
- Family beliefs/culture/peers/environment
- Media/legislation
- Time

Depending on the service user's circumstances and perceptions, specific areas could be identified as a strength or difficulty. The terms 'strengths' and 'difficulties' are subjective. The nurse may define one area as a difficulty but others may view it as a strength. An example of this was a man referred to as 'aggressive and possibly paranoid, who may be on the periphery of criminal activity'. The referrer was concerned about the way the person expressed his anger and potential risks associated with this. When this was explored with him, he thought his perceived aggression was a strength, describing himself as assertive and able to protect himself. He also talked about his fear of being labelled as an aggressive criminal without truly understanding his way of expressing himself or taking the time to find out what he was angry about.

Another example would be that everyone has a financial position. The amount of money they have may not be particularly relevant but the way they cope with and live within their means may be either a strength or difficulty. Although generally not a symptom of a mental disorder, financial hardship can be the problem identified by the patient causing the most concern and therefore impacting on their mental health. A care plan could therefore be negotiated to facilitate them getting financial assistance.

There is a danger when specifying types of strengths and difficulties that they are viewed in a compartmentalized way instead of considering the interplay between areas and the changing nature, over time, of both strengths and difficulties. The problems or strengths could be located in any of the circles in the diagrams and, when reviewing the situation at a later date, the nurse can work with the service user to adapt the model of their situation, demonstrating changes that have taken place.

When presented with a referral it is important to notice the concerns and presenting problems, as described by the referrer, but not to consider this as the only version of the situation. The service user and carers will have their own view of what the strengths and difficulties are. The nurse will also come with their view of the situation. It is important to keep an open mind and explore all perspectives before deciding, with the service user, what the treatment objectives will be.

 ## 15.4 Developing a care plan

Writing a care plan

There are numerous examples of documented care plans. Services may have their own template on paper, or electronically, others may include their care plan in the body of a letter. Some even have standardized care plans for specific disorders, although it could be questioned how these are written in partnership with a service user.

Whatever the format, general principles apply to all of them. Goals and actions are central. Enough time should be allowed to discuss and agree the care plan and options without the service user feeling hurried. Two examples are shown below.

Both of these are examples of how care plans can be formally documented. Example one has the benefit of all the information, including the review, being easily identifiable on one sheet. In some services a similar document is created through an electronic field in patient records and the care plan is either printed out or rewritten in a

---

Box 15.1 Care plan template

Name				
Date of birth				
Date care plan written				
Created by	*Service user's name*	*Carer's name*	*Nurse's name*	*Name of any others*
Goal	*Only one goal per care plan*			
Action number	Actions		Who is responsible	Review date
1				
2				
3				
4				
5				
Care plan review date	Review details	Continue as above	Continue with changes	End
Service user signature		Printed name		
Nurse signature		Printed name		
Date		Copies given to		

Box 15.2 Care plan in the body of a letter

When we met we discussed how we can work together to achieve the goal you identified. This goal was … We thought about how this goal could be achieved and agreed actions we needed to take. Our team call this your care plan. There were actions I agreed to complete and some that you agreed to complete. These were:

1. Action 1
2. Action 2
3. Action 3

When we meet again on, *date*, we will talk about how we got on and whether we are nearing the goal. We will also think about any changes we may need to make to your care plan. In the meantime please do not hesitate to contact me if you think we need to review your plan sooner.

letter, similar to example two. The system of reviewing the care plan can make the document look messy and muddled. It can therefore be helpful to rewrite the care plan if a number of changes are needed, clearly marking it with the version number.

Example two can be adapted to suit the service user, making it very personalized. The letter should be copied to relevant parties which can cause some difficulties if the service user wants to keep some content confidential. This can be overcome by writing a letter to the other recipients with the care plan, and copying it to the service user.

Goal-setting

Once the service user has identified, in partnership with the nurse, the difficulties he or she faces and wishes to address, it is time to consider setting goals. Everyone needs to be clear about what the goals are. By having goals clearly articulated and

documented, a meaningful review and evaluation can take place both while the care plan is being implemented and at its end point. It can be difficult to effectively evaluate treatment, therefore it is helpful to have goals that are:

- **S**pecific;
- **M**easurable;
- **A**chievable;
- **R**ealistic;
- **T**ime orientated;
- **E**xplicit;
- **N**egotiated.

Once a goal is written it should be tested against these to consider whether it can be improved. There could be multiple goals for a particular problem. What the service user would like to achieve needs to be explored and then this is fine-tuned to elicit a very specific goal.

Thinking Space 15.1

Consider the following goals. Why might they present a problem when implementing the care plan? How could they be rewritten?

1. Jo to be symptom free.
2. Alice will attend to her personal hygiene regularly.

Feedback to Thinking Space 15.1

1. It is possible that Jo set the goal of being symptom free. The nurse would need to work with Jo to reframe this goal to minimize the risk of not achieving it and to understand what he means by being 'symptom free'. Also, how will Jo and his nurse know when he is symptom free? When does he want to achieve this by? The goal could be: 'Jo would like, by the end of September, to have two hours a day when he is not troubled by the voices that tell him to hurt other people and that he is a bad person.' This is a specific goal that can be measured using a rating scale, where Jo rates how troubled he is by the voices at any one time. It is achievable and realistic if Jo and the care team put in place actions to achieve the goal. It is time orientated in terms of when it will be achieved by and how long Jo will not be troubled for. The goal is explicitly stated and was negotiated between Jo and his nurse.

2. Alice attending to her personal hygiene is an action rather than a goal. It is unclear whether this was a goal set by Alice or her nurse but exploring what would be achieved if Alice attended to her personal hygiene could be the next step in generating a workable goal. The new goal could be: 'Alice is recovering from a severe depressive episode and would like to go out socially once a week, with a close friend, by the end of the month.' This may be Alice's goal, but to achieve it she needs to prepare herself for a social outing. One action needed to achieve this goal would be for Alice to attend to her personal hygiene. The specific details of the action would be discussed with Alice and broken down into achievable steps while discussing what may be obstacles to her completing the action.

Priorities are things that take precedence in position, and are considered the most important at the time. Goal-setting is a decision-making process that ranks the order of importance. The service user, carers, nurse and the rest of the multi-disciplinary team may have conflicting priorities. Decisions relating to risk and service user priorities may therefore need to be made that involve compromise from any of the parties.

When considering which goals to work on, a shared understanding between the service user and the nurse of what the difficulties and goals are and what priority they should take needs to be developed. By explaining models, such as Maslow's hierarchy of needs (Maslow 1943), and highlighting life-threatening situations, actual difficulties, rather than potential concerns, can be explored.

At times the nurse can struggle to engage the service user. Goals that are important to the service user and which also address the most pressing concerns in relation to safety may not be compatible. In addition these may or may not be something that the current evidence base suggests is the priority in relation to their primary diagnosis. Without developing the partnership and agreed goals, future collaborative relationships and treatment may be put at risk.

By setting the goals themselves, service users are saying how they wish to change the situation. To start the process the nurse can talk about the general aims or direction the service user wants to go in. They can ask how will we know the goal has been met – what will it look like? These then need to be developed into goals by the nurse and the service user, using the criteria above. The service user needs to think about what is manageable for them to achieve in a given period of time and be mindful of not setting goals that are not achievable. By doing this the goals can be expressed as an outcome, (what the target is), and as positively as possible.

Planning action

Once the goals are set, actions need to be planned in order to prevent obstacles getting in the way and to help the service user to achieve them. It could be argued that each intervention should be supported by a scientific rationale, which is the justification or reason for carrying out the intervention. This may not always be possible as there is not always an evidence-based action or the service user does not want to follow what the evidence base suggests.

The service user and, where appropriate their carer, are the experts and are best able to think about actions realistically, although the nurse can engage by exploring and suggesting alternatives. The nurse's experience and knowledge of the evidence base, and available resources, can be shared to suggest alternative actions that the service user may not have considered.

It can be tempting for the nurse to immediately suggest strategies to solve the difficulties or to achieve general aims rather than a specific goal. It can therefore be helpful to prioritize, with the service user, and keep referring back to their goals and how they think they may be achieved. Prioritizing one or two goals at any one time can be helpful and allows adequate time for review at a later date.

Initially it can be helpful to generate an extensive list of actions that may or may not be realistic. In doing this glimpses of further ideas can be generated. The ideas can be discussed and thinking around them developed. Some will be rejected, others will be put aside and eventually more appropriate ideas, that fit the service user, will be developed into specific actions. This process requires creative thinking.

Creativity often instils despair in people who think they are not 'artistic'. The word can be seen in a negative light and the process can feel chaotic and unboundaried. The nurse's role is to support and encourage the process, contribute to it, but not stifle someone's creativity even if ideas appear unrealistic.

However a care plan is written, it is important that all parties understand what they have agreed to and what is expected of them. In a survey of adults receiving mental health care the Care Quality Commission (CQC 2010) found that 48 per cent said they definitely understood their care plan, 29 per cent understood it to some extent, 9 per cent said they did not understand it and 15 per cent were not sure. If the service user is to understand then the language used is a key consideration.

The language needs to be non-judgemental, personalized and wherever possible, in the service user's own words. This is not a time for the nurse to show off their literacy skills, rather for the service user to come away with a working document that is both meaningful and useful. It can be helpful to ask the service user how they would like the action phrased and then to help them develop their words into specific, measureable, achievable, realistic and time-orientated actions. Jargon, unless generated by the service user, should be avoided.

Consideration needs to be paid to the service user's level of literacy which can be a particularly sensitive issue. In addition, where English is not the service user's first language, they may be able to speak fluently but not read confidently. Translating the care plan into their first language can increase the likelihood of them fulfilling the actions and can contribute to the service user feeling listened to and respected.

Finally the service user needs to be consulted about who should have a copy of their care plan. Minimally all those who have an action assigned to them need to have a copy. The consent the service user gives is then documented in their clinical notes and copies are given to the relevant parties.

Case Study

Sarah

Sarah, 14 years old, was referred to child and adolescent mental health services (CAMHS) as she was truanting from school and becoming 'rude'. The school wondered whether she had a 'conduct disorder' or attention deficit hyperactivity disorder (ADHD). There was a very detailed family history given. Sarah had a 21-year-old sister with challenging behaviour, autism and learning difficulties and a 5-year-old brother with autism. Their father had died two years before, unexpectedly. Sarah's behavioural difficulties were presented as the key problem.

During the initial appointment it came to light that Sarah's mother had mental health problems and was being treated for depression, having previously been admitted to hospital. The mother believed she was well and the adult mental health services believed she was stable. Sarah spoke about how she saw the 'problem'. She feared her mother may attempt suicide or not cope with her siblings and so wanted to be at home to look after her. She did not feel anyone was listening to her or telling her what was happening, despite being her mother's main carer.

For Sarah the most important area was to ensure her mother was safe. Sarah, her mother and both the adult and the CAMHS nurse met to draw up a contingency care plan that detailed what would happen if Sarah noticed her mother's mental health was deteriorating. This included what Sarah had noticed were her mother's early warning signs and what to do in a crisis.

Commentary

This case study demonstrates how services can come together to develop a care plan that is helpful for both the service user and their carer. Care plans can be reassuring to all parties, detailing what can be done in a crisis, with telephone numbers and opening hours all documented in one place.

Thinking Space 15.2

Molly is a day patient in a service for people with long-term mental health problems and has a diagnosis of paranoid schizophrenia. She attends a day centre Monday to Friday where she is frequently heard to talk about her desire to return to paid employment. She has not been in paid employment for the previous 30 years. The multi-disciplinary team's main concern is her inconsistent use of her medication and risk of relapse.

Molly and her nurse arrange a meeting to review her care plans as she has achieved the goals previously set. They decide to develop a new care plan. Molly is keen that her goal is to gain paid employment within the next year.

Consider how the nurse can develop a care plan, in partnership with Molly, that addresses both Molly's goal and the concerns of the multi-disciplinary team.

Feedback to Thinking Space 15.2

Nursing has, at its core, caring and working in partnership with service users, at the same time as understanding and implementing evidence-based practice. In your answer you may have considered breaking down the goal into manageable steps that Molly can see are achievable, at the same time as working towards her long-term goal. Writing down the stages, thinking about time frames and then drawing a time line with Molly can be a useful tool in thinking about how realistic the time frame is. It can also be revisited at the review meetings and the time frame adjusted.

The goals as specific steps might initially include:

■ One morning a week voluntary work
■ Two mornings a week voluntary work

By starting with voluntary work, Molly can test out what is achievable at the same time as gaining useful experience and references. As the steps increase in hours, part-time paid employment can be set as the goal.

Once the first goal has been defined the actions need to be considered. The nurse can think with Molly about what is needed for her to be able to participate in voluntary work. One necessity may be for her symptoms to be manageable. This could then lead to the action that Molly will take her medication, as prescribed, without missing doses.

 ## 15.5 Implementation

Implementation involves carrying out the actions to achieve the goals set when writing the care plan. It can be helpful to have follow-up sessions, phone calls or emails between formal reviews. Goals and actions may need to be changed or fine-tuned. The identified problem may differ over time because working on the actions has highlighted an alternative view of the issues.

To implement the strategies everyone needs to be clear about what is expected and what the possible outcomes might be. When writing a care plan, the actions can appear clear but, when implementing them, it may become evident that there have been miscommunications or misunderstandings. The nurse can assist the service user by being approachable and accessible as well as troubleshooting and rewriting the actions.

The nurse then provides support to the service user and carers while they implement the strategies.

It can be helpful to decide how this is done when writing the care plan and to detail what the nurse agrees to do. The nurse should then ensure they complete the tasks assigned to them.

 ## 15.6 Review

Reviews can take place throughout implementation but a formal review is usually arranged when the care plan is written. Reviews can also take place following a critical incident or a change in medication. The review formally evaluates progress but also plans the next steps. Less formal reviews can be undertaken through telephone conversations or email discussions, depending on what is practical and the service user's preference.

During reviews the originally identified problem can be considered as well as the goal and planned actions. Whether each has been completely met, partially met or completely unmet can be a useful starting block for further discussion (e.g. How were the goals met? Did the actions have the desired outcome? Were there any stumbling blocks or challenges that were not foreseen and planned for?).

As the actions and the strategies aimed at meeting the goals are explicitly stated in the care plan they provide a framework for discussions. The service user and nurse update, celebrate success, discuss what worked and what did not work and consider any new thoughts they might have as a result of implementing the care plan. New actions or goals can then be identified and the care plan continued as it is, or with changes, or ended.

 15.7 Discharge

Although the process described appears straightforward it is in fact complex and requires skill to remain focused on the task. The process could potentially become a never-ending loop so it is important the service user is involved, in partnership, and is seen as an integral part of the process. Through explicitly setting goals and actions, and taking part in the process, service users can go on to work on their goals independently.

The ending of the care plan, and the working relationship with the nurse, needs to be planned, spoken about and agreed. The ending can mean a transition to another service such as from child and adolescent services to adult services or discharge from services altogether. These transitions are critical times that need careful thought and planning.

 15.8 Conclusion

Care plans come in many formats and there is more than one way of documenting them. However, there are stages common to all. These are:

- identifying the difficulty;
- identifying the goal;

- agreeing the actions;
- implementing the actions;
- review.

Wherever possible these stages should be undertaken in partnership with the service user, using their language and ideas. This chapter has looked at this process and explored the nurse's role and some of the challenges that may be faced.

In summary, the key points of learning from this chapter are:

- **Partnership:** establishing a therapeutic relationship and shared understanding of the situation with the service user is fundamental to collaboratively writing a care plan that is both meaningful and realistic.

- **Goal:** the service user and the nurse need to decide what the goal of a care plan is. Only one goal should be documented per care plan. Care pathways for specific disorders are important when thinking about the goal of a care plan but should not detract or replace what the service user prioritizes.

- **Actions:** a care plan needs to detail the actions that individuals will take in order to work towards the goal. These need to be specific, measurable, achievable, realistic, time orientated, explicit and negotiated.

- **Review:** the care plan needs to have a fixed review date but should also be reviewed throughout the time a nurse works with a service user. The review may lead to a change in goal or actions. Changes may be needed due to a change in circumstance, a new understanding of the difficulty or a realization that the planned actions were not helping to achieve the goal.

- **Transition:** transitions to other services or teams need careful care planning to ensure risks are managed and everyone is working towards the same goals.

Annotated bibliography

Hall, A., Wren, M. and Kirby, S. (2007) *Care Planning in Mental Health: Promoting recovery.* **Oxford: Wiley-Blackwell.**
This thorough book offers a full and detailed exploration of care planning in the mental health setting. The focus is on nursing and the recovery model but it also discusses care planning across professional and organizational boundaries, as well as safeguarding children.

Jakopac, K.A. and Patel, S.C. (2009) *Psychiatric Mental Health Case Studies and Care Plans.* **Burlington, MA: Jones & Bartlett Publishers.**
A useful book that details a number of case studies with accompanying care plans.

Davis, H. and Day, C. (2010) *Working in Partnership with Parents: The Family Partnership Model,* **2nd edn. London: Pearson.**
This is an excellent book that looks in detail at building a partnership relationship with families. Although the emphasis is on families the principles and practical examples offer the reader ideas about how to engage with service users that are difficult to reach.

Barrett, D., Wilson, B. and Woollands, A. (2008) *Care Planning: A guide for nurses.* **London: Pearson.**
This book is a helpful exploration of care plans in relation to specific nursing models and theory.

References

CQC (Care Quality Commission) (2010) Supporting briefing note: community mental health survey 2010, available at: http://tinyurl.com/3xnkvaz, accessed 27 July 2011.
DH (Department of Health) (2008) *Refocusing the Care Programme Approach: Policy and positive practice guidance.* London: DH.
Engel, G. L. (1977) The need for a new medical model: a challenge for biomedicine, *Science,* 196: 129–36.
Maslow, A., H. (1943) A theory of human motivation, *Psychological Review,* 50: 4, 370–96.

Chapter 16

Admission and Discharge Planning

Charlotte Roberts and Jane Padmore

16.1 Introduction

This chapter addresses admission and discharge planning with particular emphasis on the nurse's role. Although the chapter focuses on adult patients, the processes described are transferrable with only minor revision to children and older adults.

This chapter should be read in conjunction with the other core procedure chapters, in particular, 'The therapeutic relationship: engaging clients in their care and treatment' (Chapter 12), 'Assessment' (Chapter 14), and 'Care planning' (Chapter 15). These skills are necessary for effective admission and discharge planning. Crisis and contingency planning are not discussed in detail as they are considered in Chapters 17 and 18.

In this chapter, using a case study, the following areas are explored:

- preparation for admission;
- reasons for admission;
- the nurse's role in admission;
- challenges during admission;
- admission under the Mental Health Act;
- discharge planning;
- the role of the nurse in discharge planning;
- the transition from inpatient to community;
- challenges to discharge planning.

The case of Anna will be used as this chapter explores admission and supported discharge.

Case Study

Anna

Anna is a 22-year-old white British female who has previously been diagnosed with schizoaffective disorder. She has been known to mental health services since the age of 12, when she began to report feeling low in mood and refused to attend school. Prior to age 12 she had been described as lively, popular and outgoing. Before she became unwell, Anna used to enjoy art, swimming and riding bikes.

Anna has previously attended cognitive behavioural therapy (CBT) sessions as an outpatient and been prescribed a range of antidepressants. She was reluctant, during adolescence, to comply with the medication regime due to fears that she would put on weight. She was detained under the Mental Health Act (MHA) on two occasions prior to the age of 18 due to risks she posed to herself in the form of suicidal thoughts and plans.

Since the age of 18, Anna has been known to her local community mental health team (CMHT). Over time, she has developed a good relationship with her care coordinator, Nicola. She is also supported by a support, time and recovery worker (STaR), Betty. Over the past year Anna has been attending an art evening class on a regular basis.

Anna continues to live with her mother and father. She has a 25-year-old sister who lives with her partner and child nearby. She enjoys spending time with her sister and her family, often entertaining her nephew. Anna's mother has no contact with her siblings following an argument many years ago. Anna's paternal grandparents provide some support to the family, however, their health has recently deteriorated and they require intensive support. The family have very few social networks or support systems.

The family relationships are generally positive, however, Anna's parents have struggled to talk about Anna's difficulties. They appear to feel guilty and report not being able to cope when Anna is acutely unwell. The family avoid conflict and rarely discuss any concerns. They have always presented as supportive of Anna and the professionals involved in her care but find it difficult to acknowledge their role in her recovery.

Anna left mainstream school when she was 14, after her first admission to hospital. She was home tutored until she was 16. Following this she has had little educational input. She has had three part-time jobs working as a sales assistant but found it difficult to meet the demands of the roles. She maintains regular contact with a friend who she went to school with and they occasionally meet up at the weekends. Aside from him, she has no other friends.

Anna's father recently contacted Nicola to express concerns about Anna's mental health. Her parents were concerned that she had stopped taking her prescribed medication and was spending increasingly long periods of time in her bedroom. She was refusing them entry into her bedroom and they could smell urine and faeces when the door was opened. Anna had stopped attending her art class and contacting her friend.

When Anna took food from them, at her bedroom door, her parents thought they had seen razor blades and empty packets of paracetamol on her bedroom floor, among the mess. They could not be clear about the accuracy of this or if an overdose had been taken. They also raised a concern that Anna may be responding to unseen stimuli. Anna's parents did not feel they could cope any longer, fearing that Anna may end her life, and requested an admission to hospital in order to keep Anna safe, to give them a break and an opportunity to clean her bedroom. Anna was assessed by the CMHT and admitted to Green Ward.

16.2   Pre-admission

Preparation for admission

Anna's need for admission could have been the result of a rapid or a gradual deterioration in her mental state. During the admission procedure the nurse can explore the pathway to admission with Anna to assist her, and her family, to recognize early warning signs and to encourage them to seek assistance as soon as these are spotted. Early referral may reduce the frequency of Anna's admissions to hospital in future.

Admissions to inpatient mental health wards can be either planned or unplanned. An unplanned admission refers to those which occur in an emergency situation, usually because of risks to the safety of the patient or others. Unplanned admissions include those which involve Section 136 of the MHA 2007 (see Chapter 10).

Unplanned, emergency admissions can be very distressing both for the patient and their carers. They can, without warning, severely disrupt a person's day-to-day life and impact on work, education and social life. In spite of this, unplanned admissions are often necessary. Nurses have an important role in supporting patients to address these difficulties as early as possible – for example, by helping them to let their family know where they are or by contacting, with consent, their employer. The nurse may highlight or help patients consider how their responsibilities can be managed while they are an inpatient. These responsibilities could include the care of their children and pets and communication with their employer.

Planned admissions to inpatient wards involve more communication prior to admission. Planned admissions can be appropriate for women who have a mental health problem who have relapsed previously when pregnant or following childbirth. In such cases, community professionals and the mother may liaise with a mother and baby unit to plan a timely admission to ensure support is available to prevent relapse. Other examples of planned admissions involve alcohol or substance detox units or eating disorder units, or may be appropriate for patients who are not acutely unwell but require admission to an acute ward for observation while their medication is being titrated or changed.

The benefits of a planned admission include: care plans can be devised prior to admission, the patient can be prepared for the admission by visiting the ward and the family or carers can be offered support early. In addition, all professionals, including the general practitioner (GP), can be notified in advance of the planned admission.

Thinking Space 16.1

Consider how Nicola, Anna's care coordinator, could support her and her family prior to Anna's arrival on the ward.

Feedback

- Basic details about the ward including its location, the patient group it accepts for admission, the number of patients it admits at any one time, and whether it is a gender-specific ward.
- An overview of who is in the team that will be providing care for Anna.
- Details of who Anna's parents can contact on the ward for an update of her progress and to discuss her care.
- Visiting hours for family, friends or professionals.

- Expectations or ward rules including smoking regulations, mobile phone use and attendance at a group programme.
- Details of the weekly programme including ward round times, meal times and any group or individual sessions that may be offered.
- Any relevant Care Programme Approach (CPA) information or MHA information, if appropriate.
- Contact details for the ward, the patient telephone, the chaplain and the patient advocacy and liaison service (PALs).
- A list of essential belongings that Anna will need to bring including toiletries, night clothes and underwear.
- A list of any items which are not allowed on to the ward and should therefore be left at home. For example, some wards may not allow lighters or sharp items such as razors on the ward.

You may also have noticed that familiarity with the local inpatient wards would be an advantage to Nicola and would be an essential part of orientation to her care coordinator role. Nicola has a role in assisting Anna and her family to prepare emotionally and practically for Anna's admission to the ward, by sharing her knowledge of the local inpatient wards and explaining the admission procedure and what Anna might expect from this. By preparing them in this way, Nicola lays foundations for therapeutic relationships with her and inpatient staff during the admission and post-discharge.

Nicola will need to tailor information to suit the patient's needs and mental state. It is unlikely that Anna would be able to absorb or want to hear a lot of detail. Her family, though, may want to know what is going to happen, why it may be happening, what they need to pack and how they can support Anna. Being available to answer their questions and prompt them to ensure Anna has clothes and toiletries may be all they can cope with in the short term.

It can be helpful if community nurses, like Nicola, together with the inpatient team, prepare an information pack for patients, clearly written and comprehensive, but without having so much detail that it feels overwhelming. A similar pack may be available on the ward, as an admission pack. The pack offers the patient an initial impression of the type of experience they can expect to have as well as minimizing the distress that can be caused by matters such as not having the appropriate clothing or not knowing the patients' telephone number. The pack may include a statement about the philosophy of the ward, practical information such as visiting hours and ward timetables. In addition, ward rules with regard to smoking, locked doors and aggression can be set out. The pack may offer a selection of questions a patient can ask if they are admitted to an inpatient service that the community team is unfamiliar with. A clear statement about the community team's ongoing involvement and role during the patient's admission can set the scene for a collaborative working relationship with ward staff.

Bed management

Successful admission requires collaboration between both inpatient and community staff to ensure seamless care. Given the overall change in focus from inpatient wards to community services, the limited number of available beds requires careful management to ensure these resources are used as efficiently as possible. The sparse existing evidence base indicates that having a gatekeeper to act at this interface is one way to achieve this (McEvoy 2000). In addition, a framework for formalized communication and information-sharing is required.

The gatekeeper, generally a nurse, may be referred to as the 'bed manager'. This person is the central point for communication between services and is responsible for maintaining a balance between the appropriate usage of the inpatient beds and the need for emergency admissions. A key role for the bed manager is to assess the appropriateness of patients referred for admission by community mental health services. This will usually involve scrutiny of referral forms in consultation with other members of the inpatient team. If a referral for admission is accepted, the bed manager identifies a bed and liaises with the ward to agree and arrange the admission.

Since the scope of bed managers' decisions is restricted by available funds and resources they need to work closely with inpatient staff to facilitate appropriate admissions. A key challenge of the bed manager's role is being able to successfully manage competing pressures arising from wanting to meet patients' needs, adhere to inpatient admission criteria and manage demands for admission from community teams. As a consequence, bed managers' decisions may often be criticized by patients, the assessing community professionals and also inpatient staff concerned about admissions they regard as inappropriate. Ultimately the goal should be to ensure that someone who is acutely unwell, and who is judged to pose a risk, either to themselves or others, is placed in an appropriate inpatient setting as quickly as possible. In Anna's case, it would probably be Nicola who refers her to the bed manager to request admission. Some UK National Health Service (NHS) trusts will accept direct referrals from community care coordinators; others require agreement from the community consultant psychiatrist. Factors that may influence the allocation of the bed in Anna's case would include:

- **geographical location of the bed:** close to Anna's family to enable them to visit and so support her;
- **ward demographics:** Anna requires an adult female bed on a ward for acute mental health problems;

- **Anna's past history:** wards where Anna has been admitted previously and how she progressed on them.

Once a bed is identified, the bed manager will contact the ward nursing team to discuss the referral and request that they liaise directly with Anna and her family to arrange admission.

Clearly documented bed management protocols that are shared by both community and inpatient staff can ensure admissions take place quickly and smoothly, minimizing stress to people like Anna and her family. Trends in admissions from specific teams or involving specific patients should be audited periodically to inform service development.

 ## 16.3 Admission

Reasons for admission

Staff require a clear understanding of the grounds upon which admission is justified to be able to effectively work in collaboration with community services and families when agreeing and planning an admission. Without this, tension between different parts of the mental health service is unavoidable. One way of achieving this is through the use of care pathways.

Local care pathways should be developed to promote implementation of key principles of good care (NICE 2011). They allow for a shared understanding of why people need admitting to hospital. For example, a person may have been offered several antipsychotic medications with limited success in reducing symptoms. An admission could be beneficial to enable a detailed review of their mental state and compliance with medication. Alternatively, their symptoms may have reached a level of severity where there are concerns about their vulnerability, level of self-care and engagement with services.

Although care pathways are helpful for promoting liaison between services and providing clarity for patients, it is important for nurses to always consider patients as individuals who may not fit neatly into a care pathway. Care pathways offer a framework for practice, that nurses apply their clinical expertise to, rather than a set of rules to be followed unquestioningly.

The function of inpatient wards is not explicitly defined by current national policy or legislation. National Institute for Health and Clinical Excellence (NICE) guidelines suggest when admission is indicated. A review of the literature found that the most common reasons for admission were when patients were at risk to themselves or others, for detailed assessment of complex symptoms, for medical treatment, the presence of positive or negative symptoms which cannot be managed in the community, and respite for carers. The chapters presented in Part 5 of this book examine mental disorders and identify when admission may be indicated in particular cases.

Anna presented for admission due to deterioration in her mental state, which led to behaviours that, if left, would have been both harmful to her and her family. Although there was no definitive evidence that she was suicidal, Anna's history, withdrawal from her family and friend, self-neglect and aspects suggestive of self-harm indicated that she was a risk to herself.

The nurse's role

The role of the nurse in relation to admission is complex and varies. Despite the NICE guidelines suggesting when admission is warranted, there remains a lack of clarity around the purpose of inpatient stays and consequently the role of nurses from the point of admission onwards. Psycho-education, managing anxiety, anger and self-harm, techniques for coping with specific symptoms such as hearing voices and managing medication as well as other opportunities to engage in structured activities are some aspects of care and treatment to which nurses can make a valuable contribution.

Nurses can find it a challenge to articulate what their contribution is in relation to the purpose of admissions. This has been attributed, in part, to a paucity of research in inpatient settings in recent years. Whatever the reasons, the result has been a lack of consistency in practice around both admis-sion and discharge. This section discusses some of the core roles nurses have during admission in inpatient settings.

Liaison with the bed manager

Nurses may be involved in liaising with the bed manager to discuss the appropriateness of any referrals. Ward nurses know the current mix of patients on the ward and the level of risk. They are therefore well placed to share information and provide advice about how the new patient will fit in and whether they will feel safe and secure. As well as the patient feeling safe, nurses are also responsible for ensuring the ward remains a safe environment and this should influence their decision-making when accepting referrals to a ward.

Preparation prior to arrival

Following liaison with the bed manager, and acceptance of an admission, a bedroom or bay should be prepared for the patient to be shown to when they arrive. Paperwork, such as an induction pack for both the patient and their carers, should be ready.

The rest of the team should be informed of the admission and any particular risks or clinical needs. Where possible the nurse needs to be aware of all the medication the patient is currently prescribed so that the pharmacy can be alerted to any non-stock medication required.

Allocation of a named nurse

Although practice differs between services, most wards allocate a named nurse to each patient. It is good practice to allocate this person prior to the patient arriving. Where possible, the named nurse should be someone who is on shift when the person is admitted so that they can begin to develop a relationship straight away and initial care plans can be devised.

Arrival at the ward

On arrival patients should be welcomed by a member of the nursing team and orientated to the ward. Simple things, such as asking what the patient would like to be called or whether they would like a drink can make a significant difference to the patient's experience of feeling cared for.

The admitting nurse is responsible for checking the suitability of patients' possessions prior to allowing them onto the ward. For example, sharp items or materials that could be used for arson are generally not allowed to be kept in bedrooms or on someone's person. The patient may wish to be introduced to other patients. The importance of these duties should not be underestimated as they form the patient's first impression of the service.

Contact with carers

If a carer attends with the patient, it is essential that their contact details are taken and recorded. It may be appropriate to show them around the ward. Any questions they have should be seen as important and answered accordingly. If carers are not present, their details should be sought as a priority by the care coordinator, so that they can be involved in the care of the person admitted.

Assessment

After arrival, an assessment, led by the ward doctor and joined by the admitting nurse, will take place to ascertain the patient's perception of any recent difficulties which have led to admission, their personal and family history and social situation (see Chapter 14). This is sometimes called 'clerking in'. It is an opportunity for nurses to gather information about the patient's emotional, physical, social, cultural and spiritual needs in addition to any risk factors which would guide the care the nursing team provide.

In addition a nursing assessment can take place. Nurse-specific assessment tools can be devised and implemented and these may reflect any nursing model the team utilizes to guide their practice. This focus tends to differ from the assessment described above as the nurse will focus on the patient's experience of, and day-to-day management on, the ward. Other areas that may be considered are sleep patterns, diet preferences, how the patient communicates distress, what they found helpful during any previous admissions and their hopes and fears in relation to the admission and the future.

Nurses are the only professional group who are on hand to care for patients in inpatient units 24 hours a day, seven days a week. Therefore they are in a unique position to gather information about the patient's mental state and level of functioning through interactions and observations. If the benefits of 24-hour nursing care are to be maximized it is essential that information is collated and clearly communicated to other members of the multi-disciplinary team to inform assessment, diagnosis and treatment. All of the gathered information is essential both for the development of therapeutic relationships and of care plans that are person-centred and SMART (see Chapter 15).

Risk management

Admission should provide safety for actively suicidal, behaviourally disturbed or vulnerable individuals. Risk management and assessment is considered in Chapters 17 and 18 and so only aspects specifically relating to admission will be covered here. With respect to those who present a danger to others, there is a clear role for nurses to be involved in security. For example, on admission, the nurse needs to consider the level of observation the patient should be placed under and some patients may need to be prevented from leaving the ward on safety grounds.

A full risk assessment should be carried out as early as possible and updated throughout the admission. A risk plan should be drawn up, with the patient, which makes explicit how any aggression or violence would be managed. Similarly, if someone poses a risk to themselves an assessment with a care plan should be drawn up that ensures the person's safety as well as encourages independence. In addition, the ward environment needs to be constantly risk assessed to identify any potentially harmful objects. As well as managing risk during the patient's hospital stay, nurses need to consider and document any potential risks when the patient is on leave or discharged. This information can then be communicated and incorporated into the patient's care. When leave is granted, documentation of what the person is wearing should be kept in case they do not return to the ward. If this does occur, the nurses are responsible for informing the police that the patient is currently a missing person.

Medication

A unique responsibility of nurses is dispensing medication safely. This is particularly important for those patients who have been admitted following a worsening mental state due to non-compliance with medication in the community; a contributory factor to admission in 35 per cent of cases (Abas *et al.* 2003).

Nurses need to gather information about patients' history of compliance, their understanding of the prescribed medications, their experience of whether they have been helpful and any preferences they have such as taking the medication at a particular time of day. Side-effects need also to be discussed and any that are evident recorded. This information should be shared with the doctor and used when planning care with the patient.

Physical health

Nurses are responsible, in collaboration with the medical team, for supporting patients to promote their physical health. This includes regular monitoring of their baseline observations such as temperature, pulse, respirations, blood pressure, weight and height. This is particularly important for those who are taking medications such as olanzapine, which can cause weight gain.

While in inpatient care, patients generally eat their meals on the ward. Nurses need to work with individuals to support them to take a balanced diet. Exercise is a particular issue on wards where patients have limited access to outside areas. Therefore exercise should be incorporated into the daily programme.

Diversity issues

All inpatient units should seek to provide a safe, culturally competent and supportive environment. Issues relating to the diversity needs, such as cul-

ture, spirituality, disability, gender and religion of patients need to be considered by the nurses both on an individual patient level and on the ward level. For example, there should be a policy regarding same-sex accommodation.

The Mental Health Foundation (2007) suggests that spirituality can play an important role in helping people maintain good mental health and live with or recover from mental health problems. This is discussed in relation to acute mental health admissions by NICE (2008). Religious practices such as prayer times, dietary requirements or access to a spiritual leader can be essential for some.

Communication and coordination of care

From the moment of arrival at the ward, until discharge, the nursing team is responsible for the coordination of the individual's care and liaison with outside agencies and families. This can involve regular telephone calls to community professionals to provide updates on progress, referrals to identified agencies and keeping in touch with carers.

Communication internally is also important. The named nurse is responsible for ensuring accurate information is provided in the ward's multi-professional meeting or ward round so that appropriate decisions can be made. Reports for meetings should be written in collaboration with the patient where possible to represent their views and the views of the nursing team.

Patients' rights

Nurses are responsible for making sure patients are aware of their rights while they are an inpatient. For example, if someone is an informal patient but the ward has locked doors, they need to know that they have the right to leave the unit.

If someone is detained under the MHA 2007, their rights need to be read to them and this needs to be documented. If they do not understand their rights, this needs to be repeated, and explained, until they do. In addition, carers should be made aware of the patient's rights so that they can support them in their decision-making. A referral to a local advocate for support can be helpful.

Thinking Space 16.2

Anna arrives at Green Ward accompanied by her parents and her care coordinator. She has agreed to come to the ward voluntarily and therefore her status is informal.

1. What do you consider the reasons for admission to be?
2. If you were the admitting nurse, what factors would you consider when admitting Anna to the ward?
3. What would the role of the nursing team be during Anna's admission?

Feedback

1. Understanding the reasons for admission is important to ensure the ward team is working in partnership with Anna, her family and the community team. The ward nurse should ascertain what Anna's goals for admission are, as well as the views of her family and care coordinator. Different perspectives and goals should be worked with and incorporated into Anna's care.

   - Anna's mental health has deteriorated. The community team may want the goal of her admission to be to maintain her safety and return to a stable mental state.
   - Anna's parents stated their hope for admission. This was to keep Anna safe, to give them a break and to give them an opportunity to clean her bedroom.
   - From the scenario it is unclear what Anna wants from the admission. She may have just agreed to admission for fear of being sectioned under the MHA or she may recognize that she needs help to improve how she is feeling.

2. Admissions to acute mental health wards can happen at any time, day or night. All members of the multi-disciplinary team are unlikely to be available but there will always be a nurse on duty. Each ward will have its own admission protocol, with prepared checklists and assessment tools to use. When working on a ward for the first time it can be helpful to familiarize yourself with this before a new admission arrives. When considering this question, imagine what it might feel like to be Anna, who is both unwell and is afraid of leaving her home. She will be entering a strange environment, possibly with people acting in unusual ways, while feeling vulnerable and scared herself. Central to nursing is 'care' and, above all else, the nurse should approach Anna as a fellow human being in distress, attempting to make her feel as welcome as possible without being overbearing. The roles of the nurse in admission are many and varied. In addition to welcoming Anna and orientating her to the ward the admitting nurse should prioritize:

   - Completing and documenting a risk assessment and plan, ensuring this is communicated with the ward team. This risk assessment covers risks to her, others, the ward environment and any risk arising from her leaving the ward.
   - The initial report, from the community, is that Anna has stopped taking her medication. The nurse can talk to Anna about her medication, gaining insight into why she has stopped taking it.
   - Liaison with Anna's family, ensuring contact details and best times to call them are documented. Taking time to hear their concerns and expectations of the admission can help the ward keep Anna's family involved in her care.

- It was reported that Anna was isolated in her room, with the smell of urine and faeces coming from within. Her personal hygiene would need to be attended to. Prior to this the nurse should take time to understand and talk to Anna about any fears she has of using the toilet, or washing in the bathroom.

3. Every ward and nursing team will have, to a certain extent, different ways of working and therefore varying roles. Some roles that you may have considered, in relation to Anna, are:

   - Anna has a history of self-harm and suicide attempts. There may also be other patients who pose a risk to others. Nurses have a key role in maintaining a safe environment.

   - Nurses need to develop a therapeutic relationship with Anna to form the basis of ongoing work.

   - As Anna has not been taking her medication, the nurse has an important role in relation to medication management: the safe administration of medication, monitoring and reporting or treating side-effects.

   - Providing unique insights into Anna's mental state, progress and general needs and difficulties through observation and informal talks with her.

   - Anna came to the ward informally, indicating that she may be willing to start to think about her difficulties and set goals for recovery. The nursing team is central to this process, helping her identify anything she struggles with and setting realistic and achievable goals.

   - Keeping in touch with Anna's family and her community team.

Challenges during admission

Without clarity and agreed reasons for admission, there are negative consequences for the nursing team and consequently the patients on the ward. These include increased staff stress, leading to burnout, increased conflict within the staff team and between staff and patients, and a lack of a sense of achievement in relation to job performance. Admissions can become lengthy and lack direction. A clear framework for admission increases nurses' purposefulness, leading to higher quality care.

Nurses can play a useful role in ensuring that the multi-disciplinary team understands the reasons for a person's admission and that this understanding matches that of the referrer and the patient. As a consequence the assessment and treatment plan developed will support these views. This needs to occur prior to the patient arriving on the ward. Without this, frustrations can arise from the patient and family, as well as from members of the community team who may perceive the inpatient team as unproductive, or lacking purpose or structure.

Other barriers include a lack of available beds at the time when a patient is warranting admission, poor bed management, limited staffing both in inpatient and community services, and multi-disciplinary tensions. A lack of clarity around the roles of the community staff by the inpatient team, and vice versa, further complicates working relationships.

Detention under the MHA

Occasionally patients are detained under a section of the MHA 1983 (amendments 2007), either for their own health and safety, or because they pose a risk to other people (see Chapter 10).

Thinking Space 16.3

Anna agreed to be admitted on a voluntary basis, however, if she had not and her deterioration in mental health had warranted detention she would have been brought to Green Ward under a section of the MHA, against her will.

1. What impact would this have on the role of the nurse when she arrives at the ward?
2. How would the goals of the admission be affected?

Feedback

1. All the usual tasks and responsibilities that the nurse would normally undertake apply. Anna would still need to be welcomed, orientated and treated with respect and dignity. In addition the nurse would be responsible for checking the accuracy of the MHA papers. The appropriate paperwork would need to be completed and local policy followed to ensure that the papers are sent to the correct MHA office to be processed. If this process is not completed accurately the result can be that a patient is held illegally on a secure ward.

2. Aside from the additional paperwork responsibilities, nurses also need to ensure the patient has been told and understands their rights. Even knowing their rights patients can feel powerless, with the nurse being perceived as powerful and controlling. The nurse has a responsibility to think about how they can work with the patient in a way that they will find helpful. The nurse needs to ensure that the patient is as involved as possible in making decisions about their care and treatment.

16.4 Discharge planning

Why is discharge planning necessary?

Discharge is inevitable. Planning discharge is an essential aspect of nursing care and the admission process. The latest government legislation, *No Health Without Mental Health: A cross-government mental health outcomes strategy for people of all ages* (DH 2011), highlights the need for addressing delayed discharges to reduce service inefficiency, increase the effectiveness of inpatient care and decrease the duration of inpatient stays.

With the increased pressure to release beds, discharge in recent years has often arisen from demand for a vacant bed rather than the patient being fit to leave (Watts and Gardner 2005). Negative conse-

quences have included patients being in the community with unmet needs, being poorly prepared for independent living after being in hospital, and increased likelihood of readmission within a short time period. Discharge planning is therefore a necessity for effective transition from the hospital to community.

What is discharge planning?

A number of definitions of discharge planning are found within the literature. These include 'the process of coordinating the delivery of health care services beyond the hospital services' (Anderson and Helms 1994: 69), and 'an on-going process that facilitates the discharge of the patient to the appropriate level of care. It involves a multidisciplinary assessment of patient/family needs and coordination of care, services and referrals' (McGinley *et al.*

1996: 55). There are common threads between the available definitions, however, ambiguity remains, which has led to variation in meaning within the evidence base.

What should discharge planning look like?

There is a lack of specific guidance around best practice in relation to discharge planning in mental health services. However, nurses can learn from the Department of Health's (DH) 2010 paper *Ready to Go? Planning the discharge and the transfer of patients from hospital and intermediate care*, which highlights the importance of starting to plan for discharge either before, or on, admission. This enables any anticipated difficulties to be identified early on and to be resolved in a timely manner.

The stages of discharge planning

There are four stages to effective discharge planning (Watts and Gardner 2005).

1. **Assessment of the patient's needs.** Although the pressure for briefer admissions means this can be difficult to achieve, it is important for two reasons. The assessment will guide the decision-making around when the patient will be ready for discharge – i.e. when the admission goals have been reached. It will identify needs to be followed up and met within the community.

2. **Development of the discharge plan.** Patients and their families should be involved in the discharge plan at the earliest opportunity. This ensures that their views are incorporated into the plan, helping them have realistic expectations about the length of admission.

3. **Implementation of the discharge plan.** Given that patients tend to require follow up and fur-

ther intervention after discharge, community services should be included in the planning stages so that the plan is realistic and achievable. This should enhance the effectiveness of the coordination and execution of post-discharge care.

4. **Evaluation of the discharge plan.**

The CPA and discharge planning

The CPA has been a part of mental health practice since 1990. It is a framework that aims to support and coordinate high quality mental health care for people requiring specialist mental health services. Any individual who requires multi-agency support, active engagement and intensive intervention should receive services in line with the CPA (DH 2008).

Each mental health trust has local policies around the use of the CPA. Overall, the CPA process supports discharge planning. It requires all agencies involved with a patient to meet on a regular basis to review with the individual, and their family or carers, their progress in relation to identified care plans.

As soon after the admission as possible, a CPA meeting should be arranged. At this meeting discharge plans should be formally considered. This will involve discussion about how the agencies and patient will know when discharge is appropriate. This will be closely linked to the admission goals. In addition, potential challenges that may lead to a delay in discharge should be highlighted so that they can be addressed. By doing this work at the start a shared understanding of the goals and process can be developed.

What should be included in a discharge plan?

Discharge plans will vary but should consider all aspects of a patient's needs.

Thinking Space 16.4

When writing a discharge plan for Anna, what would you need to consider in relation to her:

- mental health needs;
- physical well-being;
- social needs;
- spiritual needs?

Feedback

Some ideas you may have considered when responding to these questions are detailed but this is not an exhaustive list. It is important to remember that the views of Anna, her parents and professionals involved with Anna should be prioritized.

- **Mental health needs:** Anna will require a 'seven-day follow up'. This needs to be arranged with the community services, ensuring they have it scheduled and are aware of Anna's needs and the timescales. The appointment time and venue will have preferably been negotiated with Anna and her parents but the nurses can ensure they have the information and encourage them to keep the appointment. Consideration needs to be given to Anna's medication.

  - What medication is she prescribed on discharge?
  - Does she understand what it is for and when to take it?
  - Does she require support to ensure she requests repeat prescriptions, safe storage and administration?
  - Would Anna or her parents benefit from further psycho-education about the medication, its benefits and its side-effects prior to discharge?
  - After leaving the hospital, a plan is needed to specify who will prescribe and dispense her medication.

  Would Anna benefit from specific psychological treatment post discharge, either continuing work she was participating in on the ward or starting something new? There may be waiting lists for treatment and so referrals should be made as soon as possible. Crisis and contingency plans are a wise addition to anyone's discharge plan. It appears that Anna's mental state gradually deteriorated before reaching the crisis, meaning an admission was necessary. Anna, her parents and the community team can learn from this and put in place plans to stop deterioration and act quickly. This plan may include how they identify difficulties before they develop into a crisis, and what they should do in an emergency.

- **Physical well-being:** a full assessment of Anna's physical health needs will have been completed during the admission. Any issues identified will need to be managed on the ward. On discharge this responsibility reverts to her GP. If physical health difficulties are likely to affect Anna's ability to live independently, consideration needs to be given to involving social services or charitable organizations for support.

■ **Social needs:** although information about Anna's social circumstances is given in the initial referral it remains important to explore this fully during the admission. Anna lives with her parents. She may have unspoken desires to move out, or her parents may feel unable to have her back home. A lack of appropriate housing can lead to delayed discharges. Throughout the admission the question of where Anna will be discharged to needs to be addressed. Her parents' views may fluctuate over time. Anna had withdrawn from her social activities prior to admission. Reintegrating into these activities can start during the admission. In addition, new activities can be tried and plans made to continue on discharge. Assessment of her parents' needs and subsequent support for them will enhance the care Anna will receive from them. Anna has contact with her sister's young child. Whenever a patient has young children or contact with young children it is important to consider the needs of the children and identify any safeguarding concerns or measures that need to be put in place.

■ **Spiritual needs:** during the admission the nurse will have gained an understanding of Anna's spiritual needs. Incorporating these into her discharge planning can promote recovery and prevent relapse.

The role of the nurse in discharge planning

Discharge planning is a multi-disciplinary activity; however, nurses have a prominent role in ensuring its success. They are accountable for their practice and must work to ensure that the care of patients is their priority, according to the Nursing and Midwifery Council (NMC) *Code* (2008) They have a responsibility to ensure that when their patients leave the inpatient setting the appropriate services are in place to meet their needs.

Discharge planning is one element of the nursing care plan process. The nurse acts as an advocate for patients within the multi-disciplinary team, to ensure that their voice is heard when planning occurs. The role and expectations of nurses will vary between services. However, nurses are responsible for coordinating the care of their patients and therefore must be confident that appropriate discharge plans are being considered and implemented.

In preparation for discharge nurses often need to make referrals to other agencies, such as social services, charities or other mental health services. Ensuring that patients are consulted and consent is given increases the likelihood of them engaging with services post-discharge. Throughout the admission liaison with other professionals, both on the tele-

phone and in writing, is important to inform them of decisions made, progress the person is making and any changes to the agreed time frame for discharge. Regular contact with carers is essential to ensure they are part of the discharge planning progress, enabling them to prepare for the patient to return home.

It is important to ensure, where possible, that any specific therapeutic work is planned to end prior to discharge. This includes the therapeutic relationship between nurses and patients. Therefore, nurses need to work with their patients to reflect on and explore what the ending of their relationship will mean when the patient is discharged from hospital. This could be through individual one-to-one time or groups focused on the process of moving on from hospital.

The skills nurses need to fulfil their role in relation to discharge planning are varied. Nurses need to be able to engage a patient to work in partnership in establishing an agreed and realistic discharge plan. Skills in assessment and care planning are key to the development of an effective plan. Not only do nurses need to be able to assess people's mental states, they also need to be able to identify their ability and motivation to be involved in the process of discharge planning. Identification of barriers to their involvement requires clear communication to, and careful consideration by, the multi-disciplinary team.

Box 16.1 Nursing responsibilities in relation to discharge planning

- Engage with the patient
- Assessment and identification of needs
- Monitor progress
- Regular liaison with agencies and carers
- Act as an advocate for the patient and their family
- Draw up discharge plans with all involved in the care
- Make relevant referrals in a timely manner
- Communicate with multi-disciplinary team to evaluate plans and identify potential barriers to a successful discharge
- Ensure that when the patient is discharged their needs have been fully considered and appropriate plans are in place where any safeguarding concerns have been addressed

---

Commitment to equipping nurses with the necessary skills, and teams with appropriate systems, to improve the discharge process is shown by the NHS Institute for Innovation and Improvement's 'Releasing Time to Care: The Productive Ward Programme' which includes a module on admission and discharge planning.

The transition from inpatient to community care

Research suggests that it is the ending of supportive relationships which have been built up during the admission with inpatient staff that is most acutely felt by patients following discharge (Reynolds *et al.* 2004). This can be particularly difficult for patients to cope with if they do not have supportive relationships within the community. Discharge can leave individuals with little support at a time when they are likely to be experiencing stress due to their need to readapt to home life. Consequently, involving community staff in the individual's care early on in the admission is crucial.

Utilization of a transitional model of discharge has been found to improve quality of life and prevent readmission in several studies. This model acknowledges the difficulties associated with the transition from inpatient to community services unless appropriate support is in place. Support could include peer support from other patients or continued involvement from inpatient staff, over the phone or via a discharge group. While it is not general practice for inpatient staff to continue their involvement with discharged patients, evidence for a supportive discharge model does exist and has been implemented across the UK with a variety of groups of patients.

Discharge planning challenges

Thinking Space 16.5

A CPA meeting is held for Anna four weeks into her admission at Green Ward. In attendance are her parents and her STaR worker. Her care coordinator is unable to attend. This is the first multi-agency meeting since admission.

The ward staff have become increasingly frustrated with Anna's lack of commitment to the treatments they offered her and feel her progress has been limited. Based on their most recent risk assessment, her risk to self has decreased since admission. They propose that she should be discharged at some point over the next month. The family and STaR worker agree with this plan.

Over the next week at Green Ward, Anna's engagement with staff decreases further and a decision is made to discharge her. She is informed of this decision on a Wednesday morning. An email was sent to her STaR worker to inform her that afternoon. No other people were informed of the plan to discharge Anna.

Anna left the ward at 4 p.m. that day.

1. What are the strengths of this discharge plan?
2. Have you identified any potential problems with this discharge plan?
3. Can you think of anything which could have been done differently?

Feedback

The ward staff organized a CPA meeting for Anna. Ideally, the CPA meeting would have been earlier in Anna's admission; however, four weeks could fit the time frames of some local policies.

1. Having the right people at the meeting can maximize the chance of the plan being realistic, with key individuals knowing what is expected of them and when. In this case the ward and the community staff were invited along with Anna and her parents. On the day of discharge an email was sent to Anna's STaR worker, however, the STaR worker does not have the overall responsibility for her care. Additionally, there is no guarantee that she would have received the email – for example, if she was not in the office.

2. In the CPA meeting, ward staff expressed their concerns about Anna's lack of engagement with them. They acknowledged their own feelings of frustration about her lack of progress. By expressing the difficulty in this way it becomes centred around Anna and could be perceived as Anna being 'naughty'. This could lead to a breakdown in the therapeutic relationships Anna has with ward staff and to a challenge when developing a discharge plan. It was unfortunate that Anna's care coordinator was unable to attend the CPA meeting, but the nature of busy community teams coupled with rigid ward timetables can make this unavoidable. The absence of this key individual meant that the community services were not a part of the discharge planning process. In addition, as the care coordinator had known Anna and her family for some time she might have been able to give an alternative view to that held by the inpatient staff. It may have been appropriate to discharge Anna on that day but this should have been done in consultation with Anna, her parents and the care coordinator. Given that Anna's care coordinator would be responsible for offering a seven-day follow up and the community team would resume clinical responsibility for Anna's care, the lack of communication could have had serious negative consequences. Although her family were aware that her discharge would occur over the next month, this time frame lacked specificity and therefore they may not have been prepared for her arriving home that day.

3. The staff clearly felt frustrated by Anna's 'lack of engagement.' Inpatient staff require regular supervision, both as individuals and as a team, to process their feelings about individuals they are caring for. Given the high demands of inpatient settings, staff can often feel stress, which may lead to

burnout. The nurses might have considered, with Anna, why she had disengaged and explored with her whether staff could change their approach to support her to re-engage with treatment. In some cases, discharge following this situation is appropriate. In others, it may lead to increased risk following early discharge. Community mental health services will be responsible for Anna on her discharge from hospital. It is vital that they are involved in the discharge planning, otherwise it can be meaningless, only addressing what needs to happen on the ward rather than the continuity of care into the community. The community team could have sent a representative from the service. Following the CPA meeting the minutes should be put in writing and sent to all those involved. The nursing staff should also contact those who were unable to attend to update them on decisions. It may be necessary to allocate tasks to people who were not present. The details of this would need to be communicated and, if necessary, altered to ensure they are realistic. The discharge could have been delayed for 24 hours while appropriate plans were put in place, which would have included the seven-day follow up appointment.

The journey to discharge is likely to be different for each individual, raising other considerations. Anna may wish to discharge herself against medical advice. Her parents may feel unable to disagree with the treatment team and think she is not ready for discharge. The community and inpatient teams may have differing views about the best treatment or the most appropriate discharge date. Such situations need to be addressed as they arise so they do not have a negative impact on Anna's care.

There are also practical considerations that the nurse needs to address when a patient is discharged. These include:

- Medication to take home with them. The nurse needs to ensure the patient is able to self-administer the medication and that there is enough supplied to cover the period until the next prescription is written.
- The patient has all their belongings.
- Say goodbye. Although, for example in Anna's case, it may appear that patient is not engaging with staff they are likely to have developed relationships which require an appropriate ending. Leaving an inpatient service can, at times, feel like a loss or a rejection. The nurse can have an important role in saying goodbye

and offering some positive feedback about the staff's experience of working with the patient.
- Contingency and crisis plans that are easily understandable and written down, for the patient to take home.
- It is worthwhile checking, particularly if it is winter, or the patient is being discharged in the evening, that they have the means to get food and have heating and hot water in their house.
- Transport may need to be considered.

16.5 Conclusion

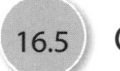

Admission and discharge planning are key components of nursing care requiring the use of the core nursing skills, in particular the ability to engage people in their care and effective coordination of care. Prior to admission, a clear reason for the admission, which is agreed by the inpatient team, the community service and the patient, needs to be established. Local care pathways can assist with this but reasons can range from the need for a secure place because of risks to self or others, assessment, a specified treatment, or respite. Without an agreed reason for admission it is difficult to set goals, leading to a lack of clarity about what the nurse's role is during the admission and discharge planning can lack clarity.

This chapter has considered the nurse's role in admission and discharge planning, including bed management, communication and working in partnership with the patient, carers and other professionals, using the case example of Anna. To facilitate an effective discharge from hospital, planning should begin before, or on, admission, considering all aspects of the individual's needs.

In summary, the key points of learning from this chapter are:

- The reason for an admission needs to be decided and articulated prior to the patient being admitted. This ensures there is a focus for the admission and that there is a way to measure the outcome of the admission. Without a defined purpose there is a risk of a prolonged admission with little improvement in the patient's mental health.

- Communication and good relationships between community and inpatient teams are essential. The transition from the community to the ward and back out into the community can be challenging. Positive outcomes are more likely to be achieved if all the professionals involved in the care pathway are involved in the care plan.

- Admission can be a frightening experience; nurses play a key role in welcoming and orientating the patient. Preparing an admission pack can assist this but should not replace a personal welcome and orientation to the ward.

- Preparation and discussion about discharge should begin as soon as possible after the admission. By starting the discharge plan at the earliest opportunity, potential challenges and blocks can be addressed by all the agencies involved in the patient's care.

Annotated bibliography

Ward, M. (1995) *Nursing the Psychiatric Emergency,* **3rd edn. Oxford: Butterworth-Heinemann Ltd.**
This book nicely balances the science of nursing with the human element of caring, while working with patients that find themselves at the receiving end of mental health services.

Hardcastle, M., Kennard, D., Grandison, D. and Fagin, L. (2007) *Experiences of Mental Health In-patient Care: Narratives from service users, carers and professionals: 2.* **London: The International Society for the Psychological Treatments of the Schizophrenias and Other Psychoses/Routledge.**
A helpful collection of first-hand accounts of mental health inpatient care.

References

Abas, M., Vanderpyl, J., Le Prou, T., Kydd, R., Emery, B. and Foliaki, S. (2003) Psychiatric hospitalisation: reasons for admission and alternatives to admission in South Aukland, New Zealand, *Australian and New Zealand Journal of Psychiatry,* 37: 620–5.
Anderson, M. and Helms, S. (1994) Quality improvement in discharge planning: an evaluation of factors in communication between healthcare providers, *Journal of Nursing and Care Quality,* 8: 62–72.
DH (Department of Health) (2008) *Refocusing the Care Programme Approach,* available at: www.dh.gov.uk/prod_consum_dh/groups/dh_digitalassets/@dh/@en/documents/digitalasset/dh_083649.pdf, accessed November 2011.
DH (Department of Health) (2010) *Ready to Go? Planning the discharge and the transfer of patients from hospital and intermediate care,* available at: www.dh.gov.uk/en/Publicationsandstatistics/Publications/PublicationsPolicyAndGuidance/DH_113950, accessed November 2011.
DH (Department of Health) (2011) *No Health Without Mental Health: A cross-government mental health outcomes strategy for people of all ages,* available at: www.dh.gov.uk/en/Publicationsandstatistics/Publications/PublicationsPolicyAndGuidance/DH_123766, accessed November 2011.
McEvoy, P. (2000) Gatekeeping access to services at the primary/secondary care interface, *Journal of Psychiatric and Mental Health Nursing,* 7: 241–7.
McGinley, S., Baus, E., Gyza, K., Johnson, K., Lipton, S., Magee, M., Moore, F. and Wojtyak, D. (1996) Multidisciplinary discharge planning, *Nurse Management,* 27: 57–60.
Mental Health Foundation (2007) *Spirituality and Mental Health,* available at: www.mentalhealth.org.uk/information/mental-health-a-z/spirituality/, accessed November 2011.

NHS Institute of Innovation and Improvement (2006–2011) *Releasing Time to Care*, available at: www.institute.nhs.uk/quality_ and_value/productivity_series/the_productive_series.html, accessed July 2011.

NICE (National Institute for Health and Clinical Excellence) (2008) *Meeting Spiritual Needs on an Acute Mental Health Admission Ward*, available at: www.nice.org.uk/usingguidance/sharedlearningimplementingniceguidance/examplesofimplementation/ eximpresults.jsp?o=236, accessed September 2011.

NICE (National Institute for Health and Clinical Excellence) (2011) *Common Mental Health Disorders*, available at: www.nice.org. uk/cg123, accessed October 2011.

NMC (Nursing and Midwifery Council) (2008) *The Code: Standards of conduct, performance and ethics for nurses and midwives*, available at: www.nmc-uk.org/Nurses-and-midwives/The-code/The-code-in-full/, accessed August 2011.

Reynolds, W., Lauder, W., Sharkey, S., Maciver, S., Veitch, T. and Cameron, D. (2004) The effects of a transitional discharge model for psychiatric patients, *Journal of Psychiatric and Mental Health Nursing*, 11: 82–8.

Watts, R. and Gardner, H. (2005) Nurses' perceptions of discharge planning, *Nursing and Health Sciences*, 7: 175–83.

Chapter 17

Assessing and Managing the Risk of Self-harm and Suicide

Ian P.S. Noonan

When I'm having a depressive episode, the whole world seems to stop around me and grow darker. I scream at the people I hold closest for no reason, all they try to do is help me, but when I start to shut down I don't see that. I see them ignoring me, ignoring my cries for help ... On occasion I find myself sat on my bed, my left arm on my lap and a razor in my right hand. I drag it across the flesh, searching for a relief from the pain, but it never comes...

Beffy94

17.1 Introduction

Self-harm and suicide are two different, yet related, phenomena and although the meaning of self-harm and attempted suicide are often very different, previous self-harm is a significant risk factor for completed suicide.

This chapter covers:

■ why people self-harm;

■ risk management of self-harm and suicide;

■ nursing interventions to promote safer self-harm, or reduce or stop it;

■ suicidal risk management;

■ promoting hope through enhanced engagement and treatment of the multi-faceted *psychache* that can underlie suicidal thoughts and actions.

17.2 What is self-harm?

Self-harm is an umbrella term used to describe a wide range of behaviours. Various terms have been used in the literature such as self-mutilation, self-cutting, self-injurious behaviours, para-suicide and deliberate self-harm. Many of these terms suggest meaning or values that are not helpful to all clients who self-harm. Furthermore, since the 2004 NICE guidelines on the short-term management of self-harm, the prefix 'deliberate' has been dropped to acknowledge that for some people they feel as if they have no choice or no other option than to self-harm, and for others the self-harm occurs in a dissociative state.

The 2011 NICE guidelines on longer-term management of self-harm provide the following definition: 'any act of self-poisoning or self-injury carried out by an individual irrespective of motivation. This commonly involves self-poisoning with medication or self-injury with cutting' (NICE 2011). The guideline provides a relatively narrow definition to be clear about to whom the recommendations apply, and excludes accidental harm to oneself, harm through excessive alcohol or drug use, and harm through starving or binge eating associated with eating disorders.

Self-harm, however, can include a wide range of behaviours that damage an individual's body, either externally or internally, with a meaning or purpose that can vary for any one client on each occasion that they self-harm, and from person to person. The act might be impulsive or planned, with immediate or long-term effect. The term describes only the behaviour and is not an illness. This does not mean that the person who self-harms will not benefit from treatment, rather that there are likely to be coexisting mental health needs which will also need to be addressed to help that person change their self-harming behaviour.

There are behaviours that are culturally congruent, such as tattooing or piercing, which involve breaking the skin; dangerous, adrenalin-fuelled sports; and long term behaviours like drinking too much alcohol which put the person's health at risk and are individual choices. The thing that distinguishes these culturally congruent behaviours that pose a risk to the individual from self-harm is often the intent and mood of the person when they take the risky action.

When considering whether or not a behaviour falls within a broad definition of self-harm we need to examine the *mechanism*, *meaning* and *motivation* to understand the degree of risk to the individual and whether they need support to help develop alternative coping mechanisms. The mechanism of injury gives a good indication of the level of risk associated with the act, but not what the act means for the person who has self-harmed. The degree of risk depends in part on how damaging and how reversible/repairable the injury or overdose is. Table 17.1 shows a continuum of self-harm and completed suicide with examples of how the mechanism, meaning and motivation might vary for each. The UK has one of the highest rates of self-harm in Europe at approximately 400 in every 100,000. At least 200,000 presentations to general hospitals in England and Wales follow an episode of self-injury or self-poisoning, and people with current mental health problems are 20 times more likely to report having harmed themselves in the past (Mental Health Foundation 2012). The ratio of women to men who self-harm is approximately equal – in their multi-centre study, Hawton *et al.* (2007) found that 57 per cent of the people presenting with self-harm were women but that the female to male ratio decreased with age. More 15–19-year-old women and 20–24-year-old men sought hospital treatment with self-injury or self-poisoning, with approximately 80 per cent of the attendances being for self-poisoning. However, the Mental Health Foundation (2006) report *Truth Hurts* found that many young people did not report self-cutting. The numbers reported as attending hospital are likely to be far lower than the true number of people who self-harm. Self-harm is not limited to young people and is an indicator of very serious risk in older adults. Murphy *et al.* (2012) studied 1,177 older adults who attended hospitals in Oxford, Manchester and Leeds with self-harm and found that 1.5 per cent had died by suicide within a year of their presentation. Men over 75 had the highest suicide rate and as a group, older adults who had self-harmed had a 67 times higher suicide risk than older adults in the general population.

17.3 Why do people self-harm?

The only way to know why the person you are working with has self-harmed is to ask them. The meaning will be different for each person and may vary on each occasion they harm themselves.

Table 17.1 Continuum of self-harm and completed suicide

	SELF-HARM → ... → COMPLETED SUICIDE								
	Any client might have suicidal thoughts, feelings or plans, whether or not they actually self-harm								
Meaning	Behaviours that may be socially acceptable, but cause harm and could result in accidental or premature death				Deliberate self-harm as a coping mechanism for psychological distress		Behaviours with varying risk of completed suicide. Remember to consider the client's view of whether an act might be lethal		
Mechanism	Tattoos, body piercing, tribal cuts or scarring	Risk-taking: driving too fast, unsafe sex	Smoking or drinking to excess	Illicit drug use or excessive use of prescribed drugs	Binge eating or starvation	Cutting or overdosing without suicidal ideation	Non-lethal cutting or overdosing with the intent to kill oneself	Overdoses, hanging, cutting or immersion with suicidal intent	Attempted suicide with lethal method resulting in death
Motivation	Boredom, thrill-seeking, frustration, experimentation, socialization, self-expression.				Feeling 'out of control', angry, guilty, low self-esteem, need to punish or purge oneself		Depressed, hopeless, unable to see a future, guilty, angry, resolved to die or apathetic about living		

McLaughlin (2007) asserts that the behaviour itself is not as important as understanding the reasons why people self-harm and that people self-harm when they have 'reached breaking point whilst trying to cope with their emotional despair' (p. 68). Thus self-harm can be regarded as a coping mechanism, but one that is often a last resort when other coping strategies (e.g. talking about their distress, fear or loss) have become ineffective. The National Self-harm Network (NSHN) (2011) identifies five broad reasons why people self-harm, each of which is illustrated with a quote from someone who self-harms:

■ As a release of tension, frustration and distress: 'I think it's somewhat of a release when you do it, you know you've not really dealt with your feelings properly but you have dealt with them in a way that's possibly the only way you can see at the time.'

■ To feel and regain control: 'When things were happening to me that I had no control over I started hurting myself, this was something that I could control, I could do as much or as little damage as I wanted, it only involved myself and I could care for the wound after.'

■ To punish: 'I would say there is a definite punishment element involved in my self-harm, a feeling that I have to take things out on myself, to drive the bad feelings away, punish myself for what I let happen to me, and to get the badness out.'

■ To feel, to ground oneself: 'When I feel numb or go to the place where I disconnect from reality I need to feel pain to bring me back to the here and now, nothing else will ground me. The pain makes me realise that I am really here.'

■ A way to express: 'It's a way of expressing negative feelings about myself that build up inside me. As someone who finds it difficult to put things into words, it can at times be the only way of expressing how I am feeling.'

Within some specific disorders there may be other reasons for self-harm. People with borderline personality disorder may experience depersonalization and derealization during periods of intense anxiety and harm themselves to reconnect with reality. In some psychotic disorders people hear voices telling them to cut themselves or attempt to remove something they perceive to be inside their bodies. In crack-cocaine withdrawal some people feel as though there is something crawling under their skin and scratch at their arms until they bleed.

People with learning disabilities may present with self-harming behaviour but without it necessarily meaning that they are experiencing psychological distress; attempting to understand the meaning may suggest behavioural interventions that could be employed to help reduce the frequency or the harm done by someone's self-injurious behaviour.

What do people who self-harm want?

In the National Inquiry into Self-harm Among Young People, *Truth Hurts* (Mental Health Foundation 2006), people who self-harmed reported a number of factors which in their experience had helped or supported them after an incident of self-harm. These included:

■ education;
■ anti-bullying strategies;
■ peer support;
■ promoting good mental health and emotional well-being;
■ diet;
■ exercise;
■ reducing social exclusion.

Many of their responses involved a request for someone to listen supportively and not to judge them. The main reason cited for not coming forward to disclose to someone that they had self-harmed was a fear of the response they might get.

Self-harm and attempted suicide

In all of the definitions given by users in the NSHN example cited above, no one expressed their intention to kill themselves: 'I don't want to die. I just want the pain to stop. The only way I can get some relief from this emotional pain is by hurting myself' (NSHN 2011). As illustrated on Table 17.1 above, people may self-harm with or without suicidal intent. Someone may have suicidal thoughts and harm themselves to cope with these thoughts – i.e. as a survival tactic. Equally, someone may have suicidal thoughts with or without any self-harming behaviour: they are overlapping phenomena. There is however a correlation between self-harm and completed suicide. A history of self-harm is associated with an increased risk of death by suicide. According to the National Institute for Health and Clinical Excellence (NICE), 'self-harm increases the likelihood that the person will eventually die by suicide between 50- and 100-fold above the rest of the population in a 12-month period' (NICE 2011). Furthermore, people with a history of self-harm are one of the targeted high-risk groups identified in the Department of Health (DH) (2012) strategy *Preventing Suicide in England*. However, it is not the self-harm that is making the person suicidal. It is much more likely to be the isolation, bullying, financial hardship, relationship breakdown, abuse or emotional distress that is the underlying cause of someone's suicidal thoughts and attempts. Consider the flow chart shown in Figure 17.1.

If the person's self-harm is *successful* – if it helps them to cope with the emotional despair, providing emotional release for example, then they will have survived. If the self-harm does not help with the emotional despair then the person is left with the intense feelings of loss, hopelessness and helplessness. If they are then feeling suicidal or attempt suicide, it would be erroneous to consider the self-harm to be the trigger factor; rather that the underlying causes of their self-harm have been overlooked. It is essential therefore that we assess

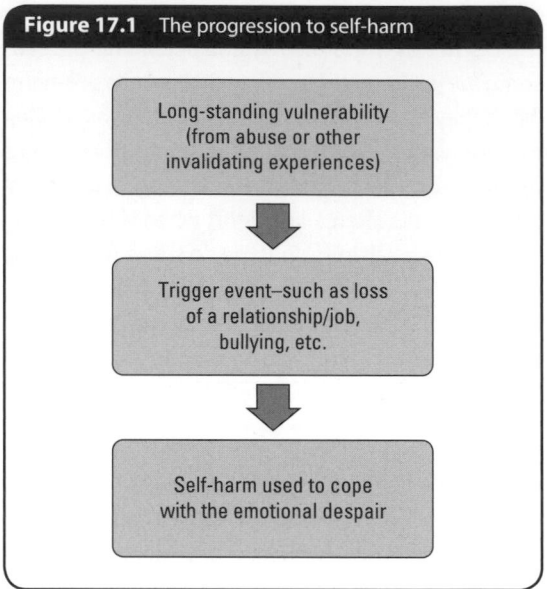

Figure 17.1 The progression to self-harm

more than just risk, but experience, meaning and coping mechanisms with people who self-harm.

A young person describing their self-harm cited in *Truth Hurts* (Mental Health Foundation 2006) said:

> *Pain works. Pain heals. If I had never cut myself, I probably wouldn't still be around today. My parents didn't help me, religion didn't help me, school didn't help me but self-harm did. And I'm doing pretty well for myself these days. Don't get me wrong, not in a heartbeat do I think that self-harm is a good or positive thing, or anything besides a heart-breaking desperate act that saddens me every time I hear about it. But there is a reason why people do it.*

Case Study

Understanding self-harm

In the early hours of a Saturday morning a young woman was referred to me in the accident & emergency (A&E) department for an assessment of her self-harm. She had required cleaning, steristripping and dressing of a laceration to her forearm.

Jess is a 19-year-old woman who had been out for the night with her boyfriend, Janek. They had both been drinking heavily and ended up getting into a heated argument in a nightclub. Janek told

Jess that he had finished with her and started to yell offensive comments in front of their other friends in the club. Jess felt out of control and just wanted everything to stop. She broke the bottle she was drinking from and cut across her left forearm. The security in the club took her outside and called an ambulance. Janek wanted to come in the ambulance and when they wouldn't let him, he punched through the window in the back door. A second ambulance was called to bring Janek to A&E.

On assessment, Jess felt embarrassed about what had happened. She described not knowing exactly what she was doing until she had cut herself, but that in that moment she suddenly felt much calmer and a huge sense of relief. She had no history of self-harm and revealed no suicidal thoughts, plans or intent. Although the self-harm had worked – functionally, it made the situation stop, got her help and got her out of there – emotionally it helped her to feel much calmer. Jess felt confident that she wouldn't do it again as it had really frightened her. She agreed to a referral to the psychologist working at her general practitioner (GP) practice for follow-up and support with the emotional distress the whole incident had caused.

Jess was however very concerned about Janek and asked whether I was seeing him next. She described a history of Janek's binge drinking, occasional drug use, impulsivity, violence to objects, threats to her, and a history of self-harm and attempted suicide. Although Janek had in essence done the same thing – damaged himself as a response to emotional distress – his action of punching the window had not been viewed by the A&E staff as self-harm and he had not been referred to me. He was awaiting review by the plastic surgeons as he needed surgical repair of damaged tendons and a broken bone in his right hand. I offered to see Janek while he was waiting as he was very angry, pacing around the department and wanting to leave. He had substantial underlying mental health needs and was ambivalent about a referral for treatment at a community mental health team. He expressed paranoid thoughts about Jess, thoughts that without her he wanted to die, and had a long-standing dysthymic mood.

Thinking Space 17.1

1. Do you think that both Jess and Janek have self-harmed?
2. Why do you think Jess's action was seen as self-harm but not Janek's by the emergency department staff?

Feedback

To understand their self-harm we need to consider the mechanism, meaning and motivation for both Jess and Janek. If only the mechanism of injury is considered we run the risk of overlooking acts which might equally well communicate significant emotional and psychological distress.

17.4 Assessing self-harm

The NICE guidelines (2004) suggest some overriding principles that should apply to all self-harm assessments.

■ **Respect, understanding and choice:** people who have self-harmed should be treated with the same care, respect and privacy as any patient. In addition, health care professionals should take full account of the likely distress associated with self-harm.

Table 17.2 Case study review

	Jess	Janek
Mechanism of injury	Cut forearm with a broken bottle. Required steristips and dressing	Punched a window breaking a bone and damaging a tendon in his right hand, requiring surgical repair
Meaning of self-harm	An impulsive act, while intoxicated in the context of feeling helpless to make a situation (the row and Janek's abusive behaviour) stop. Felt immediately more calm	An impulsive act, while intoxicated in the context of feeling helpless to influence ambulance staff to take him with them and anger/paranoia about Jess. Still very angry in the A&E department
Motivation	Embarrassed and frightened by what had happened; recognized that while it had helped, she didn't want to self-harm again; accepted a referral for psychological support at her GP practice	Remained angry and ambivalent about getting help. Expressed vague, conditional suicidal thoughts and wanted to leave hospital before surgical review of his damaged hand

- **Staff training:** clinical and non-clinical staff who have contact with people who self-harm in any setting should be provided with appropriate training to equip them to understand and care for people who have self-harmed.

- **Waiting:** if someone has to wait for assessment or treatment, a safe, comfortable and private environment should be provided with access to a named member of staff.

- **Initial assessment:** all people who have self-harmed should be offered a preliminary psychosocial assessment at their first point of contact (triage, GPs, initial assessment) that considers their capacity, level of distress, presence of any mental illness and willingness to remain for further assessment.

- **Psychosocial and risk assessment:** all people who have self-harmed should be offered an assessment of their social, psychological and mental health needs. This should be integrated with a risk assessment to evaluate their hopelessness, depression, history of self-harm or attempted suicide, and current suicidal thoughts, plans and intent.

- **Treatment:** someone who has self-harmed must be offered the same access to physical treatment and pain relief as anyone else. Staff need to provide information to the person so they can make an informed choice about the treatment they are being offered. Offers of follow-up psychological treatment should be made on the basis of the assessment and not just because someone has self-harmed.

Person-centred care

We need to find a way to achieve the goals of the assessment while remaining person-centred. If clients have a negative experience of being assessed following an episode of self-harm they may feel rejected by the service and be less likely to seek help in the future, both of which increase the risk for the person who has self-harmed.

One way to achieve this balance of a person-centred, risk-aware assessment is to structure your question around eliciting the person's mechanism of injury, the meaning of their self-harm and their motivation for the future (see Figure 17.2). This helps us to engage the client and plan short- and medium-term care.

- **Mechanism:** provides information for planning immediate care, and an opportunity to engage the person by managing any injury or pain they are experiencing. It gives the clinician an indication of risk, a sense of extent of planning, and a professional view of potential lethality.

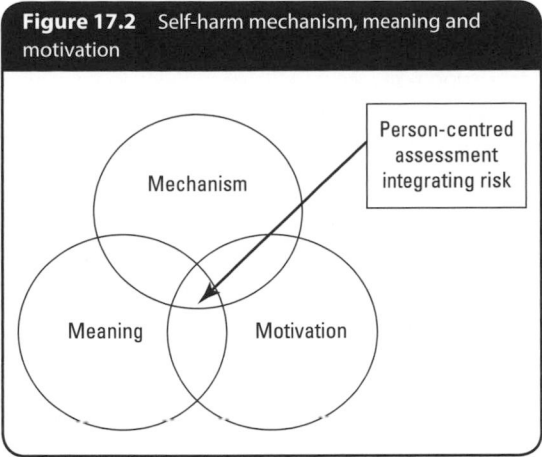

Figure 17.2   Self-harm mechanism, meaning and motivation

- **Meaning:** by asking what the self-harm meant to the client, what led up to it, what they hoped or thought would happen, and whether the self-harm helped with whatever distress they were feeling at the time, we not only elicit the client's view of what the self-harm means, but also formulate risk in terms of whether or not the acute distress remains. When asked respectfully, these questions help us to engage the client and demonstrate empathy by showing interest in what has happened to them.

- **Motivation:** this can be assessed in the very short term (is the person willing to wait to be seen, to accept further assessment and treatment, are they thinking of harming themselves now) or in the medium term (how does the client feel about their future, what help would

they like, do they want to see someone from a mental health team). It gives us an opportunity to assess feelings of hopelessness (if they cannot see a future) and any current suicidal thoughts and plans which would both be indicators of high risk. However, it also gives us the opportunity to demonstrate therapeutic optimism; to talk about their future, what they would like to achieve, and what they would find helpful from the service.

Assessment structure

The NICE guidelines for longer-term management of self-harm distinguish between the components of a needs assessment and a risk assessment. A summary of these elements is provided in Table 17.3 (NICE 2011).

Although they may be used in some services to provide a baseline for comparison pre- and post-intervention, the NICE guidelines do not recommend the use of risk assessment tools or scales to predict future repetition of self-harm or suicide.

Thinking Space 17.2

Re-read the criteria for assessment of needs and risk in Table 17.3 before reading the case study below and noting what you would need to complete a needs and risk assessment for Jenny.

Case Study

Jenny

Jenny is a 21-year-old music student training as a classical violinist. She attended the emergency department in the early hours of the morning having made 10 4 cm cuts in a row along the length of her forearm. She had played in an end-of-term concert that evening and been for a drink with her fellow students, consuming approximately 12 units of alcohol. Upon her return home she had felt an overwhelming desire to release a feeling of tension, which she described as being located in her arm. Having cut herself she felt an immediate release of this tension, but very quickly felt her anxiety levels rise again as she began to fear lest she had damaged her arm; worry about what her friends, teachers and family would think; and become angry that the tension seemed to be returning. She told one of her flatmates what she had done, and was persuaded to attend A&E.

Although this was the first time that Jenny had cut herself, she has previously taken two small paracetamol overdoses; the last time one year ago when she was doing her end-of-year exams. She made no final plans when she took these overdoses but did not seek help. She thought that the eight tablets would not do her any harm and just wanted to block out how she felt.

When she was 7 her father, who was also a professional musician and her first teacher, left her mother. From the age of 13 Jenny starved herself when feeling stressed. She would not eat for a day and enjoyed the lightheaded feeling it gave her. Jenny excelled at school and gained a place at the university of her choice, but always felt that she was somehow 'scraping by'. Since arriving at university she had struggled, and although passing her course, felt she was near the bottom of the class. She described in her own words a 'love–hate' relationship with her peers. Performing at university motivated her, but she resented doing it. As the end of her course approached she feared what would happen and was angry that she had failed to get onto a postgraduate course. Jenny seemed able only to see things as poles apart: she would either become a professional musician or she would be a failure; her teachers loved or hated her.

During her assessment with a psychiatric liaison nurse, Jenny was able to identify that when things went wrong she 'blamed' and 'hated' herself. She had a belief that she wasn't good enough for her father, her school or her university, and only felt better if she 'punished' herself by starving, taking an overdose or cutting herself. Jenny agreed that she wanted to do something to change this pattern of behaviour. She identified that drinking alcohol when she was feeling distressed made it more likely that she would do something to harm herself, or starve herself the following day because she felt guilty at having had too many calories in the alcohol. She also felt that she was 'testing' her body, and to some extent that she wanted 'it' (her body) to fail her so that she would be able to justify not becoming a professional violinist. However, she was clear that she wanted to live and that she had no current suicidal thoughts or plans.

Table 17.3 Assessment of needs and risk

Assessment of needs should include	Risk assessment should take into account
Skills, strengths and assets Coping strategies Mental health problems or disorders Physical health problems or disorders Social circumstances and problems Psychosocial and occupational functioning and vulnerabilities Recent and current life difficulties, including personal and financial problems The need for psychological intervention, social care and support, occupational rehabilitation, and also drug treatment for any associated conditions The needs of any dependent children	Methods and frequency of current and past self-harm Current and past suicidal intent Depressive symptoms and their relationship to self-harm Any psychiatric illness and its relationship to self-harm The personal and social context and any other specific factors preceding self-harm, such as specific unpleasant affective states or emotions and changes in relationships Specific risk factors and protective factors (social, psychological, pharmacological and motivational) that may increase or decrease the risks associated with self-harm Coping strategies that the person has used to either successfully limit or avert self-harm or to contain the impact of personal, social or other factors preceding episodes of self-harm Significant relationships that may either be supportive or represent a threat (such as abuse or neglect) and may lead to changes in the level of risk Immediate and longer-term risks

Feedback to Thinking Space 17.2

Table 17.4   Example of a completed needs and risk assessment for Jenny

Needs assessment component	Examples from Jenny's case
Skills, strengths and assets	Jenny is able to manage performance anxiety and play to a high standard. She is working hard and succeeding on her course even though she finds it hard to recognize her success. She has friends to confide in and has sought help for her self-harm. She is able to recognize that her behaviour poses risks. She wants to do something to change her pattern of behaviour.
Coping strategies	Jenny described a number of coping strategies: testing her body, drinking alcohol, punishing herself. Tonight she spoke to a friend about how she was feeling and what she had done. This had helped her to attend hospital.
Mental health problems or disorders	Jenny may have some standing problems with anxiety, low self-esteem and schemata that may put her at risk of depression. She has expressed herself through starving herself, but this seems to be transient and only in response to days after nights where she thinks she has consumed too much alcohol. She may benefit from a full mental health assessment.
Physical health problems or disorders	No physical health problems reported. She may need a nutritional assessment and could see her GP for this.
Social circumstances and problems	Jenny is coming towards the end of her university course. She may have financial problems and will have a major change of role soon. This needs further assessment.
Psychosocial and occupational functioning and vulnerabilities	Jenny appears to be attending her course and fulfilling her obligations: she performed in an end-of-term concert tonight. However she views herself as a failure, having not got a place on the postgraduate course she wanted and fears that she will not have a career as a violinist.
Recent and current life difficulties, including personal and financial problems	Recent feelings of tension, anxiety and fear about her future career. Struggling with the course. A love–hate relationship with her peers and tutors. Anger about not getting a postgraduate place.
Need for psychological intervention, social care and support, occupational rehabilitation, and also drug treatment for any associated conditions	No social care or rehabilitation needs identified. May benefit from screening and brief intervention for her alcohol use. Has some long-standing issues around her self-worth and anxiety that might benefit from primary care counselling or cognitive behavioural therapy (CBT) through an Improved Access to Psychological Therapies (IAPT) service.
Methods and frequency of current and past self-harm	Two previous overdoses. Eight paracetamol tablets taken without suicidal intent. No final plans made. Seem to be associated with exam stress. First episode of self-cutting tonight. Appears to be fairly controlled with low risk of accidental death.
Current and past suicidal intent	Jenny's self-harm seems to be an expression of her anxiety and tension; it is not a suicide attempt. She has no current suicidal thoughts or plans, but more information is required about her previous overdose.

Risk assessment component	Examples from Jenny's case
Depressive symptoms and their relationship to self-harm	No depressive symptoms reported. However, Jenny does have some thinking errors which may put her at risk of developing a depressive illness.
Any psychiatric illness and its relationship to self-harm	She appears to be experiencing low self-esteem and anxiety about her future. This manifests itself in tension, guilt and anger that seem strongly linked to her self-harm.
The personal and social context and any other specific factors preceding self-harm, such as specific unpleasant affective states or emotions and changes in relationships	Jenny's life as a musician seems to expose her to highly stressful situations or heightened affective states and she then uses alcohol to relax. This seems to be increasing her risk of self-harm.
Specific risk factors and protective factors (social, psychological, pharmacological and motivational) that may increase or decrease the risks associated with self-harm	Jenny is able to see herself in the future, for example she is angry about not getting a place on a postgraduate course, and is trying to work out what to do next year. Her friends seem to be supportive, but there is likely to be an increased risk if she auditions for jobs/courses and has to face rejection or failure in the months ahead.
Coping strategies that the person has used to either successfully limit or avert self-harm or to contain the impact of personal, social or other factors preceding episodes of self-harm	Jenny was worried about the damage she might have done to her arm and sought help from her flatmate. She also wants to change her pattern of behaviour and seems willing to discuss things with the psychiatric liaison nurse. She has recognized that drinking alcohol seems to make it more likely that she will harm herself.
Significant relationships that may either be supportive or represent a threat (such as abuse or neglect) and may lead to changes in the level of risk	She feels as though she has let her father and her tutors down, which appears to be contributing to her low self-esteem. She has friends at college and a flatmate who she is willing to talk to about her problems. She should be offered the opportunity for a supportive professional relationship through her GP practice or the college counselling service.
Immediate and longer-term risks	The immediate risk for Jenny is low. Her mechanism of injury is not life-threatening, she has released the tension she was feeling and wants to change her behaviour. In the longer term, if she continues to drink to excess this will increase her risk, and she may face rejection when she applies for work or further study.

17.5 Treatment for self-harm

Despite there being a wide range of interventions and studies measuring their effectiveness, systematic reviews and meta-analyses into the effectiveness of psychosocial interventions for self-harm remain equivocal. The Cochrane Review (Hawton *et al.* 1999) and the NICE guidelines (2004, 2011) found insufficient evidence to recommend one particular intervention, but noticed positive treatment effects in well-structured brief psychological interventions delivered by experienced practitioners.

Treatment may occur in primary care, in emergency departments (with psychiatric liaison teams), in community mental health teams (CMHTs), community drug and alcohol services, probation and prison services, education, and voluntary and non-statutory groups. The DH (2012) has identified 24-hour access to services for people in mental health crisis and specialist assessment of self-harm, particularly among young people, as key priorities in the ongoing strategy to reduce suicide in England.

The interventions may be delivered as a stand-alone treatment aimed at reducing or minimizing the harm of the behaviour or as part of a more holistic package of care in CMHTs where the underlying communication, relationship and cognitive factors are addressed. Everyone who presents following an incident of self-harm should have an integrated psychosocial needs and risk assessment. Following this the assessing clinician may recommend no follow-up, follow-up in primary care, follow-up within a psychiatric liaison team, referral to a CMHT or crisis resolution and home treatment team, referral for psychological treatment or inpatient admission (NICE 2011) (see Figure 17.3).

The review conducted as part of the NICE guidelines for longer-term management of self-harm

Figure 17.3 Patterns of assessment, referral and intervention for self-harm

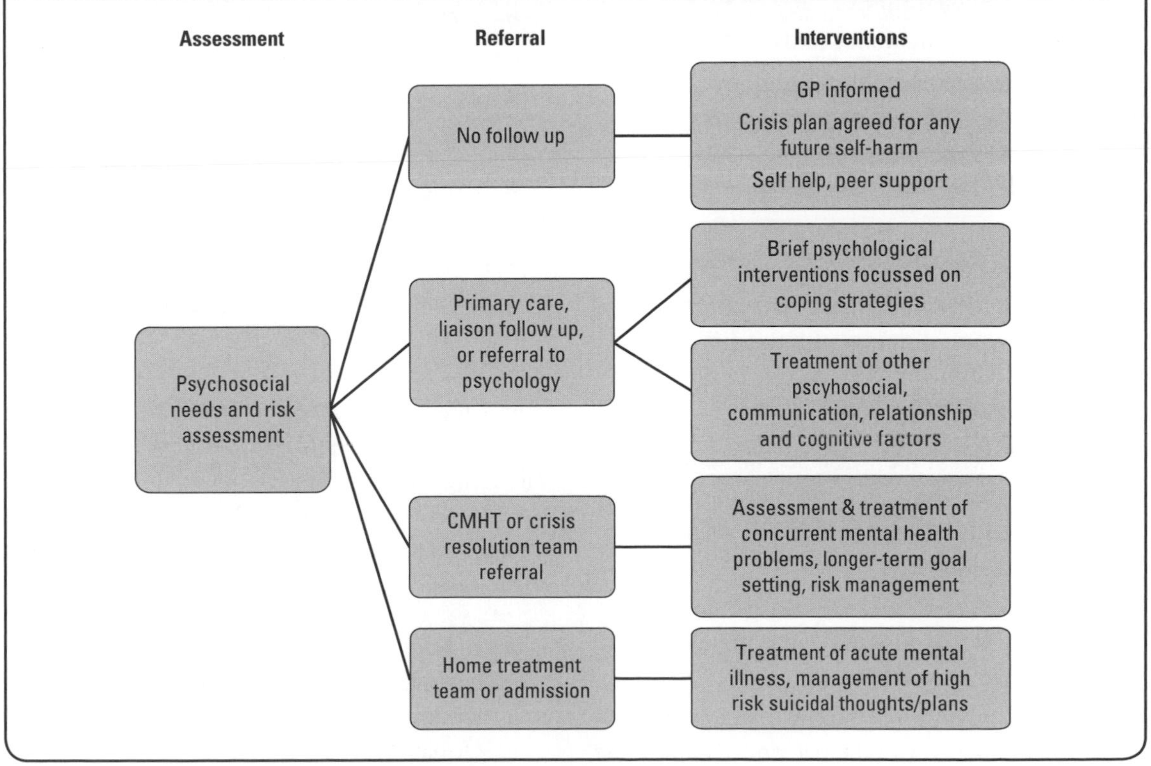

Assessment	Referral	Interventions
Psychosocial needs and risk assessment	No follow up	GP informed / Crisis plan agreed for any future self-harm / Self help, peer support
	Primary care, liaison follow up, or referral to psychology	Brief psychological interventions focussed on coping strategies / Treatment of other pscyhosocial, communication, relationship and cognitive factors
	CMHT or crisis resolution team referral	Assessment & treatment of concurrent mental health problems, longer-term goal setting, risk management
	Home treatment team or admission	Treatment of acute mental illness, management of high risk suicidal thoughts/plans

(NICE 2011) showed that psychological therapy might be effective in improving outcomes compared with treatment as usual. The outcomes considered were:

- reduced repetition of self-harm;
- suicidal ideation scores;
- depression scores;
- hopelessness scores.

This was not dependent on the type of psychological intervention. The models included:

- problem-solving interventions;
- CBT;
- psychodynamic interpersonal therapy.

The review supported the findings of Hawton *et al.* (1999) which identified other psychosocial interventions which, while supportive, did not have a statistically significant effect when compared with treatment as usual. These included:

- intensive intervention;
- provision of emergency cards;
- establishing contact by telephone support;
- follow-up postcards with contact details.

The conclusion of the review and guidelines are as follows:

- Consider offering 3 to 12 sessions of a psychological intervention specifically structured for people who self-harm, with the aim of reducing self-harm.
- In addition:
  - The intervention should be tailored to individual need, and could include cognitive-behavioural, psychodynamic or problem-solving elements.
  - Therapists should be trained and supervised in the therapy they are offering to people who self-harm.
  - Therapists should also be able to work collaboratively with the person to identify the

problems causing distress or leading to self-harm.

- Do not offer drug treatment as a specific intervention to reduce self-harm.

Harm minimization techniques

For some people, stopping self-harm may not be an achievable (or from the client's perspective, desirable) short-term goal. It is important to remember that care plans must be realistic and that we should not set our clients up to fail by creating goals they cannot achieve at the moment.

Although the evidence base is not strong, there are distraction and harm minimization techniques which people who self-harm have found helpful and reduce the risk associated with their self-harm. These include the following strategies:

- holding an ice cube for a few seconds;
- snapping an elastic band against the wrist;
- punching a cushion as hard as you can;
- smashing a watermelon;
- screaming at the top of your voice;
- tearing up a newspaper or phone directory;
- writing on or marking yourself with red pen;
- having sterile blades to minimize the risk of infection when cutting;
- taking good care of injuries;
- avoiding drugs and alcohol when self-harming (Royal College of Psychiatrists 2011).

These may help someone avoid more damaging acts of self-harm until they are able to develop alternative coping strategies.

The NICE Guidelines (2011) outline some principles that should govern harm reduction techniques:

- consider strategies aimed at harm reduction; reinforce existing coping strategies and develop new strategies as an alternative to self-harm where possible;

- consider discussing less destructive or harmful methods of self-harm with the service user, their family, carers or significant others where this has been agreed with the service user, and the wider multi-disciplinary team;

- advise the service user that there is no safe way to self-poison.

Distraction techniques

The Royal College of Psychiatrists has identified a range of techniques that people who self-harm say they find helpful to distract themselves when they feel the urge to harm themselves. Often the intense emotional distress that causes the self-harm has a limited peak and the person is able to reason with themselves and think of alternative coping strategies once they have distracted themselves enough for the peak to pass.

Distractions include leisure activities, getting out and about, being productive, using reasoning, and tactics for delaying the self-harm. There are excellent summaries and handouts you can use with clients and training updates on the website *Better Services for People who Self-harm* (Royal College of Psychiatrists 2011).

Integrated care planning for self-harm

So far this chapter has outlined psychosocial interventions, psychological interventions, harm reduction and distraction techniques as stand-alone interventions for self-harm. Longer-term treatment needs to address the self-harm in the context of both short- and long-term goals, and any other mental health, drug and alcohol, or personal problem. It may be more useful, therefore, to integrate the self-harm treatment into other care plans. The general principles of care planning apply, but the NICE (2011) guidelines suggest the following focus:

- Discuss, agree and document the aims of longer-term treatment in the care plan with the person who self-harms. These aims may be to:
  - prevent escalation of self-harm;
  - reduce harm arising from self-harm or reduce or stop self-harm;
  - reduce or stop other risk-related behaviour;
  - improve social or occupational functioning;
  - improve quality of life;
  - improve any associated mental health conditions.

Consideration of the reasons cited by service users as to why they self-harm may provide a more targeted focus for care planning and interventions. Table 17.5 shows possible interventions linked to the different meanings of self-harm.

Table 17.5 From meaning to goals

Meaning of self-harm	Possible interventions
As a release of tension, frustration and distress	Try some harm reduction techniques
To feel and regain control	Try some mindfulness techniques; breathing or meditation to help notice and acknowledge feelings
To punish	Identify someone to talk to about these bad feelings: a friend, the Samaritans, a mental health worker
To feel, to ground oneself	Harm reduction techniques or mindfulness techniques can be useful
A way to express	Try some more creative ways of expressing these negative feelings such as drawing, singing or dancing

17.6   Nursing someone who is suicidal

There are two broad approaches to nursing someone who is suicidal: risk assessment and management, and engagement and talking interventions aimed at alleviating the person's psychological distress. Ideally nurses should combine the two so that the interventions to manage risk do not seem punitive, risk assessment informs our engagement, and the person's experience of psychological distress is limited to as short a period as possible. This section outlines principles of risk assessment and management and proposes ways to engage with someone who is suicidal.

'Being suicidal' is difficult to define. Suicide is measured by outcome, and suicidal gestures or behaviours might be high risk even if someone does not intend to kill themselves. In this context, if someone is expressing suicidal thoughts, plans or intent, whether or not they feel they are going to act upon them now, they could be considered to 'be suicidal' and need a risk assessment and care to address how they feel and endeavour to keep them safe.

Sometimes people fall under the misapprehension that suicide is not preventable: 'If someone is really going to do it, they just will.' According to the 2011 National Confidential Inquiry (Appleby *et al.* 2011), over 56,000 deaths by suicide were reported in England between 1997 and 2008 (the period covered by the report), with the most common methods being hanging, self-poisoning and jumping from a height or in front of a train. Within this group there were 14,654 patient suicides (people who had been in contact with mental health services in the 12 months prior to their death). Both the national figures and 'patient' figures show a decrease in the numbers from the 2006 and 2001 National Inquiries. Importantly they found a 56 per cent decrease in inpatient suicides from 1997, and a 74 per cent decrease in the number of deaths by hanging on wards. This demonstrates that it is possible to dramatically reduce the incidence of suicide and sup-

ports the DH's (2012) focus on further reducing access to potentially lethal methods – for example, ligature points in inpatient mental health services and prisons.

Risk assessment

Risk assessment is the process of identifying 'the likelihood of an event happening with potentially harmful or beneficial outcomes for self and/or others . . . Possible behaviours include suicide, self-harm, aggression and violence, neglect: with an additional range of other positive or negative service user experiences (Morgan 2000). We need to be able to understand a hazard (risk criterion) to limit its potential negative impact and this requires more detail than just determining whether or not someone is suicidal. We need to establish:

- hazard identification (which events occur?);
- hazard accounting (how frequently?);
- scenarios of exposure (under which conditions?);
- risk characterization (conditions present?);
- risk management (which interventions?) (Morgan 2000).

This can be conceptualized as an equation where the weight of risk is estimated by multiplying the severity with the likelihood of the risk occurring:

Severity of harmful outcome x Likelihood of occurrence = Weight of risk

While statistical factors serve to increase an individual's vulnerability to suicide, the exact timing of the suicide act is often related to recent adverse events. These stressors may include interpersonal losses and conflicts, and legal problems. Ease of access to the method of suicide is also an important factor as the intensity of someone's suicidal thoughts may peak and lessen quickly. Therefore, the first part of any assessment should take a clear history which takes into account the psychological and current context risk factors identified in the best practice guidelines (DH 2007). The assessment must include:

- presenting complaint: current suicidal thoughts, plans and intent, and the presence of any major mental illness;
- history of presenting complaint: what has led up to feeling like this, recent loss events and changes in the intensity of thoughts, any preparation, collection of medications, etc., recent treatment or discharge from mental health services;
- history of self-harm or attempted suicide, including detail of what happened, how they got help and how they feel about surviving.

This forms the narrative of how the person is feeling. When asked sensitively, these questions help us to establish rapport with the client. We need to listen actively and reflectively in order to help the person tell the story of how they feel and combine this with the objective data and our observations to identify the degree of their risk. According to *Best Practice in Managing Risk* (DH 2007) the risk factors for completed suicide are:

Demographic factors

- Male
- Increasing age
- Low socioeconomic status
- Unmarried, separated, widowed
- Living alone
- Unemployed

Background history

- Deliberate self-harm (especially with high suicide intent)
- Childhood adversity (e.g. sexual abuse)
- Family history of suicide
- Family history of mental illness

Clinical history

- Mental illness diagnosis (e.g. depression, bipolar disorder, schizophrenia)
- Personality disorder diagnosis (e.g. borderline personality disorder)

- Physical illness, especially chronic conditions and/or those associated with pain and functional impairment (e.g. multiple sclerosis, malignancy, pain syndromes)
- Recent contact with psychiatric services
- Recent discharge from psychiatric inpatient facility

Psychological and psychosocial factors

- Hopelessness
- Impulsiveness
- Low self-esteem
- Life event
- Relationship instability
- Lack of social support

Current 'context'

- Suicidal ideation
- Suicide plans
- Availability of means
- Lethality of means

There are a number of structured suicide risk assessments cited in the guidelines as tools to support a clinical assessment, but there is no one tool that has sufficient evidence to recommend its use and it is concluded that 'in this case, structured assessment means a systematic assessment of key risk factors and mental state leading to an informed clinical judgement' (DH 2007). *Best Practice in Managing Risk* also outlines 16 principles to guide good practice. These include: the application of principles of evidenced-based practice; positive risk management conducted with an understanding of mental health legislation and in collaboration with the service user; appropriate use of structured clinical assessment tools to inform clinical judgement; an organizational risk management strategy to support the efforts by individual practitioners, which may involve multi-disciplinary and multi-agency working and training in risk assessment every three years; recognition that the aim may be to minimize harm as well as prevent it; a written risk management plan which covers foreseen eventualities; and continual efforts to communicate the risk management plan to others.

The DH (2012) has identified six key area for action to reduce suicide rates in England:

- reduce the risk of suicide in key high-risk groups;
- tailor approaches to improve mental health in specific groups;
- reduce access to the means of suicide;
- provide better information and support to those bereaved or affected by suicide;
- support the media in delivering sensitive approaches to suicide and suicidal behaviour;
- support research, data collection and monitoring.

The first three of these are immediately relevant to our work as mental health nurses. The groups identified as high risk include young and middle-aged men, people in the care of mental health services, including inpatients, people with a history of self-harm, people in contact with the criminal justice system, and specific occupational groups with access to potentially lethal means of ending their lives. In both the guidelines and in referring to *No Health Without Mental Health*, the DH calls for an equal emphasis and importance to be placed on both physical and mental health in terms of access to emergency services (DH 2011, 2012), and identifies children and young people and people who use drugs and alcohol as needing targeted approaches to improve their mental health. In terms of reduction of access to the means of suicide, we are challenged to continue the vigilant observation for and removal of strangulation and ligature points in psychiatric inpatient settings.

Having identified a suicide risk, one of the standard practices is to assess whether someone needs continuous close observation in order to try and minimize their risk of harm to themselves. Every UK NHS trust, private or non-statutory employer will have its own policy and regulations relating to the level of observation, how this is assessed, and the purpose and duration of the observation. It is essential to work within these policy requirements.

There is widespread agreement (e.g. Bowers *et al.* 2000) that placing a client under continuous observation provides an opportunity for the nurse to form a therapeutic relationship. However, clients' experiences of being continuously observed are often reported as being restrictive, punishing, humiliating and clearly far from therapeutic (e.g. Jones *et al.* 2000). Problems raised by continuous close observation include:

- lack of, and inconsistent application of policy, with observations often being carried out by junior or agency staff (Bowers *et al.* 2000).
- people still kill themselves while inpatients in acute admission wards (DH 2001, 2006; Appleby *et al.* 2011);
- it is stressful for the nurses doing the observation (Cutcliffe and Barker 2002);
- the nurse may be at risk if the client's impulsive behaviour becomes directed towards them (Cleary *et al.* 1999).

So the question remains, how can we nurse someone who is suicidal safely? When working with people who are experiencing suicidal thoughts, or acting on suicidal plans, there is a risk that we too can begin to feel hopeless. As practitioners, the impact of the despair felt by our clients and the depressing nature of the human drama being played out in the lives of people who are suicidal can leave us feeling impotent: only able to practise defensively in an attempt to prevent the behaviour of suicide, and hoping that the suicidal cognition and affect (or psychache) will somehow spontaneously resolve. As practitioners we need to undertake an interpersonal endeavour personified by talking and listening to be able to help the person who is suicidal rather than merely prevent the physical means of them acting on their thoughts and feelings. To engage with someone who is suicidal we need to access their experience of risk and psychache which

Shneidman (1993) defines as 'the anguish, hurt, angst, or humiliation that leads individuals to seek permanent escape from unbearable levels of psychological pain'.

Thus suicide is not necessarily as a result of any particular mental illness, but rather overwhelmingly high levels of psychache. Hopelessness is therefore a feature of feeling suicidal for the client and a risk for the practitioner when working with someone who is suicidal. We must endeavour to maintain our own hopefulness, or therapeutic optimism, and to create hope with and in our clients.

Personal security plans

Personal security plans (Barker and Buchanan-Barker 2004) are collaborative care plans negotiated with the client which:

- help the person feel more secure within him/herself and the wider social environment;
- are written in the person's own voice;
- are revised at least once daily;
- help the feeling of security become part of the person's lived experience of risk.

Case Study

Patricia

Patricia has been admitted to an acute ward for assessment of her mental health. She has rapidly become unwell again having not taken her medication for about six weeks and has increased her alcohol use to help her sleep and block out her paranoid thoughts. At the end of last week she took all the tablets she could find in the house (some olanzapine, paracetamol and ibuprofen). She was drunk when she took the overdose and thought she would rather die than live feeling like this. She sent a text message to a mate saying goodbye and her friend called the police and ambulance when he couldn't get a reply from Patricia's phone. After two days in a general hospital, she was admitted to a mental health ward.

Patricia finds it hard to see a future. She wishes that the overdose had worked and thought that the combination of alcohol, olanzapine, paracetamol and ibuprofen would kill her. On this occasion she had collected a few important belongings together in a box and left a note on the box to 'bury this with me'. On the general ward she felt too ill to think about whether or not she wanted to die. Since she has felt physically better and been moved to the mental health ward she has started to think she never wants to go through that again, and has been trying to work out what method would be guaranteed to work.

Patricia has thoughts about injecting herself with insulin. Her father is an insulin dependent diabetic and Patricia thinks she could steal enough insulin from him to put her into a coma from which she would never wake up. She has also thought about getting drunk and walking up a mountain so she would die of hypothermia. She has read about a policeman who did this and thinks it would be a good way to go.

She feels her ability to resist these thoughts is poor, and that if she went home she would do one of them. She has looked at the train times to the Lake District and thinks she could drink enough on the train journey to make sure she does it.

She thinks about death a lot on the ward, but has not made any plans to kill herself here. She thinks that it wouldn't be fair on the staff or other patients. She is distressed by her thoughts and would like help, but doesn't think anything will help her. Patricia is struggling to see herself in the future at all. She finds it hard to even envisage her next meal, let alone, tomorrow, next week, etc. She feels that life is hopeless and that she is helpless. She thinks she is a burden to the ward and the bed should be freed up for someone else.

Commentary

Patricia is at a high risk for suicide. She has a history of attempting suicide including this very recent event from which she is only just starting to recover. There is evidence too of some alcohol use. She has a major mental illness, and her symptoms (wanting to block out the voices) seem in part to be linked to her suicide attempt. She made final plans, both saying goodbye and leaving instructions for some things to be buried with her. Patricia continues to feel suicidal and has been thinking of ways more likely to work than her recent overdose. These are potentially lethal methods and she has made some realistic plans about how to organize this. Importantly, she feels hopeless, is struggling to see a future, and feels guilty about taking up a hospital bed.

The ward team would need to assess whether Patricia needs an enhanced level of observation, such as being nursed one-to-one. Her one protective factor seems to be that she is able to think of others. She contacted a friend, left instructions for whoever found her, and says she wouldn't kill herself on the ward as it wouldn't be fair on other patients and staff.

Her psychache is also profound and we need to care for her in a way that will both promote her safety and address the despair she is feeling. The idea that she wouldn't harm herself for the sake of others does not feel like a strong protective factor and she may need to be observed closely to ensure someone is with her if this feeling changes. Table 17.6 provides an example of a personal safety plan for Patricia which should be combined with efforts to listen to and engage her in her care.

Talking as the centrepiece

Patricia is experiencing profound psychache. Nurses must address, then soften and reduce this psychache to understand her suffering, psychological pain and tolerance for this pain which is now being exceeded. Patricia's risk is high but will not be reduced solely by preventing her from accessing the means to kill herself, but rather by decreasing the power of her psychache.

Cutcliffe and Stevenson (2008) conclude that this can be achieved only by asking about the person's feelings, worries and pain; finding out where it hurts; listening to and engaging with the narrative and metaphorical ways in which people express how they feel. At the heart of any treatment must be the relationship between the worker and Patricia. It is only through that relationship that the nurse can offer opportunities to reduce her psychache.

Rungapadiachy (2003) suggests that we can develop a humanistic approach to our communication by demonstrating WAGE:

Warmth

Acceptance

Genuineness

Empathy

- **Warmth:** Patricia's self-esteem is very low. She feels like a burden and is guilty about taking up a place on the ward of which someone else might have a greater need. We need to be warm and welcoming to her; available when she is able to speak; ensure that she is not dismissed or ignored; show interest in the things she does want to talk about – her friend, for example; acknowledge her thoughtfulness at not wanting to distress other clients and staff on the ward.

Table 17.6   Personal security plan

Personal security plan for Patricia	Date:	
What can I do to help myself feel more safe and secure?		
I find it hard to feel anything at the moment. I need to know that it is OK to just 'be' and that I am not letting staff down by feeling this way. I am frightened by my thoughts, which are more frightening when I am alone. I will let staff know how I am feeling I know that it is OK to ask someone to come and just sit with me I will try to occupy my time on the ward to reduce the time I spend thinking about death I will text my friend to see how she is		
What can others do to help me feel more safe and secure?		
Be with me so there is someone for me to talk to when I am frightened by these thoughts Listen to me Ask me how I am feeling Let me tell them what I am thinking, even if it sounds bad Accept that I find it hard to think about tomorrow so let me talk about now and my past Let me be quiet if I am finding it hard to talk but don't think that I am being rude or leave me alone because of it		
Client signature:	Mental health worker signature:	
Current legal status:	Leave:	Observation level: *Enhanced*
Review of personal security plan		
Date:	Time:	Client's view:
		Worker's view:
Date:	Time:	Client's view:
		Worker's view:

- **Acceptance:** we need to avoid the temptation to try and correct her suicidal thoughts – she is already distressed by them. Our work with her should not be conditional on her saying or doing the right thing. When she cannot think about or envisage her future, we need to accept that and not try to direct her to be hopeful.

- **Genuineness:** Patricia is experiencing some very distressing thoughts – we need to acknowledge when we are worried about her;

be open about the fact that her plans sound frightening; be up-front if we assess that she needs someone to be with her at all times and honest about the purpose of any enhanced observation. Although this may seem difficult it is essential to try and build trust and is one of the building blocks of the *bridging* metaphor.

- **Empathy:** we cannot feel what Patricia feels, but we can ask her, try to imagine and reflect back how her experience seems to us. We can demonstrate and establish empathy by being interested in her feelings, finding out more about how they affect her and trying to help her identify how she is managing to cope with them; how she is managing to survive.

 ## 17.7 Conclusion

This chapter has provided an overview of the different types of self-harm behaviour, explored the relationship between self-harm and suicide, and presented models for the assessment and treatment of self-harm, management of risk and nursing care for people who are suicidal. In summary, the main points are:

- Self-harm is a behaviour not an illness. However, there is a strong association between self-harm and suicide and nurses have a health-promoting role to try and help reduce

the psychological distress that underlies the behaviour.

- People who self-harm want to be treated with respect, and conveying acceptance and tolerance is a key to understanding how and why they are using self-harm as a coping mechanism.

- In all cases, the therapeutic relationship is the key to working with these client groups.

- The *science*, research evidence, suggests that techniques such as problem-solving are likely to reduce the frequency of further self-harm, though there are insufficient, large-scale, longitudinal studies to advocate one particular treatment.

- Risk assessment must combine structured clinical history-taking with an assessment of the demographic risk factors.

- The *art* is to use interpersonal skills of engagement (forming a relationship, conveying acceptance and tolerance, hearing and understanding), and inspiring hope to help clients who may be suicidal shift their position from one of hopelessness to possibility.

- Continuous observation should be used for people who are at high risk of harm to themselves, but can be effective only when the focus is on enhanced engagement with the client, so that the underlying psychache can be reduced to make the person safer.

Annotated bibliography

In practice, you must familiarize yourself with the risk management and enhanced observation policies of your employer. These will be in line with the key national guidelines: NICE 2004 (for short term) and NICE 2011 (for longer term) management of self-harm; the DH best practice guidelines for managing risk (DH 2007) and the DHstrategy *Preventing Suicide in England* (DH 2012).

Shneidman, E.D. (1996) *The Suicidal Mind.* **New York: Oxford University Press.**
This gives an excellent and authoritative insight in to the experience and motivation of people who are suicidal and makes a strong case for an engaged, humane response.

NSHN (National Self-harm Network) (2011) at www.nshn.co.uk.
The National Self-harm Network holds the person who self-harms at the centre of its work. It has excellent resources and information for people who self-harm, carers and clinicians.

Royal College of Psychiatrists (2011) *Better Services for People who Self-harm: A national quality improvement programme,* **see www.rcpsych.ac.uk/crtu/centreforqualityimprovement/servicesforself-harm.aspx.**

References

Appleby, L. *et al.* (2011) *The National Confidential Inquiry into Suicide and Homicide by People with Mental Illness: Annual report, England, Wales, and Scotland.* Manchester: The University of Manchester.

Barker, P. and Buchanan-Barker, P. (2004) *The Tidal Model: A guide for mental health professionals* London: Brunner Routledge.

Cutcliffe, J.R. and Barker, P. (2002) Considering the care of the suicidal client and the case for engagement and inspiring hope or observation, *Journal of Psychiatric and Mental Health Nursing*, 9(5): 611–21.

Cutcliffe, J.R. and Stevenson, C. (2008) Feeling our way in the dark: the psychiatric nursing care of suicidal people – a literature review, *International Journal of Nursing Studies*, 45: 942–53.

DH (Department of Health) (2001) *Safety First – Five Year Report of the National Confidential Inquiry into Suicides and Homicides by People with Mental Health Problems.* London: HMSO.

DH (Department of Health) (2007) *Best Practice in Managing Risk: Principles and evidence for best practice in the assessment and management of risk to self and others in mental health services.* London: DH.

DH (Department of Health) (2011) *No Health without Mental Health: A cross government mental health outcomes strategy for people of all ages.* London: DH.

DH (Department of Health) (2012) Preventing Suicide in England: A cross-government outcomes strategy to save lives. London: DH.

Hawton, K. *et al.* (1999) Psychosocial and pharmacological treatments for deliberate self-harm, *Cochrane Database of Systematic Reviews*, Issue 4. Art. no. CD001764. DOI:10.1002/14651858.CD001764.

Hawton, K. *et al.* (2007) Self-harm in England: a tale of three cities. Multicentre study of self-harm, *Social Psychiatry and Psychiatric Epidemiology*, 42: 513–21.

McLaughlin, C. (2007) *Suicide-Related Behaviour: Understanding, caring and therapeutic responses.* Chichester: Wiley.

Mental Health Foundation (2006) *Truth Hurts: Report of the National Inquiry into Self-harm Among Young People.* London: Mental Health Foundation/Camelot Foundation.

Mental Health Foundation (2012) *Mental Health Statistics*, available at: www.mentalhealth.org.uk/help-information/mental-health-statistics.

Morgan, S. (2000) *Clinical Risk Management: A clinical tool and practitioner manual.* London: The Sainsbury Centre for Mental Health, available at: www.centreformentalhealth.org.uk/pdfs/clinical_risk_management.pdf.

Murphy, E. *et al.* (2011) Multicentre cohort study of older adults who have harmed themselves: risk factors for repetition and suicide, *British Journal of Psychiatry*, 200: 399–404.

NICE (National Institute for Health and Clinical Excellence) (2004) *Self-harm: The short-term physical and psychological managemnt and secondary prevention of self-harm in primary and secondary care*, Clinical Guideline 16. London: NICE.

NICE (National Institute for Health and Clinical Excellence) (2011) *Self-harm: Longer-term management*, Clinical Guideline 133. London: NICE.

NSHN (National Self-harm Network) (2011) www.nshn.co.uk.

Royal College of Psychiatrists (2011) *Better Services for People who Self-harm: A national quality improvement programme*, available at: www.rcpsych.ac.uk/crtu/centreforqualityimprovement/servicesforself-harm.aspx.

Rungapadiachy, D.M. (2003) *Interpersonal Communication and Psychology for Health Care Professionals: Theory and practice.* London: Butterworth Heinemann.

Shneidman, E.S. (1993) Suicide as psychache, *Journal of Nervous and Mental Disease*, 181: 147–9.

Chapter

18

Identifying and Managing Risk of Aggression and Violence

Susan Sookoo

18.1 Introduction

The therapeutic management of violence and aggression is not separate to, but rather an integral part of, routine care. Aggressive incidents are not isolated events, but take place within a clinical, psychological, environmental and social context. Consequently, a broad range of interventions is required in order to manage violence and aggression and prevention is always more desirable than intervention. This chapter is largely concerned with methods used to safely manage anger, aggression and violence when they occur or are imminent. As such, the techniques described can be seen as 'as required' interventions aimed at short-term management. The focus is on methods used in ward environments. Although non-physical interventions may also be applicable to community settings, safe management of aggression in the community is built on effective risk assessment processes, multidisciplinary team working and attention to local policies on safety when visiting clients.

However, methods for dealing with imminent aggression alone do not constitute complete

management of violence and aggression: an understanding of the underlying factors that influence such behaviour and reduce the need for short-term intervention is also necessary. In addition, this chapter should be read in conjunction with Chapter 12 on the therapeutic relationship and Chapter 13 on the creation of a therapeutic milieu within inpatient care settings.

In summary, this chapter covers:

- the factors which influence the incidence of violence and aggression in inpatient mental health services and identification of risk;
- mechanisms underlying anger and aggression;
- observation and de-escalation techniques to manage risk;
- physical interventions.

As a starting point, some definition of commonly used terms is needed. Terms used in this chapter may be defined as follows:

- **Anger:** a subjective emotional state involving physiological arousal and associated cognitions. This can be adaptive, but frequency, intensity and duration of anger can make it dysfunctional (Novaco 1983).

- **Aggression:** a disposition to inflict harm. This may be verbally expressed in threats to harm people or objects, or result in actual harm (Wright *et al.* 2002).

- **Hostility:** a personality trait, which reflects a style of appraisal in which the actions of others are seen as harmful. This can result in anger or detachment (Novaco 1983).

- **Violence:** acts in which there is use of force to attempt to inflict physical harm (Wright *et al.* 2002).

 ## 18.2   Background

There is a public perception of the psychiatric patient as dangerous to the community at large, as well as increasing concern about the level of violence and aggression occurring within health care settings. The 2010 National Health Service (NHS) Staff Survey carried out by the Care Quality Commission (CQC) found that 8 per cent of respondents had experienced violence from patients, relatives or other members of the public – the figure for mental health NHS trusts was 15 per cent (18 per cent for ambulance workers). The Count Me In Census (CQC 2010) surveyed patient experiences and reported that 11 per cent of mental health patients had been subject to a physical assault in that year. Percentages are important, although they do not provide a qualitative picture. However, commenting on an 11 per cent rate of assaults on patients in 2006 and great local variation in this figure the then Healthcare Commission stated: 'This is simply not acceptable in a 21st century service and would not be tolerated in other walks of life' (Healthcare Commission 2008: 8).

The above figures suggest a higher than average rate of violence and aggression in mental health services but should not suggest that a relationship between mental illness and violence is inevitable. It is worth noting that mentally ill people living in the community are twice as likely to be the victim of violent abuse as the general population (NMC press release 2003). The reasons for an apparent increase in the level of violent incidents within health services are not clear but may include a higher level of violence within society in general (Wright *et al.* 2002), the reduced number of hospital beds resulting in only the most disturbed patients being admitted to inpatient units, or the effect of non-therapeutic hospital environments (Sainsbury Centre for Mental Health 1998).

 ## 18.3   The evidence base for managing violence and aggression

Violence is a complex phenomenon and it is not possible to state a theory in terms of 'violent behaviour is caused by x, y and z'. As Mason and Chandley (1999) point out, there are probably as many theories of violence as there are aggressive incidents. Neither is there definitive evidence on the effectiveness of methods to manage violence and aggression, as acknowledged by the National Institute for Health and Clinical Excellence (NICE) (2005). Most of the evidence considered by the group developing the current NICE guideline on short-term management of violence is graded Level 4 – that is, 'expert opinion or formal consensus'. However, professional bodies have produced guidance and summarized the evidence base for managing violence and aggression. The Royal College of Nursing (RCN) published a position statement on dealing with violence and aggression in 1997. In 2002, Wright *et al.* produced a report for the then UKCC (now the Nursing and Midwifery Council – NMC) providing a detailed exploration of the literature around both causes of violence and aggression and the various methods of managing them. The Royal College of Psychiatrists (RCP) Research Unit also produced *Management of Imminent Violence: Clinical practice guidelines to support mental health services* (1998) which reviewed the evidence base and made practice recommendations. In 2005 NICE produced *Violence: The short-term management of disturbed/violent behaviour in*

in-patient psychiatric settings and emergency departments (NICE 2005), a guideline which updates and replaces the RCP guideline. This chapter considers findings from all of these reports, but it must be emphasized that all staff working in mental health settings or emergency departments should be familiar with and follow the recommendations of the NICE guideline as this is the current guide to best practice and has a legal standing: 'Failure to act in accordance with the guideline may not only be a failure to act in accordance with best practice, but in some circumstances may have legal consequences' (NICE 2005: 10). The guideline has not been updated since publication but a decision was taken in February 2012 which recommended that it be reviewed to take account of more recent evidence.

18.4 Factors influencing violence and aggression

Prevention of violence requires understanding of the factors which may contribute to levels of violence and aggression and is an important part of assessment and management. Some factors are considered here, although these should always be interpreted within the context of an individual, collaborative risk assessment.

Demographic or personal factors

The NICE guidance (2005) cautiously lists several demographic or personal variables which may be risk factors for aggression (see Box 18.1).

Clinical factors

Wright *et al.* (2002) report an increased relative risk of violence in patients with psychotic illnesses, although, once again, there is not a clear relationship between specific symptoms and violence, and the relationship does not seem to be consistent. For example, one study (Lowenstein *et al.* 1990) found manic patients to have higher levels of inpatient violence than any other diagnostic group. Non-compliance with treatment and use of drugs or alcohol also complicate the picture. NICE guide-

> **Box 18.1 Demographic or personal risk factors for aggression (after NICE 2005)**
>
> - A history of violence or disturbed behaviour
> - History of substance misuse
> - Carers' reports of previous violence or anger
> - Previous expression of intent to harm
> - Previous use of weapons
> - Previous dangerous impulsive acts
> - Denial of previous (proven) dangerous acts
> - Severity of previous acts
> - Known personal trigger factors
> - Verbal threat of violence
> - Evidence of recent severe stress, particularly loss or threat of loss
> - One or more of the above plus any of the following:
>   - cruelty to animals
>   - reckless driving
>   - history of bed wetting
>   - loss of a parent before age 8

lines (2005) suggest clinical factors (listed in Box 18.2) that range across diagnoses. Wright *et al.* (2002) conclude that although symptoms may have some role in influencing violence and aggression, it is more likely that it is the effect of symptoms in reducing ability to deal with external demands and interpersonal conflict that is implicated in violent and aggressive behaviour.

Environmental factors

The Royal College of Psychiatrists Research Unit (1998) acknowledged that hospital wards are unnatural environments, which nevertheless should aim to create a safe, homely atmosphere which

> **Box 18.2 Clinical factors associated with increased risk of aggression (after NICE 2005)**
>
> - Substance abuse
> - Agitation or excitement
> - Hostility or suspiciousness
> - A preoccupation with violence
> - Poor collaboration with treatment
> - Delusions or hallucinations focused on a particular person
> - Delusions of control with a violent theme
> - Impulsive personality traits
> - Poor collaboration with treatment
> - Organic dysfunction

> **Box 18.3 Aspects of the physical and social environment affecting levels of aggression**
>
> **Physical environment should:**
> - be clean;
> - allow for daylight and fresh air;
> - avoid overcrowding;
> - have controlled noise levels (e.g. a separate TV room);
> - allow for control of temperature and ventilation;
> - provide designated smoking and non-smoking areas;[1]
> - allow for privacy in bedrooms, bathrooms and toilets;
> - provide sightlines allowing people to see what is happening in different parts of the ward.
>
> **Social environment should have:**
> - a rationale offered for ward expectations;
> - open communication processes between patients, ward staff and management;
> - patient involvement in decision-making;
> - planned, predictable activity;
> - opportunity for social and recreational activity;
> - clear staff functions;
> - adequate and consistent staffing;
> - effective multi-disciplinary working;
> - commitment to staff training and support.

allows for safety and for privacy. The supporting social environment is equally important. Patients in a US maximum security facility reported that they often did not understand the reasons for ward rules and expectations (Caplan 1993), while patients in the Sainsbury Centre for Mental Health survey of acute wards (1998) reported disliking the constant refrain from staff of 'the policy is . . . '. Boredom and lack of structured activity may also be contributory to violence and aggression. Katz and Kirkland (1990) examined levels of violence on psychiatric wards in the USA and concluded that 'violence was more frequent and extreme in wards in which staff functions were unclear, and in which events such as activities, meetings or staff–patient encounters were unpredictable' (p. 262). Shah (1993) summarized research suggesting that levels of violence increase at times when patients congregate with little structured activity (e.g. medication and meal times) (see Box 18.3.)

Staffing factors

Patients surveyed by the Royal College of Psychiatrists Research Unit (1998) emphasized that talking and listening are key interventions not to be undervalued. They focused on boredom, staff attitudes and staffing levels as factors affecting levels of violence. Patients in the Sainsbury Centre for Mental Health (1998) survey indicated that they wanted more access to staff; however, organizational and resource factors may militate against this. Shah (1993) summarized possible staff factors associated with higher levels of violence including: use of temporary staff, under-involvement of medical staff, poor communication among staff, demoralization and incompetence among staff and high staff turnover. It may be that these factors create a 'high expressed emotion' environment. Establishing an ideal number of nursing staff is complex. Owen *et al.* (1998) found an association between higher numbers of nursing staff and higher levels of violence, which may reflect increased numbers of staff as a response to violence. On the other hand, Morrison and Lehane (1995) found that over a two-year period in one psychiatric hospital, as staffing levels increased, use of seclusion fell. This study also reported that fewer seclusions took place when experienced nurses were on duty, while Owen *et al.* (1998) reported that increased violence is associated with lower levels of experience and lack of staff training in control of aggression techniques.

The Royal College of Psychiatrists Research Unit (1998), in reviewing the evidence on the influence of the physical and social environment, concluded that the quantitative evidence is too weak to draw firm conclusions about relationships between these and incidence of aggression. However, they also argue that addressing these issues makes intuitive sense. The NICE guidance (2005) concords with this and also makes recommendations about the environment in mental health wards. Box 18.3 summarizes some of the evidence on physical and social environmental factors which may influence levels of violence and aggression.

Although these points may seem self-evident, findings of a national audit of psychiatric wards for the period 1999–2000 indicated that many aspects of the physical and social environment and staff training and communication fell short of the recommendations above (Royal College of Psychiatrists Research Unit 2000). The RCP currently run the AIMS (Accreditation for Inpatient Mental Health Services) scheme, which describes a set of standards incorporating many of the regulatory requirements for wards. The standards for wards for working age adults can be found at: www. rcpsych.ac.uk/

Thinking Space 18.1

Think about wards you have worked on. Did the physical and social environment impact on levels of aggression? Were there any improvements which could have been made (consider the points in Box 18.3)?

Feedback

As well as the points made in this chapter, you may want to reflect on how you feel walking into the inpatient unit in which you work.

- Is it always too hot or too cold?
- Is it always noisy with no private spaces?
- Is there any access to fresh air?
- Do people (patients and staff) talk together or stay in their rooms or the nurses' office?
- Is there anything planned for the day or do you have no idea what might happen?
- Do you know and trust the other people you're working with that day?

It's likely that if you find the environment depressing and stressful, patients do too. Dirty, noisy or chaotic environments can increase levels of arousal which may impact on aggressive behaviour. The 2004 Ward Watch report by MIND found that 53 per cent of current or recent inpatients surveyed reported that the ward environment had not helped their recovery (see www.mind.org.uk).

18.5   Practice model

Improving services and practice in light of the factors above is likely to have a long-term and lasting impact in levels of violence. However, in the best planned environments, anger, aggression and violence will still occur, and in this case an understanding of the appropriate level of intervention matched to the phase of aggression is needed.

One model which lends itself to a range of interventions is that proposed by Novaco (1983) in his development of an anger management treatment programme. In this model, anger is seen as a state of physiological arousal leading to tension and irritability which lead to cognitions producing antagonistic thought patterns. As exposure continues, antagonistic thought patterns lead to faulty appraisal of others' behaviour or situations. Inappropriate coping mechanisms in response to increasing stress can then cause aggression. Goleman (1995), in his book on *Emotional Intelligence*, describes a similar cascade of events in which a sense of threat or danger evokes the fight or flight mechanism, in turn invoking a train of angry thoughts which in turn contribute to increased physiological arousal, rendering the person more susceptible to external triggers, each wave becoming more intense and increasing the level of physiological arousal. These models suggest that anger and aggression can often be observed to escalate, and physical harm can be prevented if the escalating situation is observed and there is early intervention.

Observation and engagement

The 2005 NICE guidelines include observation and engagement as methods for predicting and preventing escalation of anger into violence. Observation is defined in the same way as when used in the management of self-harm – i.e. on four levels from general observation through intermittent observation to 'within eyesight' and 'within arm's length'. The minimum level of observation necessary should be used and engagement with the service user is a key aim of the intervention.

It could be argued that intrusive levels of observation are both provocative to patients at risk of harm to others and place observing staff at risk. Risk assessment should be rigorous and recorded in both medical and nursing notes and consideration should be given to having more than one staff member observing the service user. All staff involved in observation should be familiar with the ward environment and methods of summoning help. In accordance with the NICE guidance, observation should be considered a short-term (72-hour) intervention. More specific methods of prediction and prevention are incorporated into de-escalation techniques.

De-escalation

The Sainsbury Centre for Mental Health (2001) includes understanding of de-escalation skills as a core capability for mental health nurses working in acute settings. The term 'de-escalation' refers to the 'processes by which a patient's expressed anger or aggression is defused, so that a calmer state ensues' (RCN 1997). In this position statement, the RCN described these short-term interventions as using a combination of immediate risk assessment together with verbal and non-verbal communication skills. Application is divided into several phases, as follows.

Understanding reasons for anger or aggression

As well as the clinical and social factors underlying aggression, the individual's specific situation has to be considered. The person may have experienced (or perceive that they have experienced) personal criticism, restriction or control, unfair treatment, frustration of intentions or the irritating behaviour of others. Nurses therefore need to be aware of what is happening both on the ward in general and for the patient in particular, which may be contributing to their anger. Stressors might also include staff behaviours. Wright *et al.* (2002) report that violent incidents are more likely when there is aversive stimulation from staff in terms of imposing limits or frustrating requests. Violence and aggression may be variously attributed to factors internal to the person or external events, but their occurrence has for some time been seen as situational. Geen (1990: 53) for example wrote that: 'Even when a person is disposed to aggress and capable of behaving aggressively, specific situations must elicit the aggression'. A study by Duxbury (2002) of three acute wards found that staff tended to attribute violence to internal factors while patients more often cited external factors. The above quotation is a reminder that incidents of aggression are generally the result of an interaction between multiple variables in a particular situation.

The NICE guideline (2005) emphasizes that staff should be aware of both general and personal factors which can provoke an individual service user. This includes an awareness of the effect of staff behaviour, both verbal and non-verbal. Staff should also encourage service users to be able to recognize and monitor their own triggers and record this in care plans. These individual factors are important to recognize as similar behaviours may mean different things when displayed by different people. A study by Whittington and Patterson (1996) matched aggressive and non-aggressive patients and found that the groups were distinguished by levels of verbal abuse, threatening gestures and either very high or very low activity. Verbal abuse was the most common behaviour and preceded two-thirds of physical attacks. However, the caveat is that in many cases key behaviours were exhibited for long periods without being followed by violence. Despite this, possible antecedents to aggression derived from the RCN (1997) and Royal College of Psychiatrists Research Unit (1998) are indicated when the person exhibits any of the behaviours listed in Box 18.4.

Having identified an increased risk of violence, maintaining safety is also necessary. Practice points drawn from the RCN (1997) and Royal College of Psychiatrists Research Unit (1998) guidelines are listed in Box 18.5.

Case Study

Richard

You arrive at work for an early shift and receive a handover about Richard. He was brought to the ward during the night by the police after throwing a brick through a neighbour's window. He felt they were secretly filming him and was trying to break the recording equipment in their house. He smelt of alcohol when admitted and looked disoriented and scared. He has only slept for a few hours. Night staff have tried on several occasions to sit down with him and talk but Richard has said that he doesn't want to do this. After the night staff leave, Richard comes into the day area. He looks agitated; pacing the day area and talking to himself.

Thinking Space 18.2

What is your assessment of any immediate risk (refer to Box 18.4)? What safety points might you consider before approaching Richard (refer to Box 18.5.)?

Feedback

From the points made so far in this chapter, you can see that Richard is showing some behavioural signs of possible anger: he's pacing and restless and, given the handover you've had, you might also think that he could feel threatened or suspicious. Try to imagine what feelings he may be experiencing other than anger: fear or worry or confusion. You might also consider your own feelings – you might feel apprehensive about approaching him. However, at this point any physical intervention wouldn't be proportional. Richard needs to be able to have the chance to talk to someone. You don't know much about his history or background at this time so a full risk assessment is not possible. You need to consider the points in Box 18.5 to maintain your own safety if necessary, but engaging Richard in conversation is your first aim.

Box 18.4 Possible indicators of anger and aggression

- Focuses attention on what is causing anger and continues to dwell on this
- Perceives threat from others or is suspicious
- Reacts in an exaggerated manner to problems
- Shows increased physical arousal – restlessness, pacing, erratic movements
- Refuses to communicate or withdraws
- Makes verbal threats or gestures
- Reports angry or violent feelings
- Shows increased volume of speech
- Has a tense facial expression – fixed stare, clenched jaw, makes constant eye contact

Box 18.5 Practice points for monitoring safety

- Don't isolate yourself – check that colleagues know your whereabouts.
- Check that you are familiar with mechanisms for calling for help and that you have access to these.
- Check escape routes – avoid corners.
- If isolated when a violent incident occurs, the priority is to get away from the situation and summon help. Do not tackle a violent person alone, whatever your or the patient's gender or size.
- Make a visual check of the immediate area for potential weapons – for example, there may be chairs, cups or glasses in the day area or dining room; if in a kitchen there may be knives or boiling water; in a bathroom razors or aerosols may be present. If identified, the priority is to maintain distance and offer the option to the person to leave the area and continue discussion elsewhere.

Once a risk assessment and safety check indicate that it is possible to approach the person safely, de-escalation techniques can be used. NICE guidelines (2005) provide specific descriptions of the techniques which should be used and recommend that one person should approach the service user and assume control of the situation (rather than several staff surrounding one service user, which can clearly be seen as threatening). Some key non-verbal and verbal interventions (derived from NICE and the RCN) are as follows.

Non-verbal communication

Key techniques include:

- Maintain an adequate distance – this is more than usual when dealing with an angry person as closeness may be interpreted as a threat or increase tension.

- Stand at an angle to the patient to avoid appearing confrontational. Do not point and do not touch the person.

- Maintain normal eye contact – staring can be threatening, avoiding can seem dismissive.

- Appear calm and speak slowly using clear and short sentences. However, avoid being patronizing (avoid telling patient to calm down!). Be courteous, and use the person's name.

- Be aware of your own reactions, which may be fear or anger, and try to consider the patient's point of view – they might be anxious as well as angry. Do not feel that you have to win any argument or that you have to deal with this situation alone and effectively in order to be a 'good nurse'. Try to show concern and attentiveness.

Verbal communication

The aim here is to continue communication and move on to problem-solving. Some key techniques are:

- Engage in conversation and most importantly acknowledge concerns, allowing the person time to express their worries or complaints. Ask the person to sit down with you or go to a quieter area (as long as other staff know where you are and your initial risk assessment indicates this is safe). Ask the person for the facts of the problem as they see them.

- Use reflective listening to acknowledge concerns. This is more skilled than it appears and is not simply stating the obvious or parroting what the person says. Be specific – 'I can see you're disappointed and upset that you won't be able to go home this weekend.'

- Convey that you want to help the person find a solution (e.g. 'Give me half an hour to try to find out what has happened'). Be realistic and do not make promises that cannot be kept. Allow the person to start generating options for dealing with the problem. Do not lecture or challenge.

- Attempt to establish rapport and emphasize cooperation.

- Negotiate realistic options and avoid using threats.

- Ask open questions.

- Listen carefully and show empathy.

Thinking Space 18.3

Richard agrees to sit down and talk to you. He doesn't understand why he is in hospital and the thinks the police may have fitted him up. He would like to go home and at least get some money and clothes. He still sounds angry when talking about his situation. What verbal interventions could you use?

Feedback

You will need to use the verbal de-escalation techniques described above. The de-escalation techniques described in this chapter are skills used when aggression seems to be imminent. The underlying attitude implied is one of willingness to engage in problem-solving if at all possible, and to be genuine about this. You might sometimes find that this is a difficult attitude to maintain because of the context in which you work. For an interesting discussion of whether humanistic models of nursing are congruent with working in a forensic setting, see Jacob *et al.* (2008).

Physical intervention

NICE guidance (2005) clearly states that de-escalation techniques should be seen as part of an ongoing response to escalation of anger and aggression. They should always be attempted before other interventions are employed. However, verbal interventions work up to a certain point of moderate anger but may fail to calm a situation. Goleman (1995) argues that after a certain stage they have no effect as people are unable to process information. Further, the relationship between anger and aggression is not straightforward. Absence of overt anger does not mean that aggression will not occur. Where aggression leads to gain – material, social or psychological – anger is not necessary to precipitate it. If, at this stage, aggression or violence occurs, physical intervention may be needed to maintain safety.

Restraint

The aim here is not to describe techniques for physical restraint. These should be taught on an approved course and involve an assessment of competence to use physical techniques. However, they should be used judiciously with an understanding of the legal, professional and ethical context. The Mental Health Act (MHA) *Code of Practice* (DH 2008) makes clear that providers of inpatient psychiatric care should have policies on the use of physical restraint, seeing it as a 'last resort' intervention. NICE place restraint, rapid tranquillization and seclusion at the end of a care pathway where prediction and prevention have failed. However, the RCN (1997) acknowledged that use of restraint should not necessarily be seen as a failure, as people in an extreme state of anger or provocation might not be able to respond to verbal interventions.

Physical intervention techniques developed from control and restraint (C&R) training used by the prison service but the term C&R should not be used within psychiatric services as techniques have been adapted for this setting. Specific techniques have also evolved and changed in the face of deaths and injuries sustained using physical intervention in mental health settings. The NICE guidance, for example, takes account of some of the findings of the 2003 inquiry into the death of David Bennett during restraint. Staff should attend regular updates to ensure that they are familiar with changes. One of the most important recommendations of the NICE guidance is the development of standardized and accredited training in both physical and non-physical management of violence and aggression. In October 2005, NHS Security Management Services published *Promoting Safer and Therapeutic Services: Implementing the national syllabus in mental health and learning disability services*. This provides learning outcomes for all non-physical aspects of training and should form the basis for physical skills training being developed by the National Institute for Mental Health in England (NIMHE) and the National Patient Safety Agency (NPSA). All relevant staff in mental health settings should have been trained in accordance with the Promoting Safer and Therapeutic Services (PSTS) curriculum by 2008. The NICE guidance makes several recommendations about the principles of use of physical restraint including:

- Staff should continue to use de-escalation techniques during physical intervention.
- Physical restraint should be avoided if possible and should not be used for prolonged periods because of risks to physical health. Rapid tranquillization or seclusion should be considered as an alternative.
- The level of force used must be justifiable and appropriate to the situation.
- The application of pain has no therapeutic value and could only be justified for the immediate rescue of others.
- Pressure should never be applied to the neck, thorax, abdomen or pelvic area. The patient's airway and breathing should be monitored throughout.

Both the Royal College of Psychiatrists Research Unit (1998) and the NMC (Wright *et al.* 2002) reviews found that studies of the effectiveness of restraint in reducing levels of violence and aggression tend to be poorly designed and descriptive in nature. Many studies are from countries other than the UK and 'restraint' may have different meanings across countries. Wright *et al.* (2002) also argue that there are significant ethical and methodological issues in conducting research in this area. There are likely to be many other intervening factors apart from restraint training which influence the incidence of violence and it is arguably unethical to withhold training from some staff in order to maintain a control group. The Royal College of Psychiatrists Research Unit (1998) concluded that evidence suggests that injury during restraint can be reduced as a result of training although the frequency of violence may not reduce. Wright *et al.* (2002: 41) concluded that 'it is reasonable to believe that the evidence base is sufficient to indicate what is likely to constitute good practice that is clinically, logically, ethically and medico-logically defensible'. What does seem clear is that the use of restraint is emotive for both patients and staff. However, patients and carers consulted by the RCP acknowledged that restraint was sometimes necessary to prevent harm to others – what was important was the judicious and rational use of physical intervention.

Seclusion

Many wards manage violence without the use of seclusion; however, its use is still widespread and remains controversial with both staff and patients expressing negative attitudes. Soliday (1985) found that patients expressed more negative feelings about seclusion than did nurses, who saw seclusion as necessary at times. As with restraint, research into the therapeutic use of seclusion lacks controlled studies. Wright *et al.* (2002) state that outcome studies are problematic because 'improvements' may be perceived as a result of a change in the patient's behaviour rather than mental state.

The MHA *Code of Practice* (DH 2008) defines seclusion as: 'the supervised confinement of a patient in a room which may be locked to protect others from significant harm. Its sole aim is to contain severely disturbed behaviour which is likely to cause harm to others' (para. 15:43: 122). In addition, it should be used as a last resort and for the shortest

possible time. It should not be used as a punishment or threat, as part of a treatment programme (it should not be confused with the use of 'time out' which is a specific behavioural intervention), because of shortage of staff or where there is any risk of suicide or self-harm. The decision to seclude should not be an automatic one following restraint. The MHA *Code of Practice* (DH 2008) states that the decision to seclude can be made by a doctor or the professional in charge (para. 15:49). If seclusion is initiated, the NICE guidelines recommend that:

- seclusion should be recorded in accordance with the MHA *Code of Practice*;
- an observation schedule should be established and the patient observed constantly by a trained person;
- seclusion must be reviewed at least every two hours and should be for the shortest time possible;
- the patient should not be deprived of clothing or personal items such as jewellery as long as there is no risk to self or others;
- if rapid tranquillization has been used, seclusion should terminate once medication has taken effect.

In addition, the seclusion room should be kept clean and free of anything that could be used as a weapon. The patient should also be checked for weapons before seclusion is initiated.

Use of seclusion is controversial and emotive. The Royal College of Psychiatrists Research Unit (1998) argued that service users should be involved in the development of local protocols and that patients who are secluded should always be given an explanation at the time, which is repeated later. Wright *et al.* (2002) also suggest that debriefing is offered afterwards to patients and that use of seclusion in principle should be discussed at ward or patient meetings.

Rapid tranquillization

Again, the decision to use medication should not be an automatic one. The aim of rapid tranquillization is to calm a situation and may or may not involve the use of anti-psychotic medication depending on the service user. The patients in the Royal College of Psychiatrists Research Unit (1998) consultation exercise expressed concern about the use of medication in people they felt were not mentally ill, but felt that informed use of medication was preferable to physical restraint.

The NICE violence guideline (2005) gives a treatment algorithm for rapid tranquillization which emphasizes the need for staff training in tranquillization protocols, in the properties of benzodiazepines, antipsychotics, flumenazil (a benzodiazepine antagonist), and in cardiopulmonary resuscitation. Use should be balanced against the risks of over-sedation causing loss of alertness or consciousness and damage to the nurse–patient relationship. If the patient is secluded and rapid tranquillization used, extra vigilance is needed. Oral medication should be offered first – lorazepam, olanzepine and haloperidol are suggested (use of the latter may also require the administration of an anticholinergic). If intramuscular (IM) administration is necessary, single use of one of the above drugs is advocated, again with the proviso that where typical antipsychotics are used, an anticholinergic should also be given. The NICE guidelines (2005) state that in urgent cases IM haloperidol and lorazepam can be given together if psychosis is indicated. There is no evidence that combining several medications of the same group or using doses above British National Formulary (BNF) limits has any better effect.

Again, the decision should be a multi-disciplinary one and a rationale clearly documented. Vital signs also need to be monitored following medication. The NICE guidelines state that staff who are involved in rapid tranquillization should be trained to the level of immediate life support and should be trained in the use of a pulse oximeter. As soon as possible, the patient should be given an opportunity to discuss the use of medication and receive an explanation for its use. At time of writing, it is important to note that the planned update of the NICE guidelines will incorporate a review of the evidence around pharmacological interventions so this guidance may change.

Post-incident management

Many nurses will be uncomfortable about using physical interventions as it is difficult to see them as 'therapeutic'. Gunn and Rodgers (2002) argue that use of restraint and seclusion cannot be justified on treatment grounds, but that the most appropriate ethical basis is in 'common law justification' – i.e. the requirement to use the least force necessary to prevent harm. The difficulty for nurses is that they may have to use these interventions while building and maintaining therapeutic relationships. It would be naive to assume that physical intervention does not affect staff–patient relationships. However, the legal, professional and ethical context which frames its use can serve to provide safety and reassurance for both patients and staff, and good post-incident management may help to reduce the longer-term effects. NICE guidance recommends both incident reporting and post-incident review following any instances of aggression or violence.

The emotional impact of coping with aggression, even if managed effectively, should not be overlooked. Wykes and Whittington (1994) found that staff reactions to assault included fear, anxiety, guilt, self-blame, anger and hatred. Crichton *et al.* (1998) suggested that staff response to aggression involves an element of moral censure of the patient related to the level of perceived threat and assessment of moral responsibility. Coping with these strong feelings has an effect on relationships with patients, possibly leading to hostility, avoidance and controlling behaviour, which feeds back to levels of violence among patients. Post-incident review is therefore vital to allow expression of difficult emotions and enable learning from the incident (critical incident analysis is one such mechanism). Patients who have been involved in or observed aggressive incidents also need support. Neither should the impact of verbal abuse be underestimated. Community staff may be particularly affected by this given that they often see clients alone and are often called on to make day-to-day practice decisions in isolation.

Thinking Space 18.4

What beliefs do you have about angry and aggressive people? Do these influence your reactions to violence and aggression?

Feedback

You may have found that your attitude to angry or aggressive individuals depends on how far you see them as responsible for their behaviour. Your reaction to aggression from an elderly woman with dementia might be different to agression from a young man with schizophrenia who has had too much to drink, for example. In some respects these judgements are essentially moral ones, but you might find it interesting to look at the issue of responsibility from a legal perspective – for example the categories of defence for criminal acts described in Dimond (2011) Chapter 2, including:

- infancy (under 10)
- insanity
- diminished responsibility and loss of control
- mistake
- necessity
- duress
- superior orders
- self-defence

18.6   Conclusion

There is no 'cookbook' approach to managing anger, violence and aggression. Interventions need to be adapted to the needs of the patient. The current NICE guidance emphasizes the recognition of the individual needs of service users including all aspects of diversity such as social, physical and spiritual needs. On a positive note, research suggests that nurses do actually use a creative mixture of techniques when dealing with violence and aggression, adopting an approach which tailors interventions to seriousness of situation. However, there is overwhelming consensus that the interventions discussed above are no substitute for competent and confident staff working as a team in a safe and therapeutic environment. The importance of supporting staff and ensuring an environment conducive to professional practice has an increasing evidence base. A recent study by Papadopoulos *et al.* (2012) found 13 themes that were associated with increased likelihood of both conflict and consequent containment measures on acute mental health wards. Eleven of these were staff related, and in particular staffing change and negative staff morale were associated with an increase in conflict and containment.

To summarize:

- The quality of the physical and social environment on mental health wards is likely to have an impact on the level of violence and aggression.
- Talking and listening to patients are fundamental interventions in preventing violence and aggression.
- Intervention should be matched to the level of anger or aggression; there is a hierarchy of methods from verbal to physical techniques. NICE (2005) guidance emphasizes that any staff response should be proportionate to the level of risk.
- Physical intervention occurs within a legal, professional and ethical framework. Staff should make sure they understand these considerations before any incident.
- Patients and staff need to be offered support after an incident of aggression.
- Supporting staff to provide positive practice may have a positive impact on levels of violence and aggression.

Annotated bibliography

Wright, S., Gray, R., Parkes, J. and Gournay, K. (2002) *The Recognition, Prevention and Therapeutic Management of Violence in Acute In-patient Psychiatry: A literature review and evidence-based recommendations for good practice.* London: UKCC.
This report, prepared for the NMC, provides a comprehensive review of the research on violence and aggression in mental health settings and discusses the evidence base for factors which influence violence as well as the effectiveness of management interventions.

NICE (National Institute for Health and Clinical Excellence) *Violence: The short-term management of disturbed/violent behaviour in in-patient psychiatric settings and emergency departments.* Clinical Guideline 25, February 2005. London: NICE.
This is the current definitive guide to practice in the management of violence or aggression. The full guideline also provides a review of the most recent evidence in the area. The guideline was developed in conjunction with service users.

Mason, T. and Chandley, M. (1999) *Managing Violence and Aggression: A manual for nurses and healthcare workers.* Edinburgh: Churchill Livingstone.
This provides a practice-based discussion of interventions used during different phases of aggression. The sections on longer-term, structured intervention such as behavioural programmes give another perspective on management of aggression.

Vaughan, P.J. and Badger, D. (1995) *Working with the Mentally Disordered Offender in the Community.* London: Chapman & Hall.
For guidance on managing aggression in the community, Chapter 4 contains practical advice on maintaining safety in community mental health centres and when visiting clients.

Note

1 This is as stated in the 2005 NICE guidance. Since then UK law on smoking in public places has changed and the forthcoming review of the NICE guideline will incorporate this.

References

Caplan, C.A. (1993) Nursing staff and patient perceptions of ward atmosphere in a maximum security forensic hospital, *Archives of Psychiatric Nursing,* 3(1): 23–9.
CQC (Care Quality Commission) (2010) *Count Me In 2010 Census,* available at: http://www.cqc.org.uk/sites/default/files/media/documents/count_me_in_2010_final_tagged.pdf.
Crichton, J., Callanan, T.S., Beauchamp, L., Glasson, M. and Tardiff, H. (1998) Staff response to psychiatric inpatient violence: an international comparison, *Psychiatric Care,* 5(2): 50–6.
DH (Department of Health) (2008) *Mental Health Act 1983 Code of Practice.* London: TSO.
Dimond, B. (2011) *Legal Aspects of Nursing,* 6th edn. Harlow: Pearson.
Duxbury, J. (2002) An evaluation of staff and patient views of and strategies employed to manage inpatient aggression and violence on one mental health unit: a pluralistic design, *Journal of Psychiatric and Mental Health Nursing,* 9: 325–37.
Geen, R. (1990) *Human Aggression.* Milton Keynes: Open University Press.
Goleman, D. (1995) *Emotional Intelligence.* London: Bloomsbury.
Gournay, K. (2000) *The Recognition, Prevention and Therapeutic Management of Violence in Mental Health Care: A consultation document.* London: UKCC.
Gunn, M. and Rodgers, M. (2002) Mental health nursing, in J. Tingle and A. Cribb (eds) *Nursing Law and Ethics,* 2nd edn. Oxford: Blackwell Science.
Haber, L.C., Fagan-Pryor, E.C. and Allen, M. (1997) Comparison of registered nurses' and nursing assistants' choices of interventions for aggressive behaviours, *Issues in Mental Health Nursing,* 18: 325–8.
Healthcare Commission (2008) *The Pathway to Recovery: A review of NHS acute inpatient mental health services,* available at: http://webarchive.nationalarchives.gov.uk/20110515082446/http://cqc.org.uk/_db/_documents/The_pathway_to_recovery_200807251020.pdf.
Independent Inquiry into the Death of David Bennett (2003) An independent inquiry set up under HSG(94) 27.
Jacob, J., Holmes, D. and Buus, N. (2008) Humanism in forensic psychiatry: the use of the tidal nursing model, *Nursing Inquiry,* 15(3): 224–30.
Katz, P. and Kirkland, F.R. (1990) Violence and social structure on mental hospital wards, *Psychiatry,* 53: 262–77.
Lowenstein, M., Binder, R.L. and McNiel, D.E. (1990) The relationship between admission symptoms and hospital assaults, *Hospital and Community Psychiatry,* 41(3): 311–13.
Mason, T. and Chandley, M. (1999) *Managing Violence and Aggression: A manual for nurses and healthcare workers.* Edinburgh: Churchill Livingstone.

Monaghan, J. (1993) Mental disorder and violence: another look, in S. Hodgins (ed.) *Mental Disorder and Crime*. London: Sage.

Morrison, P. and Lehane, M. (1995) Staffing levels and seclusion use, *Journal of Advanced Nursing*, 22: 1192–202.

NICE (National Institute for Health and Clinical Excellence) (2005) *Violence: The short-term management of disturbed/violent behaviour in in-patient psychiatric settings and emergency departments*. Clinical Guideline 25. London: NICE.

NMC (Nursing and Midwifery Council) (2003) Press release, 3 February 2003.

Novaco, R.W. (1983) *Stress Inoculation Therapy for Anger Control: A manual for therapists*. Irvine, CA: University of California.

Owen, C., Tarantello, C., Jones, M. and Tennant, C. (1998) Violence and aggression in psychiatric units, *Psychiatric Services*, 49(11): 1452–7.

Papadopoulos, C., Bowers, L., Quirk, A. and Khanom, H. (2012) Events preceding changes in conflict and containment rates on an acute psychiatric ward, *Psychiatric Services*, 63(1): 40–7.

RCN (Royal College of Nursing) (1997) *The Management of Aggression and Violence in Places of Care: An RCN position statement*. London: RCN.

Royal College of Psychiatrists Research Unit (1998) *Management of Imminent Violence: Clinical practice guidelines to support mental health services*, Occasional Paper OP41. London: RCP.

Royal College of Psychiatrists Research Unit (2000) *National Audit of the Management of Violence in Mental Health Settings 1999–2000*. London: RCP.

Sainsbury Centre for Mental Health (1998) *Acute Problems: A survey of the quality of care in acute psychiatric wards*. London: Sainsbury Centre for Mental Health.

Sainsbury Centre for Mental Health (2001) *The Capable Practitioner: A framework and list of the practitioner capabilities required to implement The National Service Framework for Mental Health*. London: Sainsbury Centre for Mental Health.

Shah, A.K. (1993) An increase in violence among psychiatric in-patients: real or imagined? *Medical Science Law*, 33(3): 227–9.

Soliday, S.M. (1985) A comparison of patients and staff attitudes toward seclusion, *Journal of Nervous and Mental Disease*, 173(5): 282–6.

Vinestock, M. (1996) Risk assessment: 'a word to the wise', *Advances in Psychiatric Treatment*, 2: 3–10.

Whittington, R. and Patterson, P. (1996) Verbal and non-verbal behaviour immediately prior to aggression by mentally disordered people: enhancing the assessment of risk, *Journal of Psychiatric and Mental Health Nursing*, 3: 47–54.

Whittington, R. and Wykes, T. (1994) An observational study of associations between nurse behaviour and violence in psychiatric hospitals, *Journal of Psychiatric and Mental Health Nursing*, 1: 85–92.

Wright, S., Lee, S., Sayer, J., Parr, A. and Gournay, K. (2000) A review of the content of management of violence policies in in-patient mental health units, *Mental Health Care*, 3(11): 373–6.

Wright, S., Gray, R., Parkes, J. and Gournay, K. (2002) *The Recognition, Prevention and Therapeutic Management of Violence in Acute In-patient Psychiatry: A literature review and evidence based recommendations for good practice*. London: UKCC.

Wykes, T. and Whittington, R. (1994) Reactions to assault, in T. Wykes (ed.) *Violence and Healthcare Professionals*. London: Chapman & Hall.

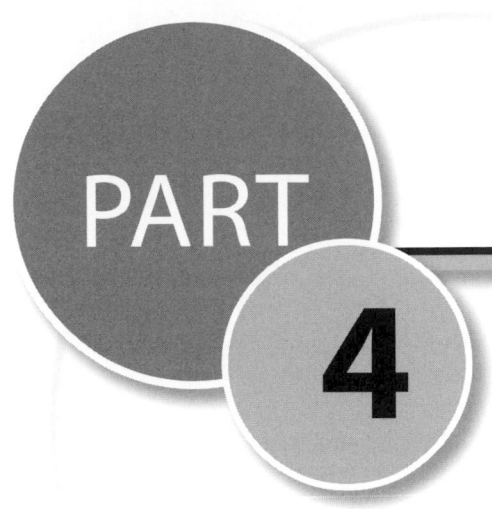

PART 4

Interventions

Chapter 19

Self-management

Mary O'Toole

The Expert Patient's Group was time for me. It helped me to focus on what I could do to help myself. Talking to others, we didn't dwell on what was wrong and what we couldn't do … I've made some very good friends.

The group situation was powerful – I came away with a sense of control over my own life.

It was always my voices that dictated the sort of day I was going to have … now it's me that decides how things are going to be!

At first I was very nervous about facing other people … the atmosphere is warm and accepting … I felt cared about and understood.

19.1 Introduction

This chapter provides an account of self-management approaches in mental health. Self-management is about people being actively involved in and engaged with their own health care. At the heart of self-management is the concept of recovery. Recovery in mental health has come to prominence in recent years and has now been adopted as the accepted paradigm for mental health service provision in the UK. One of the key characteristics of the recovery approach is that service users are acknowledged as experts in their experience. The approach recognizes the personal resourcefulness of individuals and that a person's recovery is unique, with a diverse range of views on mental distress and personally lived experiences. In terms of mental health service provision, the recovery approach emphasizes choice, autonomous action, empowerment and personal responsibility, all of which are key components in self-management. In addition, the increasing social and financial burden of chronic disease on health care services, as well as less than optimal outcomes, has led to a widespread increase in self-management initiatives and the potential for less demand on statutory services.

This chapter clarifies the different terms currently in use and describes the origins and rationale for self-management along with key policy developments relevant to self-management. Self-management approaches in mental health have progressed significantly over the past 10 years and there are a variety of recognized programmes widely available. The chapter describes these different programmes as well as the various behaviours, strategies and tools identified by service users that have been recognized as helpful in enabling people to manage their own mental health. Research evaluating the effectiveness and cost effectiveness of self-management interventions is summarized, together with implications for the role of the mental health nurse.

This chapter covers:

- terminology;
- origins and rationale for self-management;
- key policy initiatives;
- behaviours that support self-management;
- self-management programmes;
- the evidence base for self-management programmes;
- role of the nurse/mental health care professional.

Case Study

Lucy

Lucy is 28 and lives alone. She experienced her first psychotic episode aged 20, shortly after starting university and living away from home. This resulted in a four-month formal admission to an acute mental health unit where she was assessed and prescribed antipsychotic medication. She was given a diagnosis of schizophrenia at this time and although she returned to university, she quit her course two months later because she found it too stressful.

Over the last eight years Lucy has been prescribed a variety of antipsychotic medications and has been admitted to hospital five times. When she is unwell her symptoms include hearing the voice of her mother who died when she was aged 12. The voice is sometimes friendly and supportive but can, at times, become hostile and angry. Lucy often responds to the voice out loud which has caused her unwanted attention in the past. Some of the children in the neighbouring flats and houses taunt her and call her names like 'psycho'. Lucy also believes that the ghost of her mother follows her around, sometimes in a protective way, but at other times she believes she is out to harm her. When Lucy begins to feel bad she finds it difficult to deal with everyday activities, such as shopping and cooking, cleaning and personal self-care. When Lucy's voices get bad she will isolate herself; she will stop answering the door and will switch off her mobile phone. Lucy will usually drink more when she is feeling bad. She will drink up to six cans of strong lager daily and will often smoke cannabis if she can afford to buy it. Lucy says that the alcohol helps her to feel calm but often stops her having a good nights' sleep.

Lucy has a small circle of friends who she met mainly through mental health services. She has little contact with her family. Currently unemployed and in receipt of state benefits, she has not worked for eight years.

Lucy has not been admitted to hospital for over a year, although recently she reports frequently having bad days when she hears voices almost continually and resorts to isolating herself in her flat and drinking alcohol. She is under the care of the local community mental health team (CMHT) and sees her case worker, Lorraine, every three to four weeks. She has recently gained two stone in weight which she believes is a side-effect of medication and she is thinking about reducing the dose.

We will re-visit Lucy throughout the chapter and there will be opportunities to consider a number of issues relating to her care and recovery.

 ## 19.2 Origins and terminology

The origins of self-management in the UK lie in the 'expert patient' movement which began in the 1970s, culminating in the launch of the Department of Health (DH) (England) Initiative, *The Expert Patient: A new approach to chronic disease management for the 21st century* (DH 2001). This was largely based on chronic physical health conditions although mental health did feature, it was not specifically targeted. A number of programmes specific to mental health have been developed subsequently and it would be fair to say that self-management has now become an integral part of care.

In any discussion of the role of the patient in understanding and managing their own chronic health condition, a variety of terms may be used and lack of clarity between them hampers clear communication. Widely used terms include *patient education*, *self-care*, *self-help* and *self-management* which are often used interchangeably to describe different types of programme or intervention. For the purpose of this chapter the following definitions are adopted:

- **Patient education:** 'the teaching or training of patients concerning their own health needs' (DH 2005).
- **Self-care:** 'activities that individuals, families and communities undertake with the intention of enhancing health, preventing disease, limiting illness, and restoring health' (WHO 1983).
- **Self-help:** 'interventions that should guide and encourage the patient to make changes, focusing on methods that can be utilized to sustain change over time' (Faulkner and Ryrie 2009). However, such interventions should require minimal input from a health care professional beyond initial assessment and possible signposting to appropriate self-help resources.
- **Self-management:** 'the individual's ability to manage the symptoms, treatment, physical and psychosocial consequences and lifestyle changes inherent in living with a long term disorder' (DH 2005).

Rethink Mental Illness, the leading National UK mental health charity, defines self-management in the context of schizophrenia or psychosis as:

something we all do. It is whatever we do to make the most of our lives by coping with our difficulties and making the most of what we have. Applied specifically to people with a schizophrenia diagnosis, it includes the way we cope with, or manage, or minimise, the ways the condition limits our lives, as well as what we do to thrive, to feel happy and fulfilled, to make the most of our lives despite the condition.

(Martyn 2002)

Faulkner and Ryrie (2008) provide further clarification of the difference between self-help and self-management. Self-help tools are usually developed around a particular issue or diagnosis and imply that the person is doing something for themselves, either on their own or in a group of people who share similar experiences and can offer mutual support. Self-management, on the other hand, refers to a more comprehensive approach, which may include a particular diagnosis but will also take a 'whole-life approach towards managing your life with the diagnosis', including a range of different strategies, services and treatments whether or not they are themselves self-help strategies. Rather than simply providing information specific to a particular disease or condition, self-management encompasses problem-solving skills which enable individuals to take actions that may improve their health and also their general well-being.

Self-management has been linked with the concept of recovery (Davidson 2005), a complex concept in its own right, which emphasizes that:

> while people may not have full control over their symptoms, they can have full control over their lives. Recovery is not about 'getting rid' of problems. It is about seeing beyond a person's mental health problems, recognising and fostering their abilities, interests and dreams.

> (Mental Health Foundation 2011)

Davidson (2005) describes self-management as one aspect of recovery that provides the practical tools of everyday living.

Richards (2004) has suggested two distinct perspectives relating to self-management and self-care. On the one hand, self-management or self-help serves to empower the client and enables them to be in control of their health. On the other hand, self-management initiatives provide part of the solution to the huge disparity between client need and provision within current mental health services. Self-management initiatives go some way to overcoming the ongoing problems of accessing over-stretched statutory mental health services and the inherent shortages of specialist staff. Furthermore, Faulkner and Ryrie (2009) stress that care led by the users themselves enables the person to not only identify their own personal coping strategies but also develop alternative explanations for distress and become an 'expert by experience'. Self-management represents an integrative approach, which embraces complementary therapies and recognizes the interplay between the physical, emotional and mental aspects of a person's life and can often be more effective than any one single route of treatment (Cornah 2006a).

 19.3 Policy

Self-management has now become central to mainstream mental health care and is implicit to UK government health policy. *No Health Without Mental Health: A cross-government mental health outcomes strategy for people of all ages* (DH 2011) supports the concept of service users managing their own health needs. The policy recommends peer-support services, user-led self-help groups, mentoring and befriending, and time-banking schemes, to enable service users to be both providers and recipients of support. The strategy suggests that well managed and well supported volunteering opportunities can help people to develop the skills and confidence to play a more active role in their own well-being and their community, and to influence the shape and scope of local services. Furthermore, initiatives designed to involve service users and the wider community in supporting positive mental health can help break down barriers and challenge the stigma associated with mental illness. It would seem then that what started out as seemingly modest ideas about service users being in control of their own care have now become sufficiently established to change the culture and emphasis of today's mental health services.

NICE guidance

Self-management or self-care is advocated by a number of clinical guidelines from the National Institute for Health and Clinical Excellence (NICE). For example, the NICE guideline for depression (NICE 2009) advises that a person with mild to moderate depressive symptoms should engage in 'individual guided self-help based on the principles of cognitive behavioural therapy (CBT)'. The guideline states that this should consist of up to six or eight sessions (face-to-face and telephone) supported by a trained practitioner, who reviews progress and outcome, over 9–12 weeks. The programme should include behavioural activation and problem-solving techniques.

Recommended treatment for generalized anxiety disorder (NICE 2011) includes individual non-facilitated self-help, individual guided self-help and psycho-educational groups. 'Non facilitated self-help' consists of a written or electronic workbook that the client is expected to systematically work through over a period of at least six weeks. The workbook is based on the principles of CBT and there should be minimum therapist contact, apart from the occasional short telephone call. 'Individual guided self-help' consists of five to seven weekly or fortnightly face-to-face or telephone sessions, facilitated by a trained practitioner. Each session lasts 20–30 minutes and includes written or electronic materials based on the principles of CBT. The facilitator is also responsible for reviewing progress and outcome. 'Psycho-educational groups' should consist of six weekly sessions, each lasting two hours, including self-help manuals and presentations. The group should be facilitated by a trained practitioner and have a maximum of 12 participants.

19.4   Behaviours that support self-management

So far in this chapter the origins and rationale for self-management have been explored together with discussion of the terminology in use. Coster and Norman's (2009) review of Cochrane reviews of educational and self-management interventions concluded that the active ingredients of many successful self-management interventions are unclear. In other words, it is often unclear what specific factors help service users to manage their condition.

Patterson (2001) argued that a person with a long-term condition will have a shifting perspective on their illness – sometimes a person will have illness in their psychological foreground and sometimes wellness (i.e. good days and bad days). These perspectives will shift in response to external factors, such as symptoms of the illness and the amount of support that the person is receiving, and also in response to psychological factors, such as mood and fatigue. Self-management interventions should therefore aim to help clients maintain wellness as their foreground perspective. Lorig and Holman (2003) state that the self-management of a chronic disease involves three distinct tasks: medical management, role management and emotional management. Based on a model derived from Corbin and Strauss (1988), medical management of a long-term condition relates to adhering to a medication regime or a particular diet specific to the condition. Role management involves maintaining, adapting and developing roles in life. For example, a person with chronic back pain may change the type of exercise that they engage in. Applied to mental health, a person with a chronic depressive illness may reduce their working hours so they do not become too tired. Finally, emotional management refers to the management of those emotions that may often result from having a chronic health problem such as anger, fear, frustration and depression.

Self-management skills

Lorig and Holman (2003) argue that any self-management programme must be based on the patient's perceived problems. She uses an example of an arthritis self-management programme which traditionally focused on managing physical disability. It emerged, however, that the main concern for arthritis patients was not physical disability but pain. Therefore the programme needed to focus on pain management; managing disability could still be addressed, but within the context of pain management.

Lorig proposes five core self-management skills inherent in any self-management intervention: problem-solving, decision-making, resource utilization, forming partnerships with health care providers, and taking action.

- **Problem-solving skills:** these include problem definition, generation of possible solutions (including asking the opinions of others such as friends, peers, health care professionals), solution implementation and evaluation of results.

- **Decision-making skills:** these are acquired if the person has enough knowledge about their condition or at least knows where to get information. For example, if the person is aware of what to expect they are less likely to reach crisis point. Mental health problems can often be exacerbated by anxiety.

- **Resource utilization:** if the person is familiar with the day-to-day management of their condition (their symptoms) and aware of available resources, they are less likely to use emergency services unnecessarily.

■ **Forming partnerships with health care providers:** self-management training endeavours to teach the person to work collaboratively with their health care provider in partnership, discussing options for treatment and making informed decisions.

■ **Taking action:** this final core self-management skill largely involves learning the skills necessary to change behaviour, make an action plan and carry out the change. Proposed changes should be realistic and may require modifying. It may be helpful to explore self-confidence in the behaviour change and incorporate the other skills of problem-solving and decision-making before taking action.

Thinking Space 19.1

An overarching theme implicit in these self-management skills is personal responsibility. A key issue in Lucy's care would be to explore her perceptions and aspirations with her and how she would like her future to work out. It would also be important to ascertain Lucy's perception of her own self-efficacy in managing her own health.

Which areas do you think Lucy might focus on so that she can begin to make steps to improve her quality of life?

Feedback

Lucy is unhappy about her recent weight gain which she associates with her medication. She is planning to reduce her dose. It would be helpful if Lucy were to work collaboratively with her case worker, Lorraine. They might discuss her options and what resources are available to her. Lucy could start attending an exercise class or swimming. This would help with her weight loss and also provide her with a meaningful activity to engage in during the day. She may start to socialize with other people and the exercise will also help lift her mood.

Mental health self-help strategies

Several research studies have identified common themes, largely highlighted by service users, that are perceived to be important in the self-management of mental health.

Strategies for Living

The 'Strategies For Living Programme' (Faulkner and Layzell 2000) explored the expertise of mental health service users to achieve a better understanding of what it might be like to live with and manage mental ill health. Faulkner and Layzell interviewed service users about different aspects of their lives to identify what different strategies and supports people found most helpful to them overall. Some respondents identified a combination of two or three types of support, while others identified a single strategy. Examples included friends, relatives and other services users; mental health professionals; physical exercise; religion and spirituality; thinking positively and taking control; hobbies and interests and creative expression. The predominant theme throughout people's responses was the value of relationships with others, whether with family and friends, other service users or mental health professionals. There was little mention of medication or other mental health services and treatments. Further analysis enabled the researchers to identify underlying themes which included: shared experience and identity; emotional support; a reason for living; finding meaning and purpose; peace of mind and relaxation; taking control and having choices; security and safety; and pleasure. The research was useful in highlighting some of the areas that we might consider when advising someone with mental health problems about what they might find helpful. This study has also guided and influenced subsequent work on self-management programmes for mental health.

Rethink Mental Illness

A study by Rethink Mental Illness (Martyn 2002) examined how people used self-management and what part it played in their recovery journey. Fifty-two people with a diagnosis of schizophrenia or psychosis took part in the study, sharing their experiences of self-management through interviews, discussion groups and written reports. The themes that emerged are summarized in Table 19.1.

Mental Health Foundation

The Mental Health Foundation, a leading mental health research, policy and service improvement charity in the UK (www.mentalhealth.org.uk), has published a list of 10 practical ways to look after your mental health, derived from the experience of service users. These are summarized in Box 19.1.

The evidence base for self-management strategies

The strategies for self-management of mental health discussed so far have been identified by service users, and therefore by their nature rely largely on personal testimony and anecdotal evidence. Here we consider the evidence base for the effectiveness of four key self-management strategies: physical exercise, healthy eating, spirituality and religion, and complementary therapies.

Physical exercise

A recent Cochrane systematic review (Mead *et al.* 2010) examined data from 25 trials in which exercise was compared to no treatment or usual treatment (e.g. CBT) for people with a diagnosis of depression. The authors concluded that exercise seemed to improve the symptoms of depression, although there was no clear evidence as to how effective exercise was and what particular type of exercise was the most effective. However, there was evidence that exercise needs to be continued long term for the benefits on mood to be maintained. Another Cochrane review (Larun *et al.* 2009) explored exercise in the prevention and treatment of anxiety and depression among children and young people up to the age of 20. This review found that while exercise is promoted as a strategy to prevent and treat depression and anxiety, the research data was limited. However, a small number of trials indicated that exercise decreased reported anxiety and depression scores in healthy children when compared to no intervention.

Table 19.1 Self-management strategies (Martyn 2002)

Relationships with other people	Including other users and the user movement; family and friends; colleagues and community; mental health and other practitioners
Maintaining morale, finding meaning	Personal qualities, attitudes and beliefs; exploring and understanding your experience; reading; religion and spirituality
An ordinary life: coping	Interpersonal self-management; basic living skills; healthy living; personal self-management
An (extra)ordinary life: thriving	Occupation; recreation; social life
Managing having schizophrenia	Information and education; talking therapies; managing relationships with health care workers; complementary therapies; symptom management; managing medication; relapse management

Box 19.1 Ten ways to look after your mental health

1. **Talk about your feelings:** talking about your feelings and taking charge of your well-being.

2. **Eat well:** there are strong links between what we eat and how we feel – for example, caffeine and sugar can have an immediate effect. But food can also have a long-lasting effect on your mental health.

3. **Keep in touch:** friends and family can make you feel included and cared for. They can offer different views from whatever's going on inside your own head. They can help keep you active, keep you grounded and help you solve practical problems.

4. **Take a break:** a change of scene or a change of pace is good for your mental health. It could be a five-minute pause from cleaning your kitchen, a half-hour lunch break at work or a weekend exploring somewhere new. A few minutes can be enough to de-stress you.

5. **Accept who you are:** some of us make people laugh, some are good at maths, others cook fantastic meals. Some of us share our lifestyle with the people who live close to us, others live very differently. We're all different.

6. **Keep active:** experts believe exercise releases chemicals in your brain that make you feel good. Regular exercise can boost your self-esteem and help you concentrate, sleep, look and feel better. Exercise also keeps the brain and your other vital organs healthy.

7. **Drink sensibly:** we often drink alcohol to change our mood. Some people drink to deal with fear or loneliness, but the effect is only temporary.

8. **Ask for help:** none of us are superhuman. We all sometimes get tired or overwhelmed by how we feel or when things go wrong. If things are getting too much for you and you feel you can't cope, ask for help.

9. **Do something you are good at:** what do you love doing? What activities can you lose yourself in? What did you love doing in the past? Enjoying yourself helps beat stress. Doing an activity you enjoy probably means you're good at it and achieving something boosts your self-esteem.

10. **Care for others:** caring for others is often an important part of keeping up relationships with people close to you. It can even bring you closer together.

Source: Mental Health Foundation, www.mentalhealth.org.uk/help-information/10-ways-to-look-after-your-mental-health, accessed 13 October 2012

Healthy eating

There is growing evidence that nutrition can influence our mental health (Faulkner and Layzell 2000). Some foods serve to temporarily promote a neurotransmitter that we may be lacking and will make us feel better, at least in the short term. If the brain is continually flooded by an artificial influx of a neurotransmitter (e.g. adrenaline from strong coffee), the receptors will close down until the excess is metabolized away. This is called 'down regulation' and is the brain's instinctive mechanism for achieving homeostasis.

Unfortunately this down regulation of the brain in response to certain substances may prompt the individual to increase their intake of that particular substance in order to release the particular neurotransmitter that their brain is lacking (e.g. they drink more coffee). This will, in turn, lead to feelings of craving. Holford (2003) provides a useful summary of nutrients that can improve mood in a healthy way, without the consequence of unhealthy craving and subsequent over-consumption. For example, a deficiency in the neurotransmitter serotonin is associated with low mood and sleep disturbance. Its effects are exacerbated by alcohol consumption but alleviated by eating plenty of fish, fruit, eggs, low-fat cheese and poultry. A deficiency in the neurotransmitter GABA can lead a person to have difficulty relaxing, and being anxious and irritable. This is exacerbated by sugar, alcohol and caffeine but alleviated by consuming green vegetables, seeds, nuts, potatoes, bananas and eggs.

A review by Deborah Cornah (2006a) for the Mental Health Foundation shows that a balance of neurotransmitters is essential for good mental health, as they influence feelings of contentment, anxiety, memory and cognitive function. The review also identified the role of diet in relation to specific mental health problems such as depression, schizophrenia, Alzheimer's disease and attention deficit hyperactivity disorder (ADHD) and provides a comprehensive summary of the evidence.

Spirituality and religion

Cornah (2006b) conducted an extensive review of the literature examining the impact of spirituality on mental health and well-being on behalf of the Mental Health Foundation. She concluded that there was a consistent, although in some cases modest, positive relationship between spirituality and mental well-being. In particular a positive association was found between church attendance and lower levels of depression in adults and children. In addition, a positive relationship was found between spirituality and reduced levels of stress and anxiety in a number of client groups including women with breast cancer, people with cardiac problems and those recovering from spinal surgery. The links between schizophrenia and spirituality, however, are not so clear. One review (Mohr and Huguelet 2004) found that religion played an important part in the process of recovery and brought hope, comfort and meaning to the person.

In addition, religious values shared within the family can bring support and cohesion. Some research, however, has demonstrated a negative relationship between religion and schizophrenia whereby the service user who expresses strong religious beliefs has become stigmatized when health care professionals have not adequately explored the significance of religion to that person and see it as part of their illness.

Cornah (2006b) identifies a number of mechanisms through which potential benefits of spirituality and religion occur. These include coping styles, locus of control, social support and networks, psychological mechanisms (hope, contentment, love and forgiveness) and environment. Cornah also points to a number of limitations in the spirituality literature. For example, many of the studies employ quantitative methods which fail to capture the complex nature of spirituality and merely reduce it to single behaviours such as church attendance. A further limitation identified is the difficulty in defining religion and spirituality and the subsequent difficulty in measuring and comparing the concepts.

Complementary therapies

The benefits of various complementary therapies have come under more scrutiny in recent years and have subsequently become part of mainstream psychiatry in some services. There have been a number of Cochrane reviews conducted relating to the effectiveness of different complementary therapies in treating mental health problems such as depression (relaxation for depression, Jorm *et al.* 2008; acupuncture for depression, Smith *et al.* 2010), psychosis (art therapy for schizophrenia, Ruddy *et al.* 2009), substance misuse (auricular acupuncture for cocaine dependence, Gates *et al.* 2008) and anxiety (therapeutic touch for anxiety disorders, Robinson *et al.* 2009).

For some individuals, complementary therapies work in conjunction with conventional methods, whereas other people choose to use them as an alternative to prescribed or conventional treatments. Overall the research evidence is limited due to small samples and various methodological limitations. Most reviews conclude that complementary therapies should be advocated in conjunction with other treatments such as medication and psychological therapies. It would seem then that, although not necessarily underpinned by robust evidence, complementary therapy fits well with the philosophy of self-management as it is a strategy that service users can choose to engage in and continue with if found to be beneficial by the individual. Complementary therapies are discussed in detail in Chapter 29.

19.5 Self-management programmes

There are a number of well established self-management programmes in use, many of which were designed originally for people experiencing chronic physical health problems such as arthritis, asthma and diabetes, but have been adapted to suit the needs of mental health service users.

Expert Patients Programme

In the UK, the Expert Patients Programme (www.expertpatients.co.uk), originally based on the Stanford self-management programme (Lorig et al. 1997), delivers courses aimed at anyone who experiences a long-term health problem with the aim of helping them to manage their condition better. The Programme has developed in recent years and now provides a number of different courses, some aimed at general lifestyle topics (dealing with pain and extreme tiredness; coping with feelings of depression; relaxation techniques and exercise; healthy eating; communication with family, friends and professionals; planning for the future) and some that are condition specific (diabetes; mental health; pain; learning difficulties; substance and alcohol misuse). Most courses run over six weeks and consist of weekly two and a half hour sessions in which participants are encouraged to take more responsibility to self-manage their condition and work collaboratively with health care professionals. The

groups are facilitated by trained tutors who also have first-hand experience of living with a long-term condition.

'New Beginnings' is a self-management course provided by the Expert Patients Programme and aimed specifically at people who are living with, or are in recovery from, a mental health condition. The group approach is structured and uses cognitive behavioural techniques (see Chapter 21). Participants (maximum 12) are encouraged to support each other through open and positive discussion and sharing of experiences. The aim is to help group members to learn how to deal with problems of everyday living. The intended benefits for participants who complete the course include: improved quality of life; increased confidence and motivation; improved relationships with family, friends, work colleagues, and health and social care professionals; reduction in the effects of stigma and disempowerment; increased social inclusion; reduced feeling of isolation, anxiety and depression and an increased awareness of relapse symptoms.

A recent research study of the social impact of self-management (Expert Patients Programme 2011a) used the 'social return on investment approach' (SROI), a widely accepted method of measuring the social or environmental value of a project or organization which captures aspects of society that cannot be captured in economic terms (see www.thesroinetwork.org). This study found that direct outcomes of self-management included improved diet, meeting new people, better control of feelings and increased self-awareness and self-worth. Increased confidence led, in turn, to decreased anxiety, better sleep, a willingness to try new things and increased motivation. Participants subsequently felt able to make important life changes including improving the quality of their relationships, volunteering, and accessing further education and employment. A further study by the Expert Patients Programme (2011b) outlines the economic benefits of self-management, including a reduction in unplanned hospital admissions.

Thinking Space 19.2

At her next appointment, Lorraine suggests that Lucy attends a self-management course being run by the local Expert Patients Programme group. Initially Lucy is not keen as she is reluctant to mix with other people when her voices are bad. She finds it impossible to stop herself responding to her voices in public and quickly becomes very distressed.

How might you help Lucy to make her decision about whether or not to attend the self-management group?

Feedback

It would be helpful if Lucy were to talk to her case worker, Lorraine, about her concerns. Lorraine could introduce Lucy to another client who already attends the group. This may provide some reassurance for Lucy as she will come to understand that the atmosphere of the self-management groups is generally one of acceptance and support. Lucy will find out that the group is made up of other service users who may be having similar experiences to her and that it may be useful to chat together and share their stories and potential coping strategies.

Wellness Recovery Action Plan

The Wellness Recovery Action Plan (WRAP) was developed in the USA in the late 1980s by Mary Ellen Copeland and is now known and utilized worldwide (see www.mentalhealthrecovery.com). As with other similar programmes, it aims to encourage people who experience mental ill health to take responsibility for their own wellness by using a variety of self-help techniques as well as drawing on the support of family, friends and health care professionals. The key objective is for people to increase their self-confidence and self-esteem and become a valued and contributing member of their community. As its title suggests the programme is based on the concept of recovery and identifies five key areas: hope, personal responsibility, education, self-advocacy and support.

Through attendance at seminars and practical group sessions, the person is assisted to become aware of the things they need to do on a daily basis to remain well, and develop an awareness of external factors that may make them feel unwell. The person is encouraged to use wellness tools that they have identified for themselves and to devise a 'wellness recovery action plan' which comprises a number of lists, as follows:

- everyday strategies that keep you well such as eating healthy meals and exercising;
- external factors that may make you feel unwell such as substance misuse or not getting enough sleep;
- wellness tools that will prevent external factors from making you feel worse;
- early warning signs that may indicate you are starting to feel unwell and a response plan;
- signs that the situation is becoming much worse and needs stabilizing.

The wellness tools are identified by the individual and may include things such as eating three healthy meals per day, taking a nap, writing in a journal, listening to music or asking for a medication check. The person must also decide when it would be appropriate to use each wellness tool, whether every day or only in response to certain feelings and situations.

The person is also encouraged to devise a personal crisis plan that can be acted upon if and when the person becomes unwell to the point that another person needs to take responsibility for their care. The crisis plan will include details of others who are important to them and their contact details, as well as instructions about what the person would like them to do on their behalf.

A recent randomized controlled trial (Cook *et al*. 2011) involving 519 adults with severe and enduring mental health problems compared the WRAP programme with usual care. The trial found that WRAP participants reported significantly greater reduction in psychiatric symptoms and a significantly greater improvement in hopefulness and enhanced quality of life. These improvements were present immediately post-intervention and at six-month follow-up.

Bipolar Organization self-management programme

The Bipolar Organization (formerly the Manic Depression Fellowship) offers self-management training courses to give people diagnosed with bipolar disorder a thorough and comprehensive understanding of the concepts, tools and techniques involved in learning to self-manage extreme mood swings.

Based on the WRAP technique, the programme consists of six sessions for up to 14 participants, facilitated by two tutors who themselves have a diagnosis of bipolar disorder. It aims to teach the individual how to recognize the triggers for, and warning signs of, an impending episode of illness. Participants learn to take action to prevent or reduce the severity of an episode.

The first session describes principles of self-management and covers the aims and objectives of the course. Personal expectations of the participants and their experience of the nature and impact of manic depression are also addressed. Subsequent sessions cover the identification of triggers and warning signs, coping strategies and self-medication, support networks and action plans, strategies for maintaining a healthy lifestyle, advance directives (crisis plans) and finally complementary therapies, coping strategies and finalizing action plans.

Research has shown that learning to self-manage bipolar disorder (manic depression) makes an important contribution to stabilizing the condition. It can significantly improve an individual's affective perception of areas such as self-esteem and reduction in suicidal thoughts. A randomized controlled trial by Perry *et al*. (1999) concluded that teaching patients to recognize early symptoms of manic relapse and seek early treatment was associated with important clinical improvements in relapse rate, social functioning and employment.

Hearing Voices Network

The first UK Hearing Voices group was formed in 1988 in Manchester. The Network was inspired by the pioneering work of Marius Romme and Sondra Escher from Maastricht University and has since become a national network which promotes, develops and supports self-help groups for anyone who hears voices and those who support them (relatives and carers). The network also organizes and delivers training sessions for health workers and the general public. Hearing Voices groups are made up of people who share the experience of hearing voices, coming together to help and support each other, exchange information and learn from each other. They often share the same problems and may have similar life situations. Sometimes the group may include relatives and carers of people who hear voices (www.hearingvoices.org). The purpose of Hearing Voices groups is to offer a safe haven where people feel accepted and comfortable. They also offer an opportunity for people to accept and 'live with their voices', in a way that gives them some control and so increase power over their own lives. The Network acknowledges the conflicting theories from psychiatrists, psychologists and voice-hearers about why people hear voices. While the organization does not reject outright the traditional treatments of antipsychotic medication, the aim is to explore the different possible explanations for voice hearing and to try and understand the content and meaning of the voices.

Other areas of help

A number of other organizations, whilst not offering structured self-management programmes, also run self-help groups and offer general information and resources. These include the National Perceptions Forum (formerly National Voices Forum), the National Self Harm Network (www.nshn.co.uk) and the National Centre for Eating Disorders (www.eatingdisorders.org.uk).

19.6 The evidence base for self-management programmes

In their review of Cochrane reviews, Coster and Norman (2009) found that although self-management interventions in a number of settings were promising, there was inadequate evidence of effectiveness in over half of the Cochrane reviews considered. It is important, however, to apply some caution to these findings. Self-management programmes vary hugely and different studies tend to focus on different outcomes, rendering comparisons problematic. Lorig and Holman (2003) argue that there is an assumption when evaluating the effectiveness of self-management programmes that changes in health-related behaviours and engagement with self-management programmes would result in health improvements. However, they found that service users defined the success of a programme on the basis of feeling more in control of their illness irrespective of health improvements, so sensitive outcome measures are likely to be self-efficacy, confidence and empowerment rather than symptoms.

A large randomized controlled trial (Kennedy *et al.* 2007) investigated the value of the Expert Patients Programme across a range of long-term conditions and found significant improvements in patients' self-efficacy and self-reported energy. There was no significant effect on health service use over six months, but the authors concluded that the programme was cost effective. In addition, a number of individual programmes have been evaluated (Cook *et al.* 2011; Expert Patients Programme 2011a, 2011b) with promising results. Further research is needed to identify the key components of self-management programmes as well as more studies which investigate self-management initiatives for specific long-term mental health problems.

19.7 Role of the nurse/mental health care professional

An important distinction is between self-management programmes delivered by facilitators that have their own experience of mental health problems and those that are delivered by health care professionals, such as nurses and psychologists (inevitably there is sometimes an overlap between these two roles). Both forms of self-help are important. Furthermore, if mental health services are to focus more on supporting self-management, nurses need to develop their skills in comprehensive assessment, health promotion and the delivery of evidence-based psychological therapies, such as CBT. Nursing staff also need to be attaining the skills that help them to enable clients to take better personal responsibility for their health. This view is supported by the Expert Patients Programme (2011b) which argues that as self-management programmes become integrated within the British National Health Service (NHS) and form an integral part of the patient care pathway, clinicians will need further training in the core competencies of self-care and self-management.

19.8 Conclusion

This chapter has provided an account of self-management approaches in mental health. The main learning points are as follows:

■ The increasing social and financial burden of chronic disease on health care services, as well as less than optimal outcomes, has led to a significant increase in the development of educational interventions to help service users better manage chronic mental health problems. Self-management is about people being actively involved in and engaged with their own health care.

- A number of behaviours, skills and strategies have been identified that support the self-management of mental health. A variety of recognized programmes have been developed that encompass these.

- Most programmes aim to educate the person to become aware of the things they need to do on a daily basis to remain well, and develop an awareness of external factors that may make them feel unwell. Programmes explore areas such as friendship and support, managing symptoms and early warning signs, healthy eating and exercise, relaxation and having fun, getting enough sleep and substance misuse. Skills will be developed such as problem-solv-ing, decision-making, resource utilization, forming partnerships with health care providers and action planning.

- Much of the evidence for self-management is anecdotal and relies largely on personal testimony. Some studies have shown a positive link between self-management and an increase in self-efficacy, although further research is indicated to clarify whether self-management is related to improved health outcomes.

- Despite this lack of evidence, self-management programmes have been widely accepted and endorsed by national policy and guidance.

Annotated bibliography

DH (Department of Health) (2011) *No Health Without Mental Health: A cross-government mental health outcomes strategy for people of all ages,* **available at: www.dh.gov.uk/en/Publicationsandstatistics/Publications/ PublicationsPolicyAndGuidance/DH_123766.**
This is an interesting and comprehensive document and will allow the reader to relate the subject of self-management to current policy.

Wellness Recovery Action Plan (WRAP) at www.mentalhealthrecovery.com.
This is a useful website with a wealth of free resources and exercises that suit both clinician and service user. There is also a database of articles relating to recovery and recovery stories.

Mental Health Foundation at www.mentalhealth.org.uk.
This website has links to a variety of relevant publications and reviews, a section on looking after your mental health and an A–Z guide to mental health. An excellent resource and an opportunity for further reading on the subject of self-management.

Expert Patients Programme at www.expertpatients.co.uk.
This website has a number of recent publications to download looking at the impact of self-management, relating to both the individual service user and wider society.

References

Cook, J., Copeland, M., Jonikas, J. et al. (2011) Results of a randomized controlled trial of mental illness self-management using Wellness Recovery Action Planning, *Schizophrenia Bulletin*, advance access (published 14 March 2011).
Corbin, J. and Strauss, A. (1988) Unending work and care: managing chronic illness at home, in K.
Cornah, D. (2006a) *Feeding Minds: The impact of food on mental health.* London: Mental Health Foundation.
Cornah, D. (2006b) *The Impact of Spirituality on Mental Health.* London: Mental Health Foundation.
Coster, S. and Norman, I. (2009) Cochrane reviews of educational and self-management interventions to guide nursing practice: a review, *International Journal of Nursing Studies*, 46: 508–28.
Davidson, L. (2005) Recovery, self management and the expert patient: changing the culture of mental health from a UK perspective, *Journal of Mental Health*, 14(1): 25–35.
DH (Department of Health) (2001) *The Expert Patient: A new approach to chronic disease management for the 21st century.* London: DH.
DH (Department of Health) (2005) *Promoting Optimal Self Care Consultation Techniques that Improve Quality of Life for Patients and Clinicians.* London: DH.
DH (Department of Health) (2011) *No Health Without Mental Health: A cross-government mental health outcomes strategy for people of all ages.* London: DH, available at: www.dh.gov.uk/en/Publicationsandstatistics/Publications/ PublicationsPolicyAndGuidance/DH_123766, accessed 8 October 2011.

Expert Patients Programme (2011a) *Healthy Lives Equal Healthy Communities: The social impact of self-management*, available at: www.expertpatients.co.uk/sites/default/files/publications/healthy-lives-equal-health-communities-social-impact-self-management.pdf, accessed 2 September 2011.

Expert Patients Programme (2011b) *Self-care Reduces Cost and Improves Health: The evidence*, available at: www.expertpatients.co.uk/sites/default/files/files/EVIDENCE%20FOR%20THE%20HEALTH.pdf, accessed 2 September 2011.

Faulkner, A. and Layzell, S. (2000) *Strategies for Living: A report of user-led research into people's strategies for living with mental distress*. London: Mental Health Foundation.

Faulkner, A. and Ryrie, I. (2009) Strategies for living and lifestyle options, in I. Norman and I. Ryrie (eds) *The Art and Science of Mental Health Nursing: A textbook of principles and practice*, 2nd edn. Maidenhead: Open University Press.

Gates, S., Smith, L.A. and Foxcroft, D. (2006) Auricular acupuncture for cocaine dependence, *Cochrane Database of Systematic Reviews*, Issue 1. Art. No.: CD005192. DOI: 10.1002/14651858.CD005192.pub2.

Holford, P. (2003) *Optimum Nutrition for the Mind*. London: Piatkus.

Jorm, A.F., Morgan, A.J. and Hetrick, S.E. (2008) Relaxation for depression, *Cochrane Database of Systematic Reviews*, Issue 4. Art.No.: CD007142. DOI: 10.1002/14651858.CD007142.pub2.

Kennedy, A., Reeves, D., Bower, P. *et al.* (2007) The effectiveness and cost effectiveness of a national lay-led self-care support programme for patients with long-term conditions: a pragmatic randomised controlled trial, *Journal of Epidemiological Community Health*, 61: 254–61.

Larun, L., Nordheim, L.V., Ekeland, E. Hagen, K.B. and Heian, F. (2006) Exercise in prevention and treatment of anxiety and depression among children and young people, *Cochrane Database of Systematic Reviews*, Issue 3. Art. No.: CD004691. DOI:10.1002/14651858.CD004691.pub2.

Lorig, K. and Holman, H. (2003) Self-management education: history, definition, outcomes and mechanisms, *Annals of Behavioural Medicine*, 26(1): 1–7.

Lorig, K., Gonzlez, V. and Laurent, D. (1997) *The Expert Patients Programme Chronic Disease Self-Management Course: Leader's manual*. Stanford, CA: Patient Education Research Center.

Martyn, D. (2002) The experiences and views of self-management of people with a schizophrenia diagnosis, available at: www.rethink.org/recovery/self-management/Initial Report.pdf, accessed 1 October 2011.

Mead, G.E., Morley, W., Campbell ,P., Greig, C.A., McMurdo, M. and Lawlor, D.A. (2010) Exercise for depression, *Cochrane Database of Systematic Reviews*, Issue 3. Art. No.: CD004366. DOI: 10.1002/14651858.CD004366.pub4.

Mental Health Foundation (2011) www.mentalhealth.org.uk/help-information/mental-health-a-z/R/recovery, accessed 1 October 2011.

Mohr, S. and Huguelet, P. (2004) The relationship between schizophrenia and religion and its implications for care, Swiss.Med. Wkly, 134(25–6): 369–76.

NICE (National Institute for Health and Clinical Excellence) (2009) *Depression: Treatment and management of depression in adults, including adults with a chronic physical health problem*, available at: http://guidance.nice.org.uk/CG91, accessed 8 October 2011.

NICE (National Institute for Health and Clinical Excellence) (2011) *Generalised Anxiety Disorder and Panic Disorder (With or Without Agoraphobia) in Adults*, available at: http://guidance.nice.org.uk/CG113, accessed 8 October 2011.

Patterson, B. (2001) The shifting perspective model of chronic illness, *Journal of Nursing Scholarship*, first quarter, 21–6.

Perry, A., Tarrier, N., Morris, R. and Limb, K. (1999) Randomised controlled trial of efficacy of teaching patients with bipolar disorder to identify early symptoms of relapse and obtain treatment, *British Medical Journal*, 318: 149–53.

Richards, D. (2004) Self-help: empowering service users or aiding cash strapped mental health services, *Journal of Mental Health*, 13(2): 117–23.

Robinson, J., Biley, F.C. and Dolk, H. (2007) Therapeutic touch for anxiety disorders, *Cochrane Database of Systematic Reviews*, Issue 3. Art. No.: CD006240. DOI: 10.1002/14651858.CD006240.pub2.

Ruddy, R. and Milnes, D. (2005) Art therapy for schizophrenia or schizophrenia-like illnesses, *Cochrane Database of Systematic Reviews*, Issue 4. Art. No.: CD003728. DOI: 10.1002/14651858.CD003728.pub2.

Smith, C.A., Hay, P.P.J. and MacPherson, H. (2010) Acupuncture for depression, *Cochrane Database of Systematic Reviews*, Issue 1. Art. No.: CD004046. DOI: 10.1002/14651858.CD004046.pub3.

WHO (World Health Organization) (1983) *Health Education in Self-care: Possibilities and limitations*. Geneva: WHO.

Websites

Bipolar Organisation: www.mdf.org.uk
Expert Patients Programme : www.expertpatients.co.uk
Hearing Voices: www.hearingvoices.org
Mental Health Foundation: www.mentalhealth.org.uk
National Centre for Eating Disorders: www.eatingdisorders.org.uk
National Perceptions Forum (formerly National Voices Forum): www.voicesforum.org.uk
National Self Harm Network: www.nshn.co.uk
Rethink Mental Illness: www.rethink.org
Wellness Recovery Action Plan: http://www.mentalhealthrecovery.com
Expert Patients: www.expertpatients.co.uk

Chapter 20

Counselling Approaches

Tony Machin and Simon Westrip

Over the years I have gotten used to being Bipolar and I'm aware it will always be a part of my life. I complete daily exercise which helps and have also found group and individual counselling sessions to be very helpful.

Liz

 ## 20.1 Introduction

Effective communication skills are essential to all health and social care practitioners. For mental health nurses, these skills also need to be purposefully therapeutic, contributing to recovery processes for service users. Furthermore, most mental health nurses are required to employ counselling skills in a variety of settings, among people with a spectrum of mental health issues and problems of living. To fulfil these roles and to help people with different needs, mental health nurses require a 'toolbox' of interventions and need to operate from a stance we refer to here as 'eclectic pragmatism'.

This chapter explores the essence of therapeutic communication, framed as the use of 'helping', 'counselling' or 'micro' skills within mental health nursing practice. It addresses:

- core counselling approaches, including Rogers and Egan;

- essential attributes of effective practitioners;
- counselling;
- specific therapeutic communication skills required to attend and respond within therapeutic relationships.

Literature concerned with 'counselling' and 'helping' tends to use the term 'client' when referring to those seeking help, whereas more recent terminology relating to mental health nursing uses the term 'service user'. Within this chapter, the terms are used interchangeably.

 ## 20.2 Core values and principles of counselling approaches

Fundamental to most, if not all, forms of therapeutic communication are the goals, values and skills of establishing and developing therapeutic relationships.

Case Study

Daisy

Daisy (22) was unemployed and felt low in mood when she first attended a voluntary service for a counselling assessment. She had a complex history of poor relations with her parents, had found it difficult to establish relationships in her early adult life and described herself as being 'unloved and unloveable'. Not being able to find regular work exacerbated her problems and she thought of herself as a failure. Daisy attended a total of eight counselling sessions.

The most positive aspect of counselling for Daisy was that for the first time in her life she felt listened to and understood. For many years she had felt that she needed to justify herself to others, had felt judged and alone and had experienced little control of her life. She felt that her counsellor seemed to understand how she felt and what she had been through and he gave her positive feedback on what she had failed to recognise as her past achievements. In the counselling sessions Daisy explored issues from her past and came to understand how her past experiences had affected her view of herself and her life in the present. She reported gaining a better understanding of herself and a more realistic, and less negative, assessment of her life situation. Identifying and building on her strengths helped Daily gain confidence, feel less like a victim and begin to take more control of her life.

Daisy decided to stop coming to counselling after she successfully gained employment.

The goals of therapeutic communication

Carl Rogers (1902–1987), originator of 'person centred' approaches to therapeutic relationships/intervention, saw the goal of intervention as creating a climate within which the 'client' moves towards becoming a 'functioning person', which for Rogers (1961) meant: being rational, accepting personal responsibility, having self-regard, achieving good personal relationships and living ethically.

Egan (2010) frames the goals of 'helping' as facilitating clients toward 'full human functioning', specifically:

- life-enhancing outcomes: helping people to manage problems of living, developing resources and opportunities more fully;
- learning self-help: helping people become better at helping themselves within daily life; and
- prevention mentality: helping people develop preventative strategies for problems.

Many key texts concerned with 'counselling' or 'helping' outline skills of therapeutic communica-tion, and, necessarily a structural framework within which these skills are employed. Egan's (2010) model sees clients move through stages of: the present scenario, the preferred scenario, and strategies to move toward the preferred scenario.

Nelson-Jones (2009) outlines the stages of the counselling relationship as the relating stage, the understanding stage and the changing stage. The goals of all types of therapeutic communication need to reflect the values embodied in a 'recovery' oriented approach for the users of mental health services.

Core conditions for therapeutic relationships

Rogers (1957) outlined what he termed 'the necessary and sufficient conditions' required of an effective therapeutic relationship, summarized as:

- **Congruence:** implying the condition of being 'genuine'/'real'; not 'playing a role'.
- **Unconditional positive regard:** implying caring, acceptance, respect. This is not to imply accepting inappropriate aspects without

challenge. Behaviour can be rejected without rejecting the individual.

- **Empathy:** the capacity and ability to perceive another person's view/emotional response to issues/situations from the frame of reference of that other person. Furthermore, to *communicate* that understanding to that person.

The nature of empathy

The concept of empathy is central to therapeutic communication. For Rogers the central dimensions of empathy in the context of the therapeutic relationship are about observing/listening to the person, 'resonating' (feeling the person's emotions), discriminating (prioritizing what is important to the person), communicating (the perceived empathy to the person) and checking with the person that the empathic hypothesis is correct. Egan (2010) describes how empathy can be:

- **basic:** fundamental identification of emotion/perception;
- **accurate in degrees:** if basic empathy can identify a feeling/perception, then that can be attuned by degrees of accuracy to the precise effect and impact upon the individual.

Egan proposes 'advanced' empathy, whereby the helper 'digs deeper' into things 'half said', things 'hinted' at, things articulated in a confused way and apparently covert messages. Egan's basic 'formula' for an empathic response follows the format:

- 'You feel . . .' (related identified emotion)
- 'Because . . .' (summary of events/issues that have led to the emotion)

Empathy can be related via:

- single words: such as 'good', 'depressed';
- phrases: such as 'in the depths of despair', 'on cloud nine';
- behavioural statements: such as 'feel like . . . giving up on things';
- described experiences (implied): such as 'that made you feel unwanted?'

It is important to check that empathy has been accurate, and 'recover' from suggested understandings which have been inaccurate. For Rogers and Egan, empathy is central to the whole context of therapeutic communication, in terms of both attending and responding.

Thinking Space 20.1

Is it possible to empathize from the 'frame of reference' of all service users? For example:

- A 34-year-old homeless man with a chaotic lifestyle, homeless, in intermittent contact with services and with alcohol and substance use problems.
- A 70-year-old old man whose wife is progressively deteriorating with dementia before his eyes, visit by visit.
- Parents of a 22-year-old man, their only child, who have just been informed their son is suffering from psychosis, with an uncertain prognosis.
- A young first-time mother referred to services with phobic issues relating to hygiene.
- A man, encountered after a suicide attempt, who's wife has left him to establish a relationship with another man.

Look again at how Rogers and Egan describe empathy and the ways it can be communicated. What could you draw on to communicate empathically with the people outlined above? Look also at the information on attending to another person (p. 311) and reflecting back (p. 313) in this chapter to help you with this task.

20.3 Attributes of therapeutic communicators

The personal attributes required to facilitate therapeutic communication are implicit and reflected in the previous discussion regarding the nature/goals of therapeutic communication. They include:

- capacity for 'self awareness';
- capacity to use the self in a therapeutic way;
- ability not only to *listen*, but to *hear*.

Self-awareness requires more than self-disclosure and receiving feedback that we value/trust. It also requires 'self-reflection', a process defined by Casement (1992) as 'being your own internal supervisor', self-questioning and self-challenging.

Awareness of self extends into the reactive nature of therapeutic relationships, encompassing concepts of 'transference', and 'counter-transference'. These concepts derive from psychodynamic models of practice, but are worthy of note in terms of therapeutic relationships more generally. Transference refers to an 'unconscious' process whereby clients perceive within helpers some attribute similar to that possessed by a significant figure from their past (typically framed as childhood). Feelings and emotions appropriate to the significant figure are 'transferred' onto the helping figure. Within the notion of counter-transference, helpers may experience feelings or reactions towards clients which, upon reflection, seem unrelated, or disproportionate. These responses may be intruding from previous experiences/issues from the helper's personal history. There is debate regarding the validity of these concepts, whether they belong in the realm of 'psychotherapy' rather than 'counselling' or helping, and indeed where and how counselling and psychotherapy are distinct from one another. For the purposes of discussion here, awareness that therapeutic relationships can be influenced by factors impinging from outside is the important thing to recognize.

Mindfulness

Over recent years, there has been growing interest in the concept of 'mindfulness' for practitioners involved in mental health services and therapeutic relationships. Mindfulness draws upon Buddhist philosophy and a particular therapeutic meditative approach first explored by Kabat-Zinn (1990), who developed mindfulness-based stress reduction (MBSR) as a way of helping people cope with physical and emotional pain through 'acceptance'. This does not mean 'giving in' or trying to 'like' a situation which is distressing, but a willingness to be open to all aspects of self. McQuaid and Carmona (2004) describe the state of mindfulness as a 'moment to moment' awareness, stressing that it is not a mysterious mystical state, but one of heightened awareness of the reality of surroundings and context.

Mindfulness employs both formal and informal meditation techniques to develop a compassionate, non-judgemental awareness of mind. This does not mean suspending critical judgement, but becoming aware that thoughts are just that (thoughts), and not facts, and as such are open to challenge.

For advocates of mindful approaches, becoming a more mindful practitioner affords the opportunity to be more attentive in therapeutic relationships, complementing active attending and listening skills. It becomes a way to enhance therapeutic presence and self-awareness, as well as 'other awareness'. It also opens up the possibility of helping clients to become more aware of the relationship between their own thoughts, feelings and behaviour, and their impact upon self and others.

There is some evidence to suggest that incorporating mindfulness practice for clients increases the efficacy of therapeutic approaches by relieving psychological distress and helping clients to 'switch' to a state of mind in which unhelpful thoughts and feelings are viewed from a 'decentred' viewpoint (Westbrook *et al.* 2011). Importantly, if practitioners are to incorporate mindfulness techniques into their work with service users, it is a prerequisite that they engage with and practise mindfulness themselves.

Supervision

A final aspect relating to self-awareness for mental health nurses in employing therapeutic communication is that of supervision. Scaife (2009) outlines the fundamental characteristics of effective supervision:

- it is (or should be) fundamentally about securing the welfare of clients and enhancing services;
- it is usually framed as a formal relationship (or relationships) in a context of mutual respect and trust;
- it should, ideally, preclude the simultaneous existence of other role-relationships between supervisor and supervisee, or where such other role-relationships exist, they should be acknowledged and implications explicitly addressed;
- it is characterized by explicit agreement/ contract;
- it is focused upon the *supervisee*.

Inskipp and Proctor (1993) identify three main functions of supervision:

- **formative:** concerned with the supervisee's learning;
- **normative:** concerned with the managerial and ethical responsibilities of the supervisor;
- **restorative:** concerned with acknowledging the emotional effects upon the supervisee of working within therapeutic relationships.

Effective supervision is useful in terms of having a different perspective with regard to therapeutic relationships, and invaluable when these relationships become difficult or problematic, though good supervision should also draw explicit attention to the supervisee's accomplishments and positive elements within therapeutic relationships.

 20.4   Counselling

Crisis: the starting point

An important contextual factor for all therapeutic communication is the starting point of the thera-peutic relationship. The problems of living that users of mental health services present can be categorized into the three overlapping domains: *cognitive*, relating to thoughts and thought processes; *affective*, the emotional domain; and *behavioural*, the behavioural manifestation of the presenting problems/issues.

Within mental health services, behavioural and affective domain issues often present as the initial focus, but it is only by consideration of the interactive nature of all domains that the complex presenting situations of service users can be understood, and action plans prepared. 'Crisis' is a subjective term, but if we make the assumption that people accessing mental health services are experiencing crisis in some form, then the nature of crisis becomes an important consideration.

James and Guilliland (2001) depict 'crisis' using two key dimensions:

- **equilibrium:** the degree to which the balance of a person's life equilibrium is upset within a presenting crisis situation;
- **'mobility':** the degree to which a person can mobilize themselves in addressing the crisis situation.

In terms of the therapeutic relationship between the helper and the person in crisis, a continuum is suggested in terms of the degree to which the helper adopts a directive stance within the therapeutic relationship, as represented in Table 20.1.

Table 20.1 The crisis worker's continuum (after James and Guilliland 2001)

Crisis worker response to presenting service user equilibrium/mobility status	
Service user	Crisis worker
Immobile/ disequilibrium	Directive (takes more control)
Partially mobile	Collaborative (negotiated)
Mobile/ equilibrium	Non-directive (encourages autonomy)

Motivation and commitment

A central goal of mental health nursing practice is to enhance motivation and gain commitment from service users to plans developed collaboratively to address problems of living. When 'moving on' through problems of living, to what Egan (2010) calls the 'future scenario' or Nelson-Jones (2009) 'the changing stage', service users inevitably need to commit themselves to particular courses of action. In formulating strategies to elicit commitment from clients, nurses can draw on motivational interviewing principles which are discussed in Chapter 23. A central issue in understanding motivation from a motivational interviewing perspective is that motivation is *dynamic*, and not a phenomenon which is simply present or absent. Motivation can be *enhanced* within therapeutic relationships.

Skills of 'attending' to another person

Egan (2010) provides a comprehensive outline of the process of listening/attending to 'clients'. He frames this as 'tuning in and actively listening', and characterizes poor listening skills in terms of:

- **non-listening:** just not listening;
- **partial listening:** hearing some things but not others, possibly important things;
- **the 'tape recorder':** hearing all the words immaculately, but not necessarily their meanings;
- **rehearsing response:** being preoccupied within an interaction and rehearsing responses to something which has been said, thereby not hearing what the person is saying subsequently.

For Egan, 'focused listening' is hearing beyond the words expressed, listening for an 'integrated narrative' – specifically for experiences, thoughts and thought patterns, behaviours, affect; strengths and opportunities and non-verbal aspects of communication. Listening, in this sense, is about seeking to understand the person through context, identifying key messages and associated feelings, and hearing

the person's 'slant' or 'spin' on the narrative, including aspects which appear to be missing.

The physical/practical context of interaction

Many texts about 'helping' or 'counselling' are quite prescriptive about the way in which the environment of the interaction should be arranged. Egan (2010) coined the often cited mnemonic of 'SOLER' with regard to this aspect:

- **S**: face the person **S**quarely
- **O**: adopt an **O**pen posture
- **L**: **L**ean toward the other
- **E**: maintain good **E**ye contact
- **R**: be **R**elaxed or 'natural'

Referring back to the different contexts outlined in Table 20.1 above, the creation of an environment where these conditions prevail is more possible in some dimensions than others. Where the practitioner has access to opportunities to create space and time for therapeutic interactions, then the environment can be managed.

Skills of responding

Heron (2001) offers a conceptual framework that comprises six categories of therapeutic intervention which are of two types: *authoritative* (prescriptive, informative and confrontative interventions) and *facilitative* (cathartic, catalytic and supportive interventions). Heron sees an intervention 'gradient' from a prescriptive approach (practitioner directed) to a catalytic facilitation (promoting client self-discovery and problem-solving). A brief description of each of Heron's intervention categories is provided below:

- **Prescriptive interventions:** equate to the 'directive' type of interventions appropriate to situations where the client is 'immobilized' in Table 20.1.
- **Informative interventions:** involve giving relevant information which may be technical or theoretical (e.g. the nature of a panic attack). These may also involve giving interpretations

of client experience, behaviour and situation, or progress, in a non-evaluative way.

- **Confronting interventions:** encourage the client to recognize inconsistencies in behaviour, evidence of denial or avoidance of issues.
- **Cathartic interventions:** free up emotions and help the client to recognize and express difficult or uncomfortable feelings. Heron discusses a variety of approaches which can facilitate catharsis, although many such approaches (e.g. psychodrama) are beyond the scope of this chapter.
- **Catalytic interventions:** help the client to identify what is important in their life, and their future perspectives. This may involve the use of 'lifestyle maps', which can help facilitate learning from past experience and commitment for future plans.
- **Supportive interventions:** validate the person's worth and self-esteem; they include basic interventions such as greeting someone and making them feel welcome and valued.

Thinking Space 20.2

Think about your own practice and the ways in which you engage therapeutically with mental health service users. Map the approaches you use onto the categories proposed by Heron.

- Are your interventions weighted towards specific categories?
- What other therapeutic intervention categories would you like to develop skills in?

Heron's framework includes a useful consideration of how things can go wrong, or be less effective. He outlines what he calls 'degenerative interventions', which are summarized in Table 20.2. For Heron, these degenerative interventions are the products of poor awareness, lack of experience and lack of personal growth/training.

Finally, Heron identifies more disturbing forms of therapeutic intervention, which he terms 'perverted' –

Table 20.2 Degenerative interventions (after Heron 2001)

Degenerative interventions	Description
Unsolicited interventions	Practitioner takes charge without collaborating or seeking permission; practitioner controls the relationship
Manipulative interventions	The practitioner's needs take priority over the client's needs and goals. The practitioner manipulates the client to ensure they get what they want out of the relationship
Compulsive interventions	These interventions express the practitioner's unmet needs or emotional distress. The practitioner adopts the role of compulsive helper/rescuer; typically they take on excessive commitment and raise unrealistic expectations in the client
Unskilled interventions	Interventions which are not unsolicited, manipulative or compulsive but are simply unskilled and not competent

deliberately intended to belittle, control, distress and dominate. These approaches seem more synonymous with prison, torture and interrogation, rather than health and social care practice, but there are times when care fails and 'perverted' approaches have been identified. This serves to underline the importance of transparency in services, and of audit/inspection of health and social care services.

 ## 20.5   Specific skills

Principles and skills of questioning

Questions are important to elicit what Egan (2010) calls the client's 'story', but are also integral to the process of 'moving on'. Broadly, questions can be:

- closed: inviting simple yes/no responses;
- open: Inviting more elaborate descriptive responses.

Nelson-Jones (2009) outlines various functions which questions can serve within helping relationships:

- Clarification: what has the client meant?
- Elaboration: eliciting more detail.
- Eliciting specific details: who/what/where/when/how?
- Solution focused: what are the possibilities?
- Inviting clients to action: what will be done?

Alternatives to questions can be used:

- 'minimal encouragers', meaning non-verbal nodding or vocalizing ('hmm') while demonstrating attention, can act as an implied statement asking to be told more;
- reflecting statements back to clients, or summarizing an issue and reflecting back can imply a question, and relates to the notion of 'checking' from an empathic viewpoint.

Hypothetical questions, which invite a client to picture potential future goals, or anticipate action in specific circumstances, can also be used. 'Why' questions should be used with caution since clients can become preoccupied with the 'why' of the past rather than the how, where, when and who of the future.

Reflecting back

An important therapeutic communication skill is that of reflecting back to the client what has been understood using words or phrases used by the client or paraphrased summaries. Reflecting back to clients accurately demonstrates that they have been listened to and understood. The focus of the reflected content can be thoughts, feelings and behaviour, and can help to express empathy to clients.

Challenging/confronting

Challenging or confronting interventions may be used to overcome clients' resistance which hampers achievement of agreed goals. Egan (2010) suggests that to confront someone is to hold them account-

able. Often this will involve confronting individuals with discussion of what it will mean if they do not manage to achieve their goals. Confrontation should be conducted with empathy and respect. The practitioner effectively reflects back to the client inconsistencies, inviting the client to make sense of them; the contradictions revealed may then be further explored. Egan also advises that challenging should:

- Be tentative in the first instance, but not apologetic. When people are 'stuck' in problems, it is the role of the helper to help 'unstick' them. Challenging is a key skill in addressing this.
- Build upon the client's successes. Clients may need to be challenged to accept their successes and strengths (rather than dwell upon failures and lack of achievement).
- Be specific: a challenge should be related to specific issues, statements or episodes which can be cited.

Self-disclosure

Day-to-day communication involves 'turn-taking' in conversations, and reciprocity in disclosing information about self. Expectations of disclosure increase proportionately with the degree of intimacy in relationships. Therapeutic relationships involve intimacy, with different expectations than day-to-day interactions; one person within the relationship is helped in some way, and the other occupies a helping role. Within mental health services and relationships between mental health nurses and service users, self-disclosure should be carefully judged. There are degrees of intimacy, from disclosing relationship status (e.g. single, married) through to disclosing previous personal issues such as dealing with a divorce. It should be remembered that many users of mental health services may find intimacy (self-disclosure being a form of intimacy) difficult to manage. However, self-disclosure can be useful within a therapeutic relationship. Used appropriately it can help to cement the relationship, or open channels to examine issues from different perspectives. Egan (2010) outlines some parameters to consider around its use:

- the need to be appropriate: avoid 'exhibition-ism' and use no more than necessary;
- the need to be culturally sensitive/appropriate;
- the need to use careful timing: do not self-disclose prematurely (build the relationship first) and do not disclose frequently;
- be selective and purposeful: there should be a rationale for disclosure;
- avoid 'burdening' the client.

Immediacy

Within therapeutic relationships, regardless of the goal of intervention or approach, issues may arise in the moment which need to be addressed if the client is to move forward towards meeting their goals. There is little point proceeding doggedly along a particular course when an issue has arisen which is detracting from that course.

The term 'immediacy' is used to describe focusing upon issues which need to be addressed 'here and now'. Egan (2010) differentiates two forms of immediacy:

- Focus on the overall therapeutic relationship: 'How are you and I doing?'
- Focus on a specific issue: 'How are you and I doing right now?'

Immediacy is appropriate where:

- the therapeutic relationship seems to have become 'directionless';
- there is evident tension;
- there seem to be trust issues;
- 'distancing' seems to have emerged or evolved;
- inappropriate dependency seems to be developing.

Silence

Silences within communication processes are usually perceived as awkward. One or other of the people involved will usually, at some point, feel the need to 'rescue' the silence. Within therapeutic relationships, episodes of silence can be capitalized upon in relation to the overall goal of the interaction. In a basic sense, it can be a gentle way of encouraging a client to talk.

Back *et al.* (2009) suggest that silence can be classified in one of three ways:

- awkward silence, characterized by uncertainty of intent;
- invitational silence – intentional, giving the client time to focus on thoughts and feelings;
- silence as a means of conveying compassion, with meaningful attention and stable focus still present (this relates to the concept of 'mindfulness', discussed above).

Practitioners need to become 'comfortable' with episodes of silence. If the silence becomes counterproductive, then the nature and reasons for silence could be raised (an example of immediacy).

> ### Thinking Space 20.3
>
> Watch for and observe in day-to-day practice the use of:
>
> - Questions and reflection
> - Challenging
> - Immediacy
> - Silence
>
> Look for episodes where these skills were used effectively. Also look for instances where opportunities are missed, or could have been used more effectively.

 ## 20.6 Clients with cognitive impairment

Therapeutic communication within an acute phase of mental illness is of paramount importance and the principles outlined in this chapter are as applicable to people suffering from cognitive impairment or thought disorder as to clients who are rational. Behavioural aspects of communication such as touch and presence to promote feelings of security are particularly important in the crisis phase.

Later on, therapeutic communication skills will be needed to help clients maintain necessary therapeutic regimes, including medication adherence. Similarly, when individuals present with cognitive impairment relating to delirium or dementia, the fundamental principles outlined here remain paramount. A key role of mental health nurses with these clients is to act as a 'representative of reality' and non-verbal aspects of communication are particularly important where clients' cognitive abilities are impaired.

 ## 20.7 Ending therapeutic relationships

Therapeutic relationships will end at some point and this should be acknowledged from the outset, particularly in relationships which are intense and/ or enduring. Feelings about the ending of relationships should be acknowledged. Nelson-Jones (2009) points out that many problem situations have their own time frames, but that ending of therapeutic contact can be:

- a fixed agreed point from the outset;
- open-ended and negotiated between helper and client.

For Nelson-Jones, the ending of relationship, if negotiated, can draw upon evaluative information from:

- the client themselves – view of progression;
- the helper's observations;
- feedback from significant others;

- goal attainment.

A final important aspect related to the end of therapeutic relationships is 'relapse planning'. Effective process of helping should forearm service users with strategies to deal with future problems, or recurrence of issues.

 ## 20.8 Conclusion

Therapeutic communication underpins all aspects of mental health nursing practice. The use of a framework such as Heron's (2001) can be useful in a practical sense to enable a cohesive approach in the day-to-day use of communication skills. In a broader sense, an understanding of where the use of therapeutic communication skills fits with the role of mental health nursing can be fostered by reference to unifying concepts/constructions of mental health nursing, such as that offered by Peplau (1952, 1991).

The key learning points from this chapter are as follows:

- The need to match skills to the client, rather than the client to the available skills.
- The core values and skills which are common to the processes of therapeutic communication, including goals, core conditions and the importance of empathy.
- The importance of attributes such as self-awareness and the potential utility of 'mindfulness' for practitioners and service users.
- The importance of clinical supervision.
- Motivation to move towards recovery can be built within therapeutic relationships/ alliances.
- The development of therapeutic communication skills is an ongoing process, and relates to developing experience, use of effective clinical supervision processes and ongoing continuing professional development.

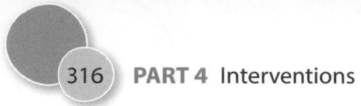

Annotated bibliography

Egan, G. (2010) *The Skilled Helper: A problem management and opportunity-development approach to helping*, 9th edn. Belmont, ??:Brooks/Cole, Cengage Learning.
Egan's seminal text outlines an eclectic and pragmatic problem-solving approach to helping. The skills involved in helping are framed usefully within his problem-solving model.

Heron, J. (2001) *Helping the Client*, 5th edn. London: Sage.
This text has been used in the field of health care, management and education and provides an extensive framework with which to devise interpersonal interventions and to reflect on and in practice, facilitating the practitioner's skill development. It covers core interventions through to the use of specialist practice such as psychodrama and is also used to structure clinical supervision in mental health nursing.

Morrissey, J. and Callaghan, P. (2011) *Communication Skills for Mental Health Nurses*. Maidenhead: Open University Press.
This text aims to offer mental health nurses a practical and friendly guide to strengthening their therapeutic communication skills with service users, families and colleagues. It covers different types of therapeutic 'talk' and gives examples from day-to-day practice to highlight how we can develop good relationships with our clients.

Nelson-Jones, R. (2011) *Theory and Practice of Counselling and Therapy*, 5th edn. London: Sage.
A readable source text exploring the theoretical positions and assumptions underpinning the most prevalent contemporary approaches to counselling and therapy.

Peplau, H. E. (1991) *Interpersonal Relations in Nursing: A conceptual framework of reference for psychodynamic nursing*. New York: Springer.
Peplau outlines a cohesive framework for the processes through which mental health nurses collaborate with their service users in moving through the stages of the therapeutic relationship towards resolution/recovery.

Williams, M. and Penman, M. (2011) *Mindfulness: A practical guide to finding peace in a frantic world*. ????: Piatkus Books.
This text draws upon a programme of mindfulness designed to help people cope with stress. It gives a readable insight into mindfulness techniques, which helps the reader to understand the experience of being more mindful.

References

Back, A. L., Bauer-Wu, S. M., Rushton, C.H. and Halifax, J. (2009) Compassionate silence in the patient–clinician encounter: a contemplative approach, *Journal of Palliative Medicine*, 10(10).
Casement, P. (1992) *Learning from the Patient*. New York: Guilford Press.
Egan, G. (2010) *The Skilled Helper: A problem management and opportunity-development approach to helping*, 9th edn. Belmont, ??: Brooks/Cole, Cengage Learning.
Heron, J. (2001) *Helping the Client*, 5th edn. London: Sage.
Inskipp, F. and Procter, B. (1993) *The Art, Craft and Tasks of Counselling Supervision Part 1: Making the most of supervision*. Twickenham: Cascade Publications.
James, R.K. and Gilliland, B.E. (2001) *Crisis Intervention Strategies*, 4th edn. Belmont, ??: Brooks/Cole.
Kabat-Zinn, J. (1990) *Full Catastrophe Living: How to cope with stress, pain and illness using mindfulness meditation*. New York: Dell Publishing.
McQuaid, J.R. and Carmona, P.E. (2004) *Peaceful Mind: Using mindfulness and cognitive psychology to overcome depression*. ????: New Harbinger Publications.
Nelson-Jones, R. (2009) *Introduction to Counselling Skills*, 3rd edn. London: Sage.
NMC (Nursing and Midwifery Council) (2008) *Standards of Conduct, Performance and Ethics for Nurses and Midwives*. London: NMC.
Peplau, H.E. (1952) *Interpersonal Relations in Nursing*. New York: G.P. Putman & Sons.
Peplau, H.E. (1991) *Interpersonal Relations in Nursing: A conceptual framework of reference for psychodynamic nursing*. New York: Springer.
Rogers, C.R. (1957) The necessary and sufficient conditions of therapeutic personality change, *Journal of Consulting Psychology*, 21: 95–103.
Rogers, C.R. (1961) *On Becoming a Person*. Boston, MA: Houghton Mifflin.
Scaife, J. (2009) *Supervision in Clinical Practice: A practitioner's guide*, 2nd edn. London: Routledge.
Westbrook, D., Kennerly, H. and Kirk, J. (2011) *An Introduction to Cognitive Behavioural Therapy Skills and Applications*, 2nd edn. London: Sage.

Chapter

21

Cognitive Behavioural Techniques for Mental Health Nursing Practice

Lina Gega and Ian Norman

A lot of the preceding points (having role models, creativity, voluntary work) helped me move along the road to recovery but it was CBT that zoomed me along that road. Basically, in a nutshell, here I found the tools to control my symptoms, rather than have them control me. Out of the CBT came my rejection of self-pity and the decision to take total responsibility for my condition and recovery, and not to expect others to 'cure' me, or wait for others to change so I could change. I had to do the work.

Dolly Sen

21.1 Introduction

This chapter seeks to meet some of the learning needs of those nurses who are not specialist cognitive or behaviour clinicians, but who are interested in the application of cognitive behavioural therapy (CBT) techniques in the course of their day-to-day nursing work. Community nurses have the opportunity to organize their work with patients to enable sessional work which reflects the traditional CBT approach. Mental health nurses working on inpatient units do not traditionally work on a sessional basis with patients but can still draw on CBT principles and techniques to build structured brief interactions with patients. The safe and effective application of CBT techniques should be guided by careful assessment and formulation of an individual's problems and needs, by ongoing professional development activities such as workshop attendance and self-directed reading, and by regular supervision from experienced practitioners. Given that nursing practice is guided by the NMC code of conduct (NMC 2012), it is the duty of each nurse to implement CBT techniques within the limitations of their professional competence.

This chapter covers:

- what CBT is;
- the CBT model;
- CBT assessment;
- CBT formulation;
- key CBT interventions.

For consistency we use the terms 'client' (patient, service user) and 'clinician' (nurse, therapist, practitioner) throughout the chapter.

 ## 21.2 What is CBT?

CBT is a form of psychological therapy which draws on two distinct therapies, cognitive therapy and behaviour therapy. Cognitive therapy is a treatment approach based on information-processing theories which explain people's emotional, physical and behavioural responses to certain experiences as arising from their perception of these experiences and the meaning they attach to them. In contrast, behaviour therapy is a treatment approach based on learning theories (classical and operant conditioning) which hold that people's behaviours are

sustained or extinguished by the presence or absence of strong associations and positive or negative reinforcements. In practice CBT practitioners draw upon techniques from both cognitive and behaviour therapy in their work with clients.

 ## 21.3 The CBT model

The basic CBT model (illustrated in Figure 21.1) hypothesizes that it is not events in themselves that cause psychological problems, but people's interpretation of them and the ways that they behave in response to them. Psychological distress arises if people interpret events or react to them negatively. CBT interventions aim to correct thinking errors which underpin these negative interpretations or behavioural responses to events that are self-defeating.

The basic CBT model comprises the three key elements of psychological distress: thoughts, feelings (which include both emotions and physical sensations) and behaviours.

Thoughts

Negative automatic thoughts (NATs) are often the cognitive aspect of distress. They are automatic (i.e. they pop into our heads without any effort), invol-

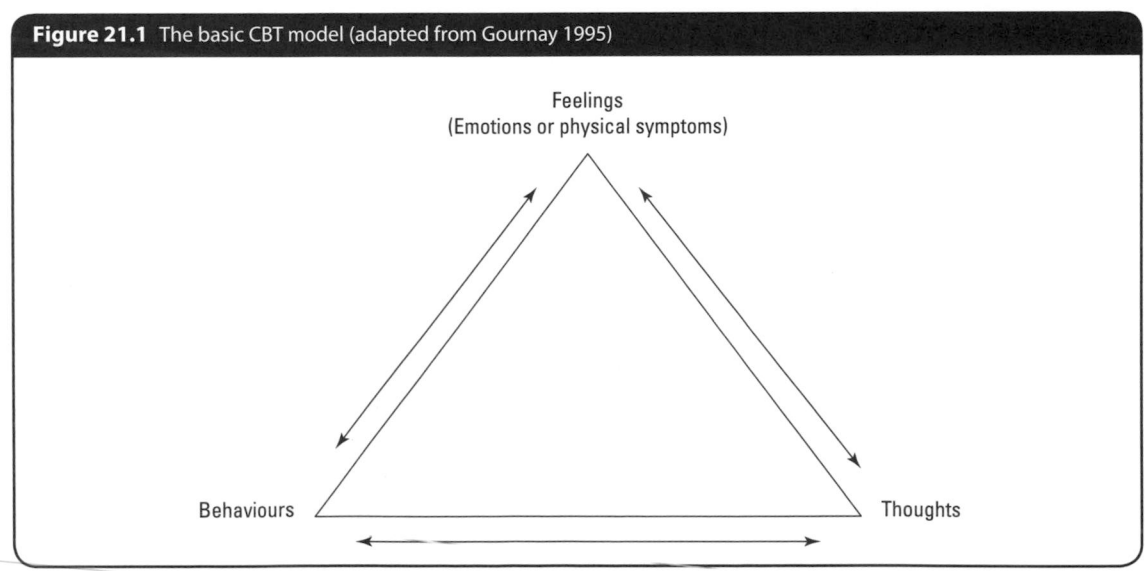
Figure 21.1 The basic CBT model (adapted from Gournay 1995)

untary (i.e. we don't choose to have them and they are difficult to stop), plausible (i.e. they are accepted as facts and are difficult to question), distorted (i.e. they do not fit all the facts, only some of them – although we don't know this at the time) and unhelpful (i.e. they make us feel bad – e.g. sad, guilty, hopeless, angry). NATs can sometimes take the form of a running commentary on the client's actions.

Feelings

■ **Emotions:** emotions (affect) are often the reason for seeking help. These can be difficult for clients to distinguish from thoughts because of our tendency in English to say 'I feel that …' when actually we mean 'I think that …'. For example, 'I felt that I would die' is a thought,

not an emotion. A rule of thumb is that an emotion is usually expressed in one word (e.g. anger, depression, sadness, fear, guilt).

■ **Physical sensations:** physical sensations and changes are often indicators of psychological distress (e.g. anxiety is indicated by increased heart rate and sweating, sadness by crying, lack of appetite, difficulty falling asleep or early morning waking).

■ **Behaviours:** psychological distress can be indicated by changes in what people do. It can be helpful to distinguish between what people do (or avoid) *because* of their problem and what they do *to make themselves feel better* (e.g. drink more alcohol, self-harm). These are sometimes called 'safety behaviours'.

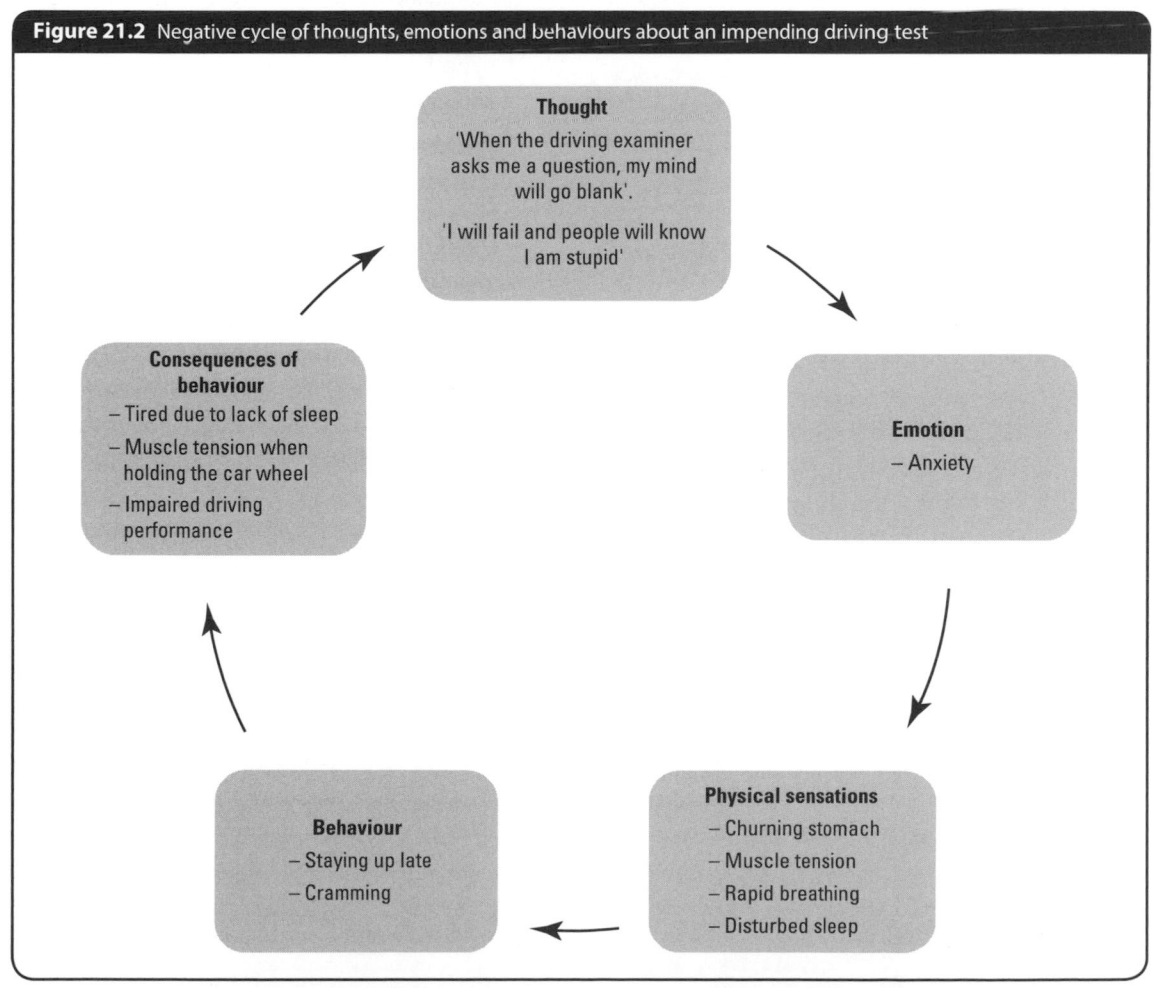

Figure 21.2 Negative cycle of thoughts, emotions and behaviours about an impending driving test

Thought
'When the driving examiner asks me a question, my mind will go blank'.
'I will fail and people will know I am stupid'

Emotion
– Anxiety

Physical sensations
– Churning stomach
– Muscle tension
– Rapid breathing
– Disturbed sleep

Behaviour
– Staying up late
– Cramming

Consequences of behaviour
– Tired due to lack of sleep
– Muscle tension when holding the car wheel
– Impaired driving performance

The CBT model suggests that the three elements of psychological distress (feelings, thoughts, behaviours) are linked so that a negative change in one element can trigger a negative change in another and a vicious cycle is created. Figure 21.2 illustrates the vicious cycle through an example which will be familiar to many readers: sitting a driving test. In this case an impending driving test examination triggers a series of negative automatic thoughts, emotions and behaviours which are likely to be self-defeating.

Thinking Space 21.1

Redraw Figure 21.2 to illustrate a virtuous circle for a client faced with a driving test who was successful at school and was always thought of as able by their parents.

Feedback

In your reformulated example the client has positive thoughts about their ability to tackle the driving test successfully. This leads to realistic positive thoughts about their performance and the likely outcome of the test, leading to emotions and behaviours that increase their chances of success.

Curwin *et al.* (2000) provide a list of characteristics of CBT, some of which require adaptation to the delivery of CBT by nurses to clients in the course of day-to-day contact with them. Morrison and Barratt (2010) also identify important ingredients of CBT for psychosis. We draw on these publications to summarize key elements of CBT below:

1. **Clinician's assumptions and normalizing symptoms:** clinicians recognize that many people experience symptoms without being distressed by them; sharing this information with clients (normalizing symptoms) can reduce stigma and improve engagement. Clinicians recognize that the amount of distress and disability caused by symptoms is a more important target for therapy than the symptoms themselves.

2. **Active, collaborative working relationship:** the clinician and client work to an open agenda to build and test hypotheses to explain how the client's problems are maintained. Both bring expertise to the partnership: the client about the particular characteristics of their problems and the clinician her/his knowledge of how similar problems are maintained and may be treated. The clinician is active in helping the client retrieve information about their problem.

3. **Psychological formulation of the problem:** the rationale for CBT is explained and demonstrated to the client through the development of an idiosyncratic (individualized) formulation. The aim is not 'diagnosis' but developing an explanation of how the client's problem is maintained, and sometimes how it developed. The client plays a key role in developing hypotheses to explain their current situation and generate potential solutions.

4. **Structured approach:** typically the CBT clinician and client meet regularly, usually weekly, for a set period, usually one hour. The sessions follow an agenda set at the start of the session and typically adopt a problem-solving approach oriented around the problems that are causing the client most distress and disability. Flexibility of delivery may be needed if nurses are to incorporate CBT techniques into their daily work with clients.

5. **Goal-directed:** the aim is to reduce the client's distress and improve quality of life. Goals should be SMART (specific, measureable, achievable and realistic, and time limited) so progress can be monitored.

6. **Identifies and examines unhelpful thinking:** clinicians use guided discovery and Socratic questioning to help clients identify key cognitions and unhelpful behaviours; partnership working and commitment to therapy is enhanced if clients draw their own insights and conclusions rather than being told about their problems.

7. **Aids and techniques:** directed by the CBT formulation (of which more later) the clinician introduces activities to help the client change inaccurate, distorted or unhelpful beliefs about situations, or signs and symptoms. The client is introduced to aids and techniques (e.g. questionnaires, activity charts, cue cards, thought records) which they can draw upon both during therapy and thereafter to address their problems and manage future threats to their mental health.

8. **Teaching the client to become their own clinician:** a key objective of the collaborative relationship is for the client to recognize their central role in overcoming their own difficulties.

9. **Homework:** homework is a standing item at each meeting between the client and clinician and acts as a bridge between therapy sessions and the real world. The client working between sessions reinforces continuity and the central role of the client in working on their own problems rather than the clinician having a magic wand. Examples of homework could be to complete a thought record, record their activities or undertake 'exposure' tasks (of which more later). Whatever the task it is important that the client monitors their progress and is able to report on this at the next session.

10. **Time-limited:** the number of sessions is negotiated at the start of therapy, typically an initial six sessions followed by review. The end of therapy is in view from the outset, which can help to avoid dependence on therapy and reinforces the primary objective which is for the client to become their own clinician.

Thinking Space 21.2

What might you say to a client to:

1. Highlight the collaborative nature of the CBT enterprise?
2. Highlight the ultimate objective which is to help the client become their own clinician?

Feedback

1. A helpful thing to say at the outset of therapy is: *You know yourself and your own problems better than anyone else, so you are an expert. My skills come from working with people who have had similar problems to you.*

2. A helpful explanation of CBT at the outset of therapy is: *The aim of CBT is not to be 100 per cent depression or fear free. It is to help you learn some skills to use in your life to help you manage your problems both now and following the end of therapy into the future.*

21.4 CBT assessment

A good approach to assessment is to ask the client to tell you about a recent occasion when she or he experienced the problem symptoms and to describe this incident from moment-to-moment, starting with what the client first noticed and its impact on the three elements of psychological distress (their thoughts, feelings and behaviour).

Where the client's problem is their behaviour (e.g. they engage in excessive avoidance or rituals) then assessment of recent incidents tend to revolve around what are referred to as the five Ws: when, where, why, with/from whom, what (happened). If, however, the client's problem is concerned with their emotions (e.g. anxiety when forced to meet people; anger towards people; low mood) then assessment is usually better focused on the emotions and the circumstances under which they are triggered.

Thinking Space 21.3

You are carrying out a recent incident analysis with a client who is depressed. What questions might you ask them to identify triggers and the three elements of psychological distress (thoughts, feelings and behaviours)?

Feedback

- Can you think of a recent incident that you remember well that made you feel really down, really bad about yourself (identification of recent incident)?
- Could you tell me more about that (probe)?
- What happened? When did this happen? Where were you at the time? Who were you with (identification of triggers)?
- Can you tell me how you felt at the time (emotions)?
- Did you notice any sensations in your body (physical reaction)?
- When this was happening, what went through your mind? What sorts of things were you telling yourself (thoughts)?
- What did you do to make yourself feel better? Did it help (safety behaviours)? Was there anything you wanted to do but couldn't? Is there anything you avoided doing (avoidance behaviours)?

Defining problems and setting therapy goals

A key outcome of CBT assessment is clear statements of the client's problems and therapy goals. Problem statements express a shared understanding between the client and the clinician of what the problems/needs are, what maintains them and what priority they should take in the care planning process. Prioritizing problems is not straightforward; we may choose to address the most severe problem first or, alternatively, a problem which could be resolved easily and have an associated effect on other areas of need.

An agreed definition and prioritization of a problem might not be feasible if the client and the clinician cannot engage in a collaborative working relationship for various reasons. Such difficulties are not a reason to exclude the patient from the care planning process, however; it is better to draw up preliminary unilateral problem statements and address the lack of a collaborative relationship as a

problem in itself. Thereafter the clinician might identify the reasons for lack of collaborative relationship (e.g. if the client is severely distressed, the clinician has not spent much time with the client, etc.), ways to facilitate collaboration (reframing the problem in different terms or with a different focus, involving the family and other members of the team, etc.), and a date by which the problem statements should be reviewed, ideally with the client's involvement.

If after discussing their understanding of the problem the clinician and client have still not reached an agreed problem statement, they may have to 'agree to disagree' or 'agree to differ' so as to avoid prolonged repetitive discussions. In this case, the client's understanding should still feature in the problem statement; it will just be different to the clinician's. Nurses tend to describe lack of agreement on problem statements as 'the patient lacking insight' but an alternative way of describing it from our client's point of view could be, 'Mrs

Smith does not agree with what the doctors/nurses/family say about what her problem is, and she feels that the only reason for being in hospital is because she has not been behaving as she was expected to.'

Language

A way to reach agreed problem statements is to use language which is user-friendly, non-judgemental and 'clientalized'. The clinician may wish to test whether their understanding and phrasing of the client's problem meets these criteria by asking him or herself:

- Would this make sense to my client?
- If this were me, would I mind someone else saying this about me?
- Would I be happy for my client to read this?
- Does this describe my client's experiences of the problem?

User-friendly language uses direct quotes or paraphrases what a client said, rather than jargon or diagnoses. Some examples of what to avoid and what to say instead are:

- 'The client is depressed' → 'Mrs Smith describes feeling low/unhappy/sad/miserable/gloomy/down.'
- 'The client exhibits bluntness of affect' → 'Mary describes feeling numb and empty, and not being able to cry even when she wanted to get some relief.'
- 'Self-neglect' → 'John has not looked after himself for several days.'
- 'Lack of motivation' → 'Mrs Smith is finding it very hard to pay the bills and do the shopping. She would like to get back to work but finds it overwhelming and does not know where to start from, so she ends up postponing and "not bothering" to fill in applications.'

Non-judgemental language describes a behaviour and the potential reasons behind it, rather than attributing a characteristic to the client based on the behaviour. The problem statement should also take into account the client's rather than the clinician's point of view. Here are some examples:

- 'The patient is acting out and is difficult to manage' → 'John swears and throws things around because he says he is fed up with being in hospital and being treated like an idiot.'
- 'The patient is non-compliant' → 'Mr Smith is unhappy about taking his medication because he is worried about not having any control over it.'

'Clientalized' statements reflect how clients experience their illness and are specific about what symptoms mean for them. Specificity can also allow for objective evaluation of any change in the problem over time. Examples of general versus 'clientalized' statements are:

- 'The patient is lethargic and has low energy levels' → 'Mary feels sluggish and slowed down in the morning, and has a two-hour sleep in the afternoon which she never used to do. She feels exhausted when she does things such as preparing dinner or going out socializing.'
- 'The patient has poor sleep and appetite' → 'Mary sleeps five hours as opposed to her eight-hour normal sleep and wakes up three to four times during the night. She has stopped enjoying her food for the past couple of months and she has lost about 10 pounds during this time. Her everyday eating and drinking includes five or six cups of coffee and a sandwich.'

Apart from the appropriate language to be used, the format of problem statements depends on the model used to explain how the problem may have developed and is maintained. If the clinician does not want to tie problem definition to a particular model, the following components can comprise a generic format for a problem statement:

- An *experience or state (physical, emotional, mental, behavioural, cognitive, social)*, which the client considers as the primary problem because it causes distress and disability.

Useful questions to ask during assessment include:

- Is anything happening at the moment that upsets you or interferes with your life?
- Is there anything that you are particularly worried about at the moment?
- What does your family think the problem is?
- If there was something that you could change to make your life better or more enjoyable, what would it be?
- What do you fear is the worst thing that might happen?
- The *occurrence* of the primary problem: relevant information on what triggers or precipitates it, how often it occurs, when and where it is more likely to occur, how long it has been going on, etc.

Useful questions to ask during assessment are:

- When is the problem more likely to happen?
- Is there anything that makes it better/worse?
- When did you start noticing that things were getting out of hand?
- How many times does it happen in a day/week/month?

- Is there anyone who helps or makes things worse?
- The client's *responses* to it and whether they are *helpful or unhelpful*.

Useful questions to ask during assessment are:

- How do you make yourself feel better? Does it help? For how long?
- Is there anything that you do more of/less of because of the problem? Is what you do effective? How long does the effect last?
- Is there anything you avoid because of the problem? Is it helpful?
- Are there any disadvantages in avoiding things?
- Do you ever blow up because of what is happening to you/around you? What exactly do you do? Do you do anything to control it?
- The primary problem's *impact on self, others and/or life*.

Useful questions to ask during assessment are:

- How does it make you feel in yourself?
- How has it been affecting your life?
- Has it affected your relationships with others? In what way?

Thinking Space 21.4

Compare the problem statements in nursing care plans for patients in your clinical setting with the problem statements below. Rate the problem statements in the nursing care plans on a scale of 0–100 per cent for: a) how 'clientalized' they are; b) how SMART they are.
What goals might the clients in the following examples wish to achieve?

Problem statement: example 1
John feels unhappy and miserable (emotional experience as the primary problem) for most days of the week and for the past month (occurrence). Ever since he stopped working, he does not go out much and sits at home (response). This makes him feel worthless and even more miserable (response is unhelpful), and he worries about being able to go back to work (impact on life).

Problem statement: example 2

Mary sleeps less than she would like to and wakes up many times during the night (physical experience of poor sleep is the primary problem for the patient). This happens mainly at night when she feels other people's presence in the house (occurrence and activating event). She tries to cope with it by telling herself that everything is OK which makes her feel better (helpful response) and she occasionally shouts at them (response) but she is not sure whether this makes them go away (unhelpful response). She feels scared and helpless during the night and tired in the morning (impact on self); she is also unable to concentrate on doing everyday things (impact on life).

Setting goals

Goals can be long or short term depending on the time and resources available, and the strengths and limitations that the patient is considered to have. Most importantly the nurse needs to identify the objectives to be achieved prior to the patient reaching their goal (i.e. what the client would be able to do and under what circumstances) to know that the problem has improved and his/her needs have been met up to a realistic point. It is helpful to include potential or actual obstacles and difficulties in meeting objectives, and to identify, also, what support or resources could assist or smooth the client's progress. Finally, both problems and goals can be documented and rated in a standard form (Marks 1986) an example of which is given in Figure 21.3.

Questions which may help elicit goals and objectives are:

1. What would you like to be able to do in the near future that you cannot do now because of the problem?
2. What sort of things can people without your problems do?
3. If you woke up tomorrow and the problem was gone, how would you know?
4. How could your family and friends tell if your problem improved?
5. How could people who know you well tell when things start getting difficult for you?
6. If there was one thing that you would like to change in your life/yourself/the world around you, what would it be?
7. What has to change in order for you to be able to … ?

Feedback to Thinking Space 21.4

Example 1

Long-term goal: to be able to go back to work part-time within three months. This could be arranged because my boss is understanding and will not have a problem with an initial trial period of part-time work for me.

Objectives

- To be able to get up in the morning at 8.00 a.m., have breakfast and then go out to buy my paper (to do this every day for two weeks and then sleep longer during the weekends).
- To be able to go out two or three days a week in the evening to see my friends.

A potential difficulty could be that my friends may expect too much too soon from me because they do not understand what is wrong with me.

Example 2

Long-term goal: to be able to sleep seven hours without waking up and, if I wake up, not be scared.

Objectives

- To be able to get back to sleep without having to shout at the people in my house and be able to do this every night for a week.
- To be able to spend one hour, without interruption, doing the housework every day for a week.

Note that although 'other people's presence in the house' could have been phrased as a problem (e.g. being a symptom of a psychotic illness), Mary chose 'sleep' as the experience that distresses her and interferes with her life more, therefore even if interventions address Mary's psychotic symptoms, this will be done within the context of improving her sleep.

 ## 21.5 CBT formulation

The process of formulation in CBT is unlike a standard diagnostic interview, in that the clinician is constantly trying to make sense of information from the client to build up a tentative explanation of how the client's problem is maintained. The clinician will represent the formulation diagrammatically and share this with the client for testing and further development as treatment proceeds and the client's problems change.

The basic CBT model shown in Figure 21.2 highlights how clients' problems can be maintained through interaction between thoughts, feelings, (emotions and physical sensations) and behaviours, is sometimes referred to as a 'maintenance formulation'.

Through the process of assessment the basic CBT model may subsequently be expanded into a developmental formulation which will, in addition to problem maintenance, address predisposing factors (such as vulnerability arising from negative childhood experiences), precipitating factors which help to explain why the problem appeared when it did (such as life changes, physical illness, unemployment) and mitigating factors (i.e. what makes the problem better or worse). A sample formulation sheet is shown in Figure 21.4. A developmental formulation also includes other key elements of an expanded CBT model: core beliefs, assumptions and triggers.

Core beliefs

There are sometimes considered to be three levels of belief in CBT. The most superficial of these are NATs which feature in the basic CBT model in Figures 21.1. and 21.2. NATs are thought to arise from maladaptive core beliefs (which are similar to what some clinicians refer to as schemas), which are absolute beliefs (about the self, others and the world) which people hold with a high degree of conviction and constitute a lens through which they see the world.

It can be helpful to think of core beliefs as coming in pairs (e.g. 'I am a success' *and* 'I am a failure'). Mental health requires that the pair is present, since in the example above the client is able to see themselves in some situations as a success and in others as a failure. Some people, particularly those with a traumatic childhood, may develop only the negative belief of the pair. Thus, a client with a core belief that they are a failure will tend to see everything through the lens of their core belief, so whatever they achieve will be viewed by them in terms of what they have *failed to achieve* rather than what they have achieved.

Fig. 21.3 Problems and goals (after Marks 1986)

PROBLEMS AND GOALS

Name: _____ Date: _____

Problem: _____

_____

_____

_____

_____

_____

_____

_____

_____

How distressing/disturbing is the problem?

0--------- 1---------- 2---------- 3---------- 4---------- 5----------- 6---------- 7----------- 8

Not at all	Slightly	Moderately	Very much	Extremely

Goal: _____

_____

_____

_____

_____

_____

_____

_____

_____

If I had to achieve this goal now, how difficult would it be?

0--------- 1---------- 2---------- 3---------- 4---------- 5----------- 6---------- 7----------- 8

Not at all	Slightly	Moderately	Very much	Extremely

Figure 21.4 Developmental formulation sheet

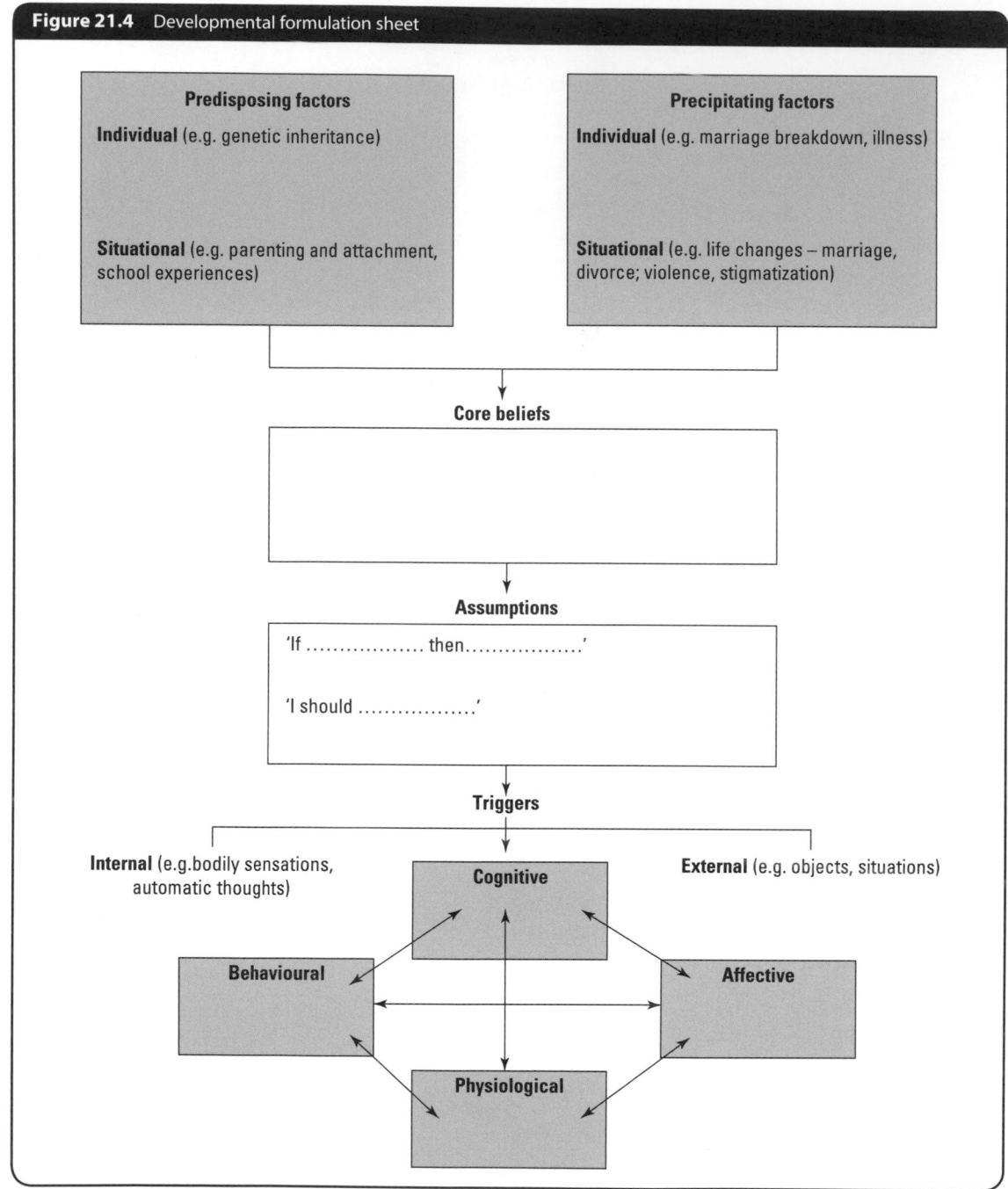

Assumptions

Assumptions, or 'rules for living' are used in an effort not to trigger our negative core beliefs. Assumptions usually take the form of 'If ... then' or 'I should ... ' statements. Rules for living are helpful most of the time, but they can lead to psychological and interpersonal problems if circumstances change and they are breached.

Thinking Space 21.5

What problems might arise for the people in the following examples?

1. A client with a core belief that they are a failure holds the assumption, 'If I do my work perfectly then people won't know I am a failure.'

2. A client with a core belief that they are unloved and unloveable holds the assumption, 'If I trust people then they will take advantage of me.'

Feedback

1. This rule for living may lead to perfectionism which could then generate anxiety, particularly if their work increases so that doing their work to their high standard is no longer possible.

2. This client may find it difficult to establish close mutually rewarding relationships with other people.

Triggers

Finally, triggers are incidents which set off the symptoms, or cause changes to one or more of the elements of psychological distress, on a regular basis. Triggers can be external to the individual (e.g. objects, situations) or internal (e.g. a bodily sensation, an automatic thought). Formulation has several functions within the therapy. It can:

- help the clinician and client make sense of what can appear to be a confusing set of symptoms and in turn encourage the client through fostering hope and motivation;

- provide a clear rationale, which is essential to the client's active engagement with therapy and identify priorities for treatment;

- individualize the client's problem, so making a link between the general CBT theories of problem development and maintenance and the client's own experience;

- open up to clients new ways of thinking about their problems which is an important first step in treatment;

- predict problems that the client may experience in carrying out the therapy which can then be planned for before they arise.

The CBT formulation is the stepping stone for appropriate interventions because it highlights that a change in any one of the elements of psychological distress can lead to changes in the others. CBT as a treatment seeks to produce change in one or more of these elements, to disrupt the vicious circle (illustrated earlier by the driving test example) which clients find themselves in. Behavioural interventions work on the assumption that if people act differently their thoughts will change; cognitive interventions assume that changing thoughts and beliefs will impact on their behaviour. Changes in thinking and behaviour impact indirectly on emotions such as anxiety, fear, anger or sadness.

We move now to consider key CBT techniques which nurses may wish to consider including within their daily nursing practice.

 ## 21.6 Key CBT interventions

Managing anxiety and panic symptoms

Techniques to manage anxiety and panic symptoms may not always be needed but can support clients' progress by reducing excessive physiological arousal (e.g. excessive hyperventilation leading to an asthma attack). Three symptom management techniques are covered briefly here: breathing retraining, tension-release exercises and coping cards.

Breathing retraining

The aim of breathing retraining is to restore the oxygen–carbon dioxide balance and acid–alkali balance which can be disrupted because of changes in the breathing rate under conditions of fear or acute stress. The key in controlled breathing is to *breathe in from the abdomen*, keep the chest still, *breathe out slowly and fully* and keep a regular pace between breathing in and out with pauses in between. This technique is being practised correctly when the abdomen moves out when you breathe in and moves in when you breathe out. This can be difficult to get used to, because most people breathe in from their chest and their stomach tends to move in as they breathe in. It is better to practise abdominal breathing when calm and comfortable in order to master the technique so that it can be used with the first warning signals of psychological arousal.

Tension-release exercises

Tension-release exercises (Gournay 1995) are part of a comprehensive applied muscle relaxation training programme for anxiety (Ost 1987). Tension-release exercises aim to control physiological arousal symptoms, such as muscle tension, sweating, pounding heart, light-headedness, 'butterflies in the stomach', etc. The client learns to recognize these symptoms early and control them before they reach their peak. This can be achieved by systematically tensing muscle groups in the body for five seconds and then releasing them for about 10 seconds. Table 21.1 summarizes how to carry out tension-release exercises. These are first practised for 20–30 minutes in comfortable conditions and then can be done in distress-provoking situations. It is important that:

- the muscles are only tensed until the client feels a sense of 'pulling'; too much pressure may cause injuries or the muscles may not be able to relax after releasing the tension;
- the release of the muscles should be immediate and *not* gradual.

Table 21.1   Tension-release exercises for anxiety

■ Tense your muscles until you feel a sense of 'pulling'; too much pressure may cause injuries, or the muscles may not be able to relax after releasing the tension. ■ Release the muscles immediately and *not* gradually.		

Muscle groups	Exercise	Time
Hands and forearms	First with right, then with left hand and forearm – Clench your fist until knuckles are white and the muscles in your forearm feel tense – Release by letting the hand fall loose	5 sec 10 sec
Arm	First with right, then with left arm – Clench your fist and bend the arm to 90° trying to make your biceps muscle bulge – Release by letting the hand and arm fall loose	5 sec 10 sec
Head *Forehead and eyebrows*	– Wrinkle the forehead by raising the eyebrows – Release the tension by letting the eyebrows relax – Bring the eyebrows close together as in frowning – Release by letting the eyebrows relax	5 sec 10 sec 5 sec 10 sec
Eyes	– Screw up your eyes and hold them tightly shut – Release by opening your eyes and letting your eyelids relax	5 sec 10 sec
Jaw	– Tense the jaw by biting the teeth together – Release by letting the jaws relax (they are *not* clenched)	5 sec 10 sec

Tongue	– Press the tongue flat against the roof of your mouth until you notice tension in your throat	5 sec
	– Release by letting the tongue rest (make sure your jaws are *not* clenched together)	10 sec
Lips	– Press the lips tightly together as in a pout	5 sec
	– Release by letting the lips relax (make sure your jaws are *not* clenched together)	10 sec
Neck	– Let the head fall back (towards the chair) without pushing it back and then let the head fall forward (your chin towards your chest without touching it)	5 sec
	– Release by bringing the head to the upright position	10 sec
Shoulders	– Hunch the shoulders up towards the ears and then rotate the shoulders	5 sec
	– Release by letting the shoulders drop	10 sec
Back	– Push your elbows into your side, push your shoulders down, push your head towards your chest and feel the big muscles across your back tense	5 sec
	– Release by letting your elbows relax, your shoulders drop, and your head in the upright position	10 sec
Chest	– Push your shoulders back, push your elbows down, tilt your head back and feel the muscles in your chest tighten	5 sec
	– Release by relaxing the shoulders and elbows and bringing the head to the upright position	10 sec
Stomach	– Tense the muscles of the stomach and push the stomach inwards	5 sec
	– Release the tension by letting the muscles relax	10 sec
Buttocks and thighs	– Squeeze your thighs and buttocks together	5 sec
	– Release by relaxing the muscles	10 sec
Calves and shins	First with right, then with left leg	
	– Keeping the leg straight, tense the calves by pushing the feet and toes downwards	5 sec
	– Release by letting the feet fall loose	10 sec
	– Keeping the leg straight, tense the shins by pulling the feet and toes upwards	5 sec
	– Release by letting the feet fall loose	10 sec
Feet	First with right, then with left foot	
	– Curl over your toes, trying to make a fist with your toes	5 sec
	– Release by letting the feet fall loose	10 sec

Coping cards

The client uses small index cards or pieces of paper, or a certain part of their diary to write a few sentences which are:

■ **Encouraging:** 'I have dealt with worse before, this is just fear and I won't let it get the best of me', 'I'm getting better at this all the time.'

■ **Challenging:** 'Don't jump to conclusions or take it personally; there might be another explanation', 'There is no need to prove myself, I am good enough as I am.'

■ **Self-instructions or reminders:** 'I must walk away now', 'Time to step back and take a breath', 'I'll make a note of this so I can take it out of my mind now and talk about it with my partner later.'

Behavioural activation

Usually motivation (desire for a bar of chocolate) preceeds action (going to the shop to buy the chocolate bar). But for many people suffering from depression, or people with negative symptoms of schizophrenia, motivation to do something does not come and will not come, no matter how long they wait. They need to kick start motivation through action ('Just do it' can be a useful cue card); because action can trigger motivation to further action. Explaining this to clients can sometimes be a helpful introduction to behavioural activation.

Behavioural activation has been used to tackle problems associated with low levels of activity and lack of pleasure or satisfaction. Its aim is to increase the levels of daily activity which could have a positive effect on energy levels and motivation and introduce pleasant, rewarding and interesting events as a positive reinforcement to daily routine. Behavioural activation comprises two main components: activity monitoring and activity scheduling (Fennell 1989; Greenberger and Padesky 1995).

Activity monitoring

The client uses a weekly or daily activity diary to record the time and type of their activities (see Figures 21.5 and 21.6). If the client's sleep pattern is interrupted, then it may be helpful for them to use a 24-hour diary to monitor their pattern of sleep and what activities take place just before they go to bed or just after they wake up in the night.

Sometimes a client may write 'doing nothing' if they consider that what they do is not productive or is not what they wanted to do in the first place. However things such as sleeping, lying in bed or looking out of the window are still activities and it is important that they are recorded to demonstrate their link with depressive feelings or negative symptoms.

In the weekly or daily activity monitoring diary, the client rates each activity using a scale 0–10 (0 = 'not at all' to 10 = 'extremely'). Intermediate ratings points could be 2 for 'slightly', 4 for 'somewhat', 6 for 'quite a lot' and 8 for 'very much'. The

client puts a P for *pleasure* with a 0–10 rating next to the activities that might be enjoyable (e.g. watching TV, eating). For example P0 would mean that the client did not enjoy the activity at all, P5 that they moderately enjoyed it and P10 that they very much enjoyed it. The purpose of pleasure ratings is to establish activities that the client used to enjoy but not any more, either because they do not have the motivation or energy to do them or because they do them but do not enjoy them, and activities that the client still enjoys to some extent, and so could be built upon.

The client puts an A for *achievement* with the 0–10 rating according to the difficulty of achievement *given how the client feels at the time* (doing the housework, taking children to school). For example A0 would show that the client found the activity quite effortless and that it did not give them a sense of achievement, A5 that the activity was moderately difficult to achieve but the client managed it, whereas A10 would represent a difficult activity that was a major achievement to complete. The purpose of achievement ratings is to demonstrate to the client that they may achieve more things than they give themselves credit for, because achievement is not what the client *wished they achieved* but what they *did achieve* considering their circumstances (e.g. low energy because of depression, no support, etc.) and, if the client does things which only require little or no effort, then there is scope to schedule activities with gradually increased effort and consequently increasingly greater sense of achievement.

Activity scheduling

Using a diary similar to the one used for daily activity monitoring, the client plans in advance their hour-by-hour activities using a daily activity schedule (see Figure 21.7).

There are two types of task which need to be scheduled: tasks the client *has* to do in balance with tasks that the client *wants* to do. The aim of activity scheduling is not to do as many things as possible in the time we have, but to plan the time we are going to spend on a particular activity in order to complete specific tasks. Sometimes clients find it easier

Figure 21.5 Weekly activity diary

Week beginning: ____________

Pleasure
How interesting and enjoyable was it?
0 -------- 2 --------- 4 --------- 6 -------- 8 -------- 10
Not at all — Extremely

Achievement
How difficult was it to do *given how I feel*?
0 -------- 2 --------- 4 --------- 6 -------- 8 -------- 10
Not at all — Extremely

Monday	Tuesday	Wednesday	Thursday	Friday	Saturday	Sunday
a.m.	a.m.	a.m.	a.m.	a.m.	a.m.	a.m.
p.m.	p.m.	p.m.	p.m.	p.m.	p.m.	p.m.

Figure 21.6 Daily activity diary

Date:

Pleasure (P)
How interesting and enjoyable was it?
0 ------- 2 -------- 4 -------- 6 ------- 8 ------- 10
Not at all   Extremely

Achievement (A)
How difficult was it to do *given how I feel*?
0 ------- 2 -------- 4 -------- 6 ------- 8 ------- 10
Not at all   Extremely

Time	Activity What did I do? Where was it? Was anyone else there? How long did it take?	P	A

to come up with the tasks that *have* to be done rather than activities that could be just pleasurable and interesting. Pleasant/interesting activities rather than chores could crop up from the activity monitoring diary (the ones with high pleasure ratings) or from a detailed history about things that the client used to enjoy in their everyday life but stopped doing because of their depression, or from questions about things that the client always wanted to do but never did.

Figure 21.7 Daily activity schedule

Date: _____

Pleasure (P)
How interesting and enjoyable was it?
0-----2-----4-----6-----8-----10
Not at all   Extremely

Achievement (A)
How difficult was it to do *given how I feel?*
0-----2-----4-----6-----8-----10
Not at all   Extremely

Time	Planned activity — What am I going to do? Where? Will anyone help/be involved?	Actual activity — What did I actually do? How did it compare with the planned activity? Was it SIMILAR, GREATER or SMALLER than planned?	P	A

The client records the planned activity in detail (including what is to be done, with whom and where) and then the actual activity which took place, including whether it was similar, greater or smaller than the planned one. Then the client records pleasure and achievement ratings as they did in the activity monitoring diary. If the planned activity was too difficult, then the client may have felt disheartened because they did not do anything at all, in which case it may be useful to break down the task to make the activity more manageable. Graded task assignment is helpful for things that the client wants to achieve but are too difficult under their current circumstances and need to be broken down before they are introduced in the activity scheduling diary. Using the daily activity schedule (Figure 21.7) the client could identify all the things they want to achieve during a certain period, always taking into consideration the balance between pleasures (things they *have to* do) and responsibilities (things they *need to* do). For each activity identified, there could be five potential actions:

1. Omit, if the activities/tasks exceed the available time.
2. Delegate, wherever possible.
3. Postpone activities which are of lower priority.
4. Seek help and support whenever possible.
5. Grade the task: if, for example, the task is 'to get the children ready for school and take them there' but the client cannot do it because he or she feels exhausted or overwhelmed, then a grading could be: 'prepare their packed lunch the night before – get up just before they go and just say goodbye – get up in the morning and make them drinks – get up in the morning and prepare drinks and breakfast – get up in the morning, prepare drinks, breakfast and take them to school'.

Thinking Space 21.6

What would you say to a client who does not complete their homework as agreed at the previous session?

Feedback

Clients not completing their homework between sessions is a frequent occurrence. The best approach is to treat this as a problem to be investigated and addressed. Asking the client, 'What stopped you doing your homework?', ensuring that they understand the contribution of the homework to their treatment and analysing a recent incident in which the good intentions to complete homework were not realized may be a helpful starting point.

Cognitive restructuring

A key assumption of CBT is that it is not events in themselves that cause psychological problems, but the meaning of these events to the client involved. Thus the emphasis of CBT on providing opportunities for people to reconsider the meaning of what happens to them and to gain a more balanced perspective.

Monitoring thoughts

The first stage in cognitive restructuring is to identify the content and occurrence of thoughts associated with a problem. This can be achieved in several ways.

- Keeping thought records (see Figure 21.8) for a period of time, detailing the situation in which

Figure 21.8 Thought record

Date	Situation What was I doing/with whom/where?	Feelings How did I feel (emotionally or physically) ?	Thoughts What thoughts/images went through my mind?	Responses What did I do because of these thoughts, or to cope?

a thought occurred, what the thought or range of thoughts was/were and how the client felt and responded at the time. The purpose of thought records is to identify the client's idiosyncratic misinterpretations or unhelpful ideas, establish a pattern of occurrence, demonstrate the link between thoughts and a client's feelings and responses, and finally rate the client's belief in them.

■ Going through a recent incident when the client experienced emotions or symptoms associated with the problem. Starting questions could be, 'When was the last time that you felt miserable/angry/anxious/scared?' or 'Looking back during the last week, which was the worst day for you? What was happening at the time that made it so bad?' Then, questions such as, 'What was going through your mind at the time?' and 'Were you saying anything to yourself at the time?' could help elicit thoughts associated with the specific incident.

■ By using the 'downward arrow technique' (also known as 'inference chaining') it is possible to to elicit the meaning of the individual's thoughts and yield potent thoughts and powerful emotions which represent the client's ultimate fears. Therefore, this technique should be used only if the practitioner is sure about 'what to do' with the statement that lies at the end of the arrows. Some useful examples of applications of the downward arrow technique are described by Greenberger and Padesky (1995) for anxiety and depression, and Turkington and Siddle (1998) for delusions. An example is given below:

The clinician starts by asking the question, *'If this were true … '*

– What would be so bad about it?
– What would this tell you about yourself/ other people/your future/your life?

and carries on by asking the same question to the patient's answer until we arrive at a statement which reflects a core belief or cliental assumption.

I am worried I am becoming mentally ill.
↓
If this were true (you became mentally ill) what would be so bad about it?
↓
I would end up in a hospital.
↓
If this were true, what would be so terrible about ending up in a psychiatric hospital?
↓
Everyone would know and also I would never work again.
↓
If this were true, what would be so bad about it?
↓
Everyone would look down on me, feel pity for me and eventually abandon me.
↓
If this were true, what would this tell you about your life?
↓
Life will not be worth living if I end up without a job and friends.

Three ways to change your mind

Stirling Moorey (personal communication) has pointed out that there are three main approaches that clients can use to obtain relief from their negative automatic thoughts: examine the evidence for and against the thought; ask oneself how helpful is it to think this way; and note the thought and let it pass by.

■ **What's the evidence?** This first approach involves the client examining the validity of the thought in relation to evidence which supports the thought and evidence which does not support the thought. This approach to cognitive restructuring is based on the assumption that people who are depressed or anxious suffer from thinking errors and selective attention which results in them seeing only the evidence which supports their negative cognitions and ignoring or discounting evidence which does not. For example, a client who thinks they are boring will not recognize instances where they have engaged the interest of others, or they will discount these as one-off random events which are unlikely to be repeated. This approach to changing your mind is the most well established strategy within CBT and is illustrated by both thought records and behavioural experiments, which are described below.

■ **How helpful is it for me to think in this way?** The second approach, which may often be used in combination with the first, involves clients recognizing the disadvanges of holding the NAT, irrespective of its validity. For example, the clinician might say to the client: 'Setting aside whether or not it is true, which it might not be, how helpful is it for you to think you are boring when going out for a drink after work with your colleagues? How is that thought likely to make you feel? (even more unconfident and frightened); How is it likely to make you behave? (I will look awkward, and won't be able to speak, I'll look at the floor, people will think I'm odd).'

■ *Note the thought and let it pass by.* The third approach involves the client noting the NAT, but not engaging with it, and simply letting it pass by, so stopping a vicious cycle of brooding and rumination on the thought which exacerbates its negative impact on emotions. This third approach to changing our mind is drawn from mindfulness-based cognitive therapy (MBCT), a treatment which helps depressed people develop their willingness to experience emotions, even painful emotions, and to allow distressing mood, thoughts and sensations come and go. Thus difficult feelings and unwanted thoughts are held in awareness, rather than battled against, so introducing a new perspective to the client which brings with it self-compassion to the suffering the client is experiencing.

Generating and testing alternative thoughts and beliefs

Generating and testing alternative thoughts and beliefs is perhaps the most difficult part of cognitive restructuring because the clinician may see the alternatives clearly, but needs to stand back and help the client to arrive at these alternatives on their own. The alternative interpretation or constructive idea is usually phrased as a *hypothesis*, i.e. a theory or assumption for which we need to come to a conclusion about how accurate it is compared to the initial interpretations and ideas, and/or how helpful it may be in changing the way we feel and behave. The objective is not to disprove the client's thought, but to introduce a bit more flexibility in the client's thinking; to help them to come to the conclusion that there are other options that could be considered. The client can then *test* the alternatives interpretations or constructive ideas by either carrying out certain activities or having guided dialogues which highlight the evidence in favour of the alternatives.

Challenging NATs with a formal thought record

Figure 21.9 is a seven-column thought record modified from Padesky (1995) which provides clients with a step-by-step procedure to challenge their NATs. Padesky's approach is to ask the client to identify the 'hot thought' that drives the other negative thoughts and to review evidence for and against that thought. The aim is not to disprove the negative thought but to develop a more balanced thought which takes account of all the evidence and not just some of it. Usually the client will be able to find plenty of evidence that supports the hot thought from their day-to-day life. A key skill of the clinician is to help the client search for evidence that does *not* support the hot thought; it may be helpful to ask the client about their life and interests before they were unwell so they can remember other points in time and other situations in which the hot thought was not true.

Figure 21.9 Evidence for and against thoughts (after Padesky 1995)

1. Situation	2. Moods	3. Automatic thoughts/images	4. Evidence that supports the hot thought	5. Evidence that does not support the hot thought	6. Alternative/ balanced thoughts	7. Re-rate mood now (0–100%)
Who were you with? What were you doing? When was it? Where were you?	Describe each mood in one word. Rate intensity of mood (0–100%)	What went through your mind? Did anything else go through your mind? Rate each of the thoughts (0–100%) to identify the 'hot thought' – the thought that drives all the others Ask yourself: 'If this thought was the only one I had how depressed/anxious would it make me feel?'	Are there things in your life experience that might make you think the hot thought? Write down the evidence that supports the hot thought	Ask yourself, 'Are there ever times when I think to myself that the hot thought isn't true?' Think about the sorts of things that interested you or that you were doing before you were depressed/anxious	A thought which takes account of all the evidence which supports and also doesn't support the hot thought Rate how much you think this balanced thought is true (0 – 100%)	If you had the hot thought now, how depressed/anxious would it make you feel?

Challenging beliefs with behavioural experiments

Behavioural experiments are among the most powerful ways of helping people to change their mind. Clients suffering from depression, anxiety or low self-esteem, for example, are likely to make negative predictions about how things will turn out. They will tend to overestimate the likelihood that bad things will happen or things will go wrong, or how bad things will be, or their ability to deal with things if they don't go well. As a result clients tend to avoid threatening situations, or engage in the situation but try to get out as soon as possible, or be cautious and engage in safety behaviours, to make themselves feel better. As a result they never actually test whether their negative prediction is accurate, and so they continue to fear the worst.

Behavioural experiments provide opportunities for clients to test their predictions against an alternative prediction with a better outcome. The nature of the experiment depends on the prediction it is designed to test and it should aim to reinforce the alternative prediction rather than undermine the old one. Experiments should be negotiated and the clinician should empower the client to design and implement appropriate behavioural experiments between sessions. A good question to guide the client towards an appropriate behavioural experiment is, '*If the alternative/belief was true, how would you behave?*'

Graded exposure and response prevention

This technique has been extensively studied and proven effective for a range of anxiety- and stress-related problems, from phobias and panic to post-traumatic stress and obsessive compulsive disorders. Graded exposure is the process of confronting anxiety and fear-provoking triggers, starting from the least unpleasant and building up to the most dreaded one. The pre-planned grading of relevant triggers for exposure is known as a 'hierarchy'. Response prevention means that the client refrains from carrying out behaviours which 'mask' or avoid fear and anxiety (safety behaviours) during and after

exposure – for example, seeking reassurance or performing rituals (Marks 1986).

A mechanism which explains how graded exposure and response prevention work is called 'habituation'. This is the reduction of anxiety over time when a client encounters an anxiety/fear-provoking trigger without the use of safety behaviours. Anxiety is the body's natural response to excessive adrenaline production when a person is faced with a situation which is threatening or is perceived as threatening. Adrenaline prepares the body for a flight-or-fight response to an actual or perceived threat. This means that the person experiences physiological changes resulting from increased oxygen flow and blood supply to the muscles, leading to increased heart and breathing rate, increased blood pressure, sweating, blurred vision, etc. Anxiety increases until it reaches a peak when the person tries to deal with it by either escaping from the situation or by doing certain reassuring or ritualistic things to 'mask' or avoid the anxiety.

With escape and avoidance, anxiety goes down rapidly but will reappear as soon as the person comes across the same trigger. If the individual remains exposed to the trigger for a certain period of time without running away or masking the symptoms of anxiety, then the excess adrenaline in the body is gradually depleted and anxiety symptoms eventually subside. Over repeated and prolonged exposure to the same or similar triggers, anxiety peaks at an increasingly lower lever and eventually fades away.

Graded exposure and response prevention involves the following steps:

1. Create a hierarchy of triggers. This is a list of all anxiety- or fear-provoking experiences with ratings of distress in a 0–8 scale (0 = not at all distressing and 8 = extremely distressing). Triggers could be anything that a client avoids altogether, or situations which the client can cope with only by using safety behaviours. Questions to ask to elicit triggers are: '*Is there anything that you avoid because of the problem?*'; '*What brings your fear/anxiety/worry on?*'; '*What places, things or people make you feel uncomfortable?*'

2. Set exposure tasks which relate to each trigger. These are exercises comprising the following components:

   - behaviours (what to do and in what order);
   - conditions (where, with whom, when, with what response prevention);
   - frequency (how often and how many times);
   - duration (a specified time period or until the anxiety subsides by 50 per cent).

   For example, an exposure task for someone who is anxious about going far from home and into public places could be to: *'travel a mile away from home to the nearest shopping centre, every day for a week, alone without carrying my mobile phone or my anxiety pills.'*

   In summary, an exposure task should be:

   - **Graded:** i.e. to start from the easiest to achieve and build up towards the most difficult task which could also be the final goal of the exposure programme.
   - **Focused:** i.e. the client should experience the whole range of anxiety without trying to mask it or avoid it with subtle behaviours.
   - **Repeated:** i.e. to carry out the same exposure task as many times as needed until it can be done with relative ease and minimal anxiety.
   - **Prolonged:** i.e. to stay with the anxiety long enough without any safety behaviours to allow habituation to take place.

3. Practise each exposure task in the list as many times as needed until the task is performed with relative ease. Keep a record of when the task is carried out, and the anxiety experienced before, during and after exposure (see Figure 21.10). Distress and discomfort are part of exposure and although they are unpleasant, they are not harmful. However, if someone finds an exposure task too difficult to achieve then:

   - Grade down the task by choosing a less distressing trigger to confront.

- Vary the task by either choosing a trigger with similar fear/anxiety rating or change some of the behaviours, conditions and frequency of the exposure (but not the duration as this would effect habituation).
- Use coping methods, such as controlled breathing, tension release and coping cards which could make the task more tolerable. Such techniques should be dropped at a later stage in exposure because they could become safety behaviours which interfere with habituation.
- Use clinician-guided exposure (such as modelling, accompanying the patient) to demonstrate how to best carry out the task and as a way of initially managing the discomfort or embarrassment that the client carrying the exposure may feel.

Moving too quickly up the hierarchy of triggers and its corresponding exposure tasks may be traumatic, and more harmful than helpful because of the excessive distress it may cause. It can also be disheartening if the client cannot achieve the task and considers they have failed. However, moving too slowly could be ineffective because the client does not experience the degree of anxiety that would allow habituation to take place. Also, having to practise two or three exposure tasks of slight anxiety could be more unpleasant than having to practise one task of moderate anxiety. In summary, the pace of exposure should be negotiated with the client who carries it out and the fine tuning of the tasks is ongoing according to the client's strengths and preferences.

Sleep hygiene

Disrupted sleep is a frequent feature of anxiety or depression and can exacerbate these conditions. Depressed people, for example, who do not sleep well at night may be tired and sleep during the day which in turn makes it difficult to sleep at night. Providing clients with information on sleep hygiene is an important part of the clinician's role and involves the following steps:

Figure 21.10 Exposure diary

EXPOSURE DIARY

Exposure task	Date	Anxiety/discomfort score 0-------2--------4--------6-------8 None Extreme		
		Before	**During**	**After**

- **Step 1, assessment of the nature of the sleep problem:** ask the client about their concerns. Is the problem: difficulty falling asleep; not staying asleep; waking early in the morning; disturbed sleep; not feeling rested following sleep; worrying about sleep?

- **Step 2, education about normal sleep and sleep problems:** highlight the variable nature of sleep patterns from one client to the next (e.g. seven to eight hours may be typical but some people need more and others less; older people tend to sleep less than younger ones) and the factors which are commonly associated with sleep problems (e.g. pain, certain medicines, drug and alcohol use, stress, anxiety and depression, environmental factors such as noise and light).

- **Step 3, provide information on sleep hygiene and promote a regular sleep routine:** provide advice which takes account of the nature of the client's sleep problem. Box 21.1 gives a list of sleep hygiene tips which are widely endorsed.

- **Step 4, monitor the effects of sleep hygiene practices:** sleep diaries can provide useful information on progress and identifying triggers for good and bad nights can be helpful to modify the treatment plan.

Problem-solving

Problem-solving is a process by which a client identifies, chooses and implements solutions to a problem. Problems can stem from the discrepancy between change and adaptation. Change can be external (e.g. loss of a job or a loved one) or internal (e.g. physical illness). If adaptation to change is poor, this may lead to distressing or disabling consequences for the client or others around them, thus creating and maintaining a problem. Solutions

---

Box 21.1 Sleep hygiene tips

Good sleep hygiene has four components: behaviour, environment, diet and exercise.

Behaviour

- Go to bed and wake up at about the same time every day, so establishing a regular schedule.
- Adopt a relaxing pre-sleep routine (e.g. have a bath, listen to relaxing music); limit stimulating activities in the hour before bedtime.
- Go to bed only when tired (or for intimacy). Don't eat, watch TV or read in bed.
- If you haven't fallen asleep after 30 minutes, get up, go to a different room and undertake a quiet activity until feeling tired and then return to bed.
- Once awake for 15–20 minutes, don't lie in bed – get up.
- Avoid naps six to eight hours prior to going to bed and naps only to retain alertness (30 minutes maximum).

Environment

- Bedroom should be dark, cool and quiet (or wear ear plugs).
- Avoid allergens that can disrupt sleep because of coughing or sneezing.

Diet

- Alcohol may help the onset of sleep but can lead to disrupted sleep; avoid alcohol three to five hours before sleep.
- Avoid going to bed having eaten too much or too little; avoid sugars and stimulants like caffeine and nicotine.

Exercise

- Regular exercise, preferably outdoors, promotes a regular sleep-wake cycle.
- Avoid raising the body temperature through exercise three to five hours prior to sleep.

to a problem are adaptive responses to change by thinking or behaving in ways that allow the client to function as well as possible, either by managing the change itself, or by reducing the distress and disability associated with the change. Problem-solving was first described by D'Zurilla and Goldfried (1971) as a component of social skills training to enhance and maintain social competence. Since then, it has been adapted and refined as a therapeutic tool for different conditions. It typically comprises the following steps:

- **Recognizing and defining the problem:** the client generates a clear statement of the problem (e.g. 'I don't have enough money to pay the bills') and a detailed account of the nature and circumstances of the problem (e.g. a financial problem is broken down into its constituents, income, expenditure, debt).

- **Identifying all possible solutions:** the client lists all possible solutions without making judgements about which are better than others at this stage. They should be encouraged to be creative.

- **Evaluating the solutions:** the client eliminates the less desirable and unreasonable solutions and places those that remain in order of preference. These are then analysed in terms of their advantages and disadvantages or their costs and benefits for the client and their carers/family.

- **Planning and implementing the preferred solution:** many solutions need careful planning, again on a step-by-step basis, taking account of available resources. The 'four Ws' (what, where, when and with whom) can provide a structure for clients to work out the implementation plan. Keep a diary of obstacles which hindered the successful implementation of the solution.

- **Evaluating the outcome:** evaluate how effective the solution was by asking questions such as *'Is the problem resolved? Do you feel differently now about the situation? Can you function*

despite the problem?' If the solution did not work, then an alternative can be tried from the list of possible solutions the client had previously identified. New information could help generate more solution options.

 ## 21.7 Conclusion

This chapter has outlined the principles of CBT and suggested a number of interventions which, with some supervision, non-specialist mental health nurses could employ in their daily work with clients who are inpatients or living in their own homes. The main points of this chapter are:

- CBT draws upon two distinct therapies: cognitive therapy which draws on information processing theories and behaviour therapy which draws on learning theories.

- CBT hypothesizes that it is not events in themselves that cause psychological problems, but people's interpretation of them and the ways they respond to them.

- The CBT model hypothesizes that the elements of psychological distress – thoughts, feelings (emotions and physical sensations) and behaviours – are linked so that a negative change in one can trigger a negative change in another and a vicious cycle is created.

- A key outcome of CBT assessment are clear statements of the client's problems and therapy goals in non-judgemental language which describes a behaviour and the potential reasons behind it, rather than attributing a characteristic to the client based on the behaviour.

- The CBT formulation provides an individualized diagrammatic description of a client's current problems, an account of why they might have developed and a tentative explanation of how they are maintained.

- A number of CBT techniques are available to non-specialist mental health nurses who are suitably trained and supervised. Behavioural interventions work on the assumption that if people act differently their thoughts will change; cognitive interventions assume that changing thoughts and beliefs will impact on their behaviour. Changes in thinking and behaviour impact indirectly on emotions such as anxiety, fear, anger or sadness.

Annotated bibliography

Hawton, K., Salkovskis, P.M., Kirk, J. and Clark, D.M. (1989) *Cognitive Behaviour Therapy for Psychiatric Problems.* **Oxford: Oxford University Press.**
A classic CBT textbook and comprehensive practical guide for students and practitioners on CBT models and methods for mental health problems. The book covers a historical overview of behavioural and cognitive treatments, and provides detailed guidelines and case examples on CBT assessment strategies, formulation and treatment methods for anxiety disorders (generalized anxiety, panic, phobias, obsessive compulsive disorder), depression, marital problems and physical problems associated with mental health factors (e.g. sleep disorders, medically unexplained symptoms, sexual problems, etc.). In addition, one chapter refers to CBT within the context of caring for patients with a high level of dependence on psychiatric services and another outlines the delivery and applicability of problem-solving.

Kingdon, D.G. and Turkington, D. (1994) *Cognitive-Behavioural Therapy for Schizophrenia.* **Sussex: Guildford Press.**
A clear and concise book which outlines the key theoretical frameworks of understanding experiences associated with schizophrenia. It also illustrates the application of specific CBT techniques with case examples, including explanations for psychotic symptoms using a normalizing rationale and stress-vulnerability model, techniques to understand and tackle delusions, and reality testing for hallucinations. Ideal as an introductory book in the field of CBT for psychosis.

Wright, J.H., Sudak, D.M., Turkington, D. and Thase, M.E. (2010) *High-yield Cognitive-behavior Therapy for Brief Sessions: An illustrated guide.* **Arlington VA: American Psychiatric Publishing.**
This book is a user-friendly and comprehensive guide on how to use specific CBT techniques during brief sessions in day-to-day clinical practice with patients who experience problems such as depression, anxiety, psychosis, suicidality, sleep problems, substance abuse and physical illness. It includes case illustrations and a CD-ROM in which the authors demonstrate the application of CBT techniques.

References

D'Zurilla, T.J. and Goldfried, M.R. (1971) Problem solving and behavior modification, *Journal of Abnormal Psychology*, 78: 107–26.

Fennell, M.J.V. (1989) Depression, in K. Hawton, P. Salkovskis, J. Kirk, and D. Clark (eds) *Cognitive Behaviour Therapy for Psychiatric Problems: A practical guide.* Oxford: Oxford University Press.

Gournay, K. (1995) *Stress Management: A guide to coping with stress.* Surrey: Asset Books.

Greenberger, D. and Padesky, C. A. (1995) *Mind Over Mood: Change how you feel by changing the way you think.* London: Guildford Press.

Marks, I.M. (1986) *Behavioural Psychotherapy: Maudsley pocket book of clinical management.* Bristol: Wright.

NMC (Nursing and Midwifery Council) (NMC) *The Code: Standards of conduct, performance and ethics for nurses and midwives.* London: NMC, available at: www.nmc-uk.org/Documents/Consultations/NMC%20Consultation%20-%20code%20of%20conduct%20-%20%20Phase%202%20draft%20code.pdf, accessed August 2012.

Ost, L.G. (1987) Applied relaxation: description of a coping technique and review of controlled studies, *Behaviour Research and Therapy*, 25: 397–410.

Turkington, D. and Siddle, R. (1998) Cognitive therapy for the treatment of delusions, *Advances in Psychiatric Treatment*, 4: 235–42.

Chapter 22

Solution-Focused Approaches

Iain Ryrie

I think it's very important for me to develop short-term, easily achievable goals which help me to reach my longer term goals, in order to accomplish everything I want to do.

Hayley (diagnosed with depression)

 ## 22.1 Introduction

Mental health nurses work with people to understand their problems and develop meaningful ways, in partnership with those people, to reduce or overcome their difficulties. This can involve articulation of the problem within the nursing process or it may involve a problem analysis in which any antecedents or causes of a problem are documented along with the problem itself and its consequences (see Chapter 21).

A different approach involves working with people to seek or evoke solutions, rather than focusing on the problem itself. This could include an exploration of times when the problem is not present, when there appear to be exceptions to problematic thoughts or behaviours, and then building on these exceptions to generate solutions.

These alternative approaches reflect fundamentally different ways of working with people and in this chapter the solution-focused approach is introduced. The content covers:

- foundations;
- practice skills.

Case Study

Mitch

Imagine that you are working with a 22-year-old man, Mitch, who has come to a substance misuse service with his sister. He had been expected to begin a university course after his gap year. This did not materialize nor did his plans for his gap year. Over the past two years Mitch has developed a liking for cannabis and alcohol. His family feels he has become increasingly dependent on drugs, staying up most nights and distancing himself from his family with whom he had been very close. They feel he is throwing his life away and creating a mountain of problems for himself that are likely to blight his life. They refer to him as their 'problem child' and are eager to point out the success with which his other siblings are progressing through life.

Thinking Space 22.1

Take a few moments to reflect on Mitch's circumstances. As a substance misuse nurse you are about to have 30 minutes of one-to-one contact with Mitch. Consider the following questions and jot down your answers:

- What do you see as the purpose or goal of your 30 minute session?
- What strategies, interventions or style of interaction might you use to achieve those goals?

You will have the chance at the end of the chapter to review your thoughts and ideas against a description of the work undertaken with Mitch in the form of a continuation of the above case study.

22.2 Foundations

Solution-focused therapy (SFT) was developed in the USA in the 1980s and was first introduced to the UK at the end of that decade. It is a form of brief therapy in that it focuses on the here and now, deals with specific, attainable goals and typically involves 20 sessions or fewer (Koss and Butcher 1986). It is brief also because solution-focused therapists deal with the problem brought by a client and rarely stray into other areas of the client's life. This means that they tend not to take full case histories that might typically be used to generate explanations of a client's problem or difficulties (O'Connell 2005).

SFT helps people to recognize what they want to be different in their lives and uncovers the strengths they have to accomplish their goals. Goals are often referred to as a person's 'preferred future'

and in this sense SFT is a future-focused, competence- or strengths-based approach. It encourages people to focus on what is attainable in their lives rather than allowing the size and complexity of a problem to overwhelm them.

Solution and problem discourse

There is an intuitive appeal to the solution-focused approach: problem-focused discourse can talk people into their problems while solution-focused discourse can talk people out of their problems (O'Connell 2005). Although this is an oversimplification it holds an important truth. When we change a behaviour or thought we don't just stop that behaviour or thought but we replace it with alternative behaviours or thoughts. Therefore, if we can find exceptions to people's problem behaviours or thoughts, and enable them to practise more of them, then we have found a potential solution.

Furthermore, this can be achieved without any analysis of the problem itself.

Solution-focused therapists do not view clients as emotionally or psychologically sick or damaged, but as unable at present to find a way around or out of their problems (Webster 2009). Focusing on problems can distort a client's experience and emphasizes their assumed deficits and pathologies, which in turn misses opportunities to learn about the unique ways in which they are able to cope – i.e. when they experience exceptions to their problem. A problem focus tends also to put the client in the role of passive recipient with the therapist acting as an expert on the analysis and management of people's problems. They might, for example, begin by asking a client 'How can I help you?'

Conversely, a solution focus seeks out and builds on what is healthy and functioning in people's lives, about which the individual client is the expert. For this reason SFT is a strengths-based approach that seeks out the competencies people have for achieving change in their lives. A solution-focused therapist might therefore begin by asking a client 'What would you like to change?'

O'Connell (2005) highlights important differences between solution and problem discourse in terms of the types of questions a counsellor or therapist might ask, some of which are presented in Table 22.1.

There is an evidence base for the solution-focused approach such as Gingerich's and Eisengart's (2000) review of 18 controlled outcome studies, 17

of which reported improved client outcomes, 10 of which were statistically significant. However, not all studies were tightly controlled and more recently O'Connell (2005) has concluded that overall there is relatively limited published research that would be acceptable to the academic community.

This chapter does not argue the merits of one approach over the other. In the author's experience there are times and contexts in which one is more suitable than the other. It is better therefore to view the approaches as complementary, each with something different to offer people who experience mental health difficulties.

Assumptions and principles

SFTs attention to solutions rather than problems is underpinned by a number of assumptions. Different solution-focused therapists tend to emphasize different assumptions as being key to their practice. Below are listed some of the more prominent assumptions from the work of O'Connell (2005) and Webster (2009):

- people are resilient, creative problem-solvers;
- as a health-oriented strengths-based approach to helping people, therapists seek evidence of competency rather than failure or weakness;
- SFT is grounded in an acceptance of multiple realities or multiple, equally plausible interpretations of any situation;
- people have a unique definition of their situation and what would be a 'solution' to any problem;
- understanding a problem does not have to precede solving it;
- people engage more with an approach that builds on their strengths than with one that highlights their deficiencies;
- it is more effective to build on 'what works' than to get someone to do something for the first time;
- small steps forward tend to be more helpful than big plans.

These assumptions imply that people attend sessions with an openness to seek solutions and a willingness

Table 22.1 Solution versus problem discourse

Solution discourse	Problem discourse
■ What would you like to change?	■ How can I help you?
■ Can we discover exceptions to the problem?	■ Can you tell me more about the problem?
■ What will the future look like without the problem?	■ How has this problem arisen in light of your past?
■ Have we achieved enough to end our contact for now?	■ How many sessions will we need to deal with this problem?

Table 22.2 Visitor, complainant and customer change agendas

Change agenda	Characteristics
Visitor	A person who does not think he or she has a problem and does not want to be in therapy, or both
Complainant	A person who is willing to discuss a problem but who sees the solution as lying elsewhere, or being someone else's responsibility
Customer	A person who recognizes that he or she has a problem and who views the session as an opportunity to do something about it

to work hard at implementing them. In reality this may not be the case. De Shazer (1988) has developed a simple model to distinguish between the different agendas that people bring to a session in respect of their readiness for change (see Table 22.2).

For SFT to work effectively clients need to be customers of the service and therapists may need to work in the first instance to support people to move from visitor or complainant to customer. Encouraging clients to see what is changeable and attainable, rather than focusing on the size and complexity of their problem, is one possible way of doing this. It is important also to review the cycle of change, which is introduced in Chapter 23 (Figure 23.1) and provides a model for the stages of change that people adopt, as well as strategies for enhancing people's motivation for change. However, some solution-focused therapists downplay the role of motivation, emphasizing instead the importance of helping clients to identify attainable goals along with the necessary solutions to realize those goals. It is this process they believe that holds potential for clients to move to the customer position (Webster 2009).

The assumptions that underpin SFT are accompanied by a number of principles to guide practice. Some are a simple reiteration of the assumptions and therapists often share these principles with clients as a basis for the work to be done. O'Connell (2005) lists five key principles:

1. **If it isn't broken don't fix it.** This principle advises against a tendency in some health care professionals to look for more and more problems in a client's life that they can help with. Many of us have been professionally trained and socialized to deal with problems and so the importance of this principle should not be underestimated. Solution-focused therapists often introduce a period of 'problem free' talk at the start of a session to avoid a problem focus. This might for example involve enquiring about what the client enjoys doing when the problem is not present. In turn this can reveal important clues as to the resources and solutions already available to a client. Most importantly this principle reminds us to avoid focusing on pathology and instead to seek out and build on what is healthy and functioning in people's lives.

2. **Small changes can lead to bigger changes.** SFT breaks down the process of change into small manageable steps on the basis that clients are more willing to make small changes in their lives. It is true also that any movement toward change, however small, can ignite hope in clients and thereby promote belief in their ability to achieve more change (Rosenbaum *et al.* 1990).

3. **If it's working, keep doing it.** Therapists seek out and encourage clients to do more of what they are already able to do – i.e. behaviours or thoughts that represent exceptions to their problem. A session might begin by the therapist asking a client about any pre-session change they have noticed or engaged in. Often, constructive behaviours or thoughts (exceptions to the problem) can begin ahead of or in anticipation of meeting a counsellor or therapist. By making enquiries of this type the therapist can uncover clues as to the solutions or resources that an individual already has at their disposal, and then explore how they can do more of them.

4. **If it's not working, stop doing it.** If clients are attempting solution behaviours that fail to bring

Table 22.3 SFT Process model – conversational themes and responses

Change discourse	Solution discourse	Strategy discourse
■ Offer genuine compliments ■ Seek out competencies ■ Explore exceptions ■ Reframe the client's experience ■ Set goals	■ Affirmation of solution opportunities ■ Ask the miracle question ■ Normalize the client's experience ■ Ask scaling questions in respect of client goals	■ Encourage utilization of learning and resources ■ Define and develop incremental solutions ■ Clarify endings and evaluate ■ Provide a key message and give homework

any relief to their problems then solution-focused therapists will encourage them to try a different strategy. Abandoning failed solutions is an important principle of SFT and opportunities to do something different have potential to break the failure cycle (O'Connell 2005).

5. **Keep therapy as simple as possible.** Therapists who look for hidden, unconscious factors or meaning behind a client's problems risk complicating the relationship. For some clients this stance implies that the therapist has a privileged view or understanding of their problems, which in turn can foster a sense of dependency on the therapist. For this reason solution-focused therapists intrude minimally into a client's life and look for opportunities to end the relationship as soon as is reasonably possible.

22.3 Practice skills

Many solution-focused therapists use a process model to understand the typical patterns that solution-focused conversations follow. The model is introduced in this section along with an abbreviated number of key solution-focused interventions that nurses can use in their work.

SFT process model

The SFT process model describes three main themes or patterns that emerge in solution-focused conversations and the interventions that the therapist might use in respect of those patterns. Table 22.3 provides an overview of the model with a select

number of interventions under each heading. The model does not depict a liner process that clients follow as there may be fluctuation between the themes over the course of a single session or multiple sessions. O'Connell (2005) also points out that the model maps out the terrain rather than being the terrain of therapy or counselling itself. Nevertheless, it remains a useful guide for understanding the themes that might emerge and how to respond to them.

Change discourse

During change discourse the therapist emphasizes the changing experience clients typically have in terms of their ability to solve a problem. Belief in change is emphasized and evidence for an already ongoing process of change in respect of a client's difficulties is explored. Seeking exceptions to the problem and a focus on competencies are both central lines of enquiry during this stage. This is important also to help clients reframe their experiences, particularly if they perceive a problem as being all-encompassing. In reality they are likely to have different experiences of a problem and its exceptions according to different contexts or circumstances (O'Connell 2005). Helping clients recognize these differences can inspire hope and increase their chances of overcoming their difficulties.

Solution discourse

Solution discourse involves interventions by the therapist to help clients progress from their current change strategies and behaviours to those they will need to achieve their desired goals. Complimenting and affirming potential solutions is important in this respect as is the 'miracle question', which represents a key SFT intervention. This question invites clients to project a possible future in which their difficulties no longer exist or are better managed. For example:

> 'Imagine you went to bed one night and while you were asleep a miracle happened so that when you woke up the problem you've brought with you today no longer existed. What would you notice that is different about your life in the morning, what would be the first things you'd notice?'

Through use of the miracle question clients are encouraged to specify realistic goals and identify the existing solutions and resources they have to move toward their goals. Solution-focused therapists use scaling techniques to help clients set these goals, measure progress and establish priorities for action. Here are some examples for a client who wants to improve their overall health by taking regular exercise (Webster 2009):

- 'On a scale of 0 to 10 how would you rate the level of exercise you take now?'
- 'If 10 represents taking regular exercise, what would you need to be doing to rate the amount of exercise you take as 10?'
- 'If you rate your current exercise as [e.g. 4] what would you need to be doing differently to rate it as 5?'

Strategy discourse

Strategy discourse reflects collaborative effort between a client and therapist to design, implement and review realistic plans to achieve client goals. This involves identifying existing, but until now devalued, strategies in the client's life (O'Connell 2005). Utilization of these resources along with learning from the session is encouraged and incremental solutions are agreed for the client to practise, typically in the form of homework. Scaling questions are used here to monitor progress and evaluate whether the work the client and therapist are doing together is proving useful. This latter

step helps clarify whether ongoing sessions are desirable.

SFT sessions always end with a concluding message from the therapist. This provides an opportunity to summarize what has been discussed, reflect back to the client the constructive strategies or exceptions to the problem they have described, to reinforce the value of those strategies and to compliment them on progress (O'Connell 2005).

SFT questioning process

The clinical team in the USA that developed SFT noticed that by a simple questioning process they could support clients to make changes in their lives. One of the originators, Steve de Shazer (1985) describes these as 'skeleton keys', which invite clients to:

- become aware of exceptions – i.e. those times when they are able to overcome their problem;
- utilize the personal and social resources they have, particularly those that are associated with 'exception' contexts;
- imagine a possible, preferred future by considering the miracle question;
- define and implement incremental solutions that reflect small, realistic steps forward.

De Shazer (1985) reports that this deceptively simple, future-oriented process empowers clients without getting them bogged down in the complexities of their problems. In other words, they make progress by imaging a preferred future rather than by analysing their problem history. Focusing on competencies and strengths was refreshing for de Shazer's team and it revolutionized their practice.

There is a parallel between their approach and the recovery model in mental health care, which supports people to develop within and beyond the limits of their condition or circumstances (see Chapter 5). Exploring exceptions to any limitations, doing more of them, imaging a preferred future and implementing small steps are useful strategies to support recovery-oriented practice.

Case Study

Mitch

A brief extract of Mitch's meeting with the nurse is presented here to demonstrate the exploration of exception and solution behaviours, and the scaling of confidence to achieve a goal. As you read through it you can review any notes you made in response to the questions that accompanied the initial case study.

NURSE: Hello Mitch, what's brought you here today?

MITCH: I didn't want to come. My family is on my back and worried about me throwing my life away.

NURSE: Oh, OK . . . well I'm pleased you came here today, it's quite a big step to take. Tell me how you feel about your family's concerns?

MITCH: Pretty angry, I've had to come here haven't I? I'm somehow responsible for how they feel, for how disappointed they are. They're a massive pain.

NURSE: It sounds like you feel you're being blamed unreasonably and don't see why you should have to do anything to change the situation.

MITCH: Yeah, too right.

NURSE: Mitch, what do you think would need to happen for your family to stop blaming you?

MITCH: No idea – they need to get over themselves.

NURSE: Can you remember a time when you were able to be yourself and your family wasn't blaming you for things? *(seeking exceptions)*

MITCH: Ummm . . . maybe when I first left school.

NURSE: What was different about then and now?

MITCH: I guess they had hopes for me then.

NURSE: What else was different, what about you? Can you think how you might have been differ-ent to have inspired hope in your family? *(specifying exceptions)*

MITCH: I was working immediately after college and I had a plan. I think they believed in me and my plan, we all did in those days.

NURSE: How did working make a difference? *(specifying exceptions)*

MITCH: I had a routine . . . and money . . . yeah, and I know those are quite useful things. I kind of paid my way in the family, you know, contributing to the cost of things but also just being about as a regular part of them all.

NURSE: Does any of that happen now?

MITCH: Well I've been 'off line' for a bit if you know what I mean . . . big decisions to make about my life and not wanting to commit . . . one challenge after another mounting up.

NURSE: You're going through a tough time. What do you think would be the first sign to your family that you're part of their life again? *(seeking solution behaviours)*

MITCH: God knows . . . ummm . . . being there for Sunday lunch maybe, each week.

NURSE: Is that something you want to do? *(specifying goals)*

MITCH: Maybe not every week.

NURSE: Yes, I understand, what do you think would be achievable?

MITCH: I haven't been for months so just turning up in the first instance would be something.

NURSE: So what would you need to do for that to happen? *(specifying solution behaviours)*

MITCH: Have a routine . . . get out of bed in time . . . get washed . . . you know, simple things.

NURSE: OK, and how confident are you that you could do that, on a scale of 0 to 10 say, with 10 representing complete confidence? *(scaling question)*

MITCH: About six.

NURSE: OK . . . is there anything you think you could do to increase that score to seven?

MITCH: I suppose I could speak to mum and agree which Sunday I'll have lunch with them. It'd feel like a commitment and she'd be pleased.

NURSE: It sounds like you know how to manage some of these difficulties between you and your family.

MITCH: Maybe, maybe not.

Mitch continued to visit the nurse over a two-month period, attending every fortnight. Most early sessions began with Mitch voicing complaints about his need to be there but invariably he moved to a customer position as each session progressed. He worked hard at exploring and implementing ways to improve his family relations with some success. By his fourth session Mitch began to talk about his drug use and how this affected his family. He had no intention of stopping his drug use but he knew that controlling it or abstaining from use while with his family was a valuable strategy for more harmonious relations. Gradually Mitch was able to make regular contact with family members without also smoking cannabis or drinking and he started to realize that these times were good for him, as well as for his family. At this point Mitch opted to end his contact with services.

22.4   Conclusion

This chapter has introduced a solution-focused approach as a style of counselling to help people recognize what they want to be different in their lives, to uncover their strengths and accomplish their goals. It includes a number of simple techniques and strategies for mental health nurses to use in their work with people who have mental health difficulties. The solution-focused approach complements recovery-oriented practice and while most mental health nurses have neither the need nor inclination to become qualified solution-focused therapists, it is possible to develop relevant skills based on the approach. In summary, the main points from this chapter are:

- SFT is a strengths-based approach to counselling that seeks out the competencies people have for achieving change in their lives.

- Helping clients identify attainable goals and uncover their own resources to generate solutions are key to its therapeutic value.

- SF conversations typically follow key themes or patterns (change, solution, strategy discourse) for which therapists use different interventions.

- A simple questioning process referred to as 'skeleton keys' can support people to make changes in their lives. The process invites people to explore exceptions to any limitations, do more of them, imagine a preferred future and implement small steps.

- SFT complements recovery-oriented practice by supporting people to realize personal goals within and beyond the limits of their illness or condition.

- SFT represents an accessible, learnable and useful counselling model for mental health nurses who are developing practice skills.

Annotated bibliography

O'Connell, B. (2005) *Solution-Focused Therapy***, 2nd edn. London: Sage.**
Now in its second edition this is an excellent introduction providing the theory, practice and skills base of the solution-focused approach. Vignettes and dialogues illustrate how to manage various scenarios with skill and sensitivity.

de Shazer, S. (1985) *Keys to Solutions in Brief Therapy***. New York: W.W. Norton.**
This is a seminal text and personal favourite. Though somewhat dated now it provides a clear and convincing exposition of the approach by one of its originators. Throughout it is enthused with the insights of a clinical team who have recently discovered a new way of working collaboratively with service users.

Ratner, H., George, E. and Iveson, C. (2012) *Solution Focused Brief Therapy: 100 key points and techniques***. London: Routledge.**
This is a concise and jargon-free guide to the thinking and practice of SFT. It is written by a team of SFT supervisors and practitioners who first introduced the approach to the UK at the end of the 1980s.

References

de Shazer, S. (1985) *Keys to Solutions in Brief Therapy*. New York: W.W. Norton.
de Shazer, S. (1988) *Clues: Investigating solutions in brief therapy*. New York: W.W. Norton.
Gingerich, W. and Eisengart, S. (2000) Solution-focused brief therapy: a review of the outcome research, *Family Process*, 39: 477–98.
Koss, M. and Butcher, J. (1986) Research on brief psychotherapy, in S. Garfield and A. Begin (eds) *Handbook of Psychotherapy and Behaviour Change*, 3rd edn. New York: Wiley.
O'Connell, B. (2005) *Solution-Focused Therapy*. London: Sage.
Rosenbaum, R. Hoyt, M. and Talmon, M. (1990) The challenge of single-session therapy: creating pivotal moments, in R. Wells and V. Gianetti (eds) *The Handbook of Brief Therapies*. New York: Plenum.
Webster, D. (2009) Using solution-focused approaches, in P. Barker (ed.) *Psychiatric and Mental Health Nursing: The craft of caring*, 2nd edn. London: Edward Arnold.

Motivational Interviewing

Iain Ryrie

I struggled with motivation and found myself allowing weeks and months to go by as though I was treading water...[then] I had a new CPN who kept teasing out my own dissatisfaction with my circumstances...she didn't tell me what to do or that I needed to change...[it was] just that eventually I couldn't ignore my own reasons to change and I gradually began to set some simple goals...my life is now progressing, albeit slowly, but it's my own efforts that are making the difference and I feel good about that

Anon

 ## 23.1   Introduction

In a typical working day most mental health nurses have many discussions with service users about behaviour change. These discussions arise whenever a nurse and a service user are considering doing something different in the interests of the service user's health. This might be to cut down on such things as long working hours or drug and alcohol use, or to increase other behaviours such as taking medication regularly, attending an employment support programme or sticking to an exercise plan. How these topics are addressed by nurses, including the style and attitudes they bring to each discussion, affects the likelihood that service users will achieve their goals.

Effective therapeutic communication as outlined in Chapter 20 remains a foundation for interpersonal relations between nurses and those with whom they work. However, these can be tailored to target particular challenges that service users face. Motivational interviewing (MI) is an example of a tailored approach. Though few of us will have the need or inclination to become qualified MI counsellors, it is possible to convey enough of the essential method to make it accessible, learnable and useful for developing practice skills. This chapter covers:

- the cycle of change;
- the foundations of MI;
- the practice of MI.

Case Study

Tom

Imagine you are working with a middle-aged man, Tom, who has been the recipient of mental health care for over 30 years and who now lives in supported accommodation. Over the past year Tom has received a lot of additional support to promote his independence and social functioning. This has included an employment support scheme, increased input from his community psychiatric nurse (CPN) and an intensive programme of rehabilitation in his own home to enhance his cooking and other domestic skills. As the year progressed Tom struggled with the support that had been put in place and gradually withdrew himself. He still sees his CPN but otherwise leads a quiet, isolated life and often complains of boredom. Tom's care providers are disappointed with his progress but still believe he has the potential to lead a much more fulfilling and independent life. His CPN has been asked to review Tom's case and to encourage him to re-engage with the support that had been made available to him.

Thinking Space 23.1

Take a few moments to reflect on Tom's circumstances. As his CPN you are about to have 20 minutes of one-to-one contact with Tom. Consider the following questions and jot down your answers:

- What do you see as the purpose or goal of your 20 minute session?
- What strategies, interventions or style of interaction might you use to achieve those goals?

You will have the chance at the end of the chapter to review your thoughts and ideas against a description of the work undertaken with Tom in the form of a continuation of the above case study.

23.2   The cycle of change

People pass through different stages in the process of changing a behaviour or aspect of their lifestyle. If someone was trying to save money or lose weight, or adhere to a new meditation regime, they would first of all need to arrive at a decision to make these changes. There will then be times when they are fully able to achieve their goals and other times when they waiver in their actions. It follows that a person's motivation for change represents an internal, psychological state that is likely to vary across time. This is a key point that underpins motivational interviewing.

A helpful model that describes the stages people pass through in the course of making changes to their lives is presented in Figure 23.1. To briefly summarize each stage of the cycle:

- **pre-contemplation:** when a person is unaware of the need to change a particular behaviour or they are so overwhelmed by their problem that any possibility of change is incomprehensible;

- **contemplation:** when someone becomes aware of a particular behaviour and begins to consider the possibility of change;

- **preparation/determination:** when a person begins to actively plan their behaviour change, perhaps calling in support from others;

- **action:** when a person puts their plan into action and takes steps to make the desired changes;

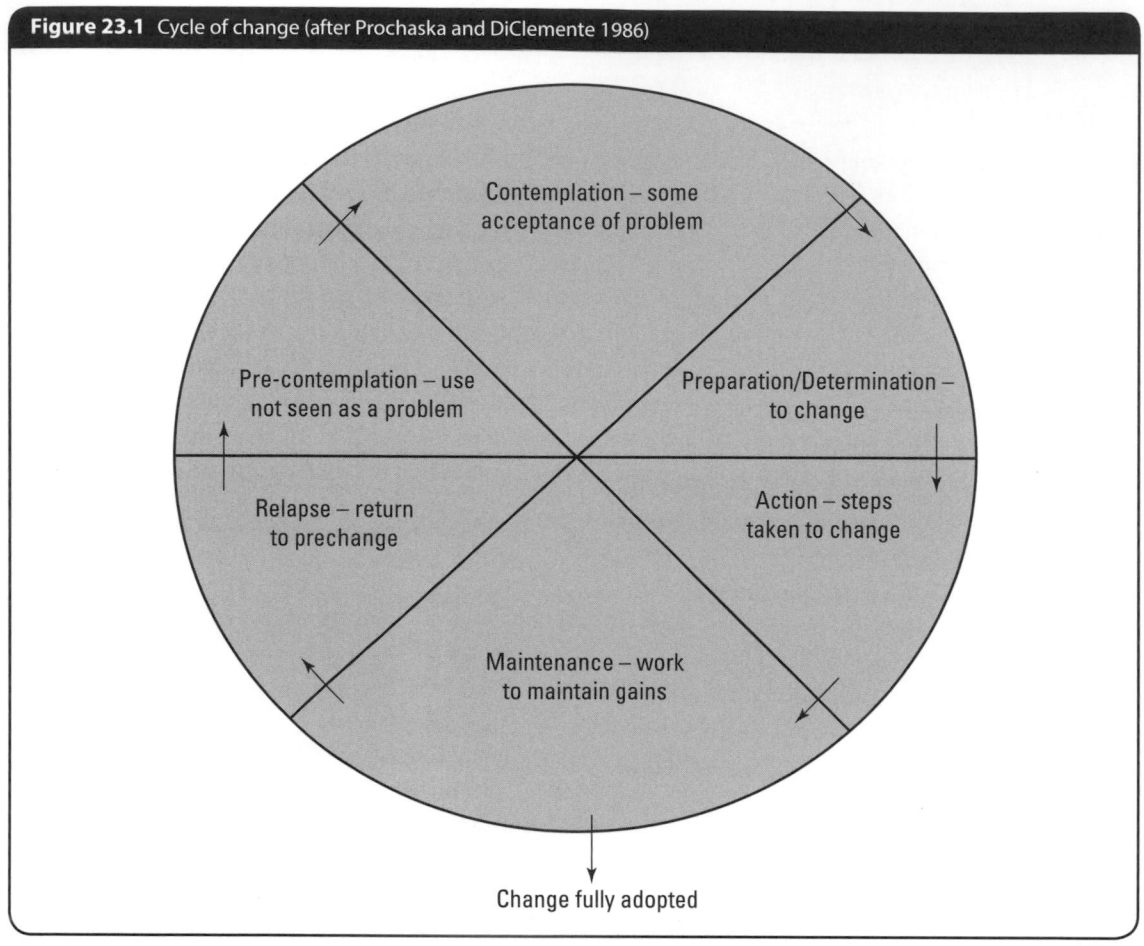

Figure 23.1 Cycle of change (after Prochaska and DiClemente 1986)

- **maintenance:** when a person has achieved change and now maintains that change and avoids relapse.

People exit the cycle at the maintenance stage after successfully consolidating any changes they have made, or they may relapse and return to an earlier stage in the cycle. It is usual for people to pass through this cycle several times when trying to change some behaviours (e.g. smokers pass through the cycle four times on average before they successfully quit – Miller and Rollnick 2002). Relapse can therefore be seen as a normal part of the behaviour change process.

MI employs the cycle of change to help develop practitioners' thinking about clients' readiness for change. Understanding a client's position in the cycle allows practitioners to tailor their interven-

tions according to that stage. For example, if someone starts to contemplate the negative consequences of an ingrained behaviour, there may be little point in offering an intervention with the aim of immediately ending the behaviour. The individual would need to be in the action stage for that to be appropriate. It may be more helpful to assist them in further exploration of their behaviour and personal circumstances, perhaps weighing up the various pros and cons of making a change and allowing their own motivation for change to develop.

Service users who are particularly resistant to nursing interventions and the possibilities of change can sometimes be labelled as unmotivated by staff. It may be thought that little can be done for them, though this type of judgement is usually wrong (Rollnick *et al.* 2008). A person's motivation is more likely to vary according to context and the types of interpersonal encounter they have. It is more useful to view resistance by service users as a critique of our own interventions. Perhaps we are offering an intervention that is at odds with a person's stage in the cycle of change. Their resistance is then understood as a mismatch between intervention and stage rather than an indication of their fundamentally unmotivated nature.

23.3 The foundations of MI

The malleable nature of people's motivation for change is an important foundation for MI and is understood to occur within the context of relationships. It follows that health care practitioners, through their contact with service users, can do much to influence motivation. The basic skills of MI that are used for this purpose are not unfamiliar to mental health nurses who typically use them in their everyday work. However, MI employs these skills in a particular spirit that follows a number of guiding principles. Before outlining some of the core skills of MI this section examines the spirit and principles of the approach, as well as introducing the concept of ambivalence.

The spirit of MI

The spirit of MI refers to the mindset with which health care practitioners approach the conversations and discussions they have with service users. This spirit has been described as collaborative, evocative and honouring patient autonomy (Rollnick et al. 2008):

- **Collaborative:** MI involves a partnership between health care practitioners and service users. This partnership is characterized by collaborative conversations and joint decision-making since it is only the client who can actually enact change.

- **Evocative:** MI seeks to evoke from service users their own reasons for change, thereby activating their motivation and any resources they have at their disposal to support the change process. It is vital that practitioners work hard to understand the service user's

perspective and to evoke from them their own arguments for change.

- **Honouring patient autonomy:** it is not unusual for practitioners to advise, tell, direct or even frighten service users into considering changes in their lives. At the end of the day, however, any change always remains the service user's choice and MI seeks to recognize and honour this autonomy.

The spirit of MI therefore involves a skilled interpersonal style for eliciting from service users their own reasons for change, which it achieves by guiding them to explore and strengthen their own motivation rather than telling them what they should be doing in the interests of their health.

Guiding principles of MI

MI has four guiding principles arranged into the acronym RULE (Rollnick et al. 2008):

- **R**esist the righting reflex – people in the helping professions often want to make things right for people, to cure them or to alleviate the pain and troubles they experience. When faced with an individual who is engaged in personally damaging behaviour we may therefore want to rush in and advise them of the need to change. While this is an understandable tendency it can have a paradoxical effect. If someone senses that their personal autonomy is under threat when asked to stop doing something they will often voice reasons why it is all right to continue the behaviour – i.e. to express the side of the argument that preserves their autonomy. This is known as 'psychological reactance' or resistance and is something that MI counsellors aim to avoid. They suppress what may seem like the obvious thing to do in the first instance and thereby resist the righting reflex.

- **U**nderstand the motivations of service users – MI places considerable emphasis on understanding service users' concerns, values and motivations since it is their reasons rather than those of staff that are most likely to trigger and sustain behaviour change. So, rather than simply telling a service user what changes they need to make an experienced MI counsellor would explore why a service user wanted to make a change and how they might go about achieving the change. Remember, it is the service user and not staff who should be voicing any arguments for change.

- **L**isten to service users – if we are to understand the motivations of service users it follows that we need to listen to them carefully. This is an active process in which MI counsellors reflect back what they think they have heard in order to check for understanding and to convey empathy. The development of empathy through active listening is considered critical for the success of MI (Miller and Rollnick 2002). This stands in contrast to the development of resistance in service users by telling them what they should be doing.

- **E**mpower service users – making a decision to change is quite different from taking action to change. MI counsellors therefore work with service users to explore *how* they can achieve the change they have decided is important to them. For example, if a service user is committed to the idea of taking up exercise an MI counsellor will explore with them all the resources they have at their disposal to make this possible. While we might all agree that exercise is important for health it is only the service user who knows how best to build exercise into their lives (Rollnick *et al.* 2008).

By following these guiding principles and enacting the spirit of MI in discussions with service users it is possible to enhance their commitment to behaviour and/or lifestyle change. The workings of this mechanism depend on the concept of ambivalence.

Ambivalence

It is not unusual for people to feel ambivalent about making changes even when those changes are likely to be good for them. Human beings are creatures of habit and the status quo is often much more appealing than an alternative that requires effort. We can all think of examples in our own lives where we feel ambivalent about changes that we know at some level are good for us (e.g. exercising, nutritious diets, quitting smoking, taking more time to relax). We certainly know the good reasons for changing but we're often more comfortable with how things are, and the users of mental health services are no different.

It is common for people to experience conflicting motivations simultaneously – i.e. to want and not want something. It is possible also for people to get stuck in ambivalence, which is often experienced as first thinking of a reason to change, then thinking of a reason not to change, and then to stop thinking about it altogether (Rollnick *et al.* 2008). Each side of the argument literally cancels out the other.

Ambivalence is presented in Figure 23.2 as a decisional balance that has arguments for and against change at its ends and a centre point that represents the status quo. It is possible for people to move towards or away from change and this can be influenced by many things including the contact people have with health care practitioners.

MI is therefore a style or approach to counselling that helps people talk about and resolve their ambivalence towards behaviour change, drawing on their own motivations and energy to achieve their goals. It avoids telling people what they should do in order to minimize the resistance that develops as people generate arguments against change to preserve their own autonomy. The principle task of an MI counsellor is to evoke reasons and motiva-

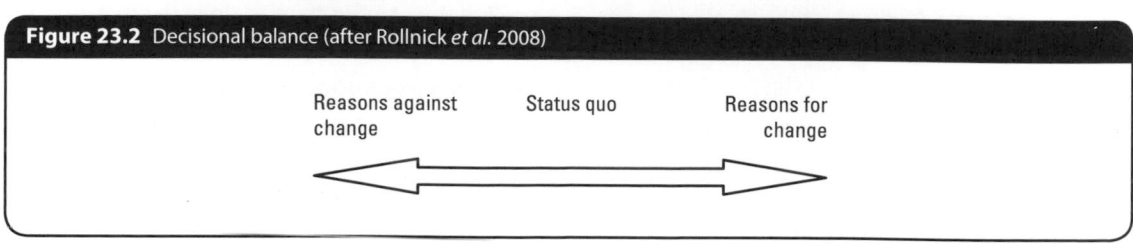

Figure 23.2 Decisional balance (after Rollnick *et al.* 2008)

Reasons against change   Status quo   Reasons for change

tions for change from service users while avoiding the development of resistance.

23.4 The practice of MI

Although experienced motivational counsellors use a wide range of techniques and strategies in their work, the basics of the approach are fairly simple. They were alluded to in the previous section of this chapter – interpersonal techniques familiar to all nurses and evoking reasons for change through the use of those techniques. This section deals with both. The former is referred to as core skills and the latter as change talk.

Core skills

The practice of MI utilizes three basic communication skills: asking, listening and informing. These will be familiar to most readers and are used in the everyday practice of mental health nursing. They reflect the core skills that MI counsellors implement following the style and guiding principles of the approach. Each is elaborated in more detail below.

- **Asking:** we ask questions to develop an understanding of a service user's context and the difficulties or challenges they face. Open questions are used for this purpose, which invite descriptive responses, rather than closed questions that invite simple yes/no responses (see Chapter 21). Open questions can be used to invite description of the experience of a problem, to clarify its extent and to provide detail on how it may have arisen in the first place. The aim is to facilitate as much sharing of knowledge as possible by the service user in order that we can understand something of their circumstances and their motivation for change. Here are some examples of opening questions:
  - May I ask you what concerns you most about your symptoms/the difficulties you face?
  - Tell me more about that experience.
  - Can I ask you to tell me some more about this particular difficulty, what actually happens to you when it occurs?

In addition to these fairly general open questions MI counsellors use more specific lines of questioning (e.g. exploring the pros and cons of a particular behaviour). The service user would be asked what is good about the way things are, followed by what's not so good. These lines of questioning facilitate direct exploration of the service user's ambivalence. Once voiced the MI counsellor would usually summarize to check they have understood correctly and offer another open question after the summary: 'So, where does this leave you now?'

- **Listening:** if we are to really understand service users' circumstances and their motivations for change, while also avoiding any resistance to change, then we need to be effective listeners. For these reasons active listening is often referred to as the core skill of MI (Miller and Rollnick 2002). Delivered effectively active listening communicates a sense that you are interested in understanding the service user, that what they have to say is important to you and that you want to hear more. It is the recognition and understanding of someone's experience by another person through attentive reflective listening that allows accurate empathy to develop. The generation of accurate empathy avoids the development of resistance in service users. This is considered critical to the efficacy of MI (Miller and Rollnick 2002). Readers are referred to Chapter 21 for more detail on listening skills.

- **Informing:** informing is used to convey information to a service user about their condition. MI counsellors use this skill very carefully. If a consultation weighs too heavily in terms of informing over asking and listening then the service user is likely to exhibit some resistance – i.e. they will voice the alternative side of the argument to that which the information points to. Typically an MI counsellor will undertake lots of open-ended asking and listening before informing. Even then they may ask permission to share information (e.g.

'Given what you have told me there is some information I'd like to share with you about the condition you describe – would that be OK?')

Although there is nothing particularly special about these core skills, MI counsellors use them in very specific ways, following the spirit and guiding principles of MI, and also for eliciting 'change talk' from service users.

Change talk

As already stated the principle tasks of an MI counsellor are to evoke reasons and motivations for change from service users while avoiding the development of resistance. This is important in terms of the decisional balance outlined in Figure 23.2. Evoking service users' own motivations is likely to tip the balance in favour of change. One technique MI counsellors use for this purpose is to listen reflectively to the service user's own change talk.

MI refers to six different themes or types of change talk (Rollnick *et al.* 2008):

- **Desire:** statements about preferences for change (e.g. 'I want to, wish, like to … ')
- **Ability:** statements about capability to make changes (e.g. 'I could, can, might be able to … ')
- **Reasons:** specific arguments or reasons for change (e.g. 'I would probably feel better if I … ')
- **Need:** statements about feeling obliged to change, out of necessity (e.g. 'I must, should, have got to … ')
- **Commitment:** statements about the likelihood of change (e.g. 'I am going to, I will, I intend to … ')

- **Taking steps:** statements about action taken (e.g. 'I tried a couple of days without smoking, I bought some healthy food … ')

Notice that the first four themes, spelt out by the acronym DARN, do not involve commitment to change or any associated actions. By themselves they do not trigger behaviour change but they are necessary precursors to action. DARN change talk indicates that the service user is in the contemplation stage of DiClemente and Prochaska's (2004) cycle of change (see Figure 23.1), while commitment and taking steps talk indicates they are in the determination and action stages.

If a service user is not particularly forthcoming with any change talk it is possible to probe for it by asking for DARN questions. For example:

- Why would you want to cut down on the hours you work? *(desire)*
- How would you go about reducing your hours if you decided to? *(ability)*
- What for you are the three best reasons for cutting down your work hours? *(reasons)*
- How important is it for you to cut down? *(need)*

It is less important to be able to accurately classify change talk than it is to recognize it, whatever its type, and affirm it with service users. An MI counsellor's task is really to collect change talk, reflecting it back, periodically reviewing it and adding to it. One analogy is to see each piece of change talk as a little weight that is being added to the pro side of the decisional balance (Figure 23.2). Over time this will gradually tip the balance in favour of change.

Case Study

Tom

As you read through this account of the CPN's meeting with Tom you can review any notes you made in response to the questions that accompanied the initial case study. Although Tom's CPN (Gisha) had been asked to encourage Tom to re-engage with support, she felt uncertain about this approach. The more staff had encouraged him in the last six months the more he withdrew. Gisha also knew that Tom was in some ways dissatisfied with his present situation, being isolated and often feeling bored. Gisha felt that a more valuable approach would be to explore Tom's feelings about these circumstances; on the one hand feeling bored and on the other rejecting the type of support that would connect him to people as well as provide meaningful activity. Gisha therefore decided that the purpose of her 20-minute contact with Tom would be to explore his ambivalence towards the proposed changes in his life. Twenty minutes is not long but Gisha knew she could make a difference if she focused on asking about and listening to Tom's experiences. She expected to hear some of Tom's own reasons for engaging with the changes as part of this process and she intended to focus on these a little more and reflect them back to him. If it felt appropriate she would then inform him of the benefits of the employment support scheme.

GISHA: Hello Tom. I know you've been working for some time now with a number of staff and were aiming to get out more and to spend less time on your own. I wanted to catch up with you about these opportunities. What would be most useful to discuss today? Where would you like to start? *(asking)*

TOM: I mostly feel depressed and haven't really got very far.

GISHA: Depressed you say? *(reflective listening)*

TOM: Well, maybe not in the sense you'd understand … you know, not as bad as really ill people but all the pressure I've been under has taken its toll.

GISHA: You feel run down by recent events? *(reflective listening)*

TOM: Yes, that's a good way of describing it, run down, that's how I feel, no gas in the tank most of the time.

GISHA: This feeling, it's with you most of the time but not always? *(reflective listening)* Can you say a little more about that? *(asking)*

TOM: Well, it's always there when I wake up and getting going is hard at the start of the day. But then … depending on what the day holds … I can forget myself and my troubles seem to lift.

GISHA: So, some parts of some days are better than others *(reflective listening)*. Can I ask what's actually happening to you to at these times to make such a difference? *(asking)*

TOM: Doing something I enjoy, like being with friends. When I'm occupied life seems OK and I feel safe. When it's just me and my head I feel very different … frightened even … empty, no energy … depressed I guess.

GISHA: OK, this seems important. Let me just check I understand. You feel down, empty and low quite a lot of the time, particularly every morning but you've also noticed times when these feelings aren't with you, like when you're with friends or doing something else you enjoy. *(reflective listening)* Is this right, have I understood you correctly? *(asking)*

TOM: Yes, that's it … do you think there is any hope for me?

GISHA: It sounds as if you'd like to change some of these experiences. *(reflective listening)* Can I ask how important it is for you to make some changes? *(asking for a DARN statement)*

TOM: Well … I've got to do something, *(need)* this can't go on.

GISHA: OK, that seems to make sense but can you help me understand a little more? What are your main reasons for wanting to change? *(asking for a DARN statement)*

TOM: Well … as we've just said I can sometimes forget my worries when I'm doing things I enjoy so I'd probably feel better if I had more to do. *(reason)*

GISHA: So how might you go about doing more things if you decided to make that change? *(asking for a DARN statement)*

TOM: I don't know.

GISHA: OK, fair enough Tom, sometimes it can be hard to find solutions to the difficulties we face. I don't know if this will make sense to you or not but I'd like to share an idea with you if that's OK?

TOM: Go on then.

GISHA: Well, on the one hand you're mood is often low and that's something to do with being on your own, being in your own head and not having things to do. On the other hand when you are doing things you enjoy you feel very different and your low mood lifts. You feel you've got to do something about this and realize that you'd probably feel better if you had more to do. *(reflective listening)* My idea is to do with the employment support scheme you've had contact with in the past. Meaningful employment makes a big difference to lots of people's lives. They make friends, have company through the day and often feel a sense of satisfaction for the work they do. *(informing)* It's just an idea Tom, what do you think? *(asking)*

TOM: You mean start attending the scheme again?

GISHA: That's certainly one possibility but I'm really interested in what you think about the general idea of structuring your day to have more contact with other people. *(asking)*

TOM: Well it does make sense but it would also be a big step.

GISHA: Yes it would and I understand that you'd need to think carefully about it. I don't think you should make a decision right now but I'd like to come back at the end of the week to pick up this discussion again. Would that be OK?

TOM: Sure … I'll try to give it some thought before then.

Gisha did not expect this session alone to make a difference but she did feel that, over time, if this style of interaction was maintained, then Tom's decisional balance might tip in favour of making some changes in his life. In fact Tom never did return to the employment support scheme but after a few months of ongoing work with Gisha he became interested in volunteering as an expert patient in local mental health services. Tom has now been trained for this role and has significantly extended his circle of contacts and has made several new friends. It is still early days but Tom is gradually finding his own path, supported by a new understanding of the pros and cons of change and fired by his own motivation to make a difference to his life.

23.5 Conclusion

This chapter has introduced the practice of motivational interviewing as a style of counselling to help people talk about and resolve their ambivalence towards behaviour change, drawing on their own motivations and energy to achieve their goals. This is a valuable counselling strategy for mental health nurses who have many discussions with service users about behaviour change as part of their everyday work. While most mental health nurses have neither the need nor inclination to become qualified MI counsellors it is possible to develop relevant skills based on the MI approach. In summary, the main points from this chapter are:

- People pass through different stages in the process of changing a behaviour from pre-contemplation to maintenance of any change.

- A person's motivation for change varies across and during the different stages of change.

- The malleable nature of people's motivation occurs within the context of relationships.

- Mental health nurses, through their contact with service users, can do much to influence motivation.

- The spirit of motivational interviewing is collaborative, evocative and honours patient autonomy by following four guiding principles: Resist the righting reflex; Understand the motivations of service users; Listen to service users, and; Empower service users (RULE).

- The practice of MI uses three core communication skills familiar to mental health nurses: asking, listening and informing.

- These skills are used to evoke change talk from service users (desire, ability, reasons, need, commitment and taking steps).

- If you hear change talk from a service user then you are practising the approach correctly.

- If you find yourself arguing for change and the service user defends the status quo, then you are off course. When service users voice arguments against change they are literally talking themselves out of changing.

- The key task of a MI counsellor is therefore to elicit change talk rather than resistance from service users.

Annotated bibliography

Arkowitz, H., Westra, H., Miller, W., and Rollnick, S. (2008) *Motivational Interviewing in The Treatment of Psychological Problems.* New York: Guilford Press.
In this text expert practitioners provide a step-by-step guide to MI with people who have a wide range of mental health problems. Vignettes and dialogues illustrate how to manage various scenarios with skill and sensitivity.

Miller, W. and Rollnick, S. (2002) *Motivational Interviewing: Preparing people to change addictive behaviour*, 2nd edn. New York: Guilford Press.
This text is written by the originators of motivational interviewing and is now in its second edition. Arguably the most detailed and expert text available, as well as outlining the methods and practice of MI the book includes a number of chapters from guest contributors who use MI across a variety of health and social care settings.

DiClemente, C. and Prochaska, J. (2004) Towards a comprehensive, transtheoretical model of change: stages of change and addictive behaviours, in W. Miller and N. Heather (eds) *Treating Addictive Behaviours*, 2nd edn. New York: Plenum.
Organized around the stages of change described in Prochaska and DiClemente's cycle of change model, this new edition provides practical, up-to-date strategies for the treatment of addictions and compulsive behaviours.

Rollnick, S., Miller, W. and Butler, C. (2008) *Motivational Interviewing in Health Care.* **New York: Guilford Press.**
This more recent update of Miller and Rollnick's original work provides a concise account of the MI style and its methods. It provides many dialogues and vignettes that bring to life the core skills of MI and how they can be incorporated into any health care setting.

References

DiClemente, C. and Prochaska, J. (2004) Towards a comprehensive, transtheoretical model of change: stages of change and addictive behaviours, in W. Miller and N. Heather (eds) *Treating Addictive Behaviours*, 2nd edn. New York: Plenum.
Miller, W. and Rollnick, S. (2002) *Motivational Interviewing: Preparing people to change addictive behaviour*, 2nd edn. New York: Guilford Press.
Rollnick, S., Miller, W. and Butler, C. (2008) *Motivational Interviewing in Health Care.* New York: Guilford Press.

Chapter 24

Working with Groups

Julie Dilallo and Jane Padmore

 ## 24.1 Introduction

People exist in groups and are shaped by them. In most instances people have learned how to behave, how to relate to others, developed ideas about self-worth, learned morals and consequences from those in their primary group – the family. Social learning extends also into schools, employment and among other groups that inform and change people's lives. It can be argued that it is the disease of these social relationships that is central to mental health difficulties. Faulkner and Layzell (2000) found that when service users were asked what had been most helpful to their recovery, relationships with others was at the top of their list. The use of groups as a medium for therapeutic change is considered in this chapter, which covers:

- a historical introduction to group therapy;
- defining a group;
- rationale for group work;
- types of group;
- research and evidence base for practice;
- setting up and facilitating a group;
- stages of group development and leadership.

 ## 24.2 A historical introduction to group therapy

Early thinkers in psychoanalysis such as Freud and Jung, writing in the late 1890s to early 1900s, focused on the internal world of individuals and the unconscious drives that might explain behaviour and mental ill health. Alfred Adler, a colleague of Freud, believed that a patient could not be seen as existing in isolation and introduced the idea of inviting the patient's family and wider contacts into therapeutic encounters.

Social psychologists, such as Kurt Lewin, similarly challenged the individual drive theorists, suggesting that an individual is greatly affected by the dynamic environment in which they live. Lewin developed field theory in his extensive work on attempting to scientifically examine group behaviours and dynamics. Much later in the 1930s, Jacob Moreno began using group interaction in his work with prison populations. Most famous as the founding father of psychodrama, he is credited with the first use of the terms 'group therapy' and 'group psychotherapy' (Ozarin 2003).

Group analysis, described by Foulkes (1964), focuses on the space between individuals; the communication between the members, aiming to deepen their insight into their own selves with a constant pressure to adapt and change towards greater maturity. Post World War II, in the UK, Wilfred Bion (1961) developed the group as a whole model. His work most notably studied the defences which groups employ, which he called 'basic assumptions', and illuminates group dynamics. It is most widely used in understanding organizations, their defences and team dynamics rather than as a therapeutic intervention per se.

Following the army's so-called Northfield Experiments during World War II, Therapeutic Communities were developed by Maxwell Jones, from 1947, and Tom Main, from 1946. They promote user empowerment to actively share responsibility for their own and each other's recovery. Studies have found that this approach to treatment is successful in substantially improving the quality of life for members. Readmission and reconviction rates have been found to drop considerably after treatment in a therapeutic community (Rethink 2011).

In present-day mental health services, group interventions are used in creative ways. Long- and short-term psychotherapy groups are offered for a range of presenting issues. Group therapists and some clinicians also combine group work with other modalities such as cognitive behavioural therapy (CBT), dialectic behavioural therapy (DBT) and psycho-education. This uses group analytic theory to assist facilitators from these various modalities to better understand and work with the group dynamics that are inevitably present.

Many clinical areas offer staff support groups to assist practitioners in their own understanding of difficult feelings that can be evoked when working with particular client groups. These are not therapy groups, instead they 'provide an opportunity for team members to reflect more openly on various aspects of their work' (Novakovic 2002).

24.3 Defining a group

Benson (2000) presents the key characteristics that define a group (see Box 24.1). Groups have bounda-

> ### Box 24.1 Definition of a group (Benson 2000)
>
> - A set of people who engage in frequent interactions
> - They identify with one another
> - They are defined by others as a group
> - They share beliefs, values and norms about areas of common interest
> - They define themselves as a group
> - They come together to work on common tasks and for agreed purposes
> - Groups are intended and organic rather than random experiences. As a result they have three crucial characteristics:
>   - There are parts
>   - There is relationship between the parts
>   - There is an organizing principle

ries, most obviously those who belong and those who do not. There are also rules that represent boundaries such as no mobile phone use, no foul language and the group starting and ending on time. These are usually given by the facilitator and are non-negotiable. There are also group-owned ground rules, often discussed in the first meeting and essential for members to develop a sense of safety. Examples include agreeing that no one leaves mid-session, or that people don't interrupt each other. Other rules are far less obvious, being implicit and slower to form. These are referred to as *group norms*.

Group norms

Norms are a set of agreed acceptable behaviours to which the group subscribes, and which develop over time. A group may develop a norm of avoiding anger or having a particular viewpoint on a given topic. Norms can be helpful in maintaining a sense of stability and predictability in the group. There is some security in knowing what might occur and what is acceptable. Norms may also be unhelpful in limiting the ability of the group to make use of material. They are usually unspoken and hence it is often difficult for new members joining to initially feel part of the group. There is variability in how strongly norms are enforced, depending on their importance to the group and some may apply to some members more than others (Stock Whitaker 1994).

Groups usually have sanctions for what is seen to be deviating from the norms. Strong reactions can be evoked, including negative evaluations and derogation by other group members (Frings *et al.* 2010). Members who are in a minority by virtue of culture, race, sexual orientation or gender may have experiences and attitudes that differ from the group norm. This may lead to increased stigmatization and negativity, both of which may serve to marginalize minority group members (Marques *et al.* 2001).

A key role for a facilitator is to pay attention to the development of norming behaviour in the early stages of group development. Supporting the group to attend to norms which restrict creativity and communication can facilitate their willingness to experiment with reflection and cognitive reframing. This could include acceptance of the minority view (Frings *et al.* 2010).

24.4 Rationale for group work

In the National Health Service (NHS), schools, prisons and many other facilities, groups are offered as a therapeutic medium, often with combined therapies, such as with CBT, family therapy, DBT and psycho-education. For any work using groups as a modality there are common therapeutic benefits.

Yalom (1985), in his seminal work on group psychotherapy, suggested that therapeutic change is an enormously complex process and occurs through an intricate interplay of various guided human experiences, which he refers to as 'therapeutic factors' (see Box 24.2).

Box 24.2 Therapeutic factors

- **Instillation of hope:** clients need to have belief in therapy working, the possibility of change. Alcoholics Anonymous (AA) uses the testimony of members at each meeting to give hope to others. In eating disorder groups, 'graduate families' meet new members to share their experience of combating the illness.

- **Universality:** many clients feel isolated by their life experiences, and may feel shame. Secrecy may have been a part of their family history (e.g. in abuse, or part of maintaining the problem such as eating disorders). Hearing others speak of similar issues can offer enormous relief.

- **Imparting of information:** both from the therapist (e.g. psycho-education groups) and from other members, who may offer information that helps others in understanding or tackling their difficulty.

- **Altruism:** clients may feel worthless or burdensome to others, but in a group have the opportunity to experience the gift of giving of themselves to help others. Clients may have become overly self-focused, and the group can help to reawaken interest in the other.

- **The corrective recapitulation of the primary family group:** members will enact their family script or position in a group (e.g. dependence on a leader or sibling rivalries). Therapy groups offer the possibility of exploring these in the here and now and experimenting with new ways of being.

- **Imitative behaviour:** clients may experiment with change and new ways of being by imitating the behaviour of others, including the facilitator.

- **Interpersonal learning:** the process of reflecting on how one is received by others in order to have more satisfying relationships.

- **Group cohesiveness:** the sense of 'we-ness', feeling accepted and approved of by the group. This sense can fluctuate at different stages of the group. Groups with high cohesiveness tend to adhere to boundaries, have sustained attendance and can tolerate a greater range of expression.
- **Development of socializing techniques:** this might occur formally, such as social skills training groups where members may role-play interactions. In any group, members may over time develop skills in giving and receiving feedback on their social interactions such as eye contact, personal boundaries, communication and listening.
- **Catharsis:** being able to 'get things off your chest' and expressing feelings.
- **Existential factors:** recognizing the mortality of life and the need to take responsibility for how individual lives are lived.

24.5 Types of group

Therapeutic groups can be grouped broadly into three types:

- **Structured groups:** typically these are skills training groups where members attend primarily to learn a prescribed set of skills such as CBT groups for anxiety management or parenting skills. Content is the major focus of this mode of working.
- **Unstructured groups:** such as analytic psychotherapy groups, prioritize the relating aspects. The unconscious processes are given greatest consideration in this mode of group work.

- **Self-help groups:** such as AA and the Hearing Voices Network. The social and supportive functions of the group is perhaps most dominant in this mode.

Membership is either *homogenous* (i.e. where members attend due to a commonality, such as alcohol misuse) or, as in the case of psychotherapy groups, a *heterogeneous* membership is sought, the intention being to select members for their differences. In such work contact outside the group is actively discouraged.

All groups have both a conscious and an unconscious life. What a facilitator chooses to attend to will depend upon their training and upon the purpose and nature of the group.

Thinking Space 24.1

Make a list of the various groups that you have encountered in your nursing practice.

- What types of group were they?
- Why was a group being used and how had it formed?
- What makes it a group rather than a collection of individuals?
- What are the rules?
- How is membership defined?
- Is it homogenous or heterogeneous?
- What are the norms of behaviour?
- How does membership of the group influence your and others' behaviour?

- What influences do you bring to bear on the group?
- Why was a group being used?

To help you think about some of these questions you might consider therapy groups in different treatment settings, inpatient and outpatient. Alternatively, reflect on groups in the staff and student domains. Thinking about colleagues as group members will help you recognize some of the behaviours, attitudes or expectations of group membership. Be curious also about positions in a group determined by individuals' histories, their personalities or hierarchical positions.

24.6 Research and evidence base for practice

Group work, which is structured and homogenous, and is combined with other therapies, such as CBT in the case of treating anxiety or depression, has robust supporting evidence from randomized controlled trials (RCTs).

For unstructured groups, with heterogeneous membership, where the focus is on the relationship and changes in interpersonal dynamics, effectiveness is much harder to measure and RCTs have yet to be conducted systematically. In this section, consideration is given to National Institute for Health and Clinical Excellence (NICE) recommendations for group work as well as other studies on the efficacy of groups.

Emotional disorders

Therapeutic groups for service users with emotional disorders have been shown to be effective. These studies have included a CBT group for older adults with depression (Welch *et al.* 2010), a multi-family psycho-educational psychotherapy group for children aged 8 to 12 years with major mood disorders (Fristad *et al.* 2009) and a structured programme followed by unstructured psychotherapy group experience to develop interpersonal skills that lead to a decrease in self-harm activity (Wood *et al.* 2001).

Personality disorder

NICE (2009a) recommends psycho-education be included in therapeutic work with clients who have

a borderline personality disorder. This can be delivered in short term groups. Barlow *et al.* (1997) suggest that these groups offer a cognitive component for new learning as well as creating momentum for change. Jacob *et al.* (2010) developed an enhance self-esteem in patients with borderline personality disorder group therapy module. Results showed a greater improvement in self-esteem in the intervention group. The findings suggest that the therapy module is an effective adjunctive treatment to help increase self-esteem for these service users.

Attention deficit hyperactivity disorder

NICE (2009b) guidance suggests group-based parent-training/education programmes should be offered to patients with attention deficit hyperactivity disorder (ADHD). Also group treatment for the young person that includes CBT and/or social skills training. This should target a range of areas known to be problematic including social skills with peers, problem-solving, self-control, listening skills, and dealing with and expressing feelings. Such group interventions are not only time efficient and educative but parents report positively on the opportunity to meet 'graduate families', hearing that they are not alone, sharing experiences, ideas and resources, and supporting each other through 'tough days'.

Obsessive compulsive disorder and body dysmorphic disorder

Nice (2005) recommends health care professionals should consider informing people with obsessive compulsive disorder (OCD) or body dysmorphic disorder (BDD) and their family or carers about local self-help and support groups, and encourage them to participate in such groups where appropriate.

Bipolar disorder

In a systematic review and meta-analysis of the efficacy of psychological therapies in bipolar disorder, including their impact in terms of an individual's previous number of illness episodes, Lam *et al.* (2009) found that 'Psychological therapy specifically designed for bipolar disorder is effective in preventing or delaying relapses in bipolar disorders, and there is no clear evidence that the number of previous episodes moderated the effect'. There is however limited evidence for the effectiveness of group therapy for bipolar disorder. Nevertheless, psycho-education is indicated in the NICE (2006) clinical guidance, which suggests groups can be an effective method for delivering this component of care.

Psychosis

There is little evidence as yet for the efficacy of group interventions for psychosis. However, in a review of the literature on the support mental health nurses can deliver to carers of clients diagnosed with schizophrenia, Macleod *et al.* (2011) found that there is some evidence that mutual support groups reduce burden and improve coping.

Substance misuse

NICE (2011) guidance for psychosis with coexisting substance misuse recommends that professionals advise families on local support groups and voluntary organizations and assist them to access these. NICE (2007) guidance for reducing substance misuse among young people recommends group-based behavioural therapy focusing on coping mechanisms, such as distraction and relaxation techniques to help develop the child's organiza-

tional, study and problem-solving skills, involving goal-setting. For parents, the group work should focus on stress management, communication skills and how to help develop the child's social-cognitive and problem-solving skills as well as advice on how to set targets for behaviour and establish age-related rules and expectations for their children.

Group work with children and young people

Children and young people can benefit from a group invention through the same therapeutic factors as described above by Yalom. There are two main theoretical orientations of group therapy offered to young people: psychodynamic or behavioural/cognitive (Reid and Kolvin 1993). Groups are offered for a range of presentations including behavioural problems, peer group difficulties and sexual abuse. Groups might be heterogeneous or homogenous depending on the clinical need, evidence and preference of the facilitators.

When conducting groups for young people additional considerations are necessary. The facilitator must be trained in understanding young people's developmental stages and their needs, and have expertise in communication with children. A particular consideration is the age range of members. In general terms young children from 5–11 years are worked with separately from older children of secondary school age. The former may work more readily with play, while the latter will manage communication through talking.

Facilitators are generally more active in establishing and holding the safety of group boundaries in comparison to adult groups, and dependency is an age appropriate need for a child when relating to an adult facilitator. Reid and Kolvin (1993) summarize by stating that 'When the boundaries of the room are firmly kept to and the adults also contain the group firmly in mind, then it is possible to allow considerable freedom of behavior, wishes, and impulses within this framework. Without this structure the therapy cannot take place'.

24.7 Setting up and facilitating a group

Before a group begins

Arguably the most important work in the life of a group takes place before anyone sits in the room. The importance of this phase is often overlooked when facilitators rush ahead, filled with enthusiasm and excitement. However, in order to have a successful experience the group needs to begin life in the facilitator's mind, and be cared for from inception to its delivery.

Foulkes (1964) coined the term 'dynamic administration' for the responsibilities and considerations the facilitator has for the creation and maintenance of the group. Creating the group boundary is essential in promoting a sense of safety in a group, a sense of being held, which will offer the possibility of thinking, creativity, honest communication and exploration.

The physical boundary is a symbol for the psychological boundary. A group where members feel safe in knowing where they will meet each week, who will be there and that it starts and ends on time is more likely to become a space where clients talk about their experience than one where people show up when they feel like it, or outsiders constantly interrupt the room. This physical boundary begins with the facilitator making decisions regarding type of group (slow, open, closed, time limited) the time, place and frequency, and the physical setting.

Case Study

Inpatient leaver's group

Mary is a staff nurse on an acute inpatient unit for adults. Through her interactions with clients, conversations with relatives and other staff members she notices that many clients have shared anxieties about being discharged from the unit, particularly those who have been hospitalized for some months. Mary decides that a leaver's group would be beneficial to clients to support and prepare them for discharge.

Informed by the Tidal Model (Barker and Buchanann-Barker 2005), Mary aims to promote a recovery ethos in the group. She aims to model enquiry among members searching for signs of resilience, hope, skills and the power to change. She decides to offer a small group on a weekly basis using psycho-education and a reflective space to talk about their experience and, through her modelling and shaping norms for the group, promote hopeful discourse. She proposes a group which allows clients to continue to attend for a limited period post-discharge.

Mary spends some time discussing the idea with the ward team. There is a mixed response with some resistance to the group. This seems linked to fears around offering something new, concerns about the leaving process changing and the time commitment needed. Mary works hard to share her ideas and the process of the group with her colleagues to gain their active support.

The inpatient leaver's group case study is referred to and developed in the pages that follow to demonstrate key points, beginning with dynamic administration tasks.

Type of group

An open group is one which allows anyone to attend with no real expectation of commitment. This would not be suitable in this case, as the leaver's group needs to have cohesion if members are to feel safe enough to share their experiences and to question or challenge each other. Closed groups are typically time-limited with a planned ending date and are structured, with specific content (e.g. CBT groups). Slow open groups tend to run for a fairly lengthy period and in so doing can afford to allow members to leave after an agreed period of time and for new members to join. This creates an overlap of new with longer-standing members.

Case Study

Mary opts to use a slow open format and an unstructured approach, with a heterogeneous membership. The group will firstly be established with a closed membership for a decided period of time, allowing a core to form, thus increasing the likelihood of the group's survival through the uncertain times of new members joining later on. In discussion with her team, Mary considers what might be an appropriate agreed maximum length of time for group membership. It is decided that it would be up to three months post-discharge. Mary aims to run the group for a period of one year which is agreed with her manager, thus she plans to stop inviting any new members after nine months as there will be insufficient time to offer three-month post-discharge support after this point.

Frequency and length of each group meeting

The frequency of a group has different effects on its members. In deciding how often to meet one must think about dependence on the group versus the need to engage in life outside of it. Analytic groups can meet two or three times weekly to intensify the experience for members. By contrast support groups may meet fortnightly.

Case Study

Mary decides a weekly group is most suitable and fits with her availability. The group will run for one and a quarter hours, which is deemed to be a manageable period of time for clients who may still be struggling with symptoms and concentration to varying degrees, while allowing sufficient time for meaningful work to take place.

Location

The location for the group needs to be easily accessible to the population and must be protected from intrusions including noise. There must be enough space to comfortably seat everyone in chairs of the same height, in a circle where they can see each other. The room must be available each week at the required time for the required duration of the group's life.

For Mary's group, discussions would be required with the ward team to agree that clients can return to the unit after discharge to attend the group. If not, the group may need to find a venue in another part of the hospital that can allow both in- and outpatients to attend.

Ethical issues

In order to be certain that the intervention offered best meets the needs of the clients and the work is conducted in an open and safe manner, a group protocol or terms of reference is required. These clearly outline the group's aims and objectives, interventions used, responsibilities of those involved, how to refer, how discharges or non-attendance are to be communicated and recording of material in clients' records. Facilitators may choose to produce a leaflet for clients and referrers that sets out these issues clearly.

Clients should be able to consent to treatment and be made aware of their right to leave if they so wish. In addition, confidentiality should be discussed in the interview stages, reinforcing that sensitive material, discussed within the group, must remain confidential to the members. For longer term psychotherapy groups, contact with members outside the meetings is discouraged. For shorter groups and other modalities the facilitator may request that outside contact is discussed with members in the next session (Mackenzie 1997).

Issues of risk and how this will be managed as well as general information-sharing with other agencies and clinical team members needs to be transparent before the group begins and may need to be repeated at times throughout the group's life span. Facilitators must be aware of destructive forces such as scapegoating, rejection and hostility that can come alive in sessions as well as premature over-disclosure from vulnerable clients in early sessions and how to manage this.

Facilitators may agree to write to referrers after the interview indicating the outcome as well as detailing what the group entails and when it will start. There may be periodic review letters and attendance at Care Programme Approach (CPA) meetings as well as a final review meeting. Details of what is included or shared outside the group can be negotiated with the clients.

Clinical record-keeping should adhere to the policy of the host organization. There needs to be a specific, agreed protocol for writing and keeping group session notes. Knauss (2006) recommends that notes be written in factual terms and related to client problems rather than opinions. Gutheil (1980) advocates recording therapist interventions and the rationale. When recording the session, no other member of the group should be named in another client's clinical records as this breaches third-party confidentiality.

Therapists may wish to make separate process and content notes. Content notes involve the spoken exchanges in the session whereas process notes are everything else including non-verbal communi-

cation, themes and dominance, which is useful material to discuss in supervision.

Group facilitation

When starting out in group work it is advisable for the facilitator to select a client group within their remit of expertise and confidence. The nurse should also consider co-facilitation with a more experienced colleague. The co-conductor relationship needs to be carefully developed by considering the following:

- Is there a joint understanding of what is being offered?
- Is there respect for each other's position and contribution to the work?
- How will the work be divided (e.g. setting up the room, writing notes)?
- Are there predetermined roles such as who presents a topic?

For some groups, where there are perceived safety risks, several facilitators may be required. This was the case in a group for young people with ADHD and anger management issues where it was agreed that there would be three facilitators. This allowed young people to leave the room, with an escort, if they became overwhelmed, while leaving the group with two facilitators in the room.

When conducting a group alone the clinician has the disadvantage of having one single perspective on events. With more than one, colleagues will often pick up on events and meaning missed by others, or offer different perspectives on a group event. Facilitators will need to discuss whether or not to conduct the groups alone in the event of sickness or annual leave, and how this will be managed or reported in the group. For longer-term group interventions, planned breaks are advisable with ample notice given.

Supervision

In order to safely run a group and make best use of material brought by members, even where this is in combination with therapies such as CBT, supervision should be at least in part focused on the group dynamics and the responses of facilitators.

Conversations in supervision before starting a group can assist facilitators in clarifying their understanding of what their aims are and how they hope to achieve them. Having a 'holding mind' of a supervisor can also help to allay some of the inevitable anxiety facilitators will have on starting a new group. Specialist supervision from a group psychotherapist will inform facilitators' thinking regarding the dynamics and thus enable them to understand unconscious communications and how to respond. This can promote greater cohesion and deeper sharing and learning, unblocking areas of stuckness and improved attendance.

Selection of group members

Having decided on the purpose, type, frequency and location of the group, attention can turn to referrals and selection. Not everyone referred may be suitable, and not everyone suitable will be referred.

Firstly, the client needs to be able to communicate in the language of the group (although some groups do work via interpreters). The client must have a wish to engage in the work. It is perfectly acceptable for clients to have anxieties about the group, particularly if they have had no previous experience in groups or poor experiences of peer relationships such as bullying at school or in the workplace. Careful preparation of members, through an interview, will help determine reluctance due to uncertainty and anxiety as opposed to not wishing to join. An interview will also assist the facilitator to understand whether the client has sufficient strength to manage any potential challenges in a group. Careful consideration needs also to be given to:

■ Those who are acutely unwell, particularly those prone to feeling paranoid or persecuted. It is likely that they would not be able to join the group until they are more stable.

■ Intellectual impairment that would prevent the use of the therapy.

■ Those who present with a high level of restlessness or agitation.

■ Those with a potential for violent outbursts.

■ Those who are in crisis, such as very recent bereavement. Their current circumstances may not allow any mental energy for thinking of themselves in relation to others.

■ The mix of people who are group members. The facilitator must hold in mind a realistic view of how much the group is able to tolerate in terms of disturbance in any one member, particularly when selecting those who may have a personality disorder.

■ The client's presentation in terms of defences and social behaviour – for example, it would be advisable to avoid selecting eight members whose coping strategy is to remain silent. A selection of extroverts and introverts will give more scope to a group.

■ The cultural, socioeconomic and language diversity of their population, selecting sufficient numbers to ensure no one is isolated on any one dimension such as a single female or single black person, or an adolescent in an otherwise middle-aged group. Members are much more likely to stay in a group that they feel part of.

■ Confidentiality will be a serious concern for most group participants. In selecting members there may be a need to ensure they are not selected from the same housing estate, workplace or school. Rules around contact outside the group need to be clear; it may be that this is allowed and even encouraged in support groups, while in other groups it may be detrimental to the therapy. It is an issue for careful consideration as it can split the group into subgroups which work against the therapy, evoking feelings of exclusion, anger or rejection for those not included in outside meetings.

Pre-group interviews with clients provide an opportunity to:

■ Discuss the aims of the group.

■ Answer questions.

- Invite the client to think about how they wish to use the work.

- Explore ways to combat the initial anxiety in the first few sessions while the group is forming. This can include explanation of what to expect and asking them to think about themselves in the group, imagining how they might experience it and behave.

- Discuss the need for commitment to the group for a minimum period.

- Discuss 'giving notice' if they should decide to leave.

- Discuss expectations of work outside the group such as 'homework tasks' in combined therapy groups.

Case Study

Having discussed the group with the ward team and gained their support, Mary invites another nurse colleague, Jo, to join as co-facilitator. She has worked with Jo for some time and feels there is a good working relationship. They find a group psychotherapist to supervise them on a fortnightly basis.

A leaflet is produced which offers practical information on the group venue, times, aims and how to contact therapists. A protocol is written for the referring ward staff outlining issues of confidentiality, clinical record-keeping and risk management. The group is discussed as a standing item on the daily ward meeting agenda. Clients on the ward are able to self-refer or be supported in this by their key worker.

In supervision it is agreed that the group will initially start with a core of six to eight members and run for six weeks before new members are invited to join. A maximum membership of eight is agreed in order to encourage a level of intimacy. Mary and Jo set time aside over a two-week period to interview potential members once an agreed start date is identified. Six clients are selected as suitable for the group:

1. Carl, a 29-year-old white British man.
2. Amrit, a 45-year-old Pakistani man.
3. Samantha, a 40-year-old mother of two.
4. Leon, a 20-year-old Afro-Caribbean student.
5. Claire, a 31-year-old white British woman.
6. Diana, a 39-year-old Irish woman.

24.8 Stages of group development and leadership

In observing group behaviour it is helpful to have a theoretical framework to make some sense of what might be going on, whether or not and how to intervene. Having an understanding of the development of a group can assist the facilitator to identify problems as well as alleviate their own feelings of confusion and anxiety.

There are several theories which guide and inform, depending on theoretical affiliation and purpose of the group. One useful model is Tuckman (1965), who suggested that groups have predictable patterns of behaviour which he described as forming, storming, norming and performing. This is not to suggest that groups move smoothly from one stage to the next in a linear fashion – they may remain fixed at one stage for a period of time, and may move backwards as well as forwards in their journey.

Forming

This stage is characterized by anxiety, uncertainty and confusion. Members are preoccupied with 'working out' fellow members, rules, expectations and other issues. Members seek guidance from the facilitators and engage in 'social chatter', with some tentative self-disclosure. Bion (1961) described three basic assumptions or defences that groups use against anxiety: dependency, pairing and fight/flight. Dependency is perhaps most visible in this stage. Members look towards the facilitator to satisfy their needs, alternating between dependency and periods of flight. It is at this stage that the facilitator is active in shaping the norms as they develop, modelling a position of enquiry and fostering conditions for trust to build.

Case Study

In the first few sessions of the leaver's group, Mary and Jo were active in their roles, encouraging reflection on the experience of being in the group. Naming and sharing the anxieties this evoked seemed to alleviate some of the stress. Diana spoke of feeling better knowing that she wasn't the only one who had been dreading the first meeting and feared others would not like her.

Issues of difference dominated with discussions about age, diagnosis, the experience of being an inpatient and the relationship with mental health professionals being common topics of conversation. The facilitators encouraged everyone to speak during each session. Amrit found it less easy to join the conversation hence, in these early meetings, the facilitators would specifically ask him for his view and make links to the conversation.

The facilitators were alert to Samantha's tendency to dominate the conversation and perhaps to disclose too much too early, which can be a shaming experience and evoke anxiety in others. Mary and Jo validated what Samantha had said, drawing out themes and diverting to others with questions such as, 'Is that different to your experience Claire?'

Jo and Mary were alert to chatter about trivial matters that could be used to avoid real contact in the group. While recognizing the need for this at some level in this early stage, they remained alert for opportunities to bring the conversation back to the focus of members' interactions in the room.

The facilitators encouraged 'between members' dialogue, shaping the discourse away from direct questions and reliance on leaders. Carl opened a later group talking about his medication side-effects and various medications that he had taken in the past, and his frustration at not yet finding the right cure. Mary resisted 'expert position' by instead asking what others thought, drawing attention to similarities and differences in their experience. She reflected on the group's questioning of their dependence on medication alone to make a difference.

Storming

The feature of this stage appears to be the expression of strong feelings by the group members, defined by issues of power and control (Garland et al. 1973). Conflict and competition among members about issues of safety in the group, authority and the facilitator are common concerns.

Subgroups and hierarchies may form, confrontation with the facilitator is common and the facilitator must differentiate between an attack on themselves as a person and an attack on their role. A balance needs to be reached between healthy conflict, which is developmental, and scapegoating. Facilitators need to be prepared to intervene to protect the safety of an individual and the group.

This stage of conflict ultimately serves to increase cohesion, solidarity and openness in the group. The facilitator's task is to steer the group through this phase, encouraging interpersonal learning between members.

Case Study

After not attending one week Claire arrived late to the group, having been discharged from the ward. Leon accused the facilitators of not doing their job, and wondered why they were bothering to attend. Samantha answered a call on her mobile phone and said that she had to step outside to talk.

Mary reflected on what was happening in the room. She suggested that the group was struggling with the task of coming together and remaining in the room to do some useful work. They were struggling to establish the rules of play and their positions in the group. She commented on angry feelings towards facilitators not being able to 'make everything OK'.

Jo questioned whether it was all right to be upset, to be angry, and wondered how much emotion the group could tolerate and how they could work together. She asked the group to consider if it was the facilitators who should demand adherence to certain rules or whether it should be the group itself that takes responsibility for this. A conversation developed between members about attendance, and expectations in the room, with some disagreements, which the group seemed able to tolerate.

Norming

Having successfully negotiated a period of storming the group moves into a phase of greater intimacy and cohesiveness, with deepening trust. The group feels like a group, with behaviour and norms becoming more established. It is less reliant on the facilitators and more able to define problems and solutions. Members are increasingly able to offer feedback to each other and develop insight. A balance is achieved between support and challenge among group members.

Case Study

A conversation was under way between Diana and Carl. Claire started to cry. Leon became angry, accusing Claire of trying to grab attention through her lateness and her tears. The group seemed split in defending or being angry with Claire. Leon was encouraged to talk about his experience of Claire arriving late and her tears directly to her. He recognized that he found it hard to share feelings, tending to engage in more practical conversations, and he wasn't sure how to respond.

Performing

This stage is a sign of a mature group that engages in the real work. There is greater openness between members who are more skilled and able to work in the group, with little intervention from the facilitator. Individual differences can be appreciated and explored.

Case Study

The group challenged Leon about his need to be in control, either through his silence, which was experienced as dismissive, or through his outbursts, which led others to feel wary of him.

Ending

Each member will, at some point, have to work through the ending of their time in the group, or the ending of the group itself. Time is needed for clients to process this, which may evoke feelings of disappointment, despair, separation anxiety, rejection, sadness and anger, especially where the group has become an important source of support. The facilitator needs to be observant for signs of flight or denial regarding the reality of the ending, promoting expression of the true feelings and attending to any unfinished business.

Case Study

Leon decided to leave the group after three months in order to return to his university studies. Despite having announced this the previous week, the group had not mentioned it this week. Leon had two more session before ending.

Mary and Jo started the session by commenting on the news from the previous week regarding Leon's departure and noticing that it has not been talked about. They wondered what Leon made of this, inviting the group to talk about what it would be like for the first member to leave. Leon spoke of feeling unimportant as it had been ignored; he felt angry and disappointed in the group. He had considered not attending for his last session. This led to the exploration of how messages can be skewed in conversations and opportunities missed.

A mix of responses became apparent and could be processed together. Feelings of loss and abandonment, hope for the future, as well as envy about Leon no longer needing them or the group and having a bright future were expressed. Leon was encouraged by the group not to avoid saying goodbye but to have an experience of a healthy ending which he tended to avoid in relationships. He was offered feedback by Diana on how he had changed over the course of the group – initially defensive and at times arrogant in his manner, he had become more open to listening and valuing others and in turn this seemed to make him more approachable.

24.9 Conclusion

This chapter has highlighted the valuable contribution group work and group theories continue to play in modern-day mental health practice where social inclusion is paramount to recovery. Group work is diverse in its application, joining with other modalities, such as CBT, in delivering evidence-based treatments. Psychodynamic and analytic group therapies face a challenge in relation to developing a robust evidence base for effectiveness, however many support their efficacy in a wide variety of clinical settings.

By understanding both theory and group processes nurses can successfully deliver group interventions in both inpatient and community settings.

The chapter has provided a guide to putting groups into practice through careful dynamic administration and selection of members. Emphasis was given to the importance of using supervision to develop an understanding of what is observed in a group and techniques for skilled intervention.

In summary the key points of learning from this chapter are:

- Group therapies are evidenced-based interventions. Most commonly combined with other modalities groups can be an effective intervention for a range of presenting mental health difficulties across the age span.

- When considering a group intervention careful pre-planning is required to prepare the physical and psychological space and boundary. Obtaining the support of the host organization and team is required. Supervision is essential for safe practice and developing a group protocol will give clarity for all involved. This process is known as 'dynamic administration' and attending to it will increase the likelihood of a successful group.

■ There are a number of different types of groups: open, closed, slow open, heterogeneous and homogenous. In the selection of potential members facilitators must attend to the purpose of the group and select members accordingly. They should select those who have the ability to cope with group situations, and a willingness to participate in the work.

They should avoid alienating members in terms of race or gender etc., and, in group dynamic or analytic therapy achieve a range of temperament types for maximum benefit.

■ Behaviour in a group is influenced by the very experience of being in it. Groups develop norms which shape behaviour and expectations. Facilitators must guide this process of development towards healthy creativity and exploration of difference.

■ Group theories such as stages of group development, therapeutic factors in groups, theories of group defences and group processes can all help facilitators recognize and respond skillfully to what is observed.

Annotated bibliography

Barnes, B., Ernst, S. and Hyde, K. (1999) *An Introduction to Group Work.* **London: Palgrave.**
A really helpful, easy to read text with practical and theoretical points clearly made. Each chapter includes a summary of learning points. The text is a good source of further reading about contemporary and historical group psychotherapy literature.

Blackmore, C., Tantam, D., Parry, G. and Chambers, E. (2012) Report on the systematic review of the efficacy and clinical effectiveness of group analysis and analytic/dynamic group psychotherapy, *Group Analysis,* **45(1).**
This is an interesting article that gives an overview of the systematic review. The authors note that the review concluded that group therapies are more effective than waiting list or standard care control across a diverse range of clinical needs and demographics. The authors discuss the current state of the evidence base, with careful explanation of the specific issues for research in group therapies. The references are particularly useful for clinicians in supporting arguments for using group interventions as well as in designing and reporting their own work.

Yalom and Leszcz (2005) *The Theory and Practice of Group Psychotherapy,* **5th edn. New York: Basic Books.**
This is a standard and very readable text that uses many detailed clinical examples to demonstrate theory and research. Now in its fifth edition it draws on nearly a decade of new research.

American Group Psychotherapy Association, at www.agpa.org.
Gives detailed practice guidelines for working with groups, and covers theory (such as stages of groups) as well as offering practical guides for the facilitator on observing and intervening, including the use of questioning techniques.

References

Barker, P. and Buchanan-Barker, P. (2005) *The Tidal Model: A guide for mental health professionals.* London: Brunner-Routledge.
Barlow, S., Burlingham, G., Harding, J. and Berham, J. (1997) Therapeutic focusing in time-limited group psychotherapy, *Group Dynamic: Theory, Research and Practice,* 1(3): 254–66.
Benson, J. (2000) *Working More Creatively with Groups.* London: Routledge.
Bion, W.R. (1961) *Experiences in Groups.* New York: Basic Books.
Faulkner, A. and Layzell, S. (2000) *Strategies for Living: A report of user-led research into people's strategies for living with mental distress.* London: Mental Health Foundation.
Foulkes, S.H. (1964) *Therapeutic Group Analysis.* New York: International Universities Press.
Frings, D., Abrams, D., Randsley de Moura, G. and Marques, J. (2010) The effects of cost, normative support, and issue importance on motivation to persuade in-group deviants, *Group Dynamics: Theory, Research and Practice,* 14(1): 80–91.
Fristad, M.A., Verducci, J.S., Walters, K. and Young, M. (2009) Impact of multifamily psycho-educational psychotherapy in treating children aged 8 to 12 years with mood disorders, *Arch Gen Psychiatry,* 66(9): 1013–21.
Garland, J., Jones, H. and Kolodny, R. (1973) A model for stages of development in social work groups, in S. Bernstein (ed.) *Explorations in Group work: Essays in theory and practice.* Boston, MA: Milford House.

Gutheil, T. (1980) Paranoia and progress notes: a guide to forensically informed psychiatric record keeping, *Hospital and Community Psychiatry*, 13: 479–82.

Jacob, A., Gabirel, S., Roepke, S., Stoffers, J., Lieb, K. and Lammers, C. (2010) Group therapy module to enhance self-esteem in patients with borderline personality disorder: a pilot study, *International Journal of Group Psychotherapy*, 60(3).

Knauss, L. (2006) Ethical issues in record keeping in group psychotherapy, *International Journal of Group Psychotherapy*, 56(4): 415–31.

Lam, D., Burbeck, R., Wright, K.A. and Pilling, S. (2009) Psychological therapies in bipolar disorder: the effect of illness history on relapse prevention – systematic review, *Bipolar Disorders*, 11: 474–82.

MacKenzie, K.R. (1997) *Time Managed Group Psychotherapy*. **????** American Psychiatric Press.

Macleod, S.H., Elliott, L. and Brown, R. (2011) What support can community mental health nurses deliver to carers of people diagnosed with schizophrenia? Findings from a review of the literature, *International Journal of Nursing Studies*, 48(1): 100–20.

Marques, J. M., Abrams, D., Páez, D., Hogg, M.A. (2001) Social categorization, social identification, and rejection of deviant group members, in M.A. Hogg and R.S. Tindale (eds) *Blackwell Handbook of Social Psychology, Volume 3: Group processes*. Oxford: Blackwell.

NICE (National Institute for Health and Clinical Excellence) (2005) *Core Interventions in the Treatment of Obsessive-compulsive Disorder and Body Dysmorphic Disorder*, available at: http://guidance.nice.org.uk/CG31.

NICE (National Institute for Health and Clinical Excellence) (2006) *Bipolar Disorder: The management of bipolar disorder in adults, children and adolescents, in primary and secondary care*, available at: www.nice.org.uk.

NICE (National Institute for Health and Clinical Excellence) (2007) *Interventions to Reduce Substance Misuse Among Vulnerable Young People*, available at: www.nice.org.uk.

NICE (National Institute for Health and Clinical Excellence) (2009a) *Borderline Personality Disorder: Treatment and management*, available at: www.nice.org.uk/CG78.

NICE (National Institute for Health and Clinical Excellence) (2009b) *Attention Deficit Hyperactivity Disorder: Diagnosis and management of ADHD in children, young people and adults*, available at: http://guidance.nice.org.uk/CG72.

NICE (National Institute for Health and Clinical Excellence) (2011) *Psychosis with Coexisting Substance Misuse: Assessment and management in adults and young people*, available at: www.nice.org.uk.

Novakovic, A. (2002) Psychotic patients in a rehabilitation unit: a short term staff support group with a nursing team, *Group Analysis*, 35(4): 560–73.

Ozarin, L. (2003) J.L. Moreno, MD: founder of psychodrama, *Psychiatric News*, 38(10): 60.

Reid, S. and Kolvin, I. (1993) Group psychotherapy for children and adolescents, *Archives of Disease in Childhood*, 69: 244–50.

Rethink (2011) www.rethink.org/living_with_mental_illness/treatment_and_therapy/other_treatments/therapeutic_communit.html, accessed 2 September 2011.

Stock Whittaker, D. (1994) *Using Groups to Help People*. London: Tavistock/Routledge.

Tuckman, B.W. (1965) Developmental sequences in small groups, *Psychological Bulletin*, 63: 384–99.

Welch, T., Welch, M., Baer, J., Dias, J., Gurney, C. and Van Dale, B. (2010) Removed but not out of reach: seniors with depression in smaller center, rural, and remote communities, *Psychiatric Annals*, 40(12): 616–23.

Wood, A., Trainor, G., Rothwell, J., Moore, A. and Harringston, R. (2001) Randomized trial of group therapy for repeated deliberate self-harm in adolescents, *Journal of the American Academy of Child and Adolescent Psychiatry*, 40: 1246–53.

Yalom, I. (1985) *The Theory and Practice of Group Psychotherapy*. New York: Basic Books.

Yorke, S. and Gaylard, M. (2003) A CBT-based group for people with enduring psychotic symptoms, *Mental Health Practice*, 6: 10.

Chapter 25

Working with Families and Carers

Helen Wilde

25.1 Introduction

Working with services users' families in care planning and treatment is often thought of as the domain of family therapists. However, it can also be a key role for the mental health nurse. A wealth of information can be gathered from service users' families and other social networks to improve the quality of their assessments. In turn, this may lead to an increased likelihood of improved recovery, sustained for longer periods. Clinical experience suggests that this is best achieved by adopting a systemic perspective to understand the needs of service users in relation to their families and the wider social contexts in which they live.

Family practice is not a stand-alone approach but one that enhances other forms of treatment and care, for example, individual therapies and use of medication. Working with families to engage them in care can be challenging due to time limitations and other organizational priorities. Also, from time to time nurses will encounter families who hold values and motivations that they find difficult to understand. For these reasons regular clinical supervision, ideally from a systemic psychotherapist, is recommended for nurses involved in family work. This chapter covers:

- the case for working with families and carers;
- contexts and levels of intervention;
- principles of practice.

25.2 The case for working with families and carers

To recognise carers as expert care partners is to value both their role in providing support and the wider knowledge and skills they possess as individuals. Doing so greatly increases the likelihood of more personalised, responsive, and high-quality outcomes for those being supported, and makes carers' valuable and informed contribution available to other carers, service providers and commissioners.

(DH 2010)

How will taking time out of an already busy day to meet with a service user's family make a difference to the care being provided by a patient's care team? At first the idea of meeting with a service user's family can seem somewhat daunting. Families sometimes ask difficult or challenging questions, can be distressed or confused, can try to engage you in conversation that leads to you taking on more tasks and on occasion are, for various reasons, unhappy or angry.

In an inpatient setting making time to stop and talk with a family during visiting time when there are also ward round summaries to write and a group activity to plan all in the next hour is a challenge. It may be difficult to decide which of these tasks should take priority. In a community setting you may have back-to-back appointments, endless emails to respond to and a team meeting to attend when you receive another call from a family member. These frequent day-to-day demands on nursing time may make providing family inclusive care appear a noble goal, but one that is very difficult to achieve.

To collate well informed, well matched care plans for the treatment and recovery of a service user the care team needs to have gathered and considered information about more than how the service user presents in the hospital or clinic setting. Engagement, assessment, treatment and recovery planning need to include an appreciation of home life, school or work, general interests, cultural and religious influences, in essesnce looking beyond the treatment of symptoms.

Involvement of a service user's family will increase the likelihood of care plans being relevant and of having the best chance of success. This will require the care team to have skills for enquiring about and sometimes managing varying opinions held by different people around one issue and then help the service user and their family to make decisions and agree plans.

From the perspective of families as well as service users, the onset of mental health problems is likely to be a time of distress, confusion, disruption and adjustment. It may also bring relief to a family that has sought for some time to have their relative's mental health problems recognized by profession-

als. In either case families can be helped to come to terms with and understand what is taking place by addressing a number of matters:

- offering emotional support in dealing with distress, anxiety and or anger/fear, feelings which are commonly experienced by families in these circumstances;

- providing information/psycho-education about the condition – explaining symptoms and behaviours and providing information about medication options;

- providing information and access to supports such as benefits, legal rights information and support groups for both carers and service users.

(Stanbridge and Burbach 2007)

Some families will be faced with challenges of coming to terms with the service user's long-term illness or recurrent relapses. In these circumstances families may have to make more significant adjustments such as one of them becoming a carer. This could lead to a reduction in working hours, loss of income, loss of social status and often being faced with prejudice and unequal opportunities due to stigma by association with mental health problems. Families can be supported through making links with a number of well established support groups for families and carers such as The Princess Royal Trust for Carers (see 'Useful resources', p. 391).

Children and young people

One in 12 children has a parent who suffers with a mental health problem. These children frequently have responsibilities that are normally seen as those which should be taken up by an adult and, as such, are known as 'young carers'. They may have a role in ensuring a parent takes their medication, and responsibilities for shopping, managing money, cooking meals and helping their parent with daily living tasks, such as washing and dressing. This can lead to the child missing school, becoming isolated or being bullied by peers. Financial problems may arise when a parent is unable to work and bills are unpaid. Mental health problems often lead to social isolation for both the parent and child/ren. These issues can lead to children being placed under so much pressure that they in turn develop mental health problems.

That a child or adolescent is a young carer often only comes to light when there is a crisis. Furthermore, families are often very frightened that talking about such matters will lead to children being 'taken away' or children may fear a parent being admitted to hospital if they talk to someone about their parent's mental health issues.

Attitudes towards children as young carers have become more positive over time. It is now recognized that the role of a child being involved in the care of a parent can be a positive one if it is not detrimental to their own well-being. Mental health professionals are advised to approach the issue of dependent children with a positive stance that does not assume such an arrangement is unacceptable. Support groups and services for young carers are provided by many local authorities and voluntary agencies.

Policy and evidence

There are legal and evidence-based principles that promote the involvement of families and carers. For example, the Carers Act 2004 makes specific provision for carers including the right to be offered and/or request a carer's assessment and the right to receive direct payments. Carers' rights to be involved in treatment are also contained in the Mental Health Act 1983 and the Mental Capacity Act 2005 (see Chapter 10).

The National Service Framework for Mental Health and associated policy guidance acknowledge the importance of including families and carers, and support the practice of designing interventions and services which enable this. Specific involvement of families is advised, not least because of the long-term impact of caring for someone with mental health problems (DH 2002a, 2002b). Kenitner et al. (1992) examined factors that improved patient recovery from depression. They found that five key elements contributed to recovery, among these being improved family functioning and support. Family therapy and psycho-education approaches have been found to reduce relapse rates in adults with schizophrenia when combined with medication and follow-up care (Falloon et al. 1985; Tarrier and Barrowclough 1995).

Kurtz and James (2003), looking at effective treatment for psychosis, found that for inpatient care to be shorter, more intense and with higher levels of support for discharge, the involvement of families in care and recovery planning was a necessary element. Including families in these processes has been found to reduce the length of stay in hospital, reduce the likelihood of readmission to hospital and increase the likelihood of treatment concordance (Kuipers 2006).

The National Institute for Health and Clinical Excellence (NICE) provides guidelines for specific family therapies and for family and carer involvement for a number of mental health conditions.

Case Study

Bill

Bill, aged 20, was admitted to hospital from accident and emergency (A&E) following a suicide attempt. On admission he told the admitting nurse that he had been depressed for some time following a relationship breakdown and that he could not see a way out of his current state of mind as he felt completely powerless and hopeless. This had led to Bill's suicide attempt, which he now regrets.

At a multi-disciplinary meeting, during which Bill was not present, the team decided that he could be discharged fairly quickly if he had support at home and so a member of the team spoke with Bill about inviting his parents to a multi-disciplinary team meeting to plan for his discharge. Bill was uncertain initially about this contact but did eventually agree to his parents' involvement.

At the multi-disciplinary meeting Bill's family were not confident about talking to 'professionals'; they did not feel it was 'their place' to ask questions or give information unless it was directly sought. The team picked up on the family's apprehensions. It was explained that their views were important to ensure that whatever treatment plan was developed would work well for Bill and also for his family.

Bill's father, Tom, said that he was concerned about his son being on antidepressants because he did not see him to be 'really depressed' as his own brother had been 25 years ago. The team explored this issue and found that Tom was encouraging Bill not to use medication as he feared that his son would follow the same pathway as his brother, who had not worked for years and had experienced relationship breakdowns and financial problems. The team acknowledged Tom's fears for his son's future, engaged the family in drawing distinctions between Bill's situation and that of his uncle, and further explained the use of medication in the overall treatment plan, which also included 'talking therapy'.

At the meeting the team suggested that Bill temporarily move back home to live with his parents. This was agreed and a plan made for Bill and one of the nurses to visit his parents' home together in preparation for discharge. During this home visit the nurse discovered that Bill would be sleeping in the sitting room. Bill's sister, who was pregnant, also lived at home and Bill would be returning home at about the same time as his sister was due to give birth.

This home visit alerted the team to circumstances that the family had not felt able to discuss at the meeting, which would have placed increased pressure on Bill and the family. Discharge plans were reviewed with the family. Bill returned to his own home with daily support from both his extended family, his peers and the community team.

Thinking Space 25.1

What features of Bill's case demonstrate the value of working with families and carers? Jot down your ideas now – feedback is provided at the end of chapter.

25.3 Contexts and levels of intervention

Nursing practices and contexts for care present many opportunities to include families in the care of a service user. These include:

- admission to hospital;
- care planning and Care Programme Approach (CPA) reviews;
- home visits;
- informal contact and introductions via waiting rooms/during visiting times;
- provision of specific family therapy interventions;
- provision of family and carer support groups;
- inclusion of service users and their families in service reviews and development;
- use of feedback forms/audit methods for gathering information about service users' and their families' experiences of care provided.

Some inpatient services have appointed a member of staff as a patient carer liaison or 'family champion', with responsibility for ensuring good communication between the ward and patients' families. Such posts can reduce the chance of regular contact between ward and family being 'missed' in the busy and unpredictable day-to-day activities that take place. As a matter of routine child and adolescent services include families in processes such as admission to hospital and care planning reviews, but this is not always the case in adult services.

Levels of intervention

Family and carer involvement differs in intensity according to its context and purpose. On the one hand it might involve formal systemic therapy interventions. On the other, it can be quite informal following general principles for involving families and carers. Gamble and Brennan (2006) propose three levels:

- **Level 1:** engagement and communication support plus introduction to service provision and personnel. Usually managed by a care coordinator who liaises with all key stakeholders and establishes pathways for two-way communication.

- **Level 2:** communication support plus tailor-made information to maintain current coping strategies and develop relapse prevention plans. Typically delivered by one or more team members with some family-work training.

- **Level 3:** full family intervention to enhance communication and coping styles. Delivered by trained family workers.

Family and carer types

All individuals with mental health problems, their families and carers should receive Level 1 interventions. It may be difficult to know at the outset, before thorough assessments are complete, which individuals and their families/carers might benefit from Level 2 and 3 interventions. However, Kuipers *et al.* (2002) provide a general 'rule of thumb' for which families it may be valuable to work with:

- carers living with clients who relapse more than twice a year despite taking regular medication;

- those who frequently contact staff for reassurance or help;

- home environments where there are repeated arguments, violence and/or the police are called;

- any carer who is looking after a client unaided.

25.4 Principles of practice

Systemic practice

Family inclusive practice requires a move from thinking about individual service users in isolation to understanding them in relation to their social and family links, cultural identity, home life and significant influences. This approach to understanding service users is known as systemic practice.

One simple, much cited, definition of systemic practice is 'any way of working that aims to bring out, share, and respect the views and stories of all involved, so to integrate a constructive way forward' (Childs 2011). In the context of mental health care it involves paying attention to and having an awareness of the relevance of a person's social, cultural, economic and family background, and of how these layers of influence interact within the life of an individual. Systemic thinking in the context of working with families means paying attention to the layers or contexts that surround a person and how these influence and inform their beliefs and behaviour. This is illustrated by Figure 25.1 which shows that each of the layers or contexts has an influence on the other and all interact with and have an influence on the individual. Some individuals will be aware of these influences and of possible personal conflicts and supports which accompany each interacting layer. Others will be less aware of conflicts and strengths created within the layers and may benefit from work to help bring such issues and their relevance to their mental health needs to awareness.

Seeking and responding to feedback from the patient and their family throughout care planning is a key feature of systemic practice. Through feedback the clinician checks out and clarifies his or her understanding of the family's views and beliefs, and can incorporate their perspective when designing care and treatment approaches. Working systemically with an individual and/or their family involves developing an understanding of the individual by engaging them in collaborative conversations about:

- the contexts in which they live and work;
- significant relationships they have with others; and
- how these contexts and relationships might influence their health problem.

Collaborative working

Systemic practice involves clinicians moving away from their traditional expert role to working in collaboration with service users and their families. For example, rather than simply providing the service user and his or her family with information about a specific disorder, treatment and medication, nurses who adopt a systemic approach would provide this information, then explore with the family how this has been understood and how the information 'fits' with their cultural or personal beliefs. Consideration would then be given to making changes or adapta-

Figure 25.1 Systemic thinking in the context of working with families

- Service user
- Immediate family/ carers
- Extended family/ friends/work/local community
- Government/economy

tions that are a 'good fit' for the family as well as the service user. This process is known as using a *feedback loop*. Working collaboratively with families requires the care team to:

- respect and value the family's point of view;
- avoid blame and passing judgement;
- work flexibly (e.g offering to meet with families at a time that suits them);
- dedicate time to engage families in treatment and care planning;
- plan in ways that facilitate joint decision making rather than making a plan and then 'telling' the family what is going to happen;
- be aware of issues and skills relevant to working across cultures.

Engaging families in care and treatment

Whether working with adults or adolescents the inclusion of the family initially needs to be discussed and agreed with the service user. It is not unusual for adolescents to go through periods of not wanting their parents to be included in meetings and treatment planning, due to relationship difficulties associated with their stage of development. Further, parents may have been the ones to raise concerns and request that their child be admitted to hospital against his or her wishes, and this may lead to the young person refusing contact. However, this should not exclude the parent from being kept in touch with and consulted about progress, treatment needs and care planning. The young person needs to be engaged in negotiations around what information can be shared and support given with rebuilding relationships.

When planning family or carer involvement with adolescents or adults mental health professionals should consider the following:

- explaining why including their family is important;
- exploring what the service user would like to gain from family meetings and how these would be helpful to them;

- ask who they see as needing to be included and why;
- consider when the best time to meet would be for all those involved;
- consider the best location for you to all meet and why;
- explore any areas of potential conflict and plan how these can be managed.

The service user and his or her family may be stressed and anxious when they initially meet with the care team; engaging with families who are under stress requires giving attention to in how meaning is attributed to behaviour and how stress and anxiety are responded to. How a family's behaviour is interpreted and the meanings given to individual family members' actions need to be explored by the care team so that any negative connotations or disagreements, blame and associated responses, can be avoided. Engagement skills that nurses need to employ at this stage include:

- expressing warmth, understanding and openness;
- acceptance;
- adopting a non-judgemental/blame stance;
- ensuring all family members are given a chance to express their personal views;
- being responsive to concerns and questions;
- establishing a collaborative approach to problem-solving and care planning.

How the suggestion of involving a family in treatment is perceived by the family needs to be addressed at the time of inviting them to meet. Explaining the rationale for including the family, the benefits to treatment outcomes of including them, the wish to understand their concerns and share knowledge of the person being cared for will all contribute toward building a trusting relationship. The aim is for the family to have an experience of being respected and valued by the care team and to allay any concerns they may have about being judged to be in some way responsible for or seen as 'part of the problem'; which is frequently an issue that concerns parents and families at some stage when a family member experiences mental health problems.

Planning and review meetings

When inviting families to attend reviews and planning meetings time needs to be set aside for explaining processes and agreeing on if/how information that may be sensitive will be shared with professionals due to attend. For example, prior to a CPA review a member of the service user's care team should alert the family to the aims of the meeting, and share with them any summary reports to be presented in which they are referred to. This will ensure the information being reported is accurate and that family members consent to it being shared with other professionals attending the meeting. During the meeting there needs to be sufficient time for identifying and working through any differences of opinion about care and treatment that come to light between family, service user and team. The team needs to take account of the family's wishes, while considering the client's care and treatment needs and adapt plans to find an acceptable compromise.

Organizations with high levels of family and carer involvement in mental health care are characterized by:

- policy that routinely expects and promotes clinical teams to include families in assessment, treatment and recovery planning;
- flexible working practices – meetings with families in their homes and at a time that suits them;
- appointment of 'family liaison' staff in inpatient settings;
- provision of written information about services provided, medication to be considered and relevant mental health problems and models of treatment being proposed.

Cross-cultural working

Working with families using a systemic framework promotes practice in cross-cultural work where there may be differences between families' and professionals' understanding of problems, and feasible solutions, and differences between cultures in how mental health is understood and treated.

How we make sense of the world around us can be understood as being socially constructed (Dallos and Draper 2000). Central to the theories of social constructionism is the view that, over time, societies create meanings/explanations for events and behaviours. A given culture will hold ideas about issues such as what is socially acceptable and unacceptable behaviour, what the social rewards are for acceptable behaviour and what the consequences are for behaving in unacceptable ways. Social expectations, laws, beliefs and practices may be strongly connected with religion as well as cultural influences.

These social and cultural expectations vary from one community to the next and in working with families the clinician/nurse will need to have an awareness of these potential differences in order to engage families and help them make sense of issues such as medical advice, diagnosis and advisable care.

Clinicians working across cultures need to be aware of their own cultural beliefs and associated 'acceptable' behaviour. In systemic practice this is described as *reflexive practice*; the art of being aware of personal beliefs and what influences our thinking about what is socially acceptable behaviour. Clinicians can be helped to develop skills in cross-cultural work by exploring such issues with colleagues to become more aware of their cultural

assumptions about issues such as what is acceptable/expected behaviour at a given stage in life.

25.5 Conclusion

In summary, the main learning points from this chapter are:

- Care providers need to understand service users from a perspective that includes curiosity for the contexts in which they live and which have an impact on their lives.

- Research evidence and best practice guidelines underpin the practice of family inclusive treatment approaches in community and hospital settings.

- There are different levels of family/carer involvement from informal information-sharing to formal structured interventions.

- Engaging families may initially appear time consuming and hard to accommodate but has value and benefits for all in the long-term recovery of the service user.

- A systemic approach highlights issues which arise when working across cultures and provides tools and skills that may be drawn on to identify and acknowledge differences in perspective and find common ground.

- Professionals need to consider the role of young carers not only with regard to safeguarding issues but also how they might be best aided to support their parent's recovery.

Feedback to Thinking Space 25.1

The family had been hesitant to disagree with the team or to express the concerns they had about plans for Bill's discharge and treatment. However, the multi-disciplinary team became aware of the family's lack of confidence in expressing their views and possible concerns about appearing to challenge 'professionals' advice'. Treatment and ongoing care plans were collaboratively made with Bill and his family, which gave time and support to his parents to ask questions and express their concerns. Plans for discharge took in to consideration Bill's family circumstances at home and were adapted accordingly.

The case also illustrates that there are occasions when a service user will not want family or friends included in any part of work and support offered. Bill reluctantly agreed to his family meeting with the team. In other cases clients may refuse to have their families involved. In such cases health professionals need to find other ways of gaining a picture of the service user within a systemic framework; understanding a person and their needs beyond their presenting problems and understanding what role their family and social circumstances may play in maintaining or alleviating their difficulties.

Annotated bibliography

Bailey, F.R., Burbach, F. and Lea, S. (2003) The ability of staff trained in family interventions to implement the approach in routine clinical practice, *Journal of Mental Health,* **12(2): 131–41(11).**
This paper reports challenges to organizations in implementing family inclusive mental health services, drawing on the experiences of a family therapy team in Somerset Partnership National Health Service (NHS) Trust.

Burnham, J.B. (1998) *Family Therapy.* **London: Routledge.**
An easy to read and sound introduction to ideas and skills used in working therapeutically with families, including a useful chapter on the use of genograms.

Falicov, C. J. (1995) Training to think culturally: a multidimensional comparative framework, *Family Process,* **34: 373–88.**
This paper provides a framework for understanding issues relevant to cross-cultural working. It emphasizes the need for practitioners to develop understanding of their own cultural influences and how these may impact on working to engage and understand another's perspective.

Goldenberg, H. and Goldenberg, I. (2011) *Family Therapy: An overview,* **8th edn. Belmont CA Cengage Learning Inc.**
A review of family intervention in clinical practice from a range of cultural perspectives. Includes a comparative view of family theories in a range of contexts in mental health practice.

NICE recommends systemic, couple or family therapy in the treatment of bipolar disorder (2006), depression in adults (2009), eating disorders (2004), post-traumatic distress (2005) and schizophrenia (2009): **www.nice.org.uk.**

NICE recommends the inclusion of family and carers, not specifically family therapy, in the treatment of self-harm (2004), attention deficit hyperactivity disorder (ADHD) (2008), dementia (2006), obsessive compulsive disorder (OCD) (2005), borderline personality disorder (2009) and post-natal mental health care (2007): **www.nice.org.uk.**

Useful resources

Barnardo's mental health research, policy and resources is an online resource including current research and resources in the field of children and family mental health – for example, research into parenting matters and young carers: www. barnardos.org.uk/what_we_do/policy_research_unit/research_and_publications/mental_health_policy_research.htm.

The Children's Society National Young Carers Initiative provides information, advice and training on young carers for professionals including principles of practice: http://www.youngcarer.com.

The Family Therapy and Systemic Research Centre is a good resource for up-to-date evidence and research in the 'pipeline', offering a comprehensive database of current research and information regarding family inclusive practice, family therapy, research seminars and conferences. Includes links to information related to evaluation and outcome studies and evidence-based research into family-based interventions in mental health practice: www.uel-ftsrc.org/research.htm.

The Princess Royal Trust for Carers provides quality information, advice and support services to nearly a quarter of a million carers, including 13,000 young carers: http://www.carers.org; http://www.youngcarers.net.

Youngcarer.com provides children's perspective of parents with mental health needs. Children whose parents have mental health problems present a video of their work with a mental health team on understanding mental health problems and their impact on family relationships: www.youngcarer.com/pdfs/Whole%20Family%20Pathway%2010th.pdf.

The Young Carers Inititiative website has been designed with input from young carers and is aimed at young carers: young-carers-initiative@childrenssociety.org.uk.

References

Childs, N. (2011) www.forallthat.com/systemic-practice.html, accessed 17 December 2011.
Dallos, D. and Draper, R. (2000) *An Introduction to Family Therapy.* Maidenhead: Open University Press.

DH (Department of Health) (2002a) *Mental Health Policy Implementation Guide: Community mental health teams.* London: HMSO.

DH (Department of Health) (2002b) *Mental Health Policy Implementation Guide: Adult acute inpatient care.* London: HMSO.

DH (Department of Health) (2010) *Carers and Personalization: Improving outcomes.* London: HMSO.

Falloon, I., Boyd, J., McGill, C. *et al.* (1985) Family management in the prevention of morbidity of schizophrenia, *Archives of General Psychiatry*, 42: 887–96.

Gamble, C. and Brennan, G. (2006) Working with families and informal carers, in C. Gamble and G. Brennan (eds) *Working with Serious Mental Illness: A manual for clinical practice*, 2nd edn. Philadelphia, PA: Elsevier.

Keitner, G.I., Ryan, C.E., Miller, I.W. *et al.* (1992) Recovery and major depression: factors associated with 12-month outcome, *American Journal of Psychiatry*, 149: 93–9.

Kuipers, E. (2006) Family interventions in schizophrenia: evidence for efficacy and proposed mechanisms of change, *Journal of Family Therapy*, 28: 73–80.

Kuipers, E., Leff, J. and Lam, D. (2002) *Family Work for Schizophrenia: A practical guide*, 2nd edn. London: Gaskell Press.

Kurtz, Z. and James, C. (2003) *What's New: Learning from the CAMHS innovation projects.* London: DH.

Stanbridge, R. and Burbach, F. (2007) Developing family inclusive mainstream mental health services, *Journal of Family Therapy*, 29: 21–43.

Tarrier, N. and Barrowclough, C. (1995) Family interventions in schizophrenia and their long term outcomes, *International Journal of Mental Health*, 24: 38–53.

Chapter 26

Psychopharmacology

Caroline Parker

Considering I presented in hospital, locked in my own reality, floridly psychotic and hallucinating, I had a long way from which to recover. Luckily, I responded to antipsychotic medication promptly and, although I had been sectioned, I was allowed to go home on leave after just one week in hospital.

Catherine

 ## Introduction

This chapter focuses on medicines which are licensed for use in the UK and widely used for the treatment of mental health disorders. The general management of specific psychiatric illnesses is described in Part 5 of this book. For further information regarding the choice of medicines in the management of each illness or patient group, refer to the relevant clinical guideline from the National Institute for Health and Clinical Excellence (NICE). For further details regarding individual medicines, refer to the current edition of the *British National Formulary* (BNF) or to the medicines Summary of Product Characteristics (SPC) accessible via www.medicines.org.uk.

This chapter covers the following groups of medicines:

- antipsychotics;
- antidepressants;
- mood stabilizers;
- anxiolytics and hypnotics;
- medicines for dementia;
- medicines for attention deficit hyperactivity disorder (ADHD);
- medicines in rapid tranquilisation;
- medicines for alcohol and opioid withdrawal and abstinence;
- adverse effects and monitoring requirements.

 ## Antipsychotics

Antipsychotics are considered first-line pharmacotherapy and are a key treatment for most individuals with schizophrenia (NICE 2009). Antipsychotics are used to both treat acute psychotic symptoms and as a maintenance treatment to prevent acute relapse and help keep the person as well and stable as possible. While antipsychotics are a core treatment of schizophrenia they are just one part of a package of care and are not effective in all cases.

Antipsychotics have been in wide use in the UK since the 1950s, during which time there have been an increasing number available, in a range of formulations. The development of antipsychotics has focused on finding agents of greater efficacy with a lower side-effect burden. Currently there are around 30 antipsychotics licensed for use in the UK, all of which are listed in the current British National Formulary (BNF) (Joint Formulary Committee 2011). Early antipsychotics were commonly known to cause extrapyramidal movement disorders as a side-effect, and it was not until clozapine was developed in the 1980s that it was established that antipsychotic efficacy (via D_2 receptors in the mesolimbic pathway) could be achieved without inducing these extrapyramidal side-effects (EPS) (via D_2 receptors in the nigrostriatal pathway). Since clozapine, antipsychotic development has focused on increasing antipsychotic efficacy without causing movement disorders, or blood dyscrasias (such as those which limit the use of clozapine). From clozapine onwards, newer antipsychotics were termed 'atypical' antip-

sychotics, while the older antipsychotics which 'typically' caused EPS became known as the 'typical' antipsychotics. In some literature these two groups of antipsychotic are termed 'first generation' and 'second generation'. The BNF classification of 'typical' and 'atypical' reflects the manufacturers' marketing authorization, which is based on the submission to the UK licensing authorities by the manufacturer. There is no definitive criteria for this classification, however it is generally accepted that when used at therapeutic doses atypical antipsychotics:

- tend not to cause EPS;
- tend not to disturb prolactin regulation.

This is not without exception, some so-called atypical antipsychotics can cause EPS and disturb the regulation of prolactin even at therapeutic doses (e.g. risperidone, amisulpride). Consequently these two classifications are probably better viewed as 'rules of thumb' which merely summarize the continuum shown in Figure 26.1.

All antipsychotics (with the exception of aripiprazole) antagonize dopamine D_2 receptors in the mesolimbic area of the brain, and it is hypothesized that this is their main mode of antipsychotic action (Joint Formulary Committee 2011) (often referred to as the 'dopamine hypothesis'). Numerous trials have shown that all antipsychotics have similar effi-

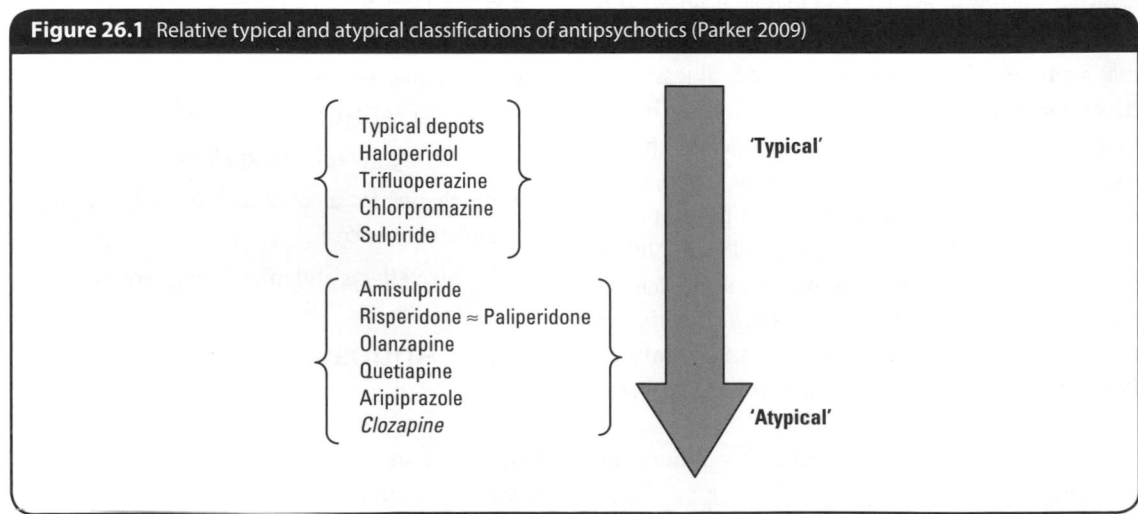

Figure 26.1 Relative typical and atypical classifications of antipsychotics (Parker 2009)

cacy in the treatment of positive symptoms of schizophrenia, that they are all poorer at treating negative symptoms, and there is little or no difference between typicals and atypicals with respect to patient preference and cognitive performance. Antipsychotics vary considerably in their pattern of activity at receptors which are not involved in the therapeutic efficacy, leading to a range of predictable side-effects (refer to Table 26.1). Clozapine is the single exception, with notable greater efficacy, and this is discussed later in the chapter.

In addition to the core hypothesized mechanism of action, with the exception of amisulpride, all atypical antipsychotics also have varying but greater degrees of activity at serotonergic receptors (i.e. $5HT_{2ac}$). It is thought possible that antipsychotic activity may also be related to the ratio of activity at $D_2/5HT_{2ac}$ receptors, and that glutamate is also involved.

Aripiprazole, a more recently developed atypical, has been described as a third generation of antipsychotic due to its slightly different mode of action. It acts as a partial agonist at D_2 dopamine and $5HT_{1a}$ serotonin receptors, and as an antagonist at $5HT_2$ serotonin receptors. It has been postulated that through these actions it stabilizes the dopamine and serotonin system. A partial D_2 agonist would be able to act as an antagonist in pathways where abundant dopamine led to psychosis, yet it would stimulate receptors as an agonist at sites in which low dopaminergic tone would produce side-effects (such as areas in the brain where low dopamine can produce side-effects such as movement disorders). Despite this postulated mechanism of action a Cochrane review (Bhattacharjee and El-Sayeh 2008) concluded that aripiprazole was as equally effective as typical and atypical antipsychotics.

Antipsychotic choice

No single antipsychotic is routinely recommended as first choice in the treatment of schizophrenia or psychosis (NICE 2009), as (excluding clozapine) no single antipsychotic has superior efficacy. Rather, when selecting an antipsychotic, prescribers should take into account the patient's clinical presentation, concurrent medical co-morbidities and treatments, the antipsychotic side-effect profile, previous response to and tolerance of other antipsychotics, and the patient's preference. The adverse effects of particular note are the propensity for typical antipsychotics to cause EPS (including akathisia), and the propensity for many of the atypical and some typical antipsychotics to cause weight gain and metabolic sequalae. This will often mean that an oral atypical antipsychotic that is less likely to induce weight gain and metabolic sequalae is used first in the treatment of people with newly diagnosed schizophrenia. NICE (2009) also encourages the use of clozapine as early as possible, for patients with treatment resistant schizophrenia.

Antipsychotic monotherapy

It is recommended that only one antipsychotic should be used at a time and that regular combinations of multiple antipsychotics should be avoided. The two exceptions are temporary and short periods when switching from one antipsychotic to another and the augmentation of clozapine in treatment resistant schizophrenia where optimized clozapine monotherapy is still insufficient (NICE 2009).

Clozapine

In a groundbreaking trial by Kane in 1988, clozapine demonstrated superior efficacy over other antipsychotics in the treatment of positive symptoms of schizophrenia for patients with a treatment resistant illness defined as a lack of response to two other antipsychotics. This is in addition to the fact that clozapine does not 'typically' induce EPS (and hence the coining of the term 'atypical'). More recent studies have also confirmed its greater efficacy compared to typical and other atypical antipsychotics and it has been shown to reduce the incidence of suicide in schizophrenia (McEvoy et al. 2006). Despite this greater efficacy, clozapine's adverse effects mean that it is not suitable to be recommended as a first-line antipsychotic. However, as the only antipsychotic with superior efficacy and demonstrated efficacy in treatment resistant individuals its use is encouraged for these patients.

Table 26.1   Relative side-effects of common antipsychotics (after Lieberman *et al.* 2005; Taylor *et al.* 2009; Joint Formulary Committee 2011)

Drug	Effect on QTc	Sedation	Weight gain	EPS	Hyper-prolactinaemia	Postural hypotension[‡]	Anti-cholinergic	Additional information/comments
Typical antipsychotics								
Chlorpromazine hydrochloride	++	+++	++	++	+++	+++	++	Class: phenothiazine Short-acting injection not recommended Patients should be warned about potential skin photosensitivity and advised to use sunscreen
Flupentixol	+	+	+	++	+++	+	++	Class: thioxanthine
Fluphenazine	+	+	+	+++	+++	+	++	Class: phenothiazine
Haloperidol	+	+	+	+++	+++	+	+	Class: butyrophenone
Pimozide	+++	+	+	+	+++	+	+	Class: diphenylbutylpiperidine CSM warning 1990 regarding ECG monitoring
Pipothiazine	+++	++	+	++	+++	++	+++	Class: phenothiazine
Sulpiride	+	–	+	+	+++	–	–	Class: substituted benzamide
Trifluoperazine	?	+	+	+++	+++	+	–/+	Class: phenothiazine
Zuclopenthixol	?	++	+	++	+++	+	++	Class: phenothiazine

(Continued)

Atypical antipsychotics							
Amisulpride	−	+	+	+++	−	−	
Aripiprazole	−	+	−/+ (akathisia)	−	−	−	
Clozapine	+	+++	−	−	+++	+++	Mandatory regular FBC and registration with a clozapine monitoring agency, due to risk of blood dyscrasias
Olanzapine	+	+++	−	−/+	−/+	+	
Quetiapine	++	++	−	−	++	+	
Risperidone/ paliperidone	+	++	+	+++	++	+	Paliperidone (hydroxy-risperidone) is the principle active metabolite of the parent drug risperidone

EPS: extrapyramidal side-effects; ‡ this effect is dose related Incidences: +++ high, ++ moderate, + low, − little or minimum, ? unknown

Clozapine can cause neutropenia which may develop into agranulocytosis (cumulative incidence of agranulocytosis is 0.78 per cent, according to the UK Clozaril Patient Monitoring Service lifetime registry database), which if left unchecked can be fatal. In view of this its use is tightly regulated, all patients and prescribers must be registered with an official clozapine monitoring service before it can be initiated, and a baseline full blood count (FBC) reported. Throughout treatment regular FBC checks are mandatory prior to medicine supply in order to ensure patient safety. The FBC must be performed weekly for the first 18 weeks, fortnightly for the remainder of the first 52 weeks, and four-weekly thereafter. Blood samples are rated according to a traffic light system according to the values of white bloods cells, neutrophils and platelets:

- green – continue monitoring as usual;
- amber – increase monitoring frequency to twice-weekly and monitor patient for signs of neutropenia;
- red – STOP clozapine and monitor patient for signs of infection.

Depot antipsychotics

There may be circumstances where oral (tablets/capsules/liquids) formulations of antipsychotics may not be suitable (e.g. for patients who struggle to remember to take medicines regularly, for those who do not like to take tablets and for those with swallowing problems). 'Depot' formulations of antipsychotics can be an alternative strategy for such patients. These long-acting formulations for intramuscular administration are given at intervals of a few weeks. Some patients simply prefer to have a depot as this avoids the daily routine of taking oral medicines.

Three atypical and five typical antipsychotics are currently licensed in the UK as long-acting depot formulations for intramuscular injection. These are given at between one- and five-week intervals. Aside from the varying drug release profile and pharmacokinetics of each depot, there is little to choose between them in terms of efficacy. Therefore other factors become more pertinent when choosing a depot (e.g. the fre-

quency of injection – two-weekly vs four-weekly, side-effects, the need for refrigeration for risperidone Consta and price – the newer atypical depots are significantly more expensive than typical depots). For a comparison of depots, refer to Table 26.2.

 26.3 Antidepressants

NICE, the British Association of Psychopharmacology and others have published up-to-date national evidence-based guidelines regarding the use of antidepressants for the treatment of unipolar depression in various populations (NICE 2005a, 2010a, 2010b; Anderson *et al.* 2008). In all these guidelines antidepressants are not routinely recommended for the initial treatment of mild or subthreshold depression as the evidence does not demonstrate that the benefits outweigh the risks. This changes with moderate to severe depression where there is evidence for the effectiveness of antidepressants. Antidepressants should only be considered for patients with mild depression if it is complicating the care of the coexisting physical health problems, or if the patient has a past history of moderate or severe depression, or if the depression persists and doesn't respond to non-drug treatments.

A generic selective serotonin reuptake inhibitor (SSRI) is recommended as the first choice antidepressant, but as when selecting other medicines, the exact choice of antidepressant should be based on:

- patient's clinical presentation including associated psychiatric disorder and general medical problems;
- response to previous treatment;
- side-effect profile;
- tolerability and adverse effects to previous treatment;
- likelihood of overdose/suicide risk;
- patient preference/past experience of treatment;
- concurrent medication and potential interactions.

Table 26.2 Depot and long-acting antipsychotic Injections (after Joint Formulary Committee 2011; Electronic Medicines Compendium: http://emc.medicines.org.uk)

Drug	Trade name	Test dose for adults‡	Usual dose range*	Usual dosing interval	Comments
Typical antipsychotics					
Flupentixol decanoate	Depixol, Psytixol	20 mg	12.5–400 mg per week	2–4 weekly	
Fluphenazine decanoate	Modecate	12.5 mg	6.25–50 mg per week	2–5 weekly	Contains sesame oil
Haloperidol decanoate	Haldol	No test dose stated by manufacturer Suggest 25 mg	12.5–75 mg per week	4 weekly	Haloperidol short-acting injection also available Contains sesame oil
Pipothiazine palmitate	Piportil	25 mg	12.5–50 mg per week	4 weekly	EPS less common than with other depots Contains sesame oil
Zuclopenthixol decanoate	Clopixol	100 mg	100–600 mg per week	2–4 weekly	Intermediate-acting injection also available (Zuclopenthixol acetate: Acuphase), lasting for 3 days Contains sesame oil
Atypical antipsychotics					
Olanzapine pamoate	Zypadhera	None, assess tolerance first orally	150–300 mg every 2 weeks	2 weekly or 4 weekly	Risk of post injection syndrome Reconstitute with an aqueous solution to form a suspension
Paliperidone palmitate	Xeplion	None, assess tolerance first orally	5–150 mg every 4 weeks	4 weekly	Pre-filled syringes of an aqueous suspension Shake well for 10 seconds before use Deltoid loading doses required initially
Risperidone	Risperdal Consta	None, assess tolerance first orally	25–50 mg every 2 weeks	2 weekly	Must be stored in a fridge, otherwise 7-day shelf life After administration there is a 3-week lag till risperidone is released

* Doses stated are for adults. Lower doses are required in the elderly.
‡ After the test dose, wait 4–10 days before starting treatment.

Generally, antidepressants act at serotonin (5HT) receptors, though some also act at noradrenaline (NA) receptors. Activity at both 5HT and NA receptors together has not been shown to be of greater benefit than only activity at 5HT receptors alone. Antidepressants are grouped together either in relation to common pharmacology or common chemical structure. No single antidepressant clearly has superior efficacy to others, they vary in their side-effect profiles and individual patients' response varies considerably.

As their name suggests the SSRIs selectively inhibit the reuptake of the neurotransmitter serotonin from the neuronal space into the neurons. There are five commonly used SSRIs: fluoxetine, paroxetine, citalopram, escitalopram and sertraline. Paroxetine use can be more problematic due to its short half life and ensuing propensity for inducing withdrawal symptoms (described later) if even a few doses are missed. A sixth, fluvoxamine, is rarely used due to its incompatibility and interactions with numerous other medicines. SSRIs (and in particular fluoxetine, citalopram and sertraline) are the antidepressants recommended as first-line choice for the treatment of moderate to severe depression as they are as effective as other antidepressants (such as tricyclic antidepressants – TCAs), better tolerated, have lower rates of discontinuation due to side-effects, and are not toxic in overdose.

To differing extents the various TCAs have activity at both 5HT and NA receptors. The TCAs are grouped together on the basis of their chemical structure, having three rings. In addition to their intended clinical activity most TCAs are also active at a variety of other receptors, such as muscarinic, alpha-1 and histamine receptors, leading to a range of side-effects.

The TCAs have dose-related arrhythmogenic potential and can increase the QTc interval on the ECG. The exception to this is lofepramine which seems to lack the arrhythmogenicity of other TCAs. TCAs can be fatally cardiotoxic especially if large quantities are taken as an overdose. As a result of this risk, balanced against no additional benefit,

TCAs (excluding lofepramine) are no longer widely used or recommended (NICE 2010a). TCAs should be avoided in patients at risk of serious arrhythmia. If a TCA other than lofepramine is used, the patient's blood pressure and ECG should be monitored periodically throughout treatment.

Venlafaxine and duloxetine have similar clinical activity as TCAs in that they are active at both the NA and 5HT receptors, but are not tricyclic in chemical structure, and have a different side-effect profile to the TCAs (although similar to each other). Similar to the TCAs, venlafaxine can alter the QTc as well as increase the diastolic blood pressure when used at higher doses (>200 mg/day). As a result it has been associated with a greater risk of death from overdose compared to other routinely used antidepressants (i.e. SSRIs), and at higher doses it may exacerbate cardiac arrhythmias (NICE 2010a). It is contraindicated in patients with an identified high risk of a serious cardiac ventricular arrhythmia and uncontrolled hypertension. If it is used at higher doses (>200 mg/day), patients' blood pressure should be routinely monitored and a baseline ECG should be considered, and in patients with cardiac risk factors a baseline ECG should be considered.

Mirtazapine is another antidepressant that acts on both 5HT and NA, but it is in a class of its own; it is a centrally active presynaptic α2-antagonist, and it is this action which increases both central noradrenergic and serotonergic neurotransmission. Its common side-effects include sedation and weight gain, as opposed to the insomnia and nausea which is are often seen with SSRIs.

Reboxetine is in a group of its own as a selective inhibitor of noradrenaline and is the only antidepressant without effects on the serotonin system. It has not been widely used in the UK. A recent large systematic review and meta-analysis of published and unpublished placebo and controlled trials showed no significant differences in remission or response rates between reboxetine and placebo (Eyding et al. 2010).

Agomelatine has a different mechanism of action to other antidepressants. It is an agonist at melatonin (MT_1 and MT_2) receptors and a $5HT_{2C}$ antagonist. Agomelatine increases noradrenaline and dopamine release specifically in the frontal cortex and has no influence on the extracellular levels of serotonin. There is no data to suggest that it has any greater efficacy than established antidepressants, but it has a different side-effect profile which may be of great benefit.

The mono-amine oxidase inhibitor (MAOI) antidepressants are included in this section for completion. These are effective antidepressants, but their place in therapy is extremely limited by their potentially fatal predictable adverse effects. They act by inhibiting the enzyme mono-amine oxidase which acts to break down mono-amine neurotransmitters in the brain. This inhibition leads to a central accumulation of mono-amines. The addition of substrates to this pathway, through food or other medicines leads to a potentially dangerous accumulation of these amines and a potentiation of their pressor effects. Consequently patients taking MAOIs are advised to be extremely careful to avoid eating foodstuffs that contain substrates of the mono-amine neurotransmitter metabolic pathway in order to avoid precipitating a hypertensive crisis. These foods include mature cheese, alcohol, Bovril, Oxo, Marmite and other similar substances containing meat or yeast extract. In the light of this MAOIs are now rarely used or recommended.

An initial response to an antidepressant may begin within two weeks. Once the patient is in remission, it is advisable to continue the antidepressant at the same treatment dose for a minimum of 6 months in adults, and 12 months in older adults, as doing so has shown to reduce the proportion of people who relapse.

Treatment resistant depression

Treatment resistant depression is defined as the failure to respond to two or more antidepressants given sequentially, at an adequate dose, for an adequate period of time. In such circumstances, as no antidepressant has clearly demonstrated superior efficacy to another, the treatment strategy is to con-

sider either augmenting the antidepressant with another (non-antidepressant) medicine, or use a combination of two antidepressants. For depression with psychotic symptoms, augmentation with an antipsychotic such as olanzapine, aripiprazole, quetiapine or risperidone is recommended (NICE 2010a). For treatment resistant depression without psychotic symptoms, augment with either lithium or an antipsychotic (refer to the section on mood stabilizers). Lithium augmentation should continue for at least six months after remission; it reduces the risk of suicide. If antidepressants are combined, this should only be cautiously done by specialists. Antidepressants with different mechanisms of action should be combined, such as mirtazapine and an SSRI or venlafaxine.

If an antidepressant is stopped suddenly or abruptly after it has been taken for several weeks, some patients may experience symptoms that are known as a withdrawal or discontinuation syndrome. Antidepressants are not addictive, they are not associated with tolerance and craving. Withdrawal or discontinuation symptoms can include imbalance, gastrointestinal and influenza-like symptoms, sensory and sleep disturbance, agitation, dizziness, anxiety and irritability. If symptoms are mild the patient should be reassured and symptoms should be monitored. If symptoms are severe, the antidepressant should be reintroduced and the dose reduced more gradually (e.g. over four weeks). Withdrawal or discontinuation symptoms are more likely with paroxetine and venlafaxine due to their short half-lives and care should be taken when stopping these. Antidepressants with a long half-life and active metabolites such as fluoxetine are less likely to precipitate withdrawal or discontinuation symptoms.

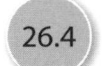 ## 26.4 Mood stabilizers

Pharmacological treatments are the primary therapy in the management of bipolar affective disorder (BPAD), although psychological and psychosocial interventions can also have an impact. Medicines can help to minimize the severity of symptoms, stabilize the mood and prevent relapses. Mood stabilizers are used in the acute and maintenance treatment of BPAD. As their name suggests they are used to stabilize mood, preventing extreme fluctuations to either pole – mania or depression. Few medicines are equally useful at protecting against both such relapses, and therefore much literature (including the BNF) classes these medicines as antimanic agents – an important distinction. Furthermore, some agents are very beneficial in the acute treatment of mania/hypomania, but not so useful or more problematic in the longer-term prophylaxis of recurrent manic/hypomanic episodes.

Medicines referred to as mood stabilizers include:

- lithium;
- valproate (valproic acid and valproate salts);
- carbamazepine.

Other relevant agents are:

- lamotrigine;
- olanzapine;
- quetiapine.

The exact medication or combination of medicines used will be tailored to the patient's previous response, their side-effects and their potential harms (e.g. the teratogenic potential of valproate limits its use in women of child-bearing potential). For severely ill patients and for patients whose symptoms are inadequately controlled with optimized doses of first-line monotherapy, combination therapy may be required:

- valproate + atypical antipsychotic; or
- lithium + atypical antipsychotic.

Combination therapy is more effective than monotherapy with either lithium, valproate or an atypical antipsychotic. If the burden of the disease is mania, the recommendation is to consider combining predominately anti-manic agents (e.g. lithium, valproate, an antipsychotic). Conversely, if the burden

of the disease is depressive, adding lamotrigine or quetiapine is recommended. All these medicines possess an array of side-effects and several have a high potential for toxicity, and are commonly needed in combinations. Therefore it is essential that patients should be adequately monitored for side-effects and toxicity as well as therapeutic benefit.

Lithium

Lithium should be considered as an initial monotherapy in BPAD as it has the best empirical evidence for maintenance treatment and is thought to be effective against both mania and depression, although it is more effective in preventing manic rather than depressive relapses. Unlike most psychotropic medicines lithium is not hepatically metabolized; it is renally excreted unchanged. It has a narrow therapeutic window and demonstrates linear kinetics. This means that there is a narrow range in lithium serum levels between clinical benefit and toxicity. Levels above the specified range put the patient at risk of toxicity, and levels below this range mean the lithium is not of any therapeutic benefit. Clinical benefit is derived with levels in the range of 0.4–1 mmol/L (ranges vary slightly between reporting laboratories), and higher levels within this range are possibly of more benefit for acutely manic patients.

Because lithium excretion is dependent on renal clearance, it should only be prescribed for people with satisfactory and stable renal function. Lithium is affected by changes in renal function and fluid balance, and altered fluid distribution such as seen in obesity and in pregnancy, as well as fluid intake such as forgetting to drink. Older adults should be carefully monitored for symptoms of lithium toxicity as this may develop even at moderate lithium levels in this population. Renal function and lithium levels should be monitored throughout treatment, usually 3-monthly or more often if clinically indicated. If serum concentrations of lithium are above the therapeutic range, signs of toxicity may be observed; these include blurred vision, muscle weakness, coarse tremor, slurred speech, confusion, seizures and renal damage. Any medicines that alter the fluid or salt balance will interact with lithium; this includes diuretics, ACE-inhibitors and non-steroidal anti-inflammatories (e.g. diclofenac, ibuprofen), and leads to increased lithium concentration and the possibility of toxicity. It is very important to inform patients of the signs of toxicity as well as of the side-effects that may occur at standard doses and serum levels.

As a drug with a narrow therapeutic window, lithium is not suitable for all patients. It is suitable for those who have a regular and reliable medicine-taking habit, and who do not vastly change diets or drinking habits. From the nature of the illness, many BPAD sufferers do not have regular routines so preclude the safe use of lithium.

Long-term lithium therapy can adversely affect the thyroid function, usually inducing hypothyroidism, which can be treated by thyroxine supplementation. In addition to monitoring renal function and lithium levels, patients taking long-term lithium should also have their thyroid function monitored.

Valproate

Sodium valproate was initially used and licensed for the treatment of various forms of epilepsy. However in recent decades its use as an anti-manic has been established, although only the valproic acid formulation is actually licensed (and therefore listed in the BNF) for this indication (Joint Formulary Committee 2011). It should be remembered that doses of sodium valproate and semi-sodium valproate are not exactly equivalent.

Valproate prevents manic and probably depressive relapses, and unlike lithium is not a medicine with a narrow therapeutic index. Against this significant advantage it can be teratogenic, and probably more so than lithium. This reduces its usefulness in women of child-bearing age and potential, and careful consideration should be given before prescribing it in such cases. Wherever possible the balance of teratogenic risks and therapeutic benefits should be discussed with the patient.

Valproate serum levels can be measured but optimum dosage should be determined mainly by clinical response rather than serum levels. If patients display adverse effects such as tremor, rash and hair loss, these may be a sign of toxicity. Measuring serum levels may be beneficial and it would be likely that a dose reduction or discontinuation of valproate would be necessary. Commonly noted side-effects include weight gain and gastrointestinal disturbances (particularly on initiation). Blood dyscrasias (e.g. thrombocytopenia and platelet dysfunction) and hepatic damage have been reported with the use of valproate, therefore periodic monitoring of full blood counts and liver function tests is recommended.

Carbamazepine

Carbamazepine has been used as a mood stabilizer, however this is not routinely recommended; it is less effective than lithium. However, if lithium has failed, or is not an appropriate choice, or the patient has previously had a good response to carbamazepine as a prophylactic agent carbamazepine may be tried. Carbamazepine has been studied more for mania and prophylaxis; there is limited data for bipolar depression. Like valproate, carbamazepine was initially used and licensed for the treatment of various forms of epilepsy, and it is listed in the BNF as an antiepileptic (Joint Formulary Committee 2011).

Carbamazepine undergoes significant hepatic metabolism and is a potent inducer of hepatic microsomal enzymes (P450 system), thus causing increased metabolism of many other medicines which are hepatically cleared, as well as inducing its own metabolism (auto-induction). Consequently pharmacokinetic interactions are particularly problematic with carbamazepine; an awareness of these and the appropriate monitoring required is necessary to help prevent precipitation or potentiation of side-effects, or reductions of plasma levels that may render the other medicines ineffective (e.g. oral contraceptives).

Like lithium, carbamazepine has a fairly narrow therapeutic window, meaning that therapeutic and toxic levels are close. This is further complicated by carbamazepine's complex pharmacokinetics, therefore measuring serum carbamazepine levels can be useful, and is routinely recommended every six months.

Lamotrigine

Lamotrigine is not routinely recommended first-line as a mood stabilizer. It has been shown to have some efficacy at preventing depressive relapses and is licensed for this indication, but not for manic relapses. Therefore it may have a role for patients whose burden of disease is depressive, more commonly in combination with another maintenance treatment that will prevent a manic relapse (e.g. lithium, valproate, an antipsychotic). It has also been shown to have some efficacy in the acute treatment of depressive relapse in BPAD. Lamotrigine should be very slowly titrated to a therapeutic maintenance dose over six weeks to minimize the risk of precipitating serious allergic dermatological reactions (such as Stephen Johnson's syndrome) that predominantly occur within the first two months of therapy. This time frame should be borne in mind if lamotrigine is initiated during an acute depressive relapse. Patients taking lamotrigine should be advised to seek urgent medical attention if any rash develops; if it does, lamotrigine should be stopped unless it is clear that the rash is not related to its use. If lamotrigine is to be initiated in a patient already taking valproate, lower doses are required as valproate significantly inhibits the clearance metabolism of lamotrigine, thereby increasing serum levels. Routine monitoring of blood levels of lamotrigine is not required as clinical response to lamotrigine appears not to be related to lamotrigine plasma levels.

Atypical antipsychotics as mood stabilizers

The atypical antipsychotics aripiprazole, olanzapine, quetiapine, and risperidone may be of use during manic relapses, and some have shown efficacy in preventing manic relapses in BPAD. An atypical antipsychotic is recommended if manic symptoms are severe, or there are marked behavioural disturbances as part of the mania and where psychotic symptoms

are also present. Olanzapine is recommended by NICE (2006) as one of the first-line antimanic agents in BPAD, either as monotherapy or in combination with other agents, both acutely and in the maintenance treatment phase. Quetiapine is also effective at preventing manic and depressive relapse.

 ## 26.5 Anxiolytics and hypnotics

The benzodiazepines as a group have four common qualities: anxiolytic potential, hypnotic or sedative effects, muscle relaxants and anti-epileptic action. Each varies in its potential for these effects, its half-life and duration of action. Thus different benzodiazepines are used for different purposes in view of these qualities. Longer acting benzodiazepines have a greater propensity to cause residual effects the following day and doses may be cumulative. Therefore, although the long-acting benzodiazepine nitrazepam has previously been used as a hypnotic it is now less used as it is not so suitable for this indication. The long acting diazepam and clonazepam are more prominently anxiolytic than sedative and therefore tend to be preferred for this indication.

Non-pharmacological strategies such as good sleep hygiene or the use of sleep diaries should be tried before medicines are considered for the treatment of insomnia. Psychological treatments, especially cognitive behavioural therapies, have also been shown to be effective in the management of persistent insomnia (NICE 2004). If it is established that non-pharmacological strategies are either inappropriate or ineffective, it may be necessary to consider using a hypnotic in the management of severe insomnia that interferes with normal daily life. Common hypnotics include the short-acting benzodiazepine temazepam, and the 'z-hypnotics' zopiclone, zolpidem and zaleplon. The 'z-drugs' are structurally unrelated to the benzodiazepines or one another, but their hypnotic effect and related adverse effects are broadly similar to those of the short-acting benzodiazepines. These all have the potential for misuse, abuse, and consequently diversion. Tolerance and dependence can develop rapidly, within 3–14 days of continuous use. They should only be prescribed for short periods of time and not for more than four weeks, and not on discharge from inpatient care (NICE 2004). Continuous benzodiazepine prescribing is associated with increased risk of hip fracture, and impairment of cognitive function and memory in older adults. This also carries increased risk of injury in road traffic accidents.

There is a lack of compelling evidence to distinguish between available hypnotics with regards to effectiveness, adverse effects, or potential for dependence or abuse. Whichever hypnotic is selected should be used at the lowest possible dose for the shortest possible period of time. Switching from one hypnotic to another should only occur when a patient experiences adverse effects directly related to a specific hypnotic (NICE 2004). Patients who have not responded to one hypnotic should not be prescribed any of the others. For those already addicted and tolerant to, or with a history of addiction to substances, it is preferable to avoid benzodiazepines and z-hypnotics. Sedating antihistamines (promethazine, diphenhydramine) can be used in preference to benzodiazepines. Table 26.3 summarizes the hypnotic properties of these antihistamines, the Z-hypnotics and benzodiazepines. If a patient is currently dependent on hypnotic or anxiolytic drugs, increasing use of addictive hypnotics should be avoided.

Melatonin (N-acteyl-5-methoxytryptamine) is a naturally occurring endogenous hormone secreted by the pineal gland, and is structurally related to serotonin. Melatonin is involved in the induction of sleep and is associated with the control of circadian rhythms and in the light-dark cycle. Secretion increases soon after the onset of darkness, peaks in the middle of the night and gradually decreases during the second half of the night. Melatonin is associated with a hypnotic effect and increased propensity to sleep, therefore exogenous melatonin can be useful in the management of primary insomnia. Melatonin's sleep-promoting properties are thought to be related to its activity at MT1 and MT2 as well as at MT3 receptors. There is a decrease in endogenous melatonin production as people age. The use of melatonin has been widely studied to aid sleep in children, particularly those with neurological (including visual impairment), developmental and neuropsychiatric disabilities. It is often used in this population when a pharmacological agent is needed in preference to an addictive hypnotic. Despite melatonin being freely available as a food supplement in some countries, it is classed as a medicine in the UK and only one brand is licensed (Joint Formulary Committee 2011).

Tolerance to the beneficial hypnotic effects of benzodiazepines develops over a few weeks, but tolerance to the anxiolytic effects can take a few

Table 26.3 Hypnotics (after Taylor *et al.* 2009; Joint Formulary Committee 2011)

Hypnotic	Time of onset (minutes)	Duration of action	Dose
Benzodiazepines			
Temazepam	30–60	Short	10–20 mg
Nitrazepam	20–60	Intermediate	2.5–10 mg
Diazepam	30–60	Long	5–15 mg
Z-hypnotics			
Zopiclone	15–30	Short	3.75–7.5 mg
Zolpidem	7–27	Short	5–10 mg
Antihistamines used as hypnotics			
Promethazine	Unclear, maybe 1–2 hours	Long	20–50 mg
Diphenhydramine	1 to 3 hours	Long	25–50 mg

months, and after regular use after as little as 3–14 days. Dependence is both physical and psychological. Stopping a benzodiazepine hypnotic or 'z-hypnotic' should be done gradually; the dose should be tapered off in order to avoid precipitating withdrawal symptoms. The exact plan should be tailored to the individual patient. Sudden cessation of benzodiazepines in those who are dependent can lead to a withdrawal syndrome that is potentially life threatening. The pharmacological mechanism of benzodiazepine tolerance and withdrawal remains unclear. Physical withdrawal symptoms include stiffness, weakness, muscle twitches, jerks, altered sensation, gastrointestinal disturbances, paraesthesia, flu-like symptoms, visual disturbances and convulsions. Psychological symptoms of withdrawal include anxiety, insomnia, depression, nightmares, depersonalization and derealization, perceptional distortions, decreased memory and concentration, delusions, visual and auditory hallucinations, confusion and delirium (Taylor *et al.* 2009).

26.6 Medicines for dementia

The most common form of dementia is Alzheimer's disease, a progressive deteriorating organic disease of the brain. The acetylcholine esterase inhibitors (AChEIs) donepezil, rivastigmine and galantamine as well as memantine are recommended in the management of dementia (NICE 2011) to enhance cognitive functioning. These do not reverse organic changes, but do slow cognitive deterioration. As their name suggests the clinical effects of AChEIs derives from their specific inhibition of the enzyme acetylcholinesterase in the brain, which is the predominant cholinesterase that acts to break down the released acetylcholine in the synapses. Inhibiting this enzyme augments the effect of acetylcholine that is released by the functionally intact cholinergic neurons. AChEIs are indicated for the symptomatic treatment of mild to moderately severe Alzheimer's dementia; increased activity in the cholinergic system is associated with improved cognitive function. This can be achieved in patients with dementia of

the Alzheimer type with sufficient acetylcholine activity to benefit from augmentation. Memantine is recommended for moderate to severe Alzheimer's disease and works via a completely different mechanism as it is a NMDA-receptor antagonist. There is increasing evidence that malfunctioning of glutamatergic neurotransmission, in particular at NMDA-receptors, contributes to both the symptoms and disease progression in Alzheimer's dementia. Anti-dementia medicines should be used as monotherapy and not combined. AChEIs should not routinely be used for mild cognitive impairment or cognitive decline in vascular dementia.

On initiation and during the first few weeks common side-effects of AChEIs include loss of appetite, nausea, vomiting and diarrhoea (Joint Formulary Committee 2011). These are directly due to the medicine's cholinergic activity and are dose-related, and may be eased by slowing the rate of titration, or dose reduction.

Dementias may present with non-cognitive symptoms such as depression, hallucinations, anxiety, delusions, marked agitation and behavioural disturbances. Behavioural disturbances or challenging behaviour include symptoms such as aggression, agitation, wandering, hoarding, sexual disinhibition, apathy and disruptive vocal activity such as shouting. The behavioural and psychotic symptoms in dementia (BPSD) can be difficult to manage. Management should initially focus on identifying any precipitating or aggravating factors, such as physical health or comfort. Once all such factors have been excluded and/or remedied and various behavioural strategies have been fully explored, only then should pharmacological options be considered. Options include initiation of AChEIs, or the short-term use of the anxiolytic lorazepam for a calming or sedative effect. Other off-label options include carbamazepine and trazodone for the management of anxiety and depression, especially where sedation is required, although there is little evidence to support the use of these two (NICE 2011).

There is growing evidence to indicate that the use of antipsychotics in patients with dementia is associated with a significantly increased risk of

stroke and death. Consequently antipsychotics are not recommended for routine use in the treatment of BPSD, unless the patient has a primary psychosis that requires antipsychotic treatment. Risperidone is the only antipsychotic licensed for the short-term treatment (up to six weeks) of persistent aggression in patients with moderate to severe Alzheimer's dementia, unresponsive to non-pharmacological approaches and when there is a risk of harm to self or others (Joint Formulary Committee 2011).

26.7 Medicines for attention deficit hyperactivity disorder (ADHD)

ADHD starts in childhood and usually subsides by adulthood in the majority of patients. Medication should be reserved for those with severe and impairing symptoms, and for those with more moderate impairment who have refused or not responded to non-pharmacological treatments. Medication should always be offered as part of a comprehensive treatment plan that includes psychological, behavioural and educational advice and interventions (NICE 2008). The most commonly used first-line medication is methylphenidate; others are atomoxetine and (much less frequently) dexamfetamine. Rarely imipramine (a TCA), clonidine, bupropion and modafinil may be considered. There is no definitive data to suggest greater efficacy of any licensed medicine over another.

Methylphenidate and dexamfetamine are central nervous system (CNS) stimulants (also known as psychostimulants) regulated under the Misuse of Drugs Act 1971 as controlled drugs (CDs). Robust evidence clearly demonstrates the efficacy of methylphenidate either alone, or in conjunction with behavioural therapy. Dexamfetamine is used far less often, as it is commonly perceived to have a greater abuse potential than methylphenidate. It is only available in an immediate-release formulation necessitating multiple daily dosing. Atomoxetine was the first non-psychostimulant to demonstrate efficacy and to be licensed for the treatment of ADHD in the UK. It is not classified as a controlled drug as it lacks the potential for abuse.

Unlike most medicines used within psychiatry, the psychostimulants usually start having an effect within a few hours, although they can take a week to gain full effect. Atomoxetine has a much slower onset of action and the initial dose titration may take several weeks. Treatment should be with a single medication, although sometimes is it necessary to combine different formulations of methylphenidate. A range of extended-release formulations are available that allow once-daily dosing, rather than twice or thrice daily with the immediate release formulation. This has a significant impact as the requirement for frequent doses often presented a practical barrier to effective medicine use. It is important that those prescribing and administering these formulations understand the differences between them, as they have a profound effect on the dosage regimen. The first (or only) daily dose of methylphenidate is usually given before breakfast to allow it to be released and take effect as the child gets up and starts their morning routine. Atomoxetine is usually given once a day in the morning, but if not tolerated this can be given as two doses. Although administered daily, it is important that the psychostimulants are used in a manner that allows serum levels to diminish to zero within the 24-hour cycle, thereby not inducing tolerance and addiction. There is a growing evidence base to support the use of methylphenidate and atomoxetine in adults with ADHD. However this data is not as robust as that for children. Medicines are not recommended nor licensed for the treatment of ADHD in pre-school children, as the diagnosis cannot be definitively clarified in this age group (NICE 2008).

26.8 Medicines in rapid tranquillization

When medicines are used to quickly calm a severely agitated patient to reduce the risk of imminent and serious violence to self or others, rather than to treat

the underlying psychiatric condition, this is referred to as rapid tranquillization (RT): 'All medication given in the short-term management of disturbed/violent behaviour should be considered as part of rapid tranquillisation (including pro re nata [PRN] medication)' (NICE 2005b). The aim of RT is for the patient to be sedated but able to participate in further assessment and treatment and able to respond to communication throughout. The medicines used for RT are usually a benzodiazepine such as lorazepam and, or, an antipsychotic, commonly haloperidol.

Principles of medicine use in RT

Violent behaviour should only be managed with medicines once non-pharmacological interventions have been explored. Medicines should only be used when it has been established that the risks of not doing so are greater than the risk of doing so. Medication should not be used to manage aggression caused by identifiable environmental factors (such as understaffing or lack of staff skills) that could be managed by non-pharmacological means. For longer-term management and prevention of violence, refer to Chapter 18.

Before giving medicine for RT, patients must be informed that medication is going to be administered, and they must be given the opportunity to voluntarily accept oral medication at all stages. All patients should be allowed to make an informed choice where at all possible. The minimum effective dose should be used, and BNF maximum doses should only be exceeded in extreme circumstances and with the advice of a consultant psychiatrist. If the maximum licensed dose is exceeded, more frequent and intensive monitoring of physical health should be conducted: 'Blood pressure, pulse, temperature and respiratory rate and hydration should be recorded regularly' post RT (NICE 2005b).

Principles of prescribing medicines for RT

All prescriptions for RT medicines should be tailored for the individual patient. The prescriber and nurse administering the medicines should consider any coexisting medical illnesses (as some may predispose the patient to agitated or dysphoric states), and any non-psychiatric causes for the disturbed behaviour (e.g. trauma, organic, psychological, intoxication or withdrawal states). Having established the need for RT, those prescribing and administering should then consider all of the medicine prescribed for the patient and any recent use of illicit substances. These may interact pharmacodynamically or pharmacokinetically with the proposed RT, leading to altered dose requirements and potential side-effects. Use of more than one medicine within a class of medication (e.g. antipsychotics) should be avoided where at all possible.

Route of administration and formulations

In general, oral medication should be offered before parenteral treatment is administered. The choice of medicine is often influenced, and limited, by the formulations available. A number of the atypical antipsychotics are available as soluble or disintegrating tablets and liquids. Several benzodiazepines are available as liquids (diazepam, clonazepam) but these as not ideal for RT due to their long duration of action. In RT it is essential to immediately determine whether a patient has swallowed an orally administered medicine, and oro-dispersible tablets and liquids aid this assessment compared to regular tablets. However, it should be noted that medicine is not buccally absorbed from oro-dispersible formulations; the tablets disperse in the saliva; which must be swallowed as the drug is absorbed from the gastrointestinal tract. Only a rather small number of benzodiazepines and antipsychotics are available as injections and this limits the choice of medicine if an injection is required.

Medication administered parenterally has a faster onset of action than oral administration, and it should not be assumed that doses given by various routes are bioequivalent. Therefore they should be prescribed separately and different doses may be needed. In routine practice if parenteral administration is required the intramuscular (IM) route is the preferred choice; although intraveous (IV) has a faster onset of action, it is hard to administer an IV injection to a struggling and restrained patient and there is a risk of inadvertent intra-arterial administration. There are very few situations in which an IM injection cannot be used.

Choice of agent in RT

Due to the acute nature of the clinical situation and the risk of violence, generating robust evidence of the clinical efficacy of medicines in RT is inherently difficult. It is notable that there are few rigorous trials directly comparing the efficacy and safety of agents in RT, with the exception of the four TREC trials (Taylor *et al.* 2009).

Medicines commonly used for RT include:

- Benzodiazepines
  - Lorazepam po & IM
- Antipsychotics
  - Haloperidol po & IM
  - Aripiprazole po & IM
  - Olanzapine po & IM
- Others
  - Promethazine IM

In general, a short-acting benzodiazepine is recommended as the first-line pharmacological treatment in RT, whether orally or parenterally (NICE 2005b). Some studies suggest that using a benzodiazepine alone is just as effective as using it in conjunction with an antipsychotic and it has a lower incidence of EPS, however other studies suggest to the contrary.

Generally, antipsychotics are not recommended as first-line or sole agents in RT. On balance, antipsychotics have greater risks over benefits compared to benzodiazepines. Various antipsychotics have a considerable risk of EPS, cardiac arrhythmia with potential cardiorespiratory collapse, and neuroleptic malignant syndrome (NMS). Furthermore, there is little difference in efficacy between using a

benzodiazepine alone or an antipsychotic alone. When parenteral haloperidol is used, an oral and parenteral antimuscarinic (e.g. procyclidine) should be immediately available to treat any acute dystonic reactions.

However, when a benzodiazepine alone is insufficient, and in more serious scenarios, it is common practice to use a benzodiazepine (commonly lorazepam) with an antipsychotic (commonly haloperidol). This combines the benefit of the sedation from the benzodiazepine, so minimizing the dose of antipsychotic required, and therefore the level of EPS experienced with typical antipsychotics. Some trials suggest that giving promethazine (a sedating antihistamine) with haloperidol is more effective and safer than using an antipsychotic alone.

When preparing to administer prescribed doses of PRN medicines for RT, nurses should also note the patient's regularly prescribed psychotropics. Giving PRN doses in addition to the regularly prescribed psychotropics may mean administration of greater than BNF maximum doses and put the patient at clinical risk.

26.9 Medicines for alcohol and opioid withdrawal and abstinence

It is key to distinguish between substance-induced mental health disorders and substance-related disorders. The influence of substance misuse (for both illicit and prescribed/over-the-counter substances) on mental health disorders is beyond the scope of this chapter; this section considers the pharmacological treatments for some substance addictions. Within the setting of mental health services, two commonly seen and pharmacologically treated addictions are alcohol and opioid addiction. For both addictions treatment focuses on two areas – firstly assisting withdrawal and managing the symptoms and secondly maintenance of longer term abstinence.

Alcohol

Withdrawal symptoms from alcohol can vary from quite mild (e.g. the commonly seen tremor), with relatively mild restlessness, agitation, anxiety, irritability and insomnia, sweating and fever, nausea and vomiting, tachycardia, systolic hypertension; to more dangerous in more severely dependent drinkers (e.g. hallucinations, seizures and life threatening delirium tremens – DT). The first symptoms of alcohol withdrawal can occur within a few hours of consumption of the last alcoholic drink (before the blood alcohol level falls to zero), peak within two to three days, and resolve within five to seven days. Long acting benzodiazepines such as chlordiazepoxide or diazepam are used as substitutes for alcohol and are prescribed as a carefully managed reducing regimen over a week or so to safely withdraw the patient. Benzodiazepines themselves have the potential for addiction, so these should not be continued long-term. The Clinical Institute Withdrawal Assessment for Alcohol scale (CIWA-Ar) is a 10-item scale that can be used to measure the severity of the withdrawal and hence inform prescribing of doses of withdrawal regimens.

It is also crucial to consider vitamin supplementation for alcoholic patients as they commonly have deficiencies particularly of thiamine (vitamin B1), which can cause Wernicke's encephalopathy. Initially Wernicke's encephalopathy is reversible but, if left inadequately or untreated can develop into Korsakoff's syndrome which is an irreversible brain damage and is associated with significant mortality. Therefore in patients at high risk of developing Wernicke's encephalopathy thiamine should be given parenterally (IM or IV) (rather than orally when it is very poorly absorbed). In the longer term, medicines such as acamprosate and disulfiram can be used alongside psychosocial interventions to assist with abstinence from alcohol use.

Opioids

Treatment of opioid addiction and dependence usually involves oral substitution with the long acting opioid methadone. This can be used as a decreasing regimen to avoid precipitating opioid withdrawal symptoms, and can be used in the longer term as an aid to abstinence from illicit opioid use, as part of a maintenance programme for individuals who are unwilling or have repetitively been unable to discontinue opioid use. Alternatively the opioid partial against buprenorphine can be used as another substitute for the misused opioids, both as a reducing regimen to avoid precipitating opioid withdrawal symptoms, and in the longer term as an aid to abstinence. This is administered sub-lingually on a daily or alternate day basis. Lastly the adrenergic agonists clonidine and lofexidine can be used to alleviate withdrawal symptoms during planned withdrawal regimens, but clonidine in particular can cause profound hypotension. Maintenance treatment minimizes some harms that would otherwise be associated with illicit opioid use; for example, doses are stable and maintained at the lowest amount reasonable, and oral administration avoids the risks associated with use of unclean injecting equipment which is associated with the transfer of blood-borne viruses.

 ## 26.10 Adverse effects and monitoring requirements

Side-effects, often more accurately described as 'adverse drug reactions' (ADRs), are unwanted or harmful reactions that a patient may experience after taking a medicine in the intended, prescribed manner, when the reaction is thought to be caused by the medicine. Such reactions are generally classified into two broad groups (Pirmohamed *et al.* 1998), which will be addressed in turn (see Box 26.1).

- **Type A reactions – predictable:** these are a result of the medicine's normal pharmacological activity, although may be unrelated to the medicine's intended clinical effect. Commonly such reactions are dose-related. These are the majority of ADRs.

■ **Type B reactions – idiosyncratic:** these are bizarre and unpredictable reactions that could not be predicted or expected from the known pharmacological activity of the medicine. They include hypersensitivity reactions mediated by immunological factors and true allergic reactions mediated by immuno-globulin E. These are not normally dose-related.

Type A reactions – pharmacologically predictable ADRs

In addition to affecting the intended receptors for their activity, nearly all psychotropics are also active at other receptors which do not contribute to their intended activity. For example, they may also antagonize or agonize other sub-types of dopamine receptors in various regions of the brain, or histamine-1 receptors, cholinergic receptors or alpha-1 receptors. The pattern of receptor blockade by individual medicines leads to pharmacologically predictable side-effects. Examples include sedation – a histaminergic effect seen with clozapine, mirtazapine, olanzapine, trazodone, and many TCAs. The following group of effects is mediated by cholinergic activity: dry mouth, blurred vision, constipation and urinary retention (seen with procyclidine, promethazine, orphenadrine and many TCAs). Postural hypotension, dizziness and syncope are alpha-1 related effects seen with chlorpromazine, clozapine, quetiapine and trazodone. The predictable and potentially dangerous pressor effects of MAOIs were described previously, and are the reason for the demise in use of these clinically effective antidepressants. It is clearly imperative to have a basic understanding of the pharmacological action of each medicine in order to understand its predictable, common and often important adverse effects. Some Type A reactions commonly seen with psychotropic medicines will now been considered.

EPS

Many antipsychotics and a few other medicines can cause EPS due to antagonism of D_2 receptors in the nigrostriatal region of the brain (whereas antipsychotic activity is attributed to antagonism of D_2 receptors in the mesolimbic pathway). EPS can be grouped as described in Box 26.2. Parkinsonian symptoms and acute dystonic reactions can be treated using antimuscarinics (e.g. procyclidine), either orally or by IM injection. The latter is needed if the patient cannot swallow a tablet (e.g. due to jaw-lock; or if a faster onset of action is needed than oral administration affords).

Electrocardiogram (ECG) changes

Several psychotropics affect the cardiac function in a number of ways. Of particular note is the association of certain antipsychotics with QTc prolongation on an ECG. This is a dose dependent effect (Taylor *et al.* 2009). An increased QTc value is a risk factor for the potentially fatal ventricular arrhythmia Torsade de Pointes. Antipsychotics that are more likely to increase the QTc include haloperidol, pimozide, sertindole and thioridazine. NICE guidelines (2009) recommend that an ECG should be offered to all inpatients prior to starting an antipsychotic. With the exception of lofepramine, TCAs also increase the QTc interval so are more cardiotoxic in overdose than other antidepressants such as SSRIs (NICE 2010a). It is recommended that if a

---

Box 26.1

Type A	Type B
Predictable	Unpredictable
Usually dose dependent	Rarely dose dependent
High morbidity	Low morbidity
Low mortality	High mortality
Responds to dose reduction	Responds to drug withdrawal

After Mhra Website: http://www.mhra.gov.uk/Safetyinformation/Reportingsafetyproblems/Reportingsuspectedadversedrugreactions/Healthcareprofessionalreporting/Adversedrugreactions/index.htm

Box 26.2 Movement disorders caused by antipsychotics (Joint Formulary Committee 2011)

EPS consist of:

1. **Parkinsonian symptoms:** (including tremor, rigidity, bradykinesia, stooping gait), which may appear gradually. These may remit if the antipsychotic is withdrawn, and may be suppressed by the administration of antimuscarinics, however, routine co-administration of antimuscarinics is not justified because not all patients are affected. Antimuscarinics are also associated with adverse effects and may unmask or worsen tardive dyskinesia.

2. **Acute dystonic reactions (abnormal face and body movements) and dyskinesia:** occurs more commonly in children or young adults and may appear after only a few doses. These are acute and painful and need immediate treatment with antimuscarinic, often in the parenteral form.

3. **Akathisia (inner restlessness):** characteristically occurs after large initial doses and may resemble an exacerbation of the condition being treated.

4. **Tardive dyskinesia (rhythmic, involuntary movements of tongue, face, and jaw):** usually develops following long-term use of antipsychotics or with high doses, but may develop on short-term treatment with low doses. It is of particular concern because it may be irreversible on withdrawing therapy and treatment is usually ineffective. However, drug withdrawal at the earliest signs may halt its full development.

patient's QTc exceeds 500 ms, the suspected causal psychotropic should be discontinued and the patient immediately be referred to cardiologist for review (Taylor *et al.* 2009). The increased risk of sudden cardiac death with antipsychotics appears to be comparable for typical and atypical antipsychotics.

Prolactin-related adverse reactions

Prolactin is a hormone released from the pituitary gland in the brain and present in the bloodstream. Some antipsychotics block dopamine receptors on the lactotroph cells in the pituitary gland preventing inhibition of prolactin secretion by dopamine. This leads to sustained raised serum prolactin, which is called hyperprolactinaemia. This is common with all typical antipsychotics, risperidone and amisulpride. Hyperprolactinaemia has acute symptoms as well as chronic effects, but may be asymptomatic. Acute symptoms include in women oligo- or amenorrhoea, loss of libido, breast tenderness and galactorrhoea, and in men impaired libido and erectile

dysfunction (Hamner and Arana 1998). Chronic effects include menstrual disturbances (including amenorrhoea) in women, gynaecomastia in men (the growth of breast tissue), infertility, obesity, acne, hirsutism and reduced bone mineral density which potentially increases the risk of osteoperosis. There may also be a risk of enhanced prolactinoma growth, breast cancer, prostate cancer and cardiovascular disease. Hyperprolactinaemia is diagnosed by measuring the level of prolactin in the blood.

Serotonin syndrome

Serotonin syndrome (SS) is a potentially life-threatening ADR, resulting from a pharmacodynamic interaction between serotonergic agents. Signs and symptoms include restlessness, diaphoresis, tremor, shivering, confusion, convulsions and death. When augmenting or combining serotonergic antidepressants there is a risk of cumulative adverse-effects including SS, so patients should be monitored even more carefully. SS is reversible on cessation of the serotonergic agent(s).

Metabolic syndrome

Metabolic syndrome has been described as a cluster of abnormalities that increase the risk of cardiovascular disease, namely:

- obesity;
- hyperlipidaemia;
- hypertension;
- hyperglycaemia.

This cluster may arise in the general population but several mental health conditions and their treatments (especially antipsychotics) may increase the likelihood. The detailed pharmacology as to why antipsychotics can precipitate metabolic syndrome is not fully understood, but they are known to increase weight and disturb lipid and glucose control (see Box 26.3). Antipsychotic induced weight gain seems to result from increased food intake and in some cases reduced energy expenditure. Most weight is gained during the first three to four months of treatment although may continue for much longer. Other psychotropics such as TCAs, mirtazapine, lithium and valproate also tend to increase appetite and lead to weight gain (see Box 26.3).

Some antipsychotics can also disturb the lipid balance potentially leading to or aggravating the onset of hyperlipidaemia (high risk: clozapine, olanzapine; moderate risk: quetiapine; minimal risk: risperidone). Some antipsychotics can also disturb the glucose balance potentially leading to or aggravating the onset of hyperglycaemia. Consequently antipsychotics have been implicated in increasing the risk of developing diabetes (NICE 2009). The mechanisms of this are unclear, but may include 5HT2A/5HT2C antagonism, increased lipids, weight gain and leptin resistance (Taylor et al. 2009).

Type B reactions – idiosyncratic ADRs

There are numerous idiosyncratic adverse effects reported with all medicines. Some are exceptional yet serious, such as fatal hepototoxicity heptatoxicity with atomoxetine. Others are still very unusual but less serious (such as alopecia with sodium valproate). In view of the likelihood, severity and pattern of onset of potential ADRs, monitoring of relevant physical health parameters may be recommended. For example, as hepatotoxicity is a very rare reaction with atomoxetine, with an acute onset, it is not considered beneficial to regularly monitor liver function tests in all children taking atomoxetine. Instead, children and carers should be advised how to recognize the clinical symptoms of hepatotoxicity and seek medical advice if these develop

---

Box 26.3 Risk of weight gain associated with antipsychotics (Allison et al. 1999; Lieberman et al. 2005; Taylor et al. 2009)

High propensity (e.g. a third or more of patients may gain >7 per cent of baseline weight)
Clozapine
Olanzapine
Moderate risk (e.g. 10–20 per cent of patients may gain >7 per cent of baseline weight)
Quetiapine
Chlorpromazine
Risperidone
Low risk (e.g. <10 per cent of patients may gain >7 per cent of baseline weight)
Amisulpride
Aripiprazole
Haloperidol
Significant weight gain has been defined as an increase >7 per cent from baseline.

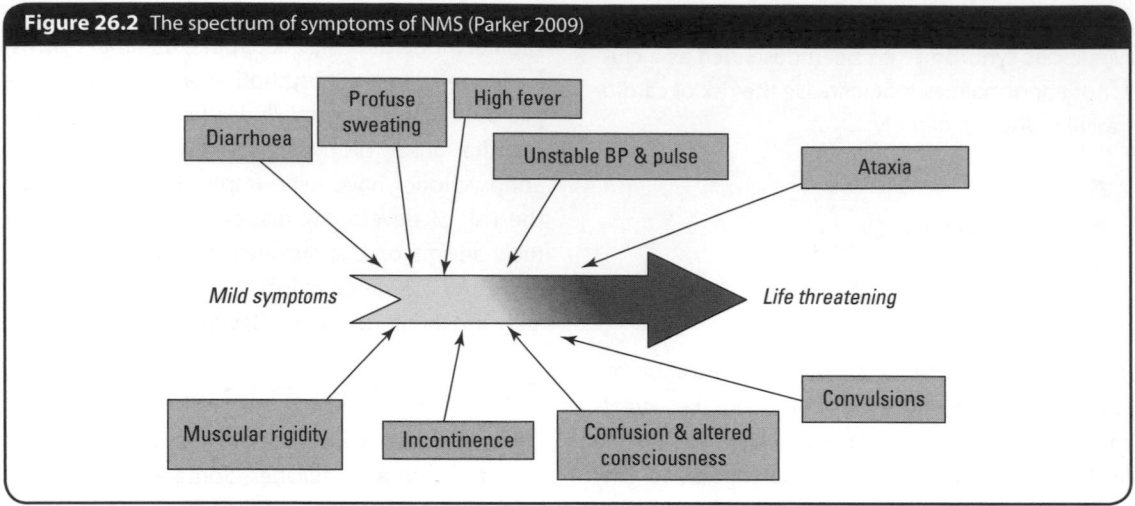

Figure 26.2 The spectrum of symptoms of NMS (Parker 2009)

(NICE 2008). For medicines where hepatic disturbances are a little more likely and have a more gradual onset, regular monitoring of liver function tests is recommended in order to identify any early signs of disturbances (e.g. valproate and carbamazepine).

Neuroleptic malignant syndrome (NMS)

NMS is a rare and potentially life-threatening disorder that (as the name suggests) is most often precipitated by 'neuroleptics' – also called antipsychotics. NMS can be complex to diagnose as there are commonly many confounding factors, and it may be confused with catatonia (Taylor *et al.* 2009). Symptoms include hyperthermia, profuse sweating, tachycardia and unstable blood pressure confusion, fluctuating levels of consciousness and stupor, catatonic muscular rigidity, incontinence and autonomic dysfunction with pallor, urinary incontinence and a raised creatine phosphokinase (CPK). Refer to Figure 26.2. There is no recognized spectrum of severity of symptoms.

It is hypothesized that NMS is due to an over-blockade of the dopaminergic system. It has been reported with all antipsychotics (both typical and atypical), and with some other agents which affect the dopaminergic system (e.g. medicines used in Parkinson's disease and related disorders, SSRI antidepressants, venlafaxine, lithium, methylphenidate, metoclopramide, tetrabenazine and zonisamide).

Because of the low incidence, the diagnostic difficulties, and the varying reports in the literature, it is not possible to confidently differentiate the incidence of NMS with various antipsychotics, but it is estimated as <1 per cent. If NMS develops it is essential to immediately discontinue the suspected causal agent(s) (i.e. any antipsychotic) and seek medical opinion. The patient's physical parameters should be closely monitored (BP, pulse, temperature) and they may need to be rehydrated. Benzodiazepines can be used as short-term sedatives, and paterneral dopaminergic agonists such as bromocriptine and dantrolene may be used in a medical setting. The symptoms of NMS usually last for five to seven days after discontinuing the suspected causal agent. If an antipsychotic depot formulation has been used, this may be considerably prolonged. Antipsychotic re-challenge is inherently associated with a risk of precipitating another episode, so should be done very cautiously. Once the diagnosis of NMS is confirmed it is recommended that antipsychotics are not re-started for about a week, and only after the symptoms have completely resolved. An alternative antipsychotic should be tried. The chosen antipsychotic should be started at a very low dose and titrated very slowly towards a therapeutic dose. Depot injections should be avoided.

26.11 Conclusion

In summary the key points of learning from this chapter are:

- All psychotropic medicines act in the CNS to exert their clinical effect, and like many medicines they can often be used for the treatment of several illnesses.

- In this chapter they are grouped and discussed according to their most common use and in line with the BNF categories.

- To use any medicine safely it is imperative that health care professionals have a working knowledge and understanding of the medicine's mode of action, common side-effects and interactions.

Annotated bibliography

Joint Formulary Committee (2011) *British National Formulary*, 61st edn. London: British Medical Association and Royal Pharmaceutical Society.
This is the essential reference text for routine use during medicine use and administration. Published six-monthly.

National Institute for Health and Clinical Excellence (NICE) clinical evidence-based guidelines, developed by consensus groups of experts in the field. These guidelines reflect optimal routine practice and should be followed in standard care.

2005: *Clinical Guideline No. 25: Violence — the short term management of disturbed/violent behaviour in in-patient psychiatric settings and emergency departments.* London: NICE.

2006: *Clinical Guideline No. 38: Bipolar disorder – the management of bipolar disorder in adults, children and adolescents, in primary and secondary care.* London: NICE.

2008: *Clinical Guideline 72: Attention deficit hyperactivity disorder – diagnosis and management of ADHD in children, young people and adults.* London: NICE.

2009: *Clinical Guideline 82: Schizophrenia – core interventions in the treatment and management of schizophrenia in primary and secondary care.* London: NICE.

2010: *Clinical Guideline 90: Depression – the treatment and management of depression in adults.* London: NICE.

2010: *Clinical Guideline 91: Depression in adults with a chronic physical health problem.* London: NICE.

2011: *Technology Appraisal 217, March 2011: Donepezil, galantamine, rivastigmine and memantine for the treatment of Alzheimer's disease – review of NICE technology appraisal guidance 111.* London: NICE.

'Stahl's Illustrated' is a series of nine short textbooks including the following titles: *Antipsychotics* (2nd edn), *Antidepressants* and *Mood Stabilizers*. These easily accessible pharmacology books are heavily illiustrated with cartoons, making the concepts of pharmacology as fun and easy to remember as they can be. The editor is Stephen M. Stahl and they are published by ?????

Taylor D. *et al.* (2012) *The Maudsley Prescribing Guidelines*, 11th edn. Informa Healthcare.
An easily accessible small textbook on medicines with comparisons and commentary.

References

Allison, D. *et al.* (1999) Antipsychotic induced weight gain: a comprehensive research synthesis, *American Journal of Psychiatry*, 156: 1686–96.

Anderson, I.M. *et al.* (2008) Evidence-based guidelines for treating depressive disorders with antidepressants: a revision of the 2000 British Association for Psychopharmacology guidelines, *Journal of Psychopharmacology*, 22(4): 343–96.

Bhattacharjee, J. and El-Sayeh, H.G.G. (2008) Aripiprazole versus typicals for schizophrenia, *Cochrane Database of Systematic Reviews*, Issue 1.

Eyding D. *et al.* (2010) Reboxetine for acute treatment of major depression: systematic review and meta-analysis of published and unpublished placebo and selective serotonin reuptake inhibitor controlled trials, *British Medical Journal*, 341: c4737.

Hamner, M.B. and Arana, G.W. (1998) Hyperprolactinaemia in antipsychotic-treated patients: guidelines for avoidance and management, *CNS Drugs*, 10: 209–22.

Joint Formulary Committee (2011) *British National Formulary*, 61st edn. London: British Medical Association and Royal Pharmaceutical Society.

Kane, J., *et al.* (1988) Clozapine for the treatment resistant schizophrenic, *Archives of General Psychiatry*, 45; 789–96.

Lieberman, J. *et al.* (2005) Clinical antipsychotics trials of intervention effectiveness (catie) investigators: effectiveness of antipsychotic drugs in patients with chronic schizophrenia, *New England Journal of Medicine*, 353(12): 1209–23.

McEvoy, J.P. *et al.* (2006) Effectiveness of clozapine versus olanzapine, quetiapine, and risperidone in patients with chronic schizophrenia who did not respond to prior atypical antipsychotic treatment, *American Journal of Psychiatry*, 163: 600–10.

NICE (National Institute for Health and Clinical Excellence) (2004) *Technology Appraisal 77: Guidance on the use of zaleplon, zolpidem and zopiclone for the short-term management of insomnia.* London: NICE.

NICE (National Institute for Health and Clinical Excellence) (2005a) *Clinical Guideline No. 28: Depression in children and young people. Identification and management in primary, community and secondary care.* London: NICE.

NICE (National Institute for Health and Clinical Excellence) (2005b) *Clinical Guideline No. 25: Violence – the short-term management of disturbed/violent behaviour in in-patient psychiatric settings and emergency departments.* London: NICE.

NICE (National Institute for Health and Clinical Excellence) (2006) *Clinical Guideline No. 38: Bipolar disorder – the management of bipolar disorder in adults, children and adolescents, in primary and secondary care.* London: NICE.

NICE (National Institute for Health and Clinical Excellence) (2008) *Clinical Guideline 72: Attention deficit hyperactivity disorder – diagnosis and management of ADHD in children, young people and adults.* London: NICE.

NICE (National Institute for Health and Clinical Excellence) (2009) *Clinical Guideline 82: Schizophrenia – core interventions in the treatment and management of schizophrenia in primary and secondary care.* London: NICE.

NICE (National Institute for Health and Clinical Excellence) (2010a) *Clinical Guideline 90: Depression – the treatment and management of depression in adults.* London: NICE.

NICE (National Institute for Health and Clinical Excellence) (2011) *Technology Appraisal 217, March 2011: Donepezil, galantamine, rivastigmine and memantine for the treatment of Alzheimer's disease – review of NICE technology appraisal guidance 111.* London: NICE.

Parker, C. (2009) Antipsychotics in the treatment of schizophrenia – review: antipsychotics, an update, *Progress in Neurology & Psychiatry*, April: 22–30.

Pirmohamed, M., Breckenridge, A.M., Kitteringham, N.R. and Park, B.K. (1998) Adverse drug reactions, *British Medical Journal*, 316: 1295–8.

Taylor, D. *et al.* (2012) *The Maudsley Prescribing Guidelines*, 11th edn. London: Informa Healthcare.

Chapter 27

Mental Health Medication in Practice

Caroline Parker

27.1 Introduction

This chapter builds on Chapter 26, focusing on the application of knowledge about medicines when using them in practice, for the benefit of patients. The chapter covers:

- the 'five rights' of medicine administration;
- The NMC standards for medicines administration;
- involving patients in medicine administration;
- assessing the benefits and adverse effects of medicines;
- psychotropics and physical health;
- medicine interactions;
- smoking and psychotropics;
- psychotropics during pregnancy and breast-feeding;
- principles of using psychotropics in children and in older adults.

The British National Formulary (BNF) is the main-stay reference text for all health care professionals involved in the use of medicines, whether pre-scribing, supplying, administering or monitoring. Published every six months (both as a hard copy and online) it lists all medicines licensed in the UK, including their indications, cautions, use in preg-nancy and breastfeeding, side-effects, dosing infor-mation, available formulations and prices. This is the primary reference source used when questions arise around the administration of any prescribed medicines. The Nursing and Midwifery Council (NMC) expects that all registered nurses be familiar with a medicine's usual dose, interactions, side-effects and intended use.

27.2 The 'five rights' of medicine administration

Medicine incidents, both actual errors and 'near misses', frequently occur across all health care set-tings, and can put patients at risk of harm. Many

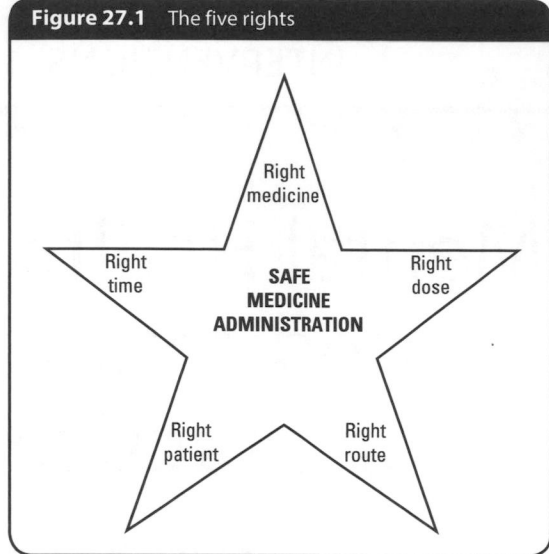

Figure 27.1 The five rights

Right medicine

Right time

Right dose

SAFE MEDICINE ADMINISTRATION

Right patient

Right route

incidents are known to be preventable, with government and professional registration bodies issuing guidance to individuals and organizations about measures to minimize the risk of medicine incidents occurring (DH 2004; NMC 2007). A frequently used aide memoir is the 'five rights' of medicine administration (see Figure 27.1) (DH 2004; Joint Formulary Committee 2011). Prior to administering any medicine a nurse should check the following: that it is the right medication, in the right dose, to the right patient, by the right route, and at the right time.

Ensuring accurate and safe administration of medicines requires cohesive working by each member of the multi-disciplinary team (pharmacists, doctors and nurses).

Right medicine

The correct medicine is selected for administration as stipulated by the prescription. This is dependent on knowledge of the medicines involved; if unsure, the nurse should check the intended medicine against other sources (e.g. the BNF and colleagues) for clarification and confirmation. Medicines with similar names are often confused (e.g. paroxetine and fluoxetine). Storing medicines in certain ways can help to minimize the risk of incorrect selection (e.g. similar packaging or names). Patients' medicine treatment plans should be clear and easily accessible for all involved health care professionals.

Right dose

Selecting the correct dose requires knowledge of the medicine involved. Appropriate doses will vary according to the indication and stage in treatment; for example, on initiation it is essential to start some antipsychotics (e.g. clozapine and quetiapine) at very low doses in order to avoid significant side-effects. Conversely, patients tolerant to the effects of opiates may require large doses (e.g. > 100 mg/day methadone), but even a few days' break in treatment can lead to decreased tolerance and the same dose can then be fatal.

Medicines are usually formulated such that, for adults, doses of oral medicines are typically one or two tablets/capsules, or 5 or 10mLs of liquid, and one ampoule/vial for injections. If when preparing a dose it appears that multiple tablets/capsules or ampoules, or a large volume of liquid, are needed this should alert the nurse to a potential error and they should seek advice to clarify the intended prescription. Errors involving injections carry potentially higher risks, therefore particular attention should be paid to their use. If there is any doubt regarding a specific dose or calculation (e.g. a dose based on mg/kg) the nurse should seek a check from another professional.

Right time

Medicines should be administered at the timing directed by the prescription (e.g. in the morning with breakfast, or at night). For some medicines the exact timing of administration is imperative (e.g. hypnotics need to be administered approximately an hour before the patient would like to go to sleep). For others, the timing is important to maintain therapeutic drug levels and/or clinical effect, (e.g. anticonvulsants, or the minimum inhibitory concentration of antibiotics). For some medicines it is the longer-term timing that is of consequence – for example, antipsychotics should be continued for one to two years following a first epi-sode of psychosis (NICE 2009a) as rates of acute psychotic relapse are high when antipsychotics are discontinued earlier (78 per cent within one year, 96 per cent within two years – Gittin *et al.* 2001). When a medicine is not given at the time pre-scribed, nurses need to apply their knowledge about the medicine, its indication, and the impact of missing a dose or giving it late, in order to decide whether to administer it at that point in time. If there is ever any doubt, advice should be sought from the prescriber or pharmacist.

Right route

As well as administering the medicine via the cor-rect route and using the correct method, it is also essential to select the correct formulation of the medicine. Doing this requires nurses to apply their knowledge of medicines and their formulations, and to refer to the BNF for clarification where there is doubt. For example, if valproate, quetiapine or methylphenidate are prescribed just once a day, the prescription should be annotated to say that a long-acting (or 'modified release') formulation is required. Administering the regular or 'immediate release' formulation of these medicines just once a day ren-ders them ineffective. The half-life of these medi-cines is relatively short, therefore the immediate release formulation needs to be given multiple times a day for therapeutic effect. For other medi-cines it is essential that they are not administered with food or antacids, as they are inactivated by these (e.g. the antibiotics flucloxacillin and ciprofloxacin).

With reference to the route of administration, the Pabrinex brand of B vitamins formulated for intramuscular (IM) use is different to the intrave-nous (IV) formulation, and each formulation must only be used for the route specified. All prepara-tions, particularly injections, should be carefully measured and prepared according to the instruc-tions supplied. Lastly, it is imperative that parenteral medicines are administered via the exact prescribed route, and sometimes even the site or muscle of administration is specified.

Right patient

Although it may be stating the obvious, all medi-cines should be given to the correct patient; unin-tentionally giving prescribed medicines to the incorrect patient is a common error which may lead to significant harm to the unintended patient receiving the medicine as well as to the intended patient who misses a medicine.

 ## 27.3 The NMC standards for medicines administration

The NMC (2007) clearly specifies the standards that registered nurses must adhere to when administer-ing prescribed medicines. The standards are help-fully specific and detailed, demonstrating that safe medicine use requires the application of theoretical knowledge about the medicine to the individual patient and their scenario. The standards set out in Box 27.1 are self-explanatory.

 ## 27.4 Involving patients in medicine administration

Patients should be given the opportunity to be involved with prescribing decisions and treatment plans (NICE 2009a). As far as possible the choice of medicine should be made jointly by the patient and prescriber based on informed discussions of the relative benefits and side-effects. Patients should be adequately informed of the potential side-effects of medicines in a suitable manner using language that they can understand. They should also be helped to understand the nature of their illness, the potential benefit of the medicines, their onset of action, the duration of treatment and the importance of taking medication as prescribed. Explanations should not assume prior knowledge or understanding, should avoid jargon and should be in lay terms that the patient can understand. To impart all this informa-tion in a meaningful way to an individual patient may take several conversations, and the information may need to be repeated or explained in a different

Box 27.1 Standards for practice of administration of medicines

Having initially checked the direction to supply or administer that a medicinal product is appropriate for your patient you may then administer medication.

Standard 8: administration

As a registrant, in exercising your professional accountability in the best interests of your patients:

- you must be certain of the identity of the patient to whom the medicine is to be administered;
- you must check that the patient is not allergic to the medicine before administering it;
- you must know the therapeutic uses of the medicine to be administered, its normal dosage, side-effects, precautions and contraindications;
- you must be aware of the patient's plan of care (care plan or pathway);
- you must check that the prescription or the label on the medicine dispensed is clearly written and unambiguous;
- you must check the expiry date (where it exists) of the medicine to be administered;
- you must have considered the dosage, weight where appropriate, method of administration, route and timing;
- you must administer or withhold in the context of the patient's condition (e.g. digoxin not usually to be given if pulse below 60) and coexisting therapies, for example, physiotherapy;
- you must contact the prescriber or another authorized prescriber without delay where contraindications to the prescribed medicine are discovered, where the patient develops a reaction to the medicine, or where assessment of the patient indicates that the medicine is no longer suitable;
- you must make a clear, accurate and immediate record of all medicine administered, intentionally withheld or refused by the patient, ensuring the signature is clear and legible; it is also your responsibility to ensure that a record is made when delegating the task of administering medicine.

In addition, where medication is not given, the reason for not doing so must be recorded. You may administer with a single signature any prescription only medicine (POM), general sales list (GSL) or pharmacy medication (P).

Guidance

Clarifying identity

- Where there are difficulties in clarifying an individual's identity, for example, in some areas of learning disabilities, patients with dementia or confusional states, an up-to-date photograph should be attached to the prescription chart(s).

Drug calculations

- Some drug administrations can require complex calculations to ensure that the correct volume or quantity of medication is administered. In these situations, it is good practice for a second practitioner (a registered professional) to check the calculation independently in order to minimize the risk of error. The use of calculators to determine the volume or quantity of medication should not act as a substitute for arithmetical knowledge and skill.

Standard 13: titration

Where medication has been prescribed within a range of dosages it is acceptable for registrants to titrate dosages according to patient response and symptom control, and to administer within the prescribed range.

Guidance

A registrant must be competent to interpret test results – for example, blood results (heparin or glucose levels (insulin)), and assess, for example, withdrawal symptoms or signs of intoxication in the management of drug or alcohol withdrawal.

way. Staff should remember that many medicines are used in the treatment of more than one condition. For example, although most antipsychotics are principally used for the treatment of schizophrenia many are also used for the treatment of other diagnoses such as bipolar affective disorder (BPAD) and (as discussed in Chapter 26) valproate, carbamazepine and lamotrigine are all widely used in the treatment of epilepsy as well as in BPAD. Therefore health care professionals should be careful when discussing the use of such medicines with patients, and ensure they are clear about the indication and the patient diagnosis, as the mention of other diagnoses can be confusing or disconcerting for some patients.

Case Study

Alex

You are working on a busy acute psychiatric ward. Alex (aged 36 years) was admitted as acutely unwell a few days ago. He has had several psychiatric admissions before. One afternoon he approaches you and asks 'Can I have one of the blue pills?'

Thinking Space 27.1

1. What does Alex want? How would you find out?
2. Once you have established this, how would you respond to his request?

Non-compliance issues

There are numerous studies and literature reviews published reporting and analysing patients' rates of non-compliance or non-adherence with psychotropics, and an even wider literature covering other prescribed medicines. The NICE clinical guideline *Medicines adherence: – involving patients in decisions about prescribed medicines and supporting adherence* (NICE 2009b) states that between a third and a half of medicines that are prescribed for any long-term condition are not used as recommended. This represents a health loss for patients and an economic loss for society. Non-adherence often results from failed communications between health care professionals and the patient. Professionals need to consider patients' beliefs and preferences that influence motivation to start and continue treatment as well as practical factors. This requires communicating in an open manner that encourages patients to discuss any doubts or concerns they may have about treatment, adapting the consultation style to the needs of the individual patient, and having an approach that encourages the patient to make informed choices.

High rates of partial or non-adherence with psychotropics is of particular concern. (Reviews of rates of non-adherence with psychotropics show that these do not vary widely from those reported with a wide range of other medicines prescribed for 'medical' conditions (60–92 per cent).) If a patient misses a dose, or takes a lower dose, or even stops the medicine completely, this does not usually lead to an immediate full-blown relapse of the psychiatric illness (although it may), but in the medium and longer term it is associated with an increased rate of psychiatric relapse, increased hospital admissions, and may lead to a poorer prognosis and self-injurious behaviour. In one study, the mortality rates among non-adherent patients with schizophrenia were 10 times higher than in those taking antipsychotics, and the risk of suicide was also increased (Tiihonen *et al.* 2006). It is imperative to emphasize these risks and longer-term effects on health outcomes and prognosis both to the patient and to the family and carers.

If a patient is, or is suspected of being, poorly adherent to the prescribed treatment plan the health care professional should skilfully interview them and discuss their views of medicines to establish the underlying reason for poor adherence. It is very difficult to develop a suitable alternative treatment plan for the patient and address the underlying issue if this is not identified. Providing the patient with straightforward factual educational sessions about medicines has not shown to be beneficial. However, providing tailored information about the benefits of medicines, their potential side-effects and disease progression may help to develop a positive alliance between the patient and the practitioner which has been shown to be beneficial. Many studies have concluded that compli-

ance or adherence therapy, which is based on motivational interviewing techniques and cognitive behavioural therapy (CBT) can be used to increase adherence rates and improve patient outcomes.

Additionally, all verbal explanations should be reinforced by written material wherever possible. For some medicines such as lithium (as well as warfarin and methotrexate to name a few), this is even more pertinent. Professionals should encourage patients to take responsibility for their medicines, and encourage understanding of their use and effects. All patients prescribed lithium should be given a specific 'lithium alert card' and 'lithium record book' in which they should record their lithium level results. Refer to the *Patient Safety Alert No. 5* (NPSANRLS 2009) for further advice about optimizing the safety of lithium treatment.

27.5 Assessing the benefits and adverse effects of medicines

Unlike using medicines in the treatment of many physical health diseases where for example a patient's blood pressure and pulse can be measured to assess the effect of an antihypertensive, or a blood glucose level can be used to assess the effects on an oral hypoglycaemic, in psychiatry there is no direct numerical measure of the impact of medicines. Alongside this, many psychotropics have a comparatively slow onset of action (two to four weeks to full effect once a dose is stabilized) and the illnesses are often chronic. Therefore unless an objective measure is used assessment of effect may be rather subjective and potentially inaccurate. Many tools have been devised to rate the severity of patients' symptoms and are designed to ask specific questions for specific illnesses. The more detailed they are the more accurate the description, but they become more lengthy and cumbersome to use.

Assessing benefit

If a patient does not adequately respond to treatment (at an appropriate dose for an appropriate duration), assuming there is clarity about the diagnosis the prescriber should assess the patient's adherence with the treatment plan and consider confounding factors (e.g. substance misuse, co-morbid conditions). As discussed previously, partial or nonconcordance is extremely common and multi-factorial and needs to be carefully explored. Similarly if misuse of alcohol and drugs is suspected an accurate history of use should be elucidated. Lack of response to one antipsychotic, antidepressant or mood stabilizer does not preclude response to another. The decision to discontinue treatments for schizophrenia or BPAD is complex and should be based on the individual's situation and diagnosis. On stopping medication the risk of relapse remains, even after a long period of remission, so where there is good clinical control treatment is usually continued long term. Where there is a clinical need to stop or change medication it should usually be slowly reduced.

Assessing adverse effects

Distressing adverse effects of medicines are associated with non-adherence and are even predictive of it. When patients are given medicines, particularly new ones, they should be informed that if they suffer any intolerable side-effects they should return and discuss this with their care coordinator, prescriber or pharmacist, and should be encouraged to do so. Health care professionals should assess and monitor patients' adverse effects, both the common and obvious ones, as well as the more subjective, unpleasant or potentially embarrassing ones. Using assessment tools adds objectivity for both the assessor and patient, establishes a logical approach to assessing a wide range of adverse effects and may reduce the chances of missing or omitting certain side-effects. In addition to lengthy and detailed tools often used in research, there are a number of short and quick-to-complete validated self-rating tools available in lay terminology.

Certain Adverse Drug Reactions (ADRs) should be reported via the UK's Yellow Card Scheme administered by the Medicines and Healthcare Products Regulatory Agency (MHRA). Reporting severe or unusual medicine ADRs from the population at large ensures that rare ADRs can be detected and potentially enables safer medicine use nationally. ADRs can be reported by patients or health care professionals online or using forms provided at the back of every BNF. Specifically the following ADRs should be reported:

- all *serious* suspected ADRs for established medicines (serious is defined as: fatal, life-threatening, disabling or incapacitating, resulting in prolonged hospitalization, and/or medically significant);
- all ADRs for new medicines (i.e. those given the black triangle symbol: ▼);
- all reactions involving children.

 ### 27.6 Psychotropics and physical health

People with schizophrenia have a 20 per cent shorter life expectancy than the general population and a greater vulnerability to several other illnesses including diabetes, coronary heart disease, hypertension and emphysema (Marder *et al.* 2004). Symptoms of schizophrenia can contribute to poor lifestyle habits such as limited physical activity, unhealthy diet and alcohol intake all of which promote weight gain which in itself is associated with diabetes, dyslipidaemia and cardiovascular disease.

Interactions between psychotropic medicines and physical health

As discussed above and in Chapter 26, all medicines have adverse effects. These may be a direct effect on the person's physical health – for example, high doses of venlafaxine can raise the blood pressure; or they may have indirect effects on physical health – for example, lithium often causes polydispia (excessive thirst) and if someone drinks a lot of sugary fizzy drinks in response this is likely to adversely affect their dental health and weight. In some cases there is both a direct and indirect effect – for example, olanzapine can disturb glucose and cholesterol balances, but it can also increase appetite and cause somnolence (daytime sedation or 'grogginess') which discourages patients from taking physical exercise. These examples start to demonstrate the complex interplay between mental health conditions and their treatments, and patients' physical health conditions and their treatments. No diagnosis should be treated in isolation – consideration should be paid to other conditions and their treatments. Response, adherence, side-effects and physical health should all be monitored regularly during treatment with psychotropics. The following are examples of physical health conditions that need to be considered when using psychotropics, but this is not exhaustive.

Metabolic syndrome

People with schizophrenia are at increased risk of premature metabolic syndrome, which has been described as a cluster of abnormalities: obesity, hyperlipidaemia, hypertension and hyperglycaemia. Metabolic syndrome increases the risk of cardiovascular disease, and has been linked with the use of antipsychotics (see Chapter 26). When prescribing antipsychotics, careful monitoring of endocrine effects, such as raised blood glucose and hyperprolactinaemia, and cardiovascular risk factors such as blood pressure, triglyceride and cholesterol levels is advised. Management of modifiable risk factors (including smoking, abnormal lipids, hypertension, diabetes, psychosocial factors and abdominal obesity) for cardiovascular disease and diabetes and advice on lifestyle changes are important ways to help reduce risk. For patients with pre-existing factors for metabolic syndrome, an antipsychotic that is least likely to worsen this cluster of effects should be selected.

Weight gain and obesity

More than half of the general adult UK population is overweight or obese, and nearly a quarter is obese (BMI >30 kg/m^2). Obesity is an important risk factor for cardiovascular disease, stroke and certain cancers, and contributes to other serious diseases such as diabetes. In addition to all the 'standard' factors affecting the wider population, there are further factors potentially increasing obesity in those with mental illnesses, such as poorer motivation, lower socioeconomic status and the prescription of psychotropic medicines. Many psychotropics, particularly antipsychotics, are known to cause significant weight gain, and this is a common reason cited by patients for discontinuing them. The mechanism by which antipsychotics induce weight gain is unclear, but it is thought to result from increased food intake and in some cases reduced energy expenditure. Most weight is usually gained during the first three to four months of treatment, although this can continue for much longer. Patients should be advised – preferably at the beginning of treatment – of the risks of weight gain with specific antipsychotics, about lifestyle changes such as healthy diets and physical exercise to prevent weight gain, and should be encouraged to monitor their own weight. In addition to the impact on general physical health, medicine-induced weight gain may also adversely affect quality of life, the individual's adjustment in the community and their self-image.

Diabetes

Risk factors for people with schizophrenia developing diabetes are the same as those in the general population, but additionally the antipsychotics may disturb the glucose balance, potentially leading to or aggravating the onset of hyperglycaemia and diabetes. This effect may be influenced by their propensity to cause weight gain but may also be a direct and independent effect on insulin function.

Cardiac disease

Schizophrenia per se can increase the risk of cardiovascular disease, and the cluster of factors that contribute to metabolic disease has already been discussed. Some psychotropics can affect other aspects of cardiac function and these possibilities guide the choice of agent in patients with pre-existing cardiac disease. For example, higher doses of venlafaxine can cause hypertension, quetiapine and clozapine can cause hypotension, tricyclic antidepressants (TCAs) can increase the heart rate and the QTc interval on the ECG which predisposes to arrhythmias.

Co-morbid bleeding disorders

In response to the injury of blood vessels, platelets release serotonin which encourages vasoconstriction and leads to their aggregation and therefore clotting. As suggested by their name, selective serotonin re-uptake inhibitors (SSRIs) inhibit the reuptake of sero-tonin into platelets, which adversely affects the ability to form clots, which in turn increases the patient's risk of bleeding. SSRIs have been shown to increase the chance of gastrointestinal (GI) bleeding and therefore should be avoided in at-risk patients such as those already taking aspirin or non-steroidal anti-inflammatory drugs (NSAIDs), as well as those with a previous history of GI bleeding. For such patients an antidepressant with a less potent effect on platelets' reuptake of serotonin should be selected, for example mirtazapine. If an SSRI needs to be used in patients at risk of a GI bleed a gastroprotective medicine should also be offered, such as a proton pump inhibitor like omperazole (NICE 2010a). SSRIs should be used cautiously in patients at risk of other types of internal bleeding, including cirrhotic patients, those post-surgery and those prescribed heparin or warfarin.

Renal dysfunction

The kidneys are frequently the organ that ensures compounds (including medicines) are filtered from the bloodstream and excreted from the body. If a patient's renal function is impaired, these processes are decreased, potentially leading to an accumulation of chemicals in the body. Most psychotropics are extensively metabolized by the liver to inactive metabolites, therefore a reduction in renal function is of little importance and the medicine can be continued at the usual dose. It is advisable to avoid very long-acting medicines (e.g. diazepam) where the risk of accumulation is greater, and only if the renal impairment is very severe would reductions of doses be recommended. For medicines that are not extensively hepatically metabolized and are therefore dependent on renal excretion (e.g. amisulpride, sulpiride and lithium), reduced renal function is very significant and use of these medicines is not recommended (Joint Formulary Committee 2011).

Renal function can be estimated by calculating the glomerular filtration rate (GFR) which is routinely done electronically by laboratories analysing blood samples. It is normal for renal function to gradually deteriorate with age, and it should be assumed that all older people have some degree of (mild) renal impairment. Renal impairment can lead to imbalances in the distribution of fluids and electrolytes, which in turn may impact on medicines used. Finally, when using medicines in patients with renal impairment it is important to consider whether any of them are renally toxic, potentially causing more renal damage – for example, lithium.

Hepatic dysfunction

The liver plays a major role in metabolizing substrates, including medicines, from the bloodstream. In hepatic dysfunction this metabolism is slowed and reduced, potentially leading to an accumulation of substrates which can put the patient at risk of increased side-effects and toxicity. Therefore, for patients with hepatic impairment it is advisable to avoid medicines that are extensively hepatically metabolized and those with long half-lives. Lower doses are required unless therapy can be changed to a psychotropic that is not significantly hepatically metabolized (Joint Formulary Committee 2011). Most psychotropics (with the exception of amisulpride, sulpiride and lithium) are hepatically metabolized before excretion. The liver also synthesizes biological materials for the body including proteins and clotting factors. In hepatic impairment this function is also reduced, leaving patients at risk of poor clotting. This needs to be considered particularly when selecting antidepressants and potentially disturbing the distribution of medicines that are highly bound to serum proteins. Lastly, psychotropics that can be directly hepatotoxic should be avoided in patients with hepatic dysfunction (e.g. agomelatine, atomoxetine, chlorpromazine).

Epilepsy

The use of psychotropics in patients with epilepsy is complicated as they commonly have some effect on the seizure threshold. Most antidepressants and antipsychotics decrease the seizure threshold in a dose-related manner, thereby making the patient more likely to have a seizure, and all benzodiazepines and z-hypnotics increase the seizure threshold, thus making a seizure less likely. Benzodiazepines can even be used in the treatment of seizures (e.g. buccal midazolam or rectal diazepam as an immediate treatment for seizures). Of the mood stabilizers carbamazepine, valproate and lamotrigine are primarily used as anticonvulsants and therefore can be used for dual effects. It is advisable not to alter psychotropics that may decrease the seizure threshold if the patient's seizures are not satisfactorily controlled.

 ## 27.7 Medicine interactions

Medicines may interact with each other (or other chemicals such as smoking, or alcohol or other substances) in two ways, either pharmacodynamically or pharmacokinetically. Pharmacodynamic interactions are when two medicines have either a similar and therefore additive effect within the body, or when they have antagonistic effects in the body. These may be their intended therapeutic effects or unrelated effects. For example, all antipsychotics antagonize the anticonvulsant effect of antepileptics; all antipsychotics enhance the response to central nervous system depressants (such as alcohol, anxiolytics, hypnotics and opioid analgesics); antipsychotics antagonize the effect of levodopa and other dopamine agonists used in the treatment of Parkinson's disease; carbamazepine can cause agranulocytosis so may interact pharmacodynamically if given with other medicines that potentially can cause agranulocytosis, such as clozapine. Pharmacodynamic interactions are usually predictable, based on knowledge of the medicines and how they work and affect bodily systems. Pharmacokinetic interactions are when two medicines directly affect each other. This may be through altering the absorption, distribution, metabolism or excretion of each other. For example, antacids can reduce the absorption of sulpiride and phenothia-

zine antipsychotics; carbamazepine undergoes significant hepatic metabolism and is a potent inducer of the hepatic microsomal enzyme (P450) system causing increased metabolism and reduced plasma levels of many other medicines that are hepatically cleared, as well as inducing its own metabolism. If used with other medicines that block its metabolism (e.g. fluoxetine), this can lead to significantly raised carbamazepine levels. Lithium has numerous and serious pharmacokinetic interactions which are related to its narrow therapeutic window and dependence on renal excretion and fluid balance – for example, ACE Inhibitors and diuretics (Joint Formulary Committee 2011).

Some medicines have hardly any potential to interact with others – for example citalopram and sertraline have few interactions (with the exception of serotonin syndrome which is a potentially life-threatening pharmacodynamic interaction between two or more serotonergic agents). In contrast some medicines have great propensity for interactions. An extensive cross-reference of medicine interactions is listed at the back of each edition of the BNF with some description and annotation of the significance. This should be the first point of reference regarding medicine interactions. For further details refer to the manufacturer's summary of product characteristics for the specific medicine.

 ## 27.8 Smoking and psychotropics

Smoking can have a direct effect on some medicines. The hydrocarbons in tobacco smoke can induce hepatic microsomal enzymes (mainly CYP1A2) in the P450 system, thereby increasing the rate of metabolism of substrates of this pathway, meaning that higher doses may be required. Conversely if a smoker is established on a medicine metabolized via this route, then stopping smoking can result in higher plasma levels and therefore side-effects, meaning that the ex-smoker may require a dose reduction. Medicines that require particular caution include clozapine, olanzapine, fluphenazine and haloperidol (Joint Formulary Committee 2011). This potential interaction should be clearly explained in lay terms to smokers prescribed such medicines.

27.9 Psychotropics during pregnancy and breastfeeding

When a woman with a mental illness becomes pregnant there are numerous and complex issues to consider in the management of her physical and mental health, as well as that of the neonate (NICE 2007). It is a slightly different, but still complex, scenario when a woman with a pre-exiting diagnosis becomes mentally unwell while pregnant. Medicines can potentially cause adverse effects at any stage in pregnancy, and this is on top of the background risk of major foetal malformations in all pregnancies and of spontaneous miscarriage. This background risk may also be increased by the presence of an untreated mental disorder. It is impossible to categorically say that any medicine is safe in pregnancy because it would be unethical to conduct trials in pregnant women to demonstrate this. Some psychotropics are known to be teratogenic (e.g. lithium, valproate, carbamazepine, lamotrigine and paroxetine), therefore exposure to these during the first three months is more likely to cause structural malformations, whereas exposure to medicines in the second and third trimester is more likely to cause growth defects. In general, when it is necessary to use medicines during pregnancy those thought to pose a lower risk to the mother and foetus should be chosen, used minimally, as monotherapy in the lowest effective dose (teratogenic effects are usually dose-dependent, such as the incidence of neural tube defects with valproate). The risks and benefits will be different in each pregnant woman depending on the nature and severity of her illness, her risk of relapse, the stage in pregnancy and her previous response to treatments. The mental health of the mother in the perinatal period influences foetal well-being, obstetric outcome and child development. The postpartum period poses an increased risk of relapse for several illnesses, therefore it is imperative to optimize the mother's mental health during the perinatal period (NICE 2007).

It is desirable that all mothers breastfeed their babies, but some medicines pass from the maternal bloodstream into breast milk and would consequently be ingested by feeding infants. Infants have a decreased capacity for drug metabolism for their first three weeks. Therefore it is important to consider prescribing medicines that will allow the mother to safely breastfeed. Where there is a high risk of relapse it is usually inappropriate to withhold the mother's psychotropic in order to allow breastfeeding.

27.10 Principles of using psychotropics in children

Currently the diagnosis of many psychiatric disorders in children and adolescents is based on criteria developed for adults, although factors within the presentations are often different in patients aged under 18 years. Consequently, evidence for the efficacy of medicines for illnesses such as schizophrenia, BPAD and depression in this population is extremely limited. With the exception of treatments for attention deficit hyperactivity disorder (ADHD), which is a psychiatric disorder with onset during childhood whose treatment has been extensively studied and is widely recommended (NICE 2008), the majority of medicines used in the management of psychiatric disorders have not been studied in detail and are not licensed for use in people under 18 years old. For details of psychotropics licensed or recommended for use in children and adolescents refer to the current *BNF for Children* (Paediatric Formulary Committee 2011).

There are NICE guidelines recommending pharmacological treatment for ADHD in school-aged children and adolescents (and adults) (NICE 2008) and depression (NICE 2005). When psychotropics are used in children or adolescents for psychiatric disorders, other than ADHD, these should be started at lower doses than used in adults, and patients should be monitored even more closely as they are more prone to side-effects such as metabolic effects with atypical antipsychotics. There is little data to clearly demonstrate the long-term effects of psychotropics on the developing brain (e.g. their impact on cognition and neurological development). Children should not be treated as 'mini-adults' – their brain development is not completed, and their response to psychotropics is not necessarily the same as that of adults. For example, fluoxetine is the only antidepressant licensed in the UK for use in children aged over 8 years for the treatment of a moderate to severe major depressive episode (Paediatric Formulary Committee 2011) because it is the only SSRI that has been shown to have a favourable balance of risks and benefits. Suicide-related behaviour (suicide attempt/self-harm and suicidal thoughts) and hostility (predominantly aggression, oppositional behaviour and anger) were observed more frequently with SSRIs compared to placebo. Tricyclic antidepressants (TCAs) are not useful in treating depression in pre-pubertal children (NICE 2005). Lastly, when using medicines in this age group the acceptability of the formulation (as a tablet or capsule or liquid) becomes even more pertinent and obviously affects adherence.

 ## 27.11 Psychotropics in older adults

The body changes as it ages and older adults (over 65 years) have increased pharmacodynamnic sensitivity, altered body fat to water ratio and altered pharmacokinetics of medicines. Due to decreased renal and hepatic function older adults generally metabolize medicines more slowly which prolongs the medicine's clearance, and potentially leads to an accumulation. Older adults are often more sensitive to the side-effects of medicines, so medicines should be started at lower doses and increased

gradually, and often the treatment dose is lower. Certain side-effects become of greater significance in this population, for example blurry vision with TCAs, as this can increase the risk of falls. The importance of such apparently mild side-effects should guide the choice of psychotropic (NICE 2010b).

Some medicines are more hazardous in this population, for example hypnotics, as older adults are more susceptible to experiencing adverse effects such as daytime drowsiness, disturbances in gait, cognitive impairment and hypotension, and these can be more debilitating in this population. Using antidepressants can be less straightforward as well. Most antidepressants have been associated with hyponatraemia – the exact mechanism is unknown but is not related to the dose. Hyponatraemia is common in older adults, thus there is an increased likelihood of developing antidepressant-induced hyponatraemia. Other risk factors for antidepressant-induced hyponatraemia include: medical co-morbidity, female gender, low baseline sodium, reduced renal function and polypharmacy; many of these also occur in this population. Older adults are also at higher risk of GI bleeding, increasing the likelihood of SSRI-induced GI bleeding (NICE 2010a, 2010b). In older adults a greater degree of co-morbid medical illness is associated with higher relapse rates of depression. Older adults usually take longer to respond to psychotropics such as antidepressants and antipsychotics, therefore a longer period of time should be given before considering the treatment to be ineffective (Joint Formulary Committee 2011). Lastly the average older adult takes at least four or more types of medicines, leading to a significant potential for drug-drug and drug-disease interactions, as well as increased chance of concurrent side-effects.

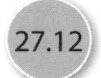 ## 27.12 Conclusion

To conclude, the main points of this chapter are summarized below:

- The BNF is the mainstay reference text for all health care professionals involved in the use of medicines.

- Medication errors and near misses occur frequently across health care settings, many of which are preventable. Prior to administering any medicine a nurse should check the following: that it is the right medication, in the right dose, to the right patient, by the right route and at the right time.

- The NMC (2007) specifies the standards that registered nurses must adhere to when administering prescribed medicines.

- As far as possible the choice of medicine should be made jointly by the patient and prescriber based on informed discussion of the relative benefits and side-effects.

- There are high rates of partial or non-adherence by patients to medicines which represents a health loss for patients and an economic loss for society.

- Non-adherence to psychotropic medicines is of particular concern because it can lead to relapse and readmission to hospital.

- Non-adherence may arise from failed communication between the patient and health care professional. Professionals need to consider patients' beliefs and preferences that influence motivation to start and continue treatment as well as practical factors.

- There is a complex interplay between mental health conditions and their treatments, and patients' physical health conditions and their treatment.

- Health care professionals should not treat a diagnosis in isolation and consideration should be paid to other conditions and their treatments.

- Response, adherence, side-effects and physical health should all be monitored regularly during treatment with psychotropics. A variety of tools have been developed to rate the severity of patients' symptoms and so assess the benefit and adverse effects of medicines.

- There are special considerations for the use of psychotropic medicines with children and older people.

Feedback to Thinking Space 27.1

1. You may already happen to know that for many years lorazepam tablets have been manufactured as blue tablets. Quite often patients who have been in a psychiatric ward before are also familiar with this fact. But this may not always be the case, so don't assume it. You should ask if he has had 'the blue pill'/'lorazepam' before and when, and if it helped. To help you identify it you could check this timing against his prescription chart and you could look at the medicines in the ward medicine trolley/cupboard to confirm their appearance. You could ask a more senior/experienced nursing colleague if they know which tablets are blue. Regardless of whether you already happen to know that lorazepam are commonly blue tablets, you should ask Alex to describe what he wants the tablet for, and why he wants it. If he is feeling anxious or agitated you are likely to also be able to see some symptoms while you talk with him.

2. In addition to discussing with Alex why he is asking for a medicine and investigating what he wants it for, you need to make your own assessment and decide whether it is appropriate to administer a dose (i.e. given the risks and benefits of this specific medicine for this specific patient) or whether something else is more suitable. You should consider whether there are any suitable non-drug

approaches (e.g. talking with Alex, time off the ward, an activity to relieve boredom, etc). Like all benzodiazepines lorazepam is addictive and so has the potential for misuse. It is commonly prescribed 'prn', but nurses should not administer this unless there is a very clear need (indication). If you were to decide this medicine was indicated and appropriate for Alex's needs, you would then need to check that it is prescribed for him on his prescription chart and follow the principles of the five rights – i.e. establish if this particular medicine is prescribed for him on a 'prn' basis, confirm the dose that you would select, consider the timing bearing in mind what Alex has already been given so far that day (particularly any other benzodiazepines and how long they act for), and lastly confirm that you are looking at the correct prescription card for this patient (note that some names are more easily confused, such as Alex, which could be a male or female).

Annotated bibliography

Joint Formulary Committee (2011) *British National Formulary*, **61st edn. London: British Medical Association and Royal Pharmaceutical Society.**
This is the essential reference text for routine use during medicine use and administration. Published six-monthly.

NMC (Nursing and Midwifery Council) (2007) *Standards for Medicines Management.* **London: NMC.**
Essential reading for all nurses who ever use medicines. It describes the standards of practice and performance expected of members of the profession.

Taylor, D. and Paton, C. (eds) (2002) *Case Studies in Psychopharmacology: The use of drugs in psychiatry*, **2nd edn. London: Dunitz Ltd.**
A short but very helpful book set out as case scenarios andworking through the potential treatment options for each individual case.

http://choiceandmedication.org/cms/subscribers.
This website draws together information about medicines, disease and general related questions, and tailors the answers for the local National Health Service (NHS) trust. It is a valuable resource for patients and health care professionals.

NICE (National Institute for Health and Clinical Excellence) clinical evidence-based guidelines, developed by consensus groups of experts in the field.
These guidelines reflect optimal routine practice and should be followed in standard care. For every guideline there is a section specifically for patients and carers, with shortened versions of the guidance written in lay terms, without jargon.

References

DH (Department of Health) (2004) *Building a Safer NHS for Patients: Improving medication safety*. London: DH.
Gittin, K. *et al.* (2001) Clinical outcome following neuroleptic discontinuation in patients with remitted recent-onset schizophrenia, *American Journal of Psychiatry*, 158: 1835–42.
Joint Formulary Committee (2011) *British National Formulary*, 61st edn. London: British Medical Association and Royal Pharmaceutical Society.
Marder S. *et al.* (2004) Physical health monitoring of patients with schizophrenia, *American Journal of Psychiatry*, 161: 1334–49.
NICE (National Institute for Health and Clinical Excellence) (2005) *Clinical Guideline No. 28: Depression in children and young people – identification and management in primary, community and secondary care*. London: NICE.
NICE (National Institute for Health and Clinical Excellence) (2007) *Clinical Guideline 45: Antenatal and postnatal mental health*. London: NICE.
NICE (National Institute for Health and Clinical Excellence) (2008) *Clinical Guideline 72: Attention deficit hyperactivity disorder – diagnosis and management of ADHD in children, young people and adults*. London: NICE.
NICE (National Institute for Health and Clinical Excellence) (2009a) *Clinical Guideline 82: Schizophrenia – core interventions in the treatment and management of schizophrenia in primary and secondary care*. London: NICE.
NICE (National Institute for Health and Clinical Excellence) (NICE) (2009b) *Clinical Guideline 76: Medicines adherence – involving patients in decisions about prescribed medicines and supporting adherence*. London: NICE.
NICE (National Institute for Health and Clinical Excellence) (2010a) *Clinical Guideline 91: Depression in adults with a chronic physical health problem*. London: NICE.

NICE (National Institute for Clinical Excellence) (2010b) *Clinical Guideline 90: Depression – the treatment and management of depression in adults*. London: NICE.

NMC (Nursing and Midwifery Council) (2007) *Standards for Medicines Management*. London: NMC.

NPSA NRLS (National Patient Safety Agency National Reporting and Learning Service) (2009) *Patient Safety Alert No. 5: Safer lithium therapy*. London.

Paediatric Formulary Committee (2011) *BNF for Children 2011–12*. London: BMJ Group, Pharmaceutical Press and RCPCH Publications.

Tiihonen, J. *et al.* (2006) Effectiveness of antipsychotic treatments in a nationwide cohort of patients in community care after first hospitalisation due to schizophrenia and schizoaffective disorder: observational follow-up study, *British Medical Journal*, 333: 224–9.

Chapter 28

Concordance, Adherence and Compliance in Medicine-taking

Sue Gurney

28.1 Introduction

Since the mid-twentieth century, compelling evidence has evolved on the efficacy of a range of psychotropic medications in reducing and managing the symptoms of an array of mental health problems. This chapter gives an overview of medication concordance, adherence and compliance and the implications for mental health nursing practice. The chapter covers:

- the concepts of concordance, adherence and compliance;
- factors affecting adherence;
- the rationale for interventions;
- reviewing the evidence;
- implications for mental health nursing practice.

The three main classes of psychotropic preparations in use for symptom relief are:

- antidepressants for treating depression;
- anxiolytics for anxiety; and
- antipsychotics for treating symptoms of psychosis (WHO 2001).

The development of new generations of psychotropic preparations, with varying profiles in both efficacy and side-effects, is adding to the range of prescribing choices (Agius *et al.* 2010). Mental health nurses are not only routinely involved in dispensing and administering medication but now actively embrace non-medical prescribing roles. Hence the concept and practice of medication adherence is central to mental health nursing practice. To reflect current practice the terms 'adherence' and 'shared decision-making' are used throughout this chapter. The phrase 'people who use services' is used to encompass the terms service user, client and patient. The chapter refers primarily to the literature on medication adherence in severe mental illness. However, many of the issues and concepts raised here are transferable to other forms of both psychotropic and generic medication adherence practice.

Case Study

Preda

Preda (56) lives with her partner Joe (64). They are both retired. Preda has a diagnosis of schizophrenia; she acknowledges this but is very opposed to medication and is now refusing to take it. Joe contacts the community mental health team (CMHT) stating that she is deteriorating. The crisis resolution team undertakes an assessment and is convinced that she needs inpatient assessment. Preda is sectioned and admitted under the Mental Health Act (MHA). Mental health professionals now face many challenges in terms of Preda's care and support.

Thinking Space 28.1

What actions can now be taken to support Preda? Jot down your thoughts in response to this question. Feedback is given at the end of the chapter.

28.2 Concordance, adherence and compliance

The use and understanding of the language in this area has significant meaning and impact for professional practice (Repper and Perkins 1998). The literature reveals an evolution in terminology, reflecting a shift in the balance of power of the relationship/alliance of the prescriber and health care worker with the person using mental health services. Overall, this describes a change in value from the individual as a passive recipient of health care to an informed partner in health care decision-making.

Psychotropic medications often need to be taken continuously over a sustained period of time to reduce symptoms and potential relapse. Conformity to prescribed medications is often referred to as adherence or compliance. Ceasing or partial conformity to the prescription is referred to as non- or partial adherence/compliance. Marland and Sharkey (1999) argue that these are value-laden terms and the emergence of the concept of concordance in promoting an equal partnership between the pre-

scriber and the user has gained prominence in the literature (NICE 2009). This implies that an equal partnership needs to exist between health care workers and the individual, before compliance/adherence is achieved, assuming the latter is appropriate.

However, the terms concordance, adherence and compliance have been and continue to be used interchangeably, resulting in some confusion. Although the term concordance is a useful construct, reflecting current social values, it is now viewed as describing the process of consultation and hence may, or may not, lead to improved adherence (Horne *et al.* 2005). The National Institute for Health and Clinical Excellence (NICE) has published recommendations, available as *Clinical Guideline 76: Medicines adherence* (2009). This guideline recommends that the term adherence should be used as it more accurately reflects medication-taking activity. In reflecting the health care professional–user/carer consultation process NICE (2009) recommends that the term 'shared decision-making' replaces the term 'concordance'. These recommendations are now followed throughout this chapter.

28.3 What is adherence?

Definitions of adherence are diverse. For Dodds *et al.* (2000) adherence is the extent to which a person's medication-taking behaviour coincides with medical or health advice. Marland and Sharkey (1999) point out that the term adherence is value-laden and that interpretation varies with each individual professional. They also propose two dimensions to the concept. The first emphasizes the process of medication-taking – that is, the degree of conformity to the prescription. The second emphasizes the outcome being determined by the maintenance of wellness.

There is a clear relationship between adherence with prescribed medication and best practice in medication management. However, it is imperative that adherence is not the main target. In fact, non-adherence for someone suffering from severe adverse reactions might be life-saving in cases of inappropriate prescription. Hence, a crucial element of best practice in medication adherence is about the health professional, the individual and carers recognizing that a problem may be medication related. Figure 28.1 summarizes why some people don't take medication as prescribed and what can be done to help them.

Measuring adherence

There are challenges in measuring adherence. Measures may include methods of observation, self-reporting, pill counts and biological assays such as urine and blood specimens; and these only

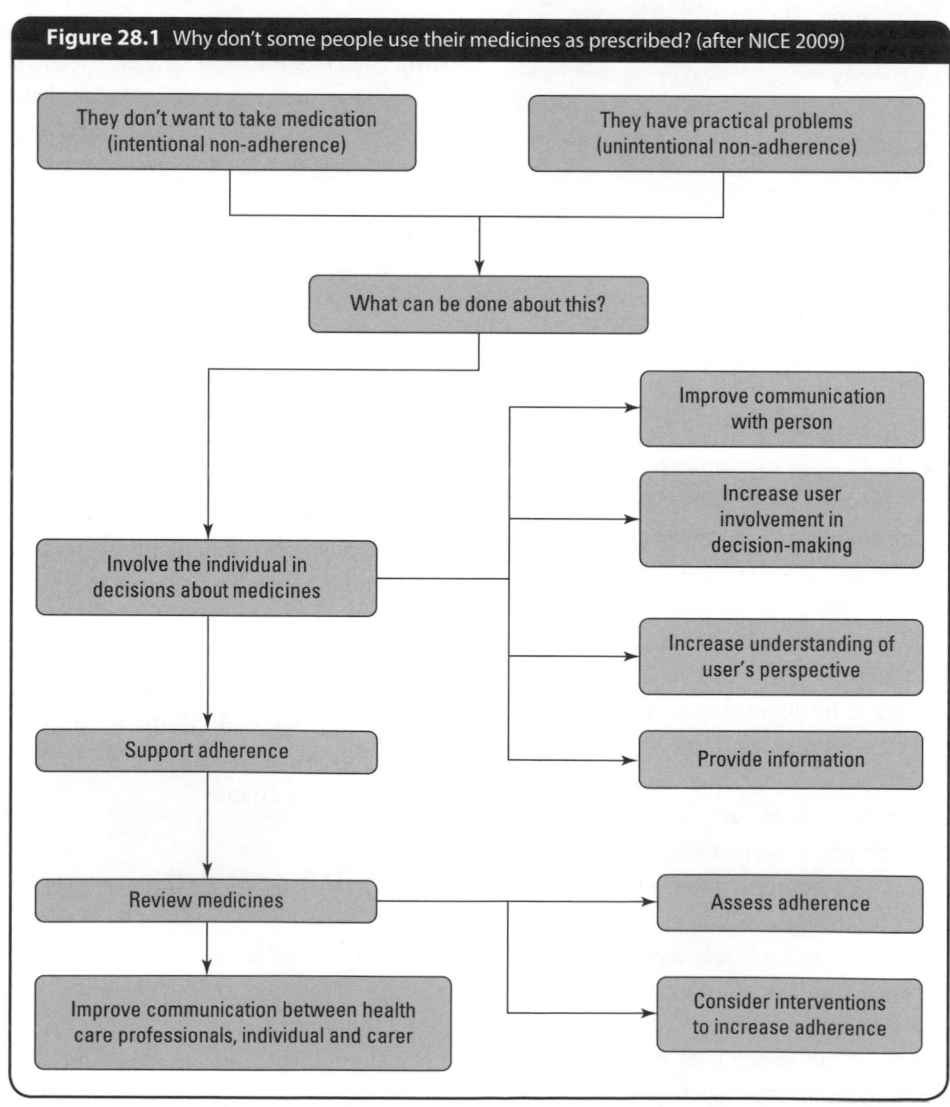

Figure 28.1 Why don't some people use their medicines as prescribed? (after NICE 2009)

determine current adherence. In clinical practice, individual and carers' reports, clinical assessment and observation are the most frequently used (subjective) measures of adherence.

Medication adherence scales or surveys are simple and low-cost approaches to identifying medication non-adherence in clinical practice. A number of validated medication adherence scales have been described in the literature, however, no gold standard exists, and no single scale is appropriate for every scenario. Issues to consider when selecting an adherence scale include: administration length, internal consistency, reliability, ability to detect barriers to adherence, validation in low-literacy clients, ability to assess self-efficacy, sensitivity and specificity as well as the 'disorder' in which it has been validated.

Adherence rates

Interpreting the literature is difficult as there is no agreed definition of non-adherence. Non-adherence with all types of medication is common with suggestions that between 30 and 50 per cent of all clients do not take or use their prescribed medicines as recommended by their prescriber (WHO 2003). Cramer and Rosenheck (1998) suggest an average adherence rate of 42 per cent for antipsychotic medication. This is similar to adherence rates for people with physical disorders (Carter *et al.* 2005). More recent work suggests non-adherence with antipsychotic medication (including the newer antipsychotic preparations) is as high as 74 per cent (Lieberman *et al.* 2005).

28.4 Factors that influence adherence with medication

Few research studies have applied theoretical models of health behaviour change to the problem of medication adherence, which might provide explanation, understanding and potential for therapeutic development (Gray *et al.* 2002). However, it is clear that adherence is linked to a complex, dynamic decision-making process. The literature identifies a range of factors that appear to influence adherence to prescribed medications. These can be categorized under the following headings:

1. **The person:** culture, values, beliefs, prejudices, experience, support networks, family and carers' involvement, personality, awareness and understanding of the problem, use of non-prescribed substances (e.g. cannabis or alcohol).
2. **The illness:** cognitive impairment, thought disorder, depression, features of hallucinations.
3. **The treatment:** value of alliance with prescriber and clinicians, complexity of the treatment, the form of treatment, the treatment setting, the experience of side-effects, stigma, effectiveness of the medication, polypharmacy, ease of accessing medications.

In summary, adherence to medication is a multifaceted issue. Decisions on whether to adhere with a prescribed medication regime can be influenced by a range of factors, the reduction/relief of symptoms being just one.

The rationale for interventions

The most important rationale for intervention to improve adherence to medication is based on moral and ethical principles of practice. This is related to symptom reduction/relief and improving and maintaining the perceived quality of life of the individual, taking into account their holistic needs, a cost-benefit analysis of the prescribed medication and awareness that improvement of health may not always be a motivating factor. Following this, interventions may be required to address the impact of side-effects or adverse reactions to medication.

There is also a strong economic case for interventions to promote medication adherence. NICE (2009a) reports that in 2007/8, £8.1 billion was spent on prescription costs and if up to 50 per cent of patients are not taking take their medicines as recommended, this implies that £4 billion of medicines are either not used correctly, or wasted and not improving health outcomes.

From this evidence there is a clear rationale for careful, individually tailored prescribing and support to improve the quality of life for people receiving prescribed medication treatments. There is also the added potential of a positive effect in reducing direct and indirect costs. As the Department of Health (DH) (2008) points out: 'Medicines management is everybody's business'.

The evidence base for adherence in medication-taking

A review of randomized controlled trials (RCTs) of both short- and long-term adherence interventions to help clients follow medication prescriptions for both physical and mental health found wide variation according to the medical condition, patient population, intervention, measures of adherence and clinical outcomes. The authors concluded that for short-term prescribing several simple interventions of counselling, written information and personal phone calls increased adherence and improved patient outcomes. For long-term treatments no simple interventions were identified and only some complex ones. These included combinations of: more convenient care; information; counselling; reminders; self-monitoring; reinforcement; family therapy; psychological therapy; mailed communications; crisis intervention; telephone follow-up calls; and other forms of additional supervision or attention (Haynes *et al.* 2008).

A meta-analysis of clinical interventions for treatment of non-adherence in psychosis reviewed 24 studies. Clinical interventions were grouped into educational strategies, psychotherapy, prompts, specific service policies and family interventions. The study concluded that interventions were positive and recommended improvements in research design (Nose *et al.* 2003).

However, no approaches that clearly increase adherence in people experiencing depression have been identified. Major reviews have drawn similar conclusions to those described above. A review of 26 studies of the effectiveness of interventions to improve antidepressant adherence concluded that the most effective adherence interventions required

complex behavioural change with multifaceted interventions (Chong *et al.* 2011). In summary, findings from the literature indicate that medication adherence is dynamic and complex and that more carefully designed and well-conducted studies are needed to clarify the effect of interventions in different patient populations and treatment settings (Haynes *et al.* 2008).

The views of people using services

Medication issues are a frequent source of tension between mental health practitioners and people using services, with some people requiring compulsory medical detention under the MHA to enforce compliance. Strategies to empower service users and carers to ask relevant questions about medication and have their views taken into account, and to help health and social care practitioners improve their person-centred approach, have emerged in the mental health policy literature (DH 2008; NICE 2009a). Increasing awareness and understanding of the views and strategies employed by service users to deal with the effects of their medications should help practitioners to engage more effectively with them when discussing their medication.

There is little in the professional literature on users' and carers' perspectives on adherence. However, there is a growing body of work that identifies a range of strategies that those suffering mental distress find useful, with a recognition that medication takes a place among them (Faulkner and Layzell 2000). Strategies employed and issues raised by users include: maintenance of a balanced lifestyle, healthy eating and sleeping routines and fostering a positive outlook on life (Meehan *et al.* 2011); the influence of the quality of the client–prescriber relationship and the user's health beliefs (Vermeire *et al.* 2001); positive perceptions about the ability to control the illness being associated with better outcomes (Broadbent *et al.* 2008); and the influence of the care environment: inpatient settings can pose particular challenges for collaborative, partnership approaches and shared decision-making (Stewart *et al.* 2010).

In a Canadian qualitative study on the meaning of recovery for people with severe mental illness, five themes related to medication emerged. These were: finding a medication that works; taking medication in combination with services and supports; complying with medication; having a say about medication; and living without medication. The researchers identified the need for users to be supported to communicate their concerns about medication and in developing self-management strategies (Piat *et al.* 2009).

Informing and working with carers is also important. Gray *et al.* (2010) raise concerns, voiced by users and carers, that mental health nurses and psychiatrists do not fully involve users in treatment decisions and want us to change how we practice. Box 28.1 summarizes some approaches that can be employed by nurses to gain greater awareness of the user perspective.

 ## 28.5 Implications for nursing practice

Medication adherence, achieved and sustained through a process of good joint decision-making, is a fundamental area of nursing practice and is increasingly so with the advent of non-medical prescribing.

The educational implications for mental health nurses are substantial. The literature suggests that nurses need greater knowledge and understanding of: users' and carers' perspectives; joint decision-making; objective assessment; pharmacology (including polypharmacy and as-needed medication); the additional needs of special groups, such as women with mental illness wishing to conceive; the care setting, particularly inpatient units; management of side-effects; and the ability to facilitate physical health care interventions in reducing physical problems.

In summary, the implications for mental health nursing practice are both dynamic and complex and involve a combination of caring, administrative, behavioural, psychological and medical approaches. The literature highlights the following key themes for clinical practice:

1. **Guiding principles:** see Box 28.2.
2. **Timing:** involvement of the user and carer at the earliest possible opportunity to ensure that they can make informed choices, when possible.

Box 28.1 Understanding the user's perspective (after NICE 2009)

Users sometimes make decisions about medicines based on their understanding of their condition and possible treatments, their view of their need for the medicine and their concerns. You can improve your understanding of the user's perspective by:

- asking users what they know and believe about medicines and their need for a medicine before prescribing and when reviewing;

- asking about general or specific concerns (such as adverse effects or dependence) and addressing these;

- bearing in mind that users may wish to minimize their medicines and to discuss:

  - what will happen if they don't take the medicine;
  - non-pharmacological alternatives;
  - reducing or stopping long-term medicines;
  - fitting medicines into their routine;
  - choosing between medicines.

If the user has specific concerns, record a summary of the discussion.

Box 28.2 Medication adherence: guiding principles (after NICE 2009)

Practitioners need to:

- Adapt their consultation style to the needs of individual patients so that all patients have the opportunity to be involved in decisions about their medicines at the level they wish.

- Establish the most effective way of communicating with each patient. Consider ways of making information accessible and understandable (e.g. use pictures, symbols, large print, different languages, an interpreter or advocate).

- Offer all patients the opportunity to be involved in making decisions about prescribed medicines and establish what level of involvement in decision-making they would like.

- Be aware that increasing patient involvement may mean that the patient decides not to take or to stop taking a medicine. If in the health care practitioner's view this could have an adverse effect, then the information provided to the patient on risks and benefits, and the patient's decision, should be recorded.

- Accept that the patient has the right to decide not to take a medicine, even if you do not agree with the decision, as long as the patient has the capacity to make an informed decision and has been provided with the information needed to make such a decision.

- Be aware that patients' concerns about medicines, and whether they believe they need them, affect how and whether they take their prescribed medicines.

- Offer patients information that is relevant to their condition, possible treatments and personal circumstances, and that is easy to understand and free from jargon.

- Recognize that non-adherence is common and that most patients are non-adherent sometimes. Routinely assess adherence in a non-judgemental way whenever you prescribe, dispense and review medicines.

---

3. **Foundation skills:** reliant on good interpersonal skills, good clinician–user relationship, relational continuity and a caring collaborative person centred-approach to providing care.

4. **Assessment:** baseline and systematic assessments of both mental and physical health, lifestyle, quality of life, syndrome, symptom and side-effects of medication. With psychiatric advance directives, providing a clinically useful conduit for communicating patient medication preferences.

5. **Pharmacology:** tailoring medication to individual needs with reference to best practice prescribing – i.e. current NICE guidance, systematic assessment of side-effects utilizing valid and reliable measures (Waddell and

Taylor 2008) and in-depth knowledge of the prescribed medication in the following areas:

- pharmacokinetics: how the medication biologically functions in the body through the process of absorption, distribution, metabolism and elimination;

- pharmacodynamics: where, how and why the medication acts;

- pharmacogenetics: awareness of the variation of ethnic and racial response.

6. **Adherence therapy techniques:**

- **Looking back: exploring the person's illness story:** experience, attitudes, beliefs, awareness and understanding; utilizing interpersonal skills and information exchange in normalizing and health-promotion opportunities. Be aware that there can be negative connotations to improved adherence and that it is important to understand the reasons for non-compliance.

■ **Looking at the future:** individuals with severe mental illness have the same aspirations as the rest of the population, including meaningful work, decent housing, financial security, friendships, health and a high quality of life.

■ **Looking at now:** exploring ambivalence towards treatment and utilizing interpersonal, problem-solving, cognitive behaviour psychotherapy and motivational interviewing approaches, skills and techniques.

■ **Providing information:** in a number of formats on medication – how it works, side-effects and the condition. Consent to treatment is the precursor to involvement in the treatment process, and information-giving is seen as a starting point in enabling people to adhere to prescribed medication.

■ **Maintaining wellness:** ensuring regular physical health checks are undertaken and exploring, promoting and supporting strategies, skills and techniques for managing health, weight gain being of particular importance.

■ **Involvement of carers:** providing information, as above.

■ **Ways of working – service protocols, designs, strategies and technology:** enhancing ways to provide support (e.g. user advanced directives, discharge protocols, telephone support, electronic records, map of medicine care pathways – www.mapofmedicine.com – and NICE guidelines, pathways and quality standards – www.nice.org.uk).

Thinking Space 28.2

Refer back to the case study at the beginning of this chapter. Having read the chapter, elaborate your answer to the question: what actions can now be taken to support Preda?

Feedback

In your answer you might have mentioned the following:

■ Preda has been admitted under the MHA for assessment. This provides a defined period of time in a safe place during which Preda's deteriorating condition can be assessed and better understood. Nursing observation of Preda's thoughts and behaviours is therefore critical in this initial assessment period. Results can be compared with what is already known about Preda's typical illness profile in order to judge the severity of her condition and to help identify appropriate interventions to support her recovery.

■ Preda's care coordinator would meet regularly to explore Preda's views of her present circumstances, including the role of medication. In this respect the care coordinator would use a range of strategies related to medication adherence best practice such as the lines of enquiry contained in Box 28.1 and the guiding principles outlined in Box 28.2.

■ The care coordinator aims to work holistically with Preda, her partner and the wider team to implement approaches that facilitate Preda's improved well-being, one of which is her treatment with medication.

- Preda's medication adherence is regularly monitored and reviewed. Clinical judgement is informed by measures such as the Beliefs about Medication Questionnaire (Horne *et al.* 1999); the Drug Attitude Inventory (Hogan *et al.* 1983); and the Glasgow Antipsychotic Side-effect Scale (Waddell and Taylor 2008).

28.6 Conclusion

This chapter has provided an overview of medication adherence achieved and sustained through a process of shared decision-making. The ideal concept of medication adherence practice is that of an equal partnership between health professionals and the person using services, which moves the relationship between service provider and user along the continuum from a paternalistic model towards a person-centred approach. How far this ideal is achieved will vary from one case to another.

Mental health nurses occupy a key and privileged position in working closely with clients to promote their recovery. Competence in medication adherence skills and techniques can help to equip nurses for this role. Applying competence in medication management to holistic care delivery, within the context of a collaborative relationship, can help clients to make informed choices that support their recovery from illness to well-being.

In summary the main points from this chapter are:

- The application of the concept of concordance to nursing practice has changed with best practice recommending the use of the term 'adherence'. Adherence is achieved and sustained through a process of shared decision-making.

- Non-adherence rates to psychotropic medication appear similar, or slightly higher, to those of generic medication prescribing.

- Adherence interventions are usually complex, composite, approaches which involve education and psychological, behavioural and socio-economic interventions.

- The literature indicates that mental health practitioners have much to learn about how to best facilitate improved adherence.

Annotated bibliography

NICE (2009) *Clinical Guideline 76: Medicines adherence,* **available at: www.nice.org.uk.**
Familiarize yourself with the range of adherence guidance for practitioners, the public and commissioners.

Taylor, D., Paton, C. and Kapur, S. (2012) *The Maudsley Prescribing Guidelines,* **11th edn. London: Informa Healthcare.**
An essential text that provides information and guidance on issues of psychotropic medication prescribing.

DH (Department of Health) (2008) Medicines *Management: Everybody's Business: A guide for service users, carers and health and social care practitioners,* **available at: www.dh.gov.uk/en/Publicationsandstatistics/Publications/ PublicationsPolicyAndGuidance/DH_082200.**
This booklet is primarily aimed to inform mental health users and carers to ask relevant questions about their medication. It is also useful for mental health practitioners in improving their person-centred approach to medications management.

National Prescribing Centre, at www.npc.nhs.uk.
This website has lots of useful information including online quizzes to test your knowledge on concordance, compliance and adherence.

Coming off psychiatric medication, at www.comingoff.com.
This website aims to give information about psychiatric medication, how it functions and the withdrawal process. It is put together by people who have been prescribed medication and withdrawn from it, and clinicians who have been involved in supporting this process.

References

Agius, M., Davis, A., Gilhooley, M., Chapman, S. and Zaman, R. (2010) What do large scale studies of medication in schizophrenia add to our management strategies? *Psychiatria Danubina*, 22(2): 323–8.

Broadbent, E., Kydd, R., Sanders, D. and Vanderpyl, J. (2008) Unmet needs and treatment seeking in high users of mental health services: role of illness perceptions, *Australian and New Zealand Journal of Psychiatry*, 42(2): 147–53.

Carter, S., Taylor, D. and Levenson, R. (2005) *A Question of Choice-Compliance in Medicine Taking: A preliminary review*, 3rd edn, available at: www.medicines-partnership.org/research-evidence/major-reviews/aquestion-of-choice.

Chong, W.W., Aslani, P. and Chen, T.F. (2011) Effectiveness of interventions to improve antidepressant medication adherence: a systematic review, *International Journal of Clinical Practice*, 65(9): 954–75.

Cramer, J.A. and Rosenheck, R. (1998) Compliance with medication regimens for mental and physical disorders, *Psychiatric Services*, 49: 196–201.

DH (Department of Health) (2008) *Medicines Management: Everybody's Business: A guide for service users, carers and health and social care practitioners*, available at: www.dh.gov.uk/health/category/publications.

Dodds, F., Rebair-Brown, A. and Parsons, S. (2000) A systematic review of randomized controlled trials that attempt to identify interventions that improve patient compliance with prescribed antipsychotic medication, *Clinical Effectiveness in Nursing*, 4: 47–53.

Faulkner, A. and Layzell, S. (2000) *Strategies for Living: A report of user-led research into people's strategies for living with mental distress*. London: Mental Health Foundation.

Gray, R., Wykes, T. and Gournay, K. (2002) From compliance to concordance: a review of the literature on interventions to enhance compliance with antipsychotic medication, *Journal of Psychiatric and Mental Health Nursing*, 9: 277–84.

Gray, R., White, J., Schulz, M. and Abderhalden, C. (2010) Enhancing medication adherence in people with schizophrenia: an international programme of research, *International Journal of Mental Health Nursing*, 19(1): 36–44.

Haynes, B.R., Ackloo, E., Sahota, N., McDonald, H.P. and Yao, X. (2008) Interventions for enhancing medication adherence, *Cochrane Database of Systematic Reviews: Issue 2*.

Horne, T., Weinman, J., Barber, N., Elliott, R., Morgan, M., Cribb, A. and Kellar, I. (2005) *Concordance, Adherence and Compliance in Medicine Taking: Report for the National Co-ordinating Centre for NHS Service Delivery and Organisation R & D*, available at: www.sdo.nihr.ac.uk.

Lieberman, J., Stroup, S., McEvoy, J. *et al.* (2005) Effectiveness of antipsychotic drugs in patients with chronic schizophrenia, *New England Journal of Medicine*, 353(12): 1209–23.

Marland, G. and Sharkey, V. (1999) Depot neuroleptics, schizophrenia and the role of the nurse: is practice evidence based? A review of the literature, *Journal of Advanced Nursing*, 30: 1255–62.

Meehan, T., Stedman, T. and Wallace J. (2011) Consumer strategies for coping with antipsychotic medication side effects, *Australasian Psychiatry*, 19(1): 74–7.

NICE (National Institute for Health and Clinical Excellence) (2009a) *Clinical Guideline 79: Medicines adherence*, available at: www.nice.org.uk.

NICE (National Institute for Health and Clinical Excellence) (2009b) *Clinical Guideline 79: Costings statement*, available at: www.nice.org.uk.

Nose, M., Barbui, C., Gray, R. and Tansella, M. (2003) Clinical interventions for treatment non-adherence in psychosis: meta-analysis, *British Journal of Psychiatry*, 183: 197–206.

Piat, M., Sabetti, J. and Bloom, D. (2009) The importance of medication in consumer definitions of recovery from serious mental illness: a qualitative study, *Issues in Mental Health Nursing*, 30(8): 1096-4673.

Repper, J. and Perkins, R. (1998) Different but normal: language, labels and professional mental health practice, *Mental Health Care*, 2: 90–3.

Stewart, D., Anthony, G.B. and Chesson, R. (2010) 'It's not my job. I'm the patient not the doctor': patient perspectives of medicines management in the treatment of schizophrenia, *International Journal of Pharmacy Practice*, 18(44): 0961–7671.

Vermeire, E., Hearnshaw, H., Van Royen, P. and Denekens, J. (2001) Patient adherence to treatment: three decades of research – a comprehensive review, *Journal of Clinical Pharmacy and Therapeutics*, 26(5): 331–42.

Waddell, L. and Taylor, M. (2008) A new self-rating scale for detecting atypical or second-generation antipsychotic side effects, *Journal of Psychopharmacology*, 22: 238–43.

WHO (World Health Organization) (2003) *Adherence to Long-Term Therapies: Evidence for action*. Geneva: WHO.

WHO (World Health Organization) (2001) *The World Health Report. Mental Health: New understanding, new hope*. Geneva: WHO.

Chapter 29

Complementary and Alternative Therapies

Hagen Rampes and Karen Pilkington

The different things that have helped me paddle on [include] learning relaxation techniques, tai chi, meditation [and] homeopathy

Penny

29.1 Introduction

This chapter describes the contribution of complementary and alternative therapies to the treatment and care of people who experience mental health problems. The chapter includes:

■ an introduction to complementary and alternative therapies;

■ specific complementary and alternative therapies.

29.2 An introduction to complementary and alternative therapies

The term *alternative medicine* was originally introduced to refer to whole medical systems that did not fit with conventional medicine and which had different ideas on causes of disease, methods of diagnosis and approaches to treatment. *Complementary medicine* or *therapies* refers to those methods which can be used alongside or to 'complement' conventional medicine. There is considerable overlap between the two areas and what is considered to be complementary or alternative in one country may be considered conventional in another. *Complementary and alternative medicine* (CAM) is often used to include both approaches and refers to any therapies, practices or approaches to health care outside mainstream conventional medicine. *Integrative or integrated medicine* is a closely related concept described as 'practice that combines both conventional and complementary and alternative medicine treatments for which there is evidence of safety and effectiveness' (NCCAM 2010).

Thinking Space 29.1

Before reading this chapter, consider each of the complementary therapies or approaches you have encountered in your practice. Could you provide a brief explanation of each of these therapies if asked by someone? Make some notes of the key points you might want to share. As you read through the chapter, review and where necessary amend or develop your notes.

Use of complementary and alternative therapies

Survey data reveal that complementary and alternative therapies are used by a sizeable proportion of the population in a number of countries: figures reported for some European countries in the early 1990s were between 20 and 50 per cent. Therapies such as herbal medicine, hydrotherapy and massage are firmly established in conventional medicine in many European countries. In 2004, a national survey revealed that 36 per cent of US adults had used complementary and alternative therapies in the previous 12 months (Barnes *et al.* 2004). Complementary and alternative therapies were most often used to treat back pain or back problems, head or chest colds, neck pain or neck problems, joint pain or stiffness, and anxiety or depression. By 2008, use had increased to approximately 38 per cent of adults and 12 per cent of children (Barnes *et al.* 2008). Natural products were the most frequently used therapies while use of breathing exercises, meditation, massage and yoga had increased significantly. In the UK, complementary and alternative therapy use was 11 per cent in 1998 (Thomas *et al.* 2001). Over 4 million UK adults made 18 million visits to practitioners of one of six therapies. The most recent survey, based on 2005 data, indicated that lifetime and 12-month prevalence of CAM use were 44 and 26 per cent respectively and 12 per cent had consulted a practitioner in the preceding 12 months (Hunt *et al.* 2010). Massage, aromatherapy and acupuncture were the most commonly used therapies.

Rationale for complementary and alternative therapies

Furnham (1996) summarized the main hypotheses relating to why people use complementary and alternative therapies. Some he described as 'push' factors. These include dissatisfaction with or outright rejection of conventional medicine through prior negative experiences or a general anti-establishment attitude. For these reasons, patients are pushed away from conventional treatment in search of alternatives. Other factors pull or attract patients towards complementary and alternative therapy. These include compatibility between the philosophy of certain therapies and patients' own beliefs and a greater sense of control over one's own treatment.

Kaptchuk and Eisenberg (1998) suggested that there are fundamental premises of most forms of complementary and alternative therapy, which contribute to its persuasive appeal. Complementary and alternative therapy is 'natural', 'pure' and 'organic', whereas conventional medicine is 'artificial', 'synthetic' and 'processed'. Another fundamental component of complementary and alternative therapy is 'vitalism'. The enhancement or balancing of 'life forces' known as *qi*, *prana* or *psychic energy* is central to many forms of complementary and alternative therapy.

Another proposed explanation is that patients using complementary and alternative therapy are essentially neurotic and are drawn towards the touching or talking approach of many therapies. While levels of psychiatric disorder are reported to be high in patients visiting complementary and alternative therapists, and higher than those visiting a general practitioner (GP), this may simply be a reflection of the nature of the conditions being treated.

Several studies (Steinsbekk & Launsφ 2005) have compared patients' views of consultations with practitioners of conventional medicine and complementary and alternative therapy. Most studies have found complementary therapy practitioners to be perceived by patients as more friendly and personal, to have treated patients more like partners in care, and provided more time for the consultation. Patients were also more satisfied with the therapeutic encounter.

In general, complementary and alternative therapy does not replace conventional medicine. Rather it serves as a substitute in some situations and as an adjunct in others, while being disregarded when not considered appropriate for the condition in question. This has been described as 'shopping for health'.

Case Study

Mrs Smith

Mrs Smith presented with feeling sad, tearfulness, irritability, poor appetite and disturbed sleep for the past four weeks. She did not have any suicidal ideation but had thoughts that she was worthless. Mrs Smith is a married lawyer. There is no family history of psychiatric disorder. Her alcohol intake is minimal. She consulted her GP who assessed her and diagnosed depressive disorder of moderate severity. She declined to take conventional antidepressant medication and preferred non-medication treatment and complementary and alternative treatment. Her doctor referred her for cognitive behavioural therapy (CBT) for the treatment of her depression.

Mrs Smith had a course of individual CBT with some improvement. However, she continued to have residual symptoms. She consulted her doctor about Hypericum (also known as St John's wort), which she had read about in the health supplement of a newspaper. Her doctor was knowledgeable about Hypericum and ensured that she was not taking any medication that had potential for interaction. Mrs Smith was on the oral contraceptive pill. She was advised that she should use an alternative form of contraception while she was on Hypericum. There is a risk of contraceptive failure and unwanted pregnancy as Hypericum can lower levels of the oral contraceptive pill.

Mrs Smith wished to take Hypericum. There are many preparations of Hypericum available, but only a few are registered with the Medicines and Healthcare Products Regulatory Agency (MHRA). She was advised to purchase a preparation registered with the MHRA, from a pharmacy. She took a Hypericum tablet daily and after two to three weeks noted improvement. She was advised to continue the Hypericum for six months. She was able to apply the CBT techniques she had learned. Her doctor had encouraged her to exercise regularly. Mrs Smith had been to yoga classes in the past which she enjoyed and she was encouraged to take up yoga again.

Commentary

Though a fictional case this is not atypical of people who present in primary care with depressive symptoms for which psychiatric medication may be indicated. Mrs. Smith's GP recognized and assessed her depression, which led to a discussion of possible treatment options including antidepressant medication and psychological treatment. The GP was able to provide advice according to Mrs Smith's preferences, who then purchased a herbal medicine antidepressant. However, though this alternative medicine is available to purchase without prescription it can interact with other medications, which the GP was able to assess with Mrs Smith and provide appropriate advice. Note also that the herbal medicine was not given in isolation but was taken alongside Mrs Smith's use of CBT, and that a further activity or intervention was now being planned to build on and complement Mrs Smith's progress to date (yoga).

Use of complementary and alternative therapies by people with mental health problems

A survey of over 16,000 people in the USA revealed that 10 per cent of those reporting a mental condition made a complementary visit, and about half of these (5 per cent) made a visit to treat the mental condition (Druss and Rosenheck 2000). Persons reporting transient stress or adjustment disorders were most likely, and those with psychotic and affective conditions least likely, to use complementary therapies to treat their mental condition. A further study revealed that individuals with panic disorder and major depression were significantly more likely to use complementary and alternative therapies than those without those disorders (Unützer *et al.* 2000).

Davidson *et al.* (1998) conducted a study to determine the frequency of psychiatric disorders in a sample of patients receiving complementary medical care in the UK and the USA. Rates of lifetime psychiatric diagnoses were 74 per cent in British patients and 61 per cent among American patients. Major depression (52 per cent of UK and 33 per cent of USA) and any anxiety disorders (50 per cent of UK and 33 per cent of USA) were the commonest lifetime diagnoses. The authors found that psychiatric disorders were not rare among patients who sought complementary medical care and that anxiety disorders were particularly represented.

Several studies have investigated which therapies are used specifically for depression. Those most frequently sought in the USA included relaxation techniques, herbal medicine, imagery and spiritual healing (Kessler *et al.* 2001). A study in Australia revealed that massage and meditation are used for mild depression, aromatherapy, St John's wort, yoga and nutritional supplements for moderate depression and relaxation therapy for moderate to severe episodes (Jorm *et al.* 2004). No complementary therapies were reported to be used for severe depression.

 29.3 ## Specific complementary and alternative therapies

Acupuncture and related therapies

Acupuncture encompasses differing philosophies and techniques. It involves the stimulation of special points on the body, usually by insertion of fine needles. How the points to be treated are selected depends on the teaching and background of the practitioner. Following insertion of needles at acupuncture points, further stimulation of the points can be achieved by manual stimulation of the needle by rotation, application of heat to the needle by burning the herb *Artemisia vulgaris* over the needle (moxibustion) or by applying an electric current to a pair of needles (electro-acupuncture). Electro-acupuncture is a modern development, which the Chinese also use. Other developments include the use of lasers to stimulate acupuncture points.

Evidence base for mental illness
Alcohol and substance misuse
Acupuncture has been used in the management of addiction. An early systematic review found encouraging evidence for efficacy of acupuncture in drug addiction and proposed that since acupuncture is

quick, inexpensive and relatively safe, it may prove to be an important component of treatment (Moner 1996). Systematic reviews since then have not found sufficient evidence to confirm efficacy (Gates et al. 2006; Jordan 2006). The evidence on acupuncture in alcohol dependence was also found to be low quality, preventing conclusions on efficacy being made (Cho and Whang 2009).

Anxiety

Anxiety is one of the most common reasons for people to visit a complementary practitioner. A systematic review of acupuncture in anxiety included 10 randomized controlled trials: four on generalized anxiety disorder or anxiety neurosis and six on anxiety in the perioperative period (Pilkington et al. 2007). There were no studies on panic disorder, phobias or obsessive compulsive disorder (OCD). It was difficult to interpret the findings because of the range of interventions against which acupuncture was compared. All trials in generalized anxiety disorder/anxiety neurosis reported positive findings but lacked many basic methodological details. There was some limited evidence from the perioperative trials in favour of auricular acupuncture in short-term anxiety, suggesting that further research may prove valuable.

Depression

In 2005, two systematic reviews were published: each included seven randomized controlled trials and concluded that there was insufficient evidence on the efficacy of acupuncture in depression (Mukaino et al. 2005; Smith and Hay 2005). A subsequent update of the latter systematic review included 30 trials with 2,812 participants (Smith et al. 2010). The majority of trials were undertaken in China and recruited participants from an inpatient hospital setting. Various forms of acupuncture were used and the control treatments included sham acupuncture, medication, standard care or placebo medication. The authors concluded that there was still insufficient evidence to recommend the use of acupuncture for people with depression. This was mainly due to the high risk of bias in the majority of trials. Randomized controlled trials car-

ried out in the USA more recently have not shown any specific beneficial effects from treating depression with acupuncture (Andreescu et al. 2011; Painovich and Herman 2012).

Smoking cessation

A Cochrane review which included 33 studies found no consistent evidence that acupuncture, acupressure, laser therapy or electrostimulation are effective for smoking cessation, but methodological problems meant that no firm conclusions could be drawn (White et al. 2011). Some researchers suggest that auricular (ear) acupuncture appears to be effective for smoking cessation, but the effect may not depend on point location (White and Moody 2006).

Other conditions

Trials of acupuncture have been conducted in a range of other conditions including attention deficit hyperactivity disorder (ADHD), dementia, restless legs syndrome, schizophrenia and sleep problems. In each case, the evidence is insufficient either in quality or quantity. Many trials are conducted in China where acupuncture is often given daily and combined with other treatments so that the results are difficult to interpret and may not be relevant to practice in western health care.

Safety considerations

A review by Rampes and James (1995) revealed that serious adverse effects of acupuncture had been reported ranging from trauma to underlying organs (e.g. pneumothorax: puncture of the lung cavity) to infections (hepatitis B). Most serious adverse effects are preventable by appropriate practitioner training. In the past, practitioners used reusable needles, which required careful sterilization. Unfortunately, poor sterilization resulted in several outbreaks of hepatitis B worldwide. Overall, the conclusion of the review was that acupuncture is relatively safe. The rate of adverse events reported by practitioners was investigated in two prospective surveys of a total of over 60,000 consultations (Macpherson et al. 2001; White et al. 2001). Eighty-six non-serious adverse events were reported, the most frequent being nausea, fainting and dizziness. The most recent study, carried out in Germany, included over 200,000 patients treated with acupuncture provided by doctors with appropriate training. Again, the results suggested that acupuncture is a relatively safe intervention if provided by trained practitioners (Witt *et al.* 2009).

Aromatherapy, massage and reflexology

Aromatherapy involves the use of essential oils from plants, which are considered to have a range of therapeutic properties. Oils may be inhaled or added to baths but are most frequently used in combination with massage. The aim of massage is to promote the circulation of blood and lymph, and relaxation of muscles, providing both physical and mental benefits. Reflexology is a method of massage in which pressure is applied to 'reflex' zones on the feet (or hands) thought to correspond to parts of the body including the major organs and glands and so connected with a range of health problems. The mechanism of action of reflexology is thought to be by stimulating the release of endorphins and enkephalins in the same way as generalized massage.

Evidence base for mental illness
Anxiety and depression
It has been suggested that improvement of depression and trait anxiety are the largest effects of massage therapy and that a course of treatment provides benefits similar to psychotherapy (Moyer *et al.* 2004). A series of randomized controlled trials of massage therapy have been conducted in a range of groups including hospitalized children and adolescents with depression, adolescent mothers with depressive symptoms and women with postnatal depression (Pilkington *et al.* 2006a). Massage therapy (regular 30–60-minute sessions) compared favourably with relaxing activities such as viewing a videotape, yoga plus progressive muscular relaxation or no treatment. Similarly, massage appeared superior to no treatment or relaxation-based control treatment based on self-assessment of anxiety: in the anxious elderly, post-traumatic stress disorder (PTSD) in children, premenstrual dysphoria disorder and preoperative anxiety (Pilkington *et al.* 2006b). There is currently insufficient research evidence on any single intervention or patient group for firm conclusions on effectiveness, role or long-term outcomes to be drawn.

The combination of aromatherapy with massage was compared with massage alone in a small study in elderly patients with anxiety and/or depression. Promising results were reported for the combined intervention. It is difficult to assess the effects of aromatherapy alone as the studies were of insufficient quality.

Several studies were found on the effects of reflexology on mood or depression in patients with conditions such as cancer but no published clinical trials specifically on anxiety disorders or depressive disorders (Pilkington *et al.* 2006c, 2006d).

Dementia
A review of evidence on massage and touch in dementia included two trials (Hansen *et al.* 2006). Both focused on specific interventions, one on hand massage for agitated behaviour and the other on addition of touch to verbal encouragement to eat. Consequently, it was not possible to draw more general conclusions on the effects of massage on dementia. In a Cochrane review of aromatherapy in dementia, data from only one trial could be included (Holt *et al.* 2003). Aromatherapy appeared to have beneficial effects on agitation and neuropsychiatric symptoms but there were concerns over randomization and that participants were taking a range of medication which may have affected the results. Thirteen studies were included in a review of aromatherapy for behavioural problems in dementia (Nguyen and Paton 2008). Most trials evaluated lavender oil and the methods for delivery included touch, massage or diffuser, but the findings were mixed.

Safety considerations
Essential oils are potent chemicals virtually all of which require dilution before use. Several oils cannot be used due to potential toxicity and many are avoided during pregnancy due to lack of information

on the possible risks. While massage is not entirely risk free, serious adverse events are probably rare and qualified massage therapists were rarely implicated in the reported problems (Ernst 2003).

Herbal medicine

Herbal medicine utilizes the healing properties of plant substances to restore health. Since antiquity, mankind has used plants for healing. In fact, many modern drugs are originally derived from plant substances but are generally administered as the pure chemical. In earlier times, plants were venerated because they were known to have valuable properties. During medieval times, the use of herbs was laden with superstition, incantation and ritual.

Modern science has analysed and studied the therapeutic effects of plants. This has led to the identification, comparison and classification of the various properties so that plants with similar effects may be grouped together, and the most effective selected for further investigation. Medicinal plants are defined as those which produce one or more active constituents capable of preventing or curing an illness. Assessing effectiveness and safety of herbal medicines is difficult because they contain mixtures of constituents which vary considerably. Nevertheless, there has been considerable research and clinical interest in their use, particularly in anxiety and depression.

Evidence base for mental illness

Hypericum for depression

St John's wort (*Hypericum perforatum*) is a flowering plant that is widely used as a herbal remedy particularly for self-treatment for depression. The extract appears to increase serotonin, noradrenaline and dopamine content in the brain but the mechanism of action is not fully understood (Mennini and Gobbi 2004).

A series of systematic reviews have been published and in most cases findings have been positive when compared with placebo for mild to moderate depression. The most recent version of the Cochrane review on this topic included 29 studies in 5,489 patients with depression (Linde *et al.* 2008). These trials compared treatment with extracts of St

John's wort for 4 to 12 weeks with placebo treatment or standard antidepressants. Several different products were tested and most patients had mild to moderately severe symptoms. The authors concluded that 'the St John's wort extracts tested in the trials were superior to placebo, similarly effective as standard antidepressants, and had fewer side effects than standard antidepressants'. The authors recommended that people with depression who wish to use a St John's wort product should consult a health professional.

Ginkgo for dementia

A Cochrane review concluded that *Ginkgo biloba* appears to be safe with no excess side-effects compared with placebo but evidence of clinically significant effects was not convincing as many of the early trials used unsatisfactory methods or were small (Birks and Grimley Evans 2009). There may also have been publication bias with a tendency to over-report positive findings. Three recent trials found no difference between gingko and placebo. One of these was the largest trial ever to investigate the effect of gingko on the development of dementia and Alzheimer's disease in older people. The Ginkgo Evaluation of Memory (GEM) study involved over 3,000 people recruited at four clinical sites who were assessed for eight years. Gingko was not found to be effective at reducing the incidence of dementia or Alzheimer's disease (DeKosky *et al.* 2008).

Kava for anxiety

Kava initially showed promise as a symptomatic treatment for anxiety although the effect size was small (Pittler and Ernst 2003). Subsequently, concerns about suspected liver toxicity caused kava to be withdrawn from the UK market in 2003, a ban that remains in place (MHRA 2006).

Passiflora for anxiety

The findings from one study suggested an improvement in job performance in favour of passiflora and one study showed a lower rate of drowsiness as a side-effect compared with mexazolam (a drug related to the benzodiazepines) (Miyasaka *et al.* 2007). However, the trials were too few in number to permit any conclusions to be drawn.

Valerian for anxiety and insomnia

Only one small study on valerian in anxiety was located providing insufficient evidence to draw any conclusions about the efficacy or safety compared with placebo or diazepam for anxiety disorders (Miyasaka *et al.* 2006). The evidence for valerian in insomnia was promising but not conclusive as not all trials reported positive findings (Bent *et al.* 2006).

Traditional Chinese herbs for schizophrenia

Traditional Chinese Medicine has been used to treat mental health disorders for more than 2,000 years. The use of Chinese herbs in a western medicine context, without incorporating traditional Chinese medicine methodology, has been evaluated in six trials (Rathbone *et al.* 2005). The results suggest that using Chinese herbs in conjunction with western antipsychotic drugs may be beneficial in terms of mental state, global functioning and decrease of adverse effects. However, because study size and length were limited, further trials are needed before the effects of Traditional Chinese Medicine for people with schizophrenia can be evaluated with any real confidence.

Safety considerations

Drugs can be measured with reliability and are tested out on animals and humans before they are allowed to be prescribed. Herbal medicines are not subject to similar scientific scrutiny although many have been widely used traditionally. Herbal medicine may be supplied by a herbalist or purchased from a pharmacy, health food shop or via the internet. Consequently, the amount of guidance on appropriate and safe use and the quality of products vary widely. Specific herbs may be contra-indicated, may need to be used with caution or may cause adverse effects which should be reported as for any medication. Often, the main safety concern relates to potential interactions with conventional treatment or other herbs and supplements. In the UK, Medicines Information Centres can advise on this. Current advice on the safe use of herbal products is provided on the MHRA website (www.mhra.gov.uk). The website also provides information on registered traditional herbal medicines.

St John's wort (*Hypericum perforatum*), one of the more widely used herbs, is well tolerated and has an incidence of adverse effects similar to that of placebo. The most frequently reported adverse effects are gastrointestinal symptoms, dizziness and sedation. The only potentially serious adverse effects are photosensitization, which is extremely rare, and precipitation of manic symptoms in pre-disposed patients. However, problems may arise when patients take hypericum with other medications as it induces a hepatic enzyme through activation of the cytochrome P450 system. Thus hypericum can decrease the plasma level of a range of prescribed drugs including anticoagulants, oral contraceptives and antiviral agents with possible clinically serious consequences. Some evidence also indicates that combining hypericum with selective serotonin inhibitors can lead to serotonin syndrome, particularly in elderly patients.

Homeopathy

Homeopathy is a school of medicine founded by Dr Samuel Hahnemann (1755–1843). The term homeopathy is derived from the Greek for 'like suffering'. It is based on the principle of 'let likes be treated with likes' or *similia similibus curentur*. This principle was known to Hippocrates but it was Hahnemann who coined the term 'homeopathy' and worked relentlessly in establishing it against much hostility from his contemporaries. Contemporary medical practice in Hahnemann's day consisted of techniques such as bloodletting, purging and prescribing toxic drugs. It was amid this background that Hahnemann developed his ideas on homeopathy. Homeopathy is used to treat a wide range of acute and chronic illness. Where a condition is beyond the scope of the body's normal self-repair mechanism, treatment is less likely to be curative, but may be palliative.

Homeopathic medicines are prepared from minerals, plant and animal substances. There are over 3,000 medicines available. For example, a commonly prescribed medicine is *lycopodium*, which is derived from the plant club moss. The plant is macerated in 95 per cent alcohol and then filtered. This juice forms the basis of medicine preparation.

A typical prescription would be *lycopodium* 30C. The number and letter refer to the degree of dilution of the original substance. One drop of the original substance is added to 99 drops of water and is then shaken vigorously. Then one drop of that is added to 99 drops of water and shaken vigorously. This is done 30 times. In fact by the laws of chemistry, lycopodium 30C is so dilute (ultramolecular) that not one atom of the original substance may be present in it. This is one of the most controversial aspects of homeopathy, which results in most people not being able to understand how homeopathic medicines may work.

Evidence base for mental illness
Anxiety
A systematic review located eight randomized controlled trials addressing test anxiety, generalized anxiety disorder and anxiety related to medical or physical conditions (Pilkington *et al.* 2006e). The trials reported contradictory results, were underpowered or provided insufficient details of methodology. It was not possible to draw firm conclusions on the effectiveness of homeopathy for anxiety.

Depression
A systematic review found only two randomized controlled trials of homeopathy in depression and one of these demonstrated problems with recruitment of patients in primary care (Pilkington *et al.* 2005a). Positive results and high levels of patient satisfaction were reported in uncontrolled and observational studies with adverse effects limited to 'remedy reactions' or 'aggravations'.

Safety considerations
Dantas and Rampes (2000) conducted a systematic review to evaluate the safety of homeopathic medicines by critically appraising reports of adverse effects published in English from 1970 to 1995. The authors found that the overall incidence of adverse effects of homeopathic medicines was higher than placebo in controlled clinical trials but effects were minor, transient and comparable. The authors concluded that pure homeopathic medicines in high dilutions, prescribed by trained professionals, are probably safe and unlikely to provoke severe adverse reactions.

Meditation, yoga and related therapies
The main types of meditation used in therapy are concentrative methods, transcendental meditation and insight forms such as mindfulness techniques, although there is some overlap between these. Transcendental meditation was introduced to the West in the 1960s and involves use of a mantra (a repeated phrase, word or sound). The aim is to 'focus attention on an object and sustain attention until the mind achieves stillness' (Krisanaprakornkit *et al.* 2006). Mindfulness meditation emphasizes an awareness of any thoughts or feelings that enter the mind or anything that arises within the field of awareness.

Yoga originated in Indian culture and consists of a system of spiritual, moral and physical practices aimed at attaining 'self-awareness'. Hatha yoga, the system on which much of Western yoga is based, has three basic components: *asanas* (postures), *pranayama* (breathing exercises) and *dhyana* (meditation). Postures involve standing, bending, twisting and balancing the body to improve flexibility and strength, the controlled breathing helps to focus the mind and achieve relaxation, while meditation aims to calm the mind. Several explanations have been proposed to account for the effects of yoga including an effect on autonomic nervous tone and an increase in the relaxation response in the neuromuscular system (Riley 2004).

Evidence base for mental illness
Anxiety
One review located 12 controlled studies of meditation in people who had an anxiety disorder, were complaining of anxiety related symptoms, had raised anxiety levels or were being treated for anxiety related to a performance or test (Kirkwood *et al.* 2005a). Various styles of meditation were used although transcendental meditation was most frequently encountered. Most of the trials found no difference between meditation and other relaxa-

tion techniques. This could be because the interventions are equally effective or due to poor methodology or a small sample size.

A subsequent Cochrane review focused only on diagnosed anxiety disorders and concluded that the small number of studies located did not permit any firm conclusions to be drawn (Krisanaprakornkit *et al.* 2006). Transcendental meditation was found to be comparable with other kinds of relaxation therapies in reducing anxiety. Adverse effects of meditation were not reported but dropout rates were high so further investigation is required.

It was not possible to say whether yoga is effective in treating anxiety or anxiety disorders because of the range of anxiety-related conditions treated and the poor quality of the majority of studies (Kirkwood *et al.* 2005b). However, there were encouraging results, particularly in OCD.

Depression

A review of meditation in depression found that there is a general lack of research in this area and so it was impossible to draw any conclusions on either its effectiveness in easing depression or its potential to exacerbate depression (Kirkwood *et al.* 2005c). Five trials of yoga interventions in depression were identified in another review (Pilkington *et al.* 2005b). Different forms of yoga were used with twice-weekly or daily practice for 20 to 60 minutes and rhythmic breathing was an important component in four trials. All trials reported positive findings. No adverse effects were reported with the exception of fatigue and breathlessness in participants in one study but participants in all the trials were under 50 years. Potentially beneficial effects of yoga interventions on depressive disorders were indicated although several of the interventions may not be feasible in those with reduced or impaired mobility. The findings should be interpreted with caution because of the variation in interventions and depression severity and the lack of some methodological details. Further investigation of which intervention is most effective, levels of severity of depression likely to respond and the effectiveness of anaerobic exercise (such as yoga) against aerobic exercise is needed.

Mindfulness-based stress reduction includes meditation and yoga components and promising results in depression have been reported (Grossman *et al.* 2004). Mindfulness-based cognitive therapy, based on aspects of CBT and of mindfulness-based stress reduction programmes may be useful in preventing relapse among people who have recovered from depression and is mentioned in current guidance for depression for people who are currently well but have experienced three or more previous episodes of depression (Segal *et al.* 2002; NICE 2009).

Other conditions

Mindfulness meditation has also been investigated as an intervention in substance abuse disorders. Conclusive evidence was not found but preliminary evidence was promising (Zgierska *et al.* 2009).

Safety considerations

A small number of cases of adverse psychological effects have been reported although these appear to be related specifically to meditation. A limited number of individual case reports of other serious adverse events have also been reported but these problems are likely to be rare and often linked to the more strenuous forms of yoga. As with other exercise programmes, yoga, particularly the more energetic forms, should only be undertaken on the advice of a health professional and practised under the supervision of skilled therapists. People with mental illness considering meditation should also consult their primary care-giver.

Box 29.1 provides a brief summary of the evidence base for the specific complementary and alternative therapies reviewed in this section of the chapter.

29.4 Conclusion

Many nurses are very interested in complementary and alternative therapies, and a number have been trained as practitioners in aromatherapy, in particular. Clinical experience suggests that there has been a move away from hands-on patient contact in nursing; complementary and alternative therapy

Box 29.1 Evidence summary

- Acupuncture may have a therapeutic role in the treatment of anxiety, depression and smoking cessation.

- The evidence base for homeopathy is currently too poor to reach firm conclusions.

- The evidence base for herbal medicines is variable but Hypericum (St John's wort) appears to be more effective than placebo for the short-term treatment of mild to moderate depression.

- There is some evidence that aromatherapy and massage reduces anxiety in the short term. It might be particularly useful as an intervention with people who are confused, have little or no preserved language, for whom verbal interaction is difficult and conventional medicine is seen as being of only marginal benefit; for example, dementia sufferers.

- Massage-related interventions can be delivered in a number of settings and may also have a potential role in, for example, mild depression where use of antidepressants as first-line treatment is discouraged particularly when their use is problematic (elderly, depressed mothers, hospitalized children). The added benefits of incorporating essential oils into the massage treatment, the selection of appropriate massage techniques and the safety of essential oils do, however, require further evaluation.

- Various forms of yoga may be helpful in anxiety and mild depression while meditation may be as helpful as relaxation in anxiety and OCD.

has perhaps filled a lacuna in nurses' professional work. There is an important potential role for nurses as providers of some complementary therapies. As researchers, nurses are particularly well placed to conduct studies to contribute to our understanding of the motivation and experiences of users of complementary and alternative therapies.

Mental health professionals need to be aware that their patients may be attending a complementary and alternative therapy provider and should enquire routinely about patients' use of complementary and alternative therapy.

The key points of learning from this chapter are:

- Complementary and alternative therapies include a broad range of 'practices and ideas which are outside the domain of conventional medicine in several countries and defined by its users as preventing or treating illness or promoting health and well-being' (Manheimer and Berman 2006).

- Survey data suggest that complementary and alternative therapy is used by a sizeable proportion of the population in a number of countries and that this proportion is increasing.

- Currently there is some provision of complementary and alternative therapy in the National Health Service (NHS), but this is not readily available to people with mental health problems. These patients are often not aware of the services and lack the finances to access them.

- Patients use complementary and alternative therapy for different reasons. The majority of people do so in addition to conventional medicine, rather than as an alternative. Complementary and alternative therapy users tend to be better educated and have a holistic orientation to health.

- Explanations for the increasing use of complementary or alternative therapy can be classified as 'push factors' – such as dissatisfaction with conventional medicine – or 'pull factors' – such as a greater sense of control over one's own treatment.

■ The question of combining therapies – i.e. what combinations of complementary and alternative therapy plus conventional treatment might be most beneficial – is one that deserves investigation. Compliance with medication is universally poor in medicine. The use of complementary and alternative therapy may improve compliance with medications.

Annotated bibliography

Boyd, H. (2000) *Banishing the Blues: Inspirational ways to improve your mood.* **London: Mitchell Beazley.**
Hilary Boyd is a qualified nurse, journalist and author. This well-presented book has a section on depression and a section on use of CAM in depression. It is aimed at patients but would be of interest to health care professionals in training as it gives pragmatic examples of how patients can help themselves. Dr Hagen Rampes was consultant editor for this book.

Ernst, E., Pittler, M.H. and Wider, B. (2006) *The Desktop Guide to Complementary and Alternative Medicine: An evidence-based approach,* **2nd edn. London: Harcourt Publishers.**
This book summarizes the extant research in the field of complementary and alternative medicine.

Frass, M., Strassl, R.P., Friehs, H., Müllner, M., Kundi, M. and Kaye, A.D. (2012) Use and acceptance of complementary and alternative medicine among the general population and medical personnel: a systematic review, *Ochsner J.,* **12(1): 45–56. Abstract on PubMed: www.ncbi.nlm.nih.gov/pubmed/22438782.**
This paper compares the use of complementary therapies in different countries. It is not specifically focused on mental health and some more recent data, for example from the UK and the USA is available, but it does provide an insight into the extent of use in the general population and several health professional groups.

Lake, J., Helgason, C. and Sarris, J. (2012) Paradigm, research, and clinical practice, *Integrative Mental Health,* **8(1): 50–7. Abstract on PubMed: www.ncbi.nlm.nih.gov/pubmed/22225934.**
This paper presents and discusses the concept of integrative mental health, which aims to incorporate pharmacologic treatments, psychotherapy and psychosocial interventions, as well as complementary therapies such as acupuncture, herbal and nutritional medicine, dietary manipulation and meditation.

Scott, S. (ed.) (2002) *Handbook of Complementary and Alternative Therapies in Mental Health.* **London: Academic Press.**
A guide which addresses topics of relevance to practice, for example, integration of complementary therapy services into mental health care.

Useful websites

BluePages Depression Information. The Centre for Mental Health Research, The Australian National University: http://bluepages.anu.edu.au.

CAMEOL (Complementary and Alternative Medicine Evidence OnLine) database. Research Council for Complementary Medicine/University of Westminster: www.rccm.org.uk/node/38.

Mental Health Information for all. Treatments. Complementary Therapy. Royal College of Psychiatrists: www.rcpsych.ac.uk/expertadvice/treatments/complementarytherapy.aspx.

National Centre for Complementary and Alternative Medicine. National Institutes of Health: www.nccam.nih.gov.

References

Andreescu, C., Glick, R.M., Emeremni, C.A., Houck, P.R. and Mulsant, B.H. (2011) Acupuncture for the treatment of major depressive disorder: a randomized controlled trial, *Journal of Clinical Psychiatry,* 72(8): 1129–35.

Barnes, P.M., Bloom, B. and Nahin, R. (2008) *CDC National Health Statistics Report #12: Complementary and alternative medicine use among adults and children,* available at: nccam.nih.gov/news/camstats.

Barnes, P.M., Powell-Griner, E., McFann, K. and Nahin, R.L. (2004) Complementary and alternative medicine use among adults: United States, 2002, *Advance Data,* 343: 1–19.

Bent, S., Padula, A., Moore, D., Patterson, M. and Mehling, W. (2006) Valerian for sleep: a systematic review and meta-analysis, *American Journal of Medicine,* 119(12): 1005–12.

Birks, J. and Grimley Evans, J. (2009) *Ginkgo biloba* for cognitive impairment and dementia, *Cochrane Database of Systematic Reviews,* Issue 1. Art. No.: CD003120. DOI: 10.1002/14651858. CD003120. pub3.

Cho, S.H. and Whang, W.W. (2009) Acupuncture for alcohol dependence: a systematic review, *Alcoholism: Clinical and Experimental Research*, 33(8): 1305–13.

Dantas, F. and Rampes, H. (2000) Do homeopathic medicines provoke adverse effects? A systematic review, *British Homeopathic Journal*, 89: S35–8.

Davidson, J., Rampes, H., Eizen, M. *et al.* (1998) Psychiatric disorders in primary care patients receiving complementary medicine, *Comprehensive Psychiatry*, 39: 16–20.

DeKosky, S.T., Williamson, J.D., Fitzpatrick, A.L. *et al.* (2008) *Ginkgo biloba* for prevention of dementia: a randomized controlled trial, *Journal of the American Medical Association*, 300(19): 2253–62.

Druss, B.G. and Rosenheck, R.A. (1999) Association between use of unconventional therapies and conventional medical services, *Journal of the American Medical Association*, 282: 651–6.

Ernst, E. (2003) The safety of massage therapy, *Rheumatology*, 42(9): 1101–6.

Furnham, A. (1996) Why do people choose and use complementary therapies? in E. Ernst (ed.) *Complementary Medicine: An objective appraisal*. Oxford: Butterworth Heinemann.

Gates, S., Smith, L.A. and Foxcroft, D.R. (2006) Auricular acupuncture for cocaine dependence, *Cochrane Database of Systematic Reviews*, Issue 1. Art. No.: CD005192. DOI: 10.1002/14651858. CD005192. pub2.

Grossman, P., Niemann, L., Schmidt, S. and Walach, H. (2004) Mindfulness-based stress reduction and health benefits: a meta-analysis, *Journal of Psychosomatic Research*, 57(1): 35–43.

Hansen, N.V., Jørgensen, T. and Ørtenblad L. (2006) Massage and touch for dementia, *Cochrane Database of Systematic Reviews*, Issue 4. Art. No.: CD004989. DOI: 10.1002/14651858. CD004989. pub2.

Holt, F.E., Birks, T.P.H., Thorgrimsen, L.M., Spector, A.E., Wiles, A. and Orrell, M. (2003) Aromatherapy for dementia, *Cochrane Database of Systematic Reviews*, Issue 3. Art. No.: CD003150. DOI: 10.1002/14651858. CD003150.

Hunt, K.J., Coelho, H.F., Wider, B., Perry, R., Hung, S.K., Terry, R., Ernst, E. (2010) Complementary and alternative medicine use in England: results from a national survey, *International Journal of Clinical Practice*, 64(11): 1496–502, doi: 10.1111/j.1742-1241.2010.02484.x.

Jordan, J.B. (2006) Acupuncture treatment for opiate addiction: a systematic review, *Journal of Substance Abuse Treatment*, 30(4): 309–14.

Jorm, A.F., Griffiths, K.M., Christensen, H., Parslow, R.A. and Rogers, B. (2004) Actions taken to cope with depression at different levels of severity: a community survey, *Psychological Medicine*, 34: 293–9.

Kaptchuk, T.J. and Eisenberg, D.M. (1998) The persuasive appeal of alternative medicine, *Annals of Internal Medicine*, 129: 1061–5.

Kessler, R.C., Soukup, J., Davis, R.B. *et al.* (2001) The use of complementary and alternative therapies to treat anxiety and depression in the United States, *American Journal of Psychiatry*, 158: 289–94.

Kirkwood, G., Pilkington, K., Rampes, H. and Richardson, J. (2005a) Meditation for anxiety: a systematic review, *Complementary and Alternative Medicine Evidence Online (CAMEOL) Database*, available at: www.rccm.org.uk/cameol/Default.aspx, accessed June 2011.

Kirkwood, G., Rampes, H., Tuffrey, V., Richardson, J. and Pilkington, K. (2005b) Yoga for anxiety: a systematic review of the research evidence, *British Journal of Sports Medicine*, 39(12): 884–91.

Kirkwood, G., Pilkington, K., Rampes, H. and Richardson, J. (2005c) Meditation for depression: a systematic review, *Complementary and Alternative Medicine Evidence Online (CAMEOL) Database*, available at: www.rccm.org.uk/cameol/Default.aspx, accessed June 2011.

Krisanaprakornkit, T., Krisanaprakornkit, W., Piyavhatkul, N. and Laopaiboon, M. (2006) Meditation therapy for anxiety disorders, *Cochrane Database of Systematic Reviews*, Issue 1. Art. No.: CD004998. DOI: 10.1002/14651858. CD004998. pub2.

Linde, K., Berner, M.M. and Kriston, L. (2008) St John's wort for major depression, *Cochrane Database of Systematic Reviews*, Issue 4. Art. No.: CD000448. DOI: 10.1002/14651858. CD000448. pub3.

MacPherson, H., Thomas, K., Walters, S. *et al.* (2001) The York acupuncture safety study: prospective survey of 34,000 treatments by traditional acupuncturists, *British Medical Journal*, 323: 486–7.

Manheimer, E. and Berman, B. (2006) *Cochrane Complementary Medicine Field: About the Cochrane Collaboration (Fields)*, Issue 1. Art. No.: CE000052.

Mennini, T. and Gobbi, M. (2004) The antidepressant mechanism of *Hypericum perforatum*, *Life Sciences*, 75: 1021–7.

MHRA (Medicines and Healthcare Regulatory Agency) (2006) *Kava Report: Report of the Committee on Safety of Medicines Expert Working Group on the safety of kava, July 2006*, available at: www.mhra.gov.uk, accessed July 2007.

Miyasaka, L.S., Atallah, A.N. and Soares, B.G.O. (2006) Valerian for anxiety disorders, *Cochrane Database of Systematic Reviews*, Issue 4. Art. No.: CD004515. DOI: 10.1002/14651858. CD004515. pub2.

Miyasaka, L.S., Atallah, A.N. and Soares, B.G.O. (2007) Passiflora for anxiety disorder, *Cochrane Database of Systematic Reviews*, Issue 1. Art. No.: CD004518. DOI: 10.1002/14651858. CD004518. pub2.

Moner, S.E. (1996) Acupuncture and addiction treatment, *Journal of Addictive Diseases*, 15(3): 79–100.

Moyer, C.A., Rounds, J. and Hannum, J.W. (2004) A meta-analysis of massage therapy research, *Psychological Bulletin*, 130(1): 3–18.

Mukaino, Y., Park, J., White, A. and Ernst, E. (2005) The effectiveness of acupunture for depression – a systematic review of randomised controlled trials, *Acupuncture in Medicine*, 23(2): 70–6.

NCCAM (National Center for Complementary and Alternative Medicine) (2010) *CAM Basics: What is complementary and alternative medicine?* NCCAM publication no. D347, available at: http://nccam.nih.gov/health/whatiscam, accessed June 2011.

Nguyen, Q. and Paton, C. (2008) The use of aromatherapy to treat behavioural problems in dementia, *International Journal of Geriatric Psychiatry*, 23(4): 337–46.

NICE (National Institute for Health and Clinical Excellence) (2009) *Depression in adults: Update CG90.* London: NICE, available at: http://guidance.nice.org.uk/CG90/Guidance.

Painovich, J. and Herman, P.M. (2012) Acupuncture in the inpatient acute care setting: a pragmatic, randomized control trial, *Evidence Based Complementary and Alternative Medicine*, 309762 (Epub 22 June).

Pilkington, K., Kirkwood, G., Rampes, H., Fisher, P. and Richardson, J. (2005a) Homeopathy for depression: a systematic review of the research evidence, *Homeopathy*, 94(3): 153–63.

Pilkington, K., Kirkwood, G., Rampes, H. and Richardson, J. (2005b) Yoga for depression: the research evidence, *Journal of Affective Disorders*, 89(1–3): 13–24.

Pilkington, K., Kirkwood, G., Rampes, H. and Richardson, J. (2006a) Aromatherapy and massage for depression: a systematic review, *Complementary and Alternative Medicine Evidence Online (CAMEOL) Database*, available at: www.rccm.org.uk/cameol/Default.aspx, accessed June 2011.

Pilkington, K., Kirkwood, G., Rampes, H. and Richardson, J. (2006b) Aromatherapy and massage for anxiety: a systematic review, *Complementary and Alternative Medicine Evidence Online (CAMEOL) Database*, available at: www.rccm.org.uk/cameol/Default.aspx, accessed June 2011.

Pilkington, K., Kirkwood, G., Rampes, H. and Richardson, J. (2006c) Reflexology for anxiety: a systematic review, *Complementary and Alternative Medicine Evidence Online (CAMEOL) Database*, available at: www.rccm.org.uk/cameol/Default.aspx, accessed June 2011.

Pilkington, K., Kirkwood, G., Rampes, H. and Richardson, J. (2006d) Reflexology for depression: a systematic review, *Complementary and Alternative Medicine Evidence Online (CAMEOL) Database*, available at: www.rccm.org.uk/cameol/Default.aspx, accessed June 2011.

Pilkington, K., Kirkwood, G., Rampes, H., Fisher, P. and Richardson, J. (2006e) Homeopathy for anxiety and anxiety disorders: a systematic review of the research evidence, *Homeopathy*, 95(3): 151–62.

Pilkington, K., Kirkwood, G., Rampes, H., Cummins, M. and Richardson, J. (2007) Acupuncture for anxiety and anxiety disorders – a systematic literature review, *Acupuncture in Medicine*, 25: 1–10.

Pittler, M.H. and Ernst, E. (2003) Kava extract versus placebo for treating anxiety, *Cochrane Database of Systematic Reviews*, Issue 1. Art. No.: CD003383. DOI: 10.1002/14651858. CD003383.

Rampes, H and James, R. (1995) Complications of acupuncture, *Acupuncture in Medicine*, 13(1): 26–33.

Rathbone, J., Zhang, L., Zhang, M. *et al.* (2005) Chinese herbal medicine for schizophrenia, *Cochrane Database of Systematic Reviews*, Issue 4. Art. No.: CD003444. DOI: 10.1002/14651858. CD003444. pub2.

Riley, D. (2004) Hatha yoga and the treatment of illness (commentary), *Alternative Therapies in Health and Medicine*, 10(2): 20–1.

Segal, Z., Teasdale, J. and Williams, M. (2002) *Mindfulness-Based Cognitive Therapy for Depression.* New York: Guilford Press.

Smith, C.A. and Hay, P.P.J. (2005) Acupuncture for depression, *Cochrane Database of Systematic Reviews*, Issue 3, Art No CD004046.. DOI: 10.1002/14651858. CD004046. pub2.

Smith, C.A., Hay, P.P.J. and MacPherson, H. (2010) Acupuncture for depression, *Cochrane Database of Systematic Reviews*, Issue 1. Art. No.: CD004046. DOI: 10.1002/14651858. CD004046. pub3.

Steinsbekk, A. and Launsø, L. (2005) Empowering the cancer patient or controlling the tumor? A qualitative study of how cancer patients experience consultations and alternative medicine practitioners and physicians respectively. *Integrative cancer Therapies*, 4(2):195-200.

Thomas, K., Nicholl, J. and Coleman, P. (2001) Use and expenditure on complementary medicine in England – a population based survey, *Complementary Therapies in Medicine*, 9: 2–11.

Unützer, J., Klap, R., Sturm, R. *et al.* (2000) Mental disorders and the use of alternative medicine: results from a national survey, *American Journal of Psychiatry*, 157(11): 1851–7.

White, A. and Moody, R. (2006) The effects of auricular acupuncture on smoking cessation may not depend on the point chosen – an exloratory meta-analysis, *Acupuncture in Medicine*, 24(4): 149–56.

White, A., Hayoe, S., Hart, A. *et al.* (2001) Adverse events following acupuncture: prospective survey of 32,000 consultations with doctors and physiotherapists, *British Medical Journal*, 323: 485–6.

White, A.R., Rampes, H., Liu, J.P., Stead, L.F. and Campbell, J. (2011) Acupuncture and related interventions for smoking cessation, *Cochrane Database of Systematic Reviews*, Issue 1. Art. No.: CD000009. DOI: 10.1002/14651858. CD000009. pub3.

Witt, C.M., Pach, D., Brinkhaus, B., Wruck, K., Tag, B., Mank, S. and Willich, S.N. (2009) Safety of acupuncture: results of a prospective observational study with 229,230 patients and introduction of a medical information and consent form, *Forschende Komplementärmedizin*, 16(2): 91–7.

Zgierska, A., Rabago, D., Chawla, N., Kushner, K., Koehler, R. and Marlatt, A. (2009) Mindfulness meditation for substance use disorders: a systematic review, *Substance Abuse*, 30(4): 266–94.

Chapter 30

Promoting Physical Health

Debbie Robson

 ## 30.1 Introduction

We have been aware for many years that people who experience a serious mental illness (SMI) such as schizophrenia, bipolar disorder or chronic depression have a higher rate of morbidity than the general population and that their life expectancy can be reduced by up to 17 years Chang *et al* 2011. Despite this knowledge and the efforts made over the past two decades to provide holistic and integrated health services for people with SMI, there is evidence that the mortality differential between the general population and people with SMI is actually increasing (Hoang *et al.* 2011). Mental health nurses face the challenge of meeting service users' mental health needs alongside their physical health needs. To meet these demands, nurses need to understand the causes of physical health problems as well as feel confident in preventing, assessing, monitoring and managing potential and existing physical health conditions. This chapter covers:

- an introduction to UK policy guidance about meeting the physical health care needs of people with SMI;

- an overview of the physical health problems people with SMI experience;

- possible reasons for these;

- suggestions for the mental health nurses' role in the promotion of physical health.

30.2 Policy guidance

A coherent approach to improve health across the lifespan, as opposed to tackling individual risk factors in isolation, is central to the UK government's drive to reduce health inequalities. Improving the physical health of the SMI population has been the focus of a range of clinical guidelines and consensus statements in Europe, the USA and Australia (Cohen and Hove 2001; De Hert *et al.* 2009). While these guidelines are helpful for synthesizing the current evidence base and provide direction for delivering high quality services, there is still a lack of consistency and agreement about who is best placed to address the physical health needs of service users with SMI. Since 2004, General practitioners (GPs) in the UK have been financially incentivized to perform annual physical health checks on patients with SMI. For the treatment of schizophrenia in primary and secondary care, the National Institute for Health and Clinical Excellence (NICE) (2009) adopts the position that it is primary care's responsibility to identify and monitor the physical health of service users with schizophrenia and recommends that mental health professionals in secondary care adopt more of a policing role to ensure that this is done. In contrast in the USA and Australia, as well as other parts of Europe, a more integrated and collaborative approach to physical health care within mental health is recommended. Essentially, the physical health care of people with SMI is the responsibility of both primary and secondary care practitioners as well as service users and their carers. The most important thing is that each of these parties knows who is responsible for doing what, when, and where, that this information is written down and all relevant parties have a copy of the plan. It is also increasingly recognized that to improve the health status of people with SMI and reduce health inequalities, ways to achieve optimal health should be of concern to all policy-makers (e.g. in housing, environment and education departments) and not simply in government health departments.

30.3 What physical health conditions do people with SMI experience?

The answer to this question is quite simple: people with SMI experience the same physical health conditions as those who don't experience mental health problems. They do however experience physical health problems more frequently and in some cases more severely. The risk of coexisting long-term conditions such as cardiovascular disease (CVD), type 2 diabetes, respiratory disease and some cancers is elevated two to three fold among people with SMI compared to those without these disorders.

Cardiovascular disease

CVD is the main cause of death in the general population in the UK, accounting for one in three of all deaths and also the leading cause of death in SMI. CVD includes conditions such as coronary heart disease, hypertension and stroke. Although increasing age and having a family history of heart disease increases the risk of having CVD, in more than 90 per cent of cases the risk of having a first heart attack is related to nine potentially modifiable risk factors all of which are more common in people with SMI. In descending order of importance they are abnormal blood lipids, smoking, psychological and social factors, such as stress and social isolation, type 2 diabetes, hypertension, abdominal obesity, low consumption of fruits and vegetables, lack of regular physical activity and low or excessive alcohol intake. The two most important risk factors are cigarette smoking and an abnormal ratio of blood lipids which together predict two-thirds of the global risk of heart attack (Yusuf et al 2004).

Respiratory disease

One fifth of the population in the UK currently dies from a respiratory related illness (British Thoracic Society 2006); these include conditions such as acute respiratory infections, pneumonia, tuberculosis, asthma and chronic obstructive pulmonary disease (COPD). Some respiratory illnesses such as COPD are mostly caused by smoking, but poor diet, poverty, environmental factors and lack of access to influenza vaccines are implicated in many of the above conditions. Social inequality, in particular, is associated with a higher proportion of deaths from respiratory diseases than in any other disease area. People with SMI are more likely than the general population to suffer from asthma, chronic bronchitis and emphysema and have poorer lung function (Samele et al. 2007).

Cancers

One in four of all deaths in the UK are due to cancer. Tobacco use is the single most important risk factor for cancer causing 22 per cent of global cancer deaths and 71 per cent of global lung cancer deaths; other causes include additional preventable lifestyle behaviours as well as physical and biological carcinogens (WHO 2008). There are more than 200 different types of cancer, but four of them, breast, lung, large bowel (colorectal) and prostate, account for over half of all new cases (Cancer Research UK 2011). Researchers have consistently reported higher rates of digestive and breast cancer in people with schizophrenia. However, rates of lung cancer in people with schizophrenia are contradictory, with some researchers reporting a decreased risk and others reporting a higher risk compared to people without a mental illness (e.g. Hippisley-Cox *et al.* 2006).

Diabetes

Diabetes occurs in approximately 15 per cent of people with schizophrenia (Holt and Pevler 2006) and possibly even higher in people with mood disorders, compared to approximately 5 per cent in the general population. It is influenced by a family history of diabetes, physical inactivity, poor diet, smoking and the metabolic effects of anti-psychotic medication. The relationship between diabetes and schizophrenia has been discussed and investigated more than any other co-occur-ring physical and mental health problem. An asso-ciation between schizophrenia and diabetes was first observed at the end of the nineteenth century by the British psychiatrist, Henry Maudsley, who noted that 'diabetes is a disease which often shows itself in families in which insanity prevails'. Insulin resistance and glucose dysregulation have been observed in psychiatric patients since the 1920s. We have therefore known that diabetes occurs independently of antipsychotic medication for over a century.

Case Study

Jane

Jane is a 35-year-old single woman who lives with her mother in rented accommodation. She has a 15-year history of schizophrenia and receives mental health care from a community mental health centre, including three-monthly appointments with a psychiatrist to monitor her mental health and psychotropic medication (risperidone 4mgs a day), along with weekly appointments with a psycholo-gist for cognitive behavioural therapy (CBT). Her physical health problems include type 2 diabetes, a gastric ulcer and asthma, all managed with medication; she has a body mass index (BMI) of 41. She smokes 50 cigarettes a day and spends 70 per cent of her welfare benefits on cigarettes. She com-plains of breathlessness and chest pain when walking up the stairs to her flat. She spends most of her time lying on the sofa watching TV, is reluctant to leave the house and often misses her CBT appoint-ments. At a recent Care Programme Approach (CPA) review, the team noted her increasing isolation and reduced activity, which compounds her mental and physical health problems. Jane is also con-cerned about her physical health. She said she wanted to stop smoking and lose weight but felt over-whelmed by these challenges and lacked confidence in using mainstream services such as her local NHS Stop Smoking Service or GP services.

Thinking Space 30.1

What do you think Jane and the team could do as the next step in her treatment plan? Jot down your ideas now, feedback is provided at the end of the chapter.

 30.4 ## Reasons for poor physical health in people with SMI

A number of reasons have been suggested for the association between SMI and poor physical health, including health behaviours, health service-related factors and the iatrogenic effects of psychotropic medication. In addition, mental disorders may influence physical health via direct physiological processes such as inflammation, immune dysfunction and decreased heart rate variability.

Health behaviours of people with SMI

The most frequently cited reasons for the increased rates of disease and death in people with SMI are their high rates of smoking, poor diet, lack of exercise, co-morbid substance use and unsafe sexual practices. In a survey of 102 service users with schizophrenia living in Scotland, McCreadie (2003) identified that 70 per cent were smokers, 86 per cent of women and 70 per cent of men were overweight, and 53 per cent had raised cholesterol, all significantly higher rates than in the general population. These behaviours are often referred in the literature as 'lifestyle choices'. Services users, however, would probably argue that these are not choices at all, but the physical, psychological, social and environmental consequences of having a severe mental illness and the treatments prescribed for them.

Smoking

Smoking is the largest preventable cause of death in the UK and is responsible for an average reduction in life expectancy of 10 years in the general population. The prevalence of daily smoking for people with major depression, bipolar disorder and schizophrenia is estimated to be 57, 66 and 74 per cent respectively, compared to approximately 21 per cent in the general population (Diaz et al. 2009). Adults with mental health problems, including those who misuse alcohol or drugs, smoke 42 per cent of all the tobacco used in England (McManus et al. 2010).

The reasons why people with SMI may have such high rates of smoking are well researched and include neurobiological, psychological, behavioural and social reasons. Qualitative studies have found that people with schizophrenia smoke for relaxation purposes, as a way of making social contact, for pleasure and as a way of gaining control in their lives (Lawn et al. 2002).

The hypothesis that people with SMI smoke to self-medicate mental health symptoms is popular among clinicians and service users, but there is actually little empirical evidence to support it. The nicotine in cigarettes causes an increase in dopamine, noradrenaline, serotonin and cortisol. Therefore as well as having rewarding properties, nicotine is also a stimulant. Service users and mental health clinicians often exaggerate the perceived benefits of smoking. They often attribute improved mood and reduced anxiety to the effects of smoking rather than the reality that smoking simply medicates the effects of nicotine withdrawal that occur several times throughout the day.

Smoke-free legislation has been introduced to ban smoking in enclosed public areas and workplaces in the UK, and in other parts of Europe, the USA and Australia. Implementation has been contentious and surveys since the ban suggest that it is only being partially implemented and mental health staff remain ambivalent about the utility and feasibility of the smoking ban (Mental Health Foundation 2009). The management of smoking behaviour on inpatient units is often a source of conflict for staff and patients and care is increasingly organized around regular smoking breaks.

Diet and physical activity

One needs to consider poor food choices made by the general population when trying to understand the dietary intake of people with SMI. The physical health consequences of a poor diet include coronary heart disease, diabetes, obesity, some cancers, osteoporosis and dental caries. Poor mental health outcomes in schizophrenia are associated with a diet high in saturated fat and unrefined sugar, whereas consumption of fish and seafood, particularly omega 3 fatty acids, is associated with better outcomes.

People with schizophrenia and bipolar disorder are less physically active than the general population and are less likely to be encouraged to exercise by health workers. In a cross-sectional survey of 120 service users with a mental illness, fatigue, mental health symptoms and lack of confidence were reported as the main barriers to regular exercise. Over half the respondents were positive about the benefits of exercise and said they were motivated to be more active (Ussher *et al.* 2007).

Substance use

People who have a dual diagnosis of schizophrenia, bipolar disorder or major depressive disorder and a co-morbid substance use problem face a greater challenge in maintaining their physical health, as the effects of substance use compound the physical health issues associated with SMI. For a full account of these co-morbidities see Chapter 39.

Health service factors

Inequalities in receiving medical care contribute to poor health outcomes in people with SMI. Elderly patients with SMI in particular have been found to be less likely to receive annual CVD screening than the general population. Although the highest number of excess deaths in schizophrenia is associated with CVD, people with psychosis have low rates of surgical interventions such as stenting and bypass grafting and are less likely to receive cerebrovascular arteriography or warfarin following stroke. They are also unlikely to receive routine cancer screening and receive poor levels of diabetes care.

As mentioned earlier, clinical guidelines are helpful for synthesizing the current evidence base and providing direction for delivering high quality services, but alone tend not to improve care. The implementation of evidence-based guidelines requires a capable workforce. Improving mental health nurses' knowledge, skills and attitudes in this aspect of care has been a key area of practice development, though there is a paucity of research in area. The attitudes of nurses are likely to affect their practice, clinical behaviour and their willingness to adopt new ways of working. In a study to develop and validate a measure of the attitudes of mental health nurses in caring for the physical health needs of patients with SMI (the PHASe), Robson and Haddad (2011) surveyed 585 qualified mental health nurses in London. Nurses who had received training in physical health

care, either through an additional Adult Nurse Qualification or post-registration training held more positive attitudes towards the physical health care of people with SMI and were more confident in their physical health care practice.

Illness-related factors

In addition to health behaviours and the limitations of health services, we need to take into account the effect of severe mental illness on help-seeking behaviour. It has been suggested that people with schizophrenia are less likely to report physical symptoms spontaneously and may be unaware of physical problems because of the cognitive deficits associated with the schizophrenia. Non-adherence with prescribed medication is common in patients prescribed for any long-term condition and has a negative effect on physical and mental health outcomes. Iwata *et al.* (2011) have recently advanced this body of literature by examining the predictors of non-adherence with physical examination in hospitalized patients with psychosis, by retrospectively examining 200 inpatient case notes. Almost 40 per cent of patients were non-compliant with physical examinations during the first 24 hours of admission and 28.4 per cent remained non-compliant after two weeks. The researchers found that lack of insight, female gender and previous history of detention were independent predictors of non-adherence with physical examination over the first 24 hours and two weeks of admission.

Treatment-related factors

Effective treatment of mental illness relies upon a clearly thought-out package of multi-disciplinary care involving pharmacological and psychosocial interventions. Psychotropic medication is often necessary for the acute management of psychosis, mania and severe depression and plays an essential role in promoting recovery. However, mental health professionals need to share information with service users and their carers about the benefits and risks of medication, particularly the impact medication may have on physical health. Treatment for mental illness has long been associated with increased morbidity and mortality, such as leucotomy and insulin coma therapy. Since antipsychotics were introduced in the 1950s they have been associated with weight gain, glucose dysregulation, cardiac abnormalities and sexual dysfunction and therefore exacerbate the poor physical health caused by unhealthy behaviours and lack of equitable health care. Chapter 26 has more details about the side-effects of medication.

Case Study

Jane

Following the CPA review, a mental health nurse trained in smoking cessation visited Jane and her mum at home to discuss her health needs further. Jane agreed to accompany the nurse to the GP surgery to review her diabetes and ulcer treatment and also to discuss her weight and smoking. Following the GP visit Jane decided she wanted to prioritize her smoking over her weight and the next couple of home visits were spent understanding the personal relevance of smoking for Jane and what her goals were. She didn't want to stop smoking immediately and preferred to cut down first with the goal of eventually quitting. She did not want to attend the local National Health Service (NHS) Stop Smoking Service, saying she was too embarrassed and afraid to go. A plan was agreed for the nurse to visit Jane and her mum weekly to offer smoking reduction and cessation support. Their next few sessions were spent exploring ambivalence about smoking and stopping smoking. They also looked ahead and discussed the problems Jane thought she may have stopping smoking. Jane's worries included:

'What am I going to do when I am climbing the walls and want a cigarette?'
'I am scared I will eat too much and put on even more weight.'
'I will get bored, what will I do with my hands?'
'How will I cope with my voices?'
'How will my mum cope with me being irritable and snappy?'

Each of these worries was discussed in turn and a personal coping plan was collaboratively developed to address each one. For example, information was exchanged regarding the reasons for nicotine withdrawal symptoms and appetite increase. Practical solutions for dealing with both nicotine and food cravings such as using the correct dose of nicotine replacement therapy (NRT) and preparing sugar-free snacks in advance were discussed.

Thinking Space 30.2

1. What could the nurse have done differently to help Jane attend the local NHS Stop Smoking Service?
2. What are your thoughts about Jane wanting to prioritize her smoking over her weight?

Feedback is provided at the end of the chapter.

30.5 What can nurses do to improve the physical health of people with SMI?

The promotion of physical health in patients with a mental illness is a collaborative endeavour between primary care, secondary care, the service user and their carer. Risk assessment of suicide and violence has, quite rightly, dominated mental health care for

Box 30.1 Examples of physical health checklists

- The Physical Health Check (Phelan *et al.* 2004)
- The Physical Health Check for Mental Health Service Users (Rethink 2007)
- The Physical Health Improvement Profile (White *et al.* 2009)

the past two decades. However, people with SMI are more likely to die at an earlier age than the general population from a physical illness than they are from suicide, therefore we need to give equal priority to the risk assessment of physical health as we do to suicide and violence. Nurses can proactively enquire about the quality and quantity of people's dietary intake, level of physical activity, any substance use including the frequency and severity of smoking behaviour. Frameworks for undertaking physical health checks are available and are helpful for the systematic assessment and profiling of common physical health problems people with SMI may experience (see Box 30.1).

Interventions to improve physical health

Identifying existing or potential health problems is an essential first step. Following this up with interventions can sometimes be more of a challenge for nurses and service users. Service users can adopt healthier lifestyles when interventions are tailored specifically to meet the complex needs associated with having a mental illness. Lifestyle interventions to improve overall health should be integrated into routine mental health care and should begin when the service user first comes into contact with mental health services, rather than waiting for someone to put on weight or develop diabetes. Most mental health services have access to dieticians, exercise instructors and smoking cessation specialists. Mental health practitioners could actively collaborate with these professionals to design specialist

health promotion programmes for people with SMI. There are also many simple interventions that mental health workers can incorporate into routine practice.

Healthy eating

We probably know from our own diets that simply knowing about the type of foods to eat and avoid has little impact on sustained change. Food choices for people with SMI are influenced not only by individual choice but also by the affordability of food, access to kitchen equipment and storage, skills and confidence in budgeting, shopping and cooking, and knowledge of nutrition. It makes sense to start by helping service users sort out practical problems they may have with kitchen equipment, storage and accessibility to nutritious food. Clinical experience suggests it is not uncommon to visit a new service user at home to discover they do not have a fridge or cooker. Acquiring skills and confidence in budgeting, shopping and cooking could be done in partnership with other members of the multi-disciplinary team, such as occupational therapists and support workers. Educational information about nutrition and portion sizes can be shared with people in a way that is understandable and meaningful to them. There are many readable and easy to follow educational leaflets (e.g. those produced by the British Heart Foundation) that are freely available to members of the public. Diets that are low in sugar, simple carbohydrates and saturated fat and high in whole-grain products, complex carbohydrates, fibre, fruit, vegetables and omega 3 fatty acids should be encouraged. Some people may need practical help with how to modify eating habits, for example suggesting recipes and menu plans and how to read food labels.

Regular physical activity

Historically exercise and physical activity were integral to mental health institutional care and given the same priority as the relief of psychiatric symptoms. A number of studies have demonstrated the positive benefits of exercise on mental health. Faulkner and Sparkes' (1999) ethnographic study examined the influence of exercise as a therapy for schizophrenia. They reported that a 10-week exercise programme of twice-weekly sessions appeared to help reduce participants' perceptions of auditory hallucinations, raise self-esteem, and improve sleep patterns and general behaviour. There is consistent evidence that moderate to vigorous physical activity reduces the risk of cardiovascular disease, type 2 diabetes, the metabolic syndrome, and some cancers. The magnitude of the health benefits of physical activity is inversely associated with baseline activity levels, with the greatest benefits occurring for inactive individuals who become moderately active. For general health benefits, at least 150 minutes a week of moderate intensity aerobic physical activity spread across the week, (e.g. at least 30 minutes on five or more days each week) is recommended. Seventy-five minutes of vigorous-intensity activity (also spread across the week) provides comparable health benefits to 150 minutes of moderate-intensity activity. Overweight and obese adults achieving the recommended weekly volume of activity will gain multiple health benefits even in the absence of reductions in body weight.

Service users may need an explanation of what is meant by 'moderate intensity' (i.e. working hard enough to be breathing more heavily than normal, becoming slightly warmer but still able to talk). People may also need explanations of the different types of exercise available to improve and maintain overall health. For example, endurance or aerobic activities that improve cardiovascular health could include brisk walking, cycling, jogging, swimming and dancing. Activities for improving flexibility and mobility could include gardening, housework and walking. Strengthening exercises can improve balance, muscle tone, bone health and increase the rate at which the body burns calories, and can be achieved by climbing stairs, carrying shopping or walking uphill.

Most inpatient mental health services have access to gyms and physical training instructors, and mental health workers can act as a link between such services. Building confidence in a hospital gym may help people feel more at ease with accessing public gyms once discharged, while acquiring tailored information about the best way to exercise. For those people who lack the confidence, motivation and finances to attend public gyms there are still many ways of increasing one's activity that can be incorporated into people's lives without any disruption or much more organization or effort. For example, breaking up the period of exercise into three 10-minute bouts of brisk walking throughout the day is initially more appealing than 30 minutes all at once and more manageable for inpatient staff trying to promote healthy behaviours on busy acute wards. Mental health workers can help people with SMI explore their beliefs about exercise and help people problem-solve barriers to increasing activity.

Smoking cessation

Primary care trusts (PCTs) in the UK have been responsible for providing Stop Smoking Services for people who want to quit. Standard NHS care includes approximately six to eight sessions of behavioural support and pharmacotherapy. Services are traditionally based on a withdrawal-orientated model, emphasizing the importance of complete abstinence, motivational support and supervision of medication use, and are clinically and cost effective (West et al. 2000).

NRT is the most widely used aid to smoking cessation. There are many products to choose from including skin patches, chewing gum, lozenges, nasal spray and inhalators. As all NRT products have similar success rates, the choice between them is a practical and personal one. Two drugs that do not replace nicotine but help the smoker by other mechanisms are buproprion and varenicline. Buproprion is an antidepressant and a nicotine antagonist. It is thought to act via doperminergic and noradrenergic pathways. Buproprion is known to lower the seizure threshold and induce mania so needs to be used with caution in service users with a history of seizures or mood disorder and also with medication that lowers the seizure threshold. Varenicline reduces the strength of the urge to smoke and the satisfaction from smoking, as well as minimizing withdrawal symptoms, though needs to be used cautiously with smokers with a history of mood disorders. Combining any of these medications with behavioural support at least doubles the chance of quitting.

Approximately half of smokers who use NHS Stop Smoking Services successfully quit within four weeks of starting treatment. However, relapse rates are very high, with approximately 75 per cent of quitters resuming smoking within 12 months (Ferguson *et al.* 2005). Despite these relapse rates, smoking cessation treatment is one of the most cost effective interventions in health care. Evidence of successfully adapting standard smoking cessation interventions to mental health services users is beginning to emerge and guidelines as well as practical advice for successfully integrating smoking cessation support in mental health settings are now available (e.g. Lawn and Campion 2010).

Case Study

Jane

Following a preparation period, Jane spent a further four weeks cutting down her cigarette intake. This was done in a planned way, with Jane deciding how many cigarettes she would cut out in the week ahead and the nurse suggesting how much NRT she should use each week. She also practised her personal coping plan. She followed the cutting down plan until she had reduced her daily intake from 50 to 25. Reducing her cigarette intake gave Jane an opportunity to increase her self-efficacy and mastery of using NRT while experimenting with her personal coping plan.

Eight weeks after the start of the home visits Jane stopped smoking. She was also given a daily nicotine transdermal patch to wear at this time but had an allergic skin reaction and stopped wearing the patches after three days. She did however continue to use the nicotine inhalator. For the next three months Jane adhered to her nicotine replacement therapy and used her personal coping plan. Her confidence and self-efficacy grew and she started going out of the house more often. There was no deterioration in her mental health symptoms, in fact there was an improvement in mood. Her attendance for CBT improved and she enrolled in a healthy living group at the local mental health centre. She also saved £2,500 in six months.

At a six-month follow-up visit, Jane reflected on her process of stopping smoking. 'All the things I worried about – not sleeping, getting ill – none of it happened ... I still don't know what to do with my hands though ... I am a lot more relaxed, calmer, I don't need it to relax, I used to rely on it to relax, any situation felt out of control ... I'm not coming down with a cold every few weeks ... everyone is proud of me, it has inspired my brother to lose weight, he's lost two stone already. I also thought if I can stop smoking, I can do anything and it gave me the confidence to focus on my weight.'

30.6 Conclusion

It is well established that people with SMI have higher rates of death and physical illness compared to the general population and die at a younger age. The causes of poor physical health in people with SMI are complex and interactive. Not only has the physical health care of people with SMI been neglected in the past, the training health professionals receive to assess, monitor and manage physical health care in people with SMI has also been lacking. Mental health nurses have an opportunity to improve the physical and mental health of people with SMI through risk assessment and collaborative health promotion interventions initiated at the onset of people's illness. Poor physical health in people with SMI does not have to be inevitable.

In summary, the main learning points from this chapter are:

- Improving the physical health of people with SMI is the focus of a range clinical guidelines and consensus statements.

- The risk of developing a long-term condition is raised two to three fold among people with SMI compared to those without these disorders, and their life expectancy is reduced by up to 17 years.

- Associations between SMI and poor physical health include personal health behaviours, health service related factors and the iatrogenic effects of psychotropic medication.

- Mental disorders may also influence physical health via direct physiological processes such as inflammation, immune dysfunction and decreased heart rate variability.

- The promotion of physical health in patients with a mental illness is a collaborative endeavour between primary care, secondary care, the service user and their carer.

- Nurses can proactively enquire about the quality and quantity of people's dietary intake, level of physical activity, and any substance use including the frequency and severity of smoking behaviour.

- Frameworks for undertaking physical health checks are available and are helpful for the systematic assessment and profiling of common physical health problems people with SMI may experience.

Feedback to Thinking Space 30.1

In your answer you might have considered how to engage Jane and enhance her motivation to change her health behaviours – for example, by asking her (and her mum) what *they* would like to do next; finding out if she would like to address her concerns about her weight and smoking at the same time or prioritize one over the other, and elicit her concerns in detail. It is often easier to deal with one problem at a time and preferably the one that Jane believes she has the most chance of success with. It's also helpful to know how ready or prepared someone is to make changes in their lifestyle. A detailed assessment of smoking behaviour/eating and activity levels should be carried out. It may also be helpful to explore the advantages and disadvantages of continuing to smoke and the same for stopping smoking; it may be helpful to ask how important is it to Jane that she stops smoking, and how confident she is about doing so. Similar questions can be asked about her weight. Once Jane has decided how she wants to move forward, it may be useful to involve her GP and encourage her to get her overall physical health checked. You, Jane, her mum and the GP can then decide on a plan of action.

Feedback to Thinking Space 30.2

1. It would be helpful to explore Jane's thoughts and feelings about going to her local NHS Stop Smoking Service and then exchange information – for example, what does she already know about the service (i.e. what is expected from her, what the success rate is) and what she would like to know? With her permission, arrange a joint appointment with local services and if possible request a home visit. If she is prepared to engage with the NHS Stop Smoking Service, close liaison

between the community team and the Stop Smoking Service is needed provide mutual support to Jane and her mum, but also for each service support to each other.

2. Addressing either smoking or weight gain will have a positive impact on Jane's health and well-being. Reflect on what thoughts immediately came to your mind when you were asked about Jane's priorities; these could have been influenced by your *own* health behaviours and beliefs and your current knowledge and clinical skills to help service users stop smoking or lose weight. Mental health workers have traditionally not encouraged service users to stop smoking – this is related to our lack of training in smoking cessation and the mistaken belief that service users' mental health will deteriorate if they stop. Jointly deciding on care and enabling Jane to feel at the centre of the choice she makes about her health is likely to lead to higher levels of satisfaction, improved health outcomes and, in turn, to more efficient use of resources. It is possible for mental health nurses to develop skills to deliver smoking cessation support and integrate this into their practice, something which is very much valued by service users.

Annotated bibliography

Meyer, J.M. and Nasrallah, H.A. (eds) *Medical Illness and Schizophrenia,* **2nd edn. Arlington, VA: American Psychiatric Publishing.**

Nash, M. (2010) *Physical Health and Well-Being in Mental Health Nursing: Clinical skills for practice.* **Maidenhead: Open University Press.**

Robson, D. and Gray, R. (2007) Serious mental illness and physical health problems: a discussion paper, *International Journal of Nursing Studies,* **44: 457–66.**

Higgins, A. (2010) *Stop Smoking Interventions in Mental Health Settings: A systems approach.* **London: DH.**
Department of Health (DH) guidance and a toolkit for integrating smoking cession support in mental health settings.

References

British Thoracic Society (2006) *The Burden of Lung Disease,* 2nd edn. ????: British Thoracic Society.

Cancer Research UK (2011) Available at: http://info.cancerresearchuk.org/cancerstats/index.htm, accessed 1 June 2012.

Chang, C-K., Hayes, RD., Perera, G., Broadbent, MTM., Fernandes, AC. et al. (2011) Life Expectancy at Birth for People with Serious Mental Illness and Other Major Disorders from a Secondary Mental Health Care Case Register in London. PLoS ONE 6(5): e19590. doi:10.1371/journal.pone.0019590

Cohen, A. and Hove, M. (2001) *Physical Health of the Severe and Enduring Mentally Ill.* London: Sainsbury Centre.

De Hert, M., Decker, J.M., Wood, D., Kahl, K.G., Holt, R.I.G. and Moller, H.J. (2009) Cardiovascular disease and diabetes in people with severe mental illness: position statement from the European Psychiatric Association (EPA), supported by the European Association for the Study of Diabetes (EASD) and the European Society of Cardiology (ESC), *European Psychiatry,* 24(6): 412–24.

Diaz, F.J. *et al.* (2009) Tobacco smoking behaviours in bipolar disorder: a comparison of the general population, schizophrenia, and major depression, *Bipolar Disorders,* 11: 154–65.

Faulkner, G. and Sparkes, A. (1999) Exercise therapy for schizophrenia: an ethnographic study, *Journal of Sport and Exercise,* 21: 39–51.

Ferguson, J., Bauld, L., Chersterman, J. and Judge, K. (2005) The English smoking treatment services: one-year outcomes, *Addiction,* 100(Suppl. 2): 59–69.

Hippisley-Cox, J., Vinogradova, Y., Coupland, C. and Parker, C. (2006) *Risk of Malignancy in Patients with Mental Health Problems.* London: Disability Rights Commission.

Hoang, U., Stewart. R. and Goldacre, M.J. (2011) Mortality after hospital discharge for people with schizophrenia or bipolar disorder: retrospective study of linked English hospital episode statistics, 1999–2006, *British Medical Journal,* 343: d5422.

Holt, R.I.G. and Peveler, R.C. (2006) Association between antipsychotic drugs and diabetes, *Diabetes, Obesity and Metabolism,* 8: 125–35.

Iwata, K., Strydom, A. and Osborn, D. (2011) Insight and other predictors of physical examination refusal in psychotic illness, *Journal of Mental Health*, 20(4): 319–27.

Lawn S. and Campion J. (2010) Factors associated with success of smoke-free initiatives in australian psychiatric inpatient units, *Psychiatric Services*, 61: 300–5.

Lawn, S.J., Pols, R.G. and Barber, J.G. (2002) Smoking and quitting: a qualitative study with community-living psychiatric clients, *Social Science and Medicine*, 54: 93–104.

McCreadie, R. (2003) Diet, smoking and cardiovascular risk in people with schizophrenia, *British Journal of Psychiatry*, 183: 534–9.

McManus, S., Howard Meltzer, H. and Campion, J. (2010) *Cigarette Smoking and Mental Health in England: Data from the Adult Psychiatric Morbidity Survey 2007*. ????: National Centre for Social Research.

Mental Health Foundation (2009) *Death of the Smoking Den*. London: MHF.

NICE (National Institute for Health and Clinical Excellence (2009) *Schizophrenia: Core interventions in the treatment and management of schizophrenia in primary and secondary care*. London: NICE.

Phelan, M., Stradins, L., Amin, D., Isadore, R., Hitrov, C., Doyle, A. and Inglis, R. (2004) The physical health check: a tool for mental health workers, *Journal of Mental Health*, 13(3): 277–85.

Rethink (2007) *The PHC: A Physical health check for mental health service users*. www.rethink.org: Rethink.

Robson, D. and Haddad, M. (2011) Mental health nurses' attitudes towards the physical health care of people with severe and enduring mental illness: the development of a measurement tool, *International Journal of Nursing Studies*, ????

Samele, C., Patel, M., Boydell, J., Leese, M., Wessely, S. and Murray, R. (2007) Physical illness and lifestyle risk factors in people with their first presentation of psychosis, *Social Psychiatry Psychiatric Epidemiology*, 42(2): 117–24.

Ussher, M., Stanbury, L., Cheeseman, V. and Faulkner, G. (2007) Physical activity preferences and perceived barriers to activity among persons with severe mental illness in the United Kingdom, *Psychiatric Services*, 58: 405–8.

West, R., McNeill, A. and Raw, M. (2000) Smoking cessation guidelines for health professionals, *Thorax*, 55: 987–99.

White J., Gray, R. and Jones, M. (2009) The development of the Serious Mental Illness Physical Health Improvement Profile, *Journal of Psychiatric and Mental Health Nursing*, 16(5): 493–8.

WHO (World Health Organization) (2008) *2008–2013 Action Plan for the Global Strategy for the Prevention and Control of Noncommunicable Diseases*. Geneva: WHO.

Yusuf, S., Hawken, S., Ounpuu, S., Dans, T., Avezum, A., Lanas, F., McQueen, M., Budai, A., Pais, P., Varigos, J., Lisheng, L. INTERHEART Study Investigators (2004) Effect of potentially modifiable risk factors associated with myocardial infarction in 52 countries (the INTERHEART study): case-control study. Lancet. 2004 Sep 11–17;364(9438):937–52.

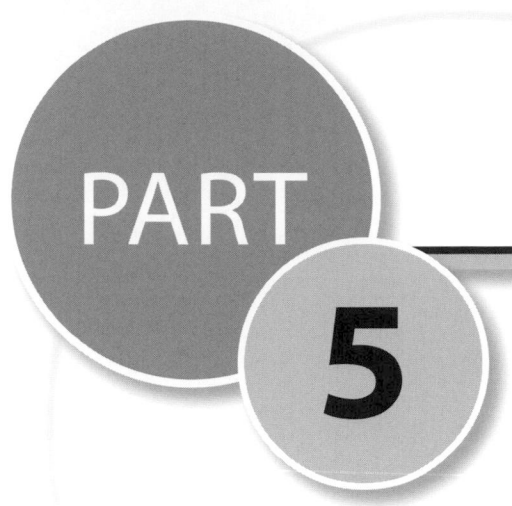

PART 5

Client Groups

Chapter 31

Children and Adolescents

Jane Padmore

I had been excluded from school and had not been back for six months. Everyone thought I was being bad and keep talking about the consequences of my behaviour. My nurse was the first person to ask me about how I felt and why I reacted as I did.

(A 12-year-old service user in the community at a care plan review meeting)

 ## 31.1 Introduction

Child and adolescent mental health services (CAMHS) are concerned with the assessment and treatment of behavioural and emotional problems in people under 18 years. Prevalence studies differ in their estimates of mental health problems in young people. Costello *et al.* (2004) found that although during a three-month period any disorder averaged 13.3 per cent; during the whole study period 36.7 per cent of participants had at least one psychiatric disorder.

People who have had mental health problems in adolescence are known to have an increase in mental health problems as adults. Long-term follow-up studies of depression in adolescents have emphasized the increased risk of adult depression. These studies have also shown that young people who have had an early onset psychosis are more likely to go on to have mental health problems as adults.

This chapter is primarily devoted to describing the manifestations of mental distress and disorder in young people that nurses may encounter in various practice settings. The chapter begins, however, with a discussion of those aspects of assessment that are particularly relevant when working with young people, since a comprehensive assessment is a prerequisite to successful treatment. In summary this chapter covers:

- assessment;
- mental health problems in young people;
- disorders;
- principles of treatment;
- the nurse's role.

31.2 Assessment and classification

Classification of disorders is increasingly important within CAMHS to ensure a young person is receiving the appropriate treatment and to inform the commissioning of services. Diagnosis should be clinically relevant and aid communication. Diagnostic labels can be seen as stigmatizing and parents often withdraw from treatment for fear of being 'labelled'. However, diagnostic labels are helpful if parents and young people have an understanding of the criteria used and the potential of a diagnosis for treatment. Moreover, diagnosis has potential benefits as it allows for special provisions to be made, such as special schooling and a statement of special education needs, which assists the school to obtain additional resources for the child.

To classify accurately a comprehensive assessment needs to take place. The essential elements of this are listed in Figure 31.1.

The two main classification systems in use are the International Classification of Diseases (ICD) (WHO 1996) and the Diagnostic and Statistical Manual (DSM) (APA 1994). These provide clear descriptive criteria that must be met before a diagnosis can be made. Multi-axial classification is an important feature of diagnosing young people. This takes into account different aspects of a person's presentation and classifies the disorder along different axes, giving a composite picture of the condition. The commonly used axes from the ICD are:

- Axis 1: psychiatric disorders;
- Axis 2: specific disorders of psychological development;
- Axis 3: intellectual level;
- Axis 4: medical conditions;
- Axis 5: associated abnormal psychosocial situations;
- Axis 6 global assessment of psychosocial disability.

The ICD-10 codes separately behavioural and emotional disorders (see Table 31.1).

31.3 Mental health problems in young people

Mental health problems can occur at any time during a person's life and the literature is increasingly taking a life course perspective with many 'adult' disorders appearing to have their origins in childhood. When considered within a developmental context, different patterns of mental health problems can be observed in young people. Typical age and gender patterns for some disorders have emerged and are detailed in Table 31.2.

There is much debate about whether it is possible or appropriate to give preschool children a mental health diagnosis. Lack of appropriate stimulation in the early years may result in language delay, which when combined with other factors such as inadequate parenting, can present as emotional or behavioural disorders (DH/DfES 2004). Adolescence is a period of transition between childhood and adulthood and, in most cultures, is heralded by the onset of puberty while termination is socially and culturally determined. The interplay of social and biological influences is important. Although often associated with a period of stress and turmoil, most adolescents manage the transition between childhood and adulthood without major problems.

> **Thinking Space 31.1**
>
> Read Daisy's case study and pay particular attention to any strategies or actions the nurse uses to engage Daisy in her care and treatment. Jot down a few notes and you can compare them with the case study commentary that follows.

Figure 31.1 CAMHS assessment framework

Presenting circumstances ■ Young person's view ■ Parent/carer's view ■ Teacher's view	Nature of the problem Onset Frequency Duration Precipitating circumstances Who is affected Sleep Appetite
Family history	Parent's personal history Relationships within the family Patterns of communication Approach to parenting Extended family Physical or mental health history Forensic history Cultural background
Personal history	Pregnancy, labour and delivery Developmental milestones (physical, social, emotional) Disruptions to and reaction to attachments/separation Preschool and education including social and academic performance and ability History of mental or physical health problems Forensic history Substance misuse Sexual history Personality prior to current difficulties including interests and hobbies

(Continued)

Figure 31.1 CAMHS assessment framework *(Continued)*

Physical health	Height
	Weight
	Immunizations
	History of physical health problems
	Dental care
Social circumstances	Diversity
	Family finances
	Accommodation
	Activities of daily living
	Relationships in and out of school
Mental state	Young person's presentation during the interview
	Appearance and behaviour
	Facial appearance
	Dress and self-care
	Manner
	Posture and movement
	Appropriateness
	Speech
	Mood and affect
	Thoughts – form and content
	Orientation
	Attention and concentration
	Memory
	Insight
Risk assessment	Self-intentional self-injury, suicide, risk taking behaviour, self-neglect
	Others – physical, sexual and emotional abuse and neglect, peer group
	Environmental
	Physical health

Case Study

Daisy

Fifteen-year-old Daisy was referred to community CAMHS following a serious overdose. The referral letter, from the Emergency Department, stated she left before a full assessment could be completed. Daisy had not had any previous contact with CAMHS and very little else was known.

The CAMHS nurse spent a significant period attempting to engage with Daisy and her family and discussing with her family how to manage the risks she posed. This resulted in an initial appointment at her home. Daisy was reluctant to speak to the nurse but agreed to stay in the room and listen while her mother and the nurse spoke. She remained silent but indicated she would read the report once completed. It was discovered that Daisy had not been in school for six months after being excluded for bullying. Since then Daisy had withdrawn from her friends and become increasingly irritable with her parents. This was having a significant impact on her younger sibling and the home atmosphere.

The nurse shared her report, written in age-appropriate language, which contained the history detailed by the mother, her current mental state and the provisional diagnosis of a moderate depressive episode. Daisy agreed to meet with the nurse after reading the report. At the meeting she decided her main goal was to return to school. The nurse then worked with partner agencies to find her a place at the local Pupil Referral Unit (PRU) (a school for excluded children).

The school agreed Daisy could be seen there, in a room that ensured her privacy was respected, by the nurse. Over the 12 weeks the nurse worked with Daisy it became clear that she had been experiencing a period of depression that was manifesting itself in conduct problems. Her father had become unwell physically and mother, as a way of coping, had spent more time at work. Simultaneously Daisy had been bullied at school and had then started to bully others, truant from school, shoplift and not return home when expected. Her appetite had declined resulting in her losing 10kg and her sleep had become disturbed. She no longer wrote songs.

The nurse worked with Daisy on the following:

1. Watchful waiting (NICE 2005a)
2. Behaviour reactivation
3. Relapse prevention
4. Developing a narrative to explain her absence from school
5. Liaising with the school nurse to monitor her weight

Daisy returned to her mainstream school after eight weeks at the PRU and, as her depression lifted, her social and home life improved. She was discharged back to the care of her general practitioner (GP) and the school.

Commentary

This case highlights some of the challenges faced by CAMHS nurses but also the rewards. An adolescent can find 'mental health' services both frightening and insulting. The nurse needed to give time and attention to engaging with Daisy and her parents. A flexible approach was needed with the nurse negotiating where to meet the family. Although Daisy initially indicated she did not want to participate it was important for the nurse to include her in an unobtrusive way while talking to her mother and giving her the first draft of the assessment for comments. Including her and respecting her views built the foundation for future work.

Prior to the referral Daisy's only contact with professionals was to discuss her unacceptable behaviour and exclusion from school. Challenging behaviours can mask underlying emotional difficulties and attending to emotional needs, not condoning behavioural difficulties and being an advocate for Daisy at school required the nurse to see the situation from a number of perspectives.

Daisy's diagnosis of a moderate depressive episode indicated a clear treatment pathway. This would have been meaningless if the nurse had only concentrated on watchful waiting and not worked in partnership with Daisy and identified her goal – to return to school. Supporting the family to approach education services became a priority. A CAMHS nurse's familiarity and relationship with the local education services are useful and can make school-based appointments achievable.

Daisy's peers were curious about her long absence from school and she was concerned about what she would say. The nurse was able to role-play with Daisy how to respond to her peers, developing her own words to explain her absence. Daisy had also withdrawn from her friends and stopped attending her street dance classes. She was fearful of returning, but the nurse worked with Daisy to implement strategies to assist her return and increase her social activity. Simultaneously the nurse worked with Daisy to understand her signs and symptoms and put in place a relapse prevention plan, with her family. Liaison between the school nurse and the CAMHS nurse provided weight monitoring and nutritional advice.

Finally the nurse supported Daisy's transition back to mainstream school. Having seen Daisy and her family through a very difficult period the nurse took time to review treatment, plan contingencies and say goodbye.

Table 31.1 Behavioural and emotional disorders with onset usually occurring in childhood and adolescence (WHO 1996)

F90	Hyperkinetic disorders
F91	Conduct disorders
F92	Mixed disorders of conduct and emotions
F93	Emotional disorders with onset specific to childhood
F94	Disorders of social functioning with onset specific to childhood and adolescence
F95	Tic disorders
F98	Other behavioural and emotional disorders with onset usually occurring in childhood and adolescence

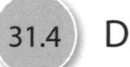

31.4 Disorders

Disorders of attention

Attention deficit hyperactivity disorder (ADHD) is a complex, multi-faceted condition with many associated risk factors. Causes remain unclear but include genetics, pre-, peri- and post-natal influences, negative parent–child relationships, poor social support, and speech and language difficulties. Food additives and watching television are not associated with ADHD. The essential features are developmentally inappropriate degrees of inattention, impulsiveness and hyperactivity which have a significant impact on functioning across different settings.

Hyperkinesis, with the more stringent criteria (ICD 10), is used by the British whereas North Americans use the wider criteria for ADHD (DSM-IV).

Table 31.2 Development of mental health problems in children by age and gender

	Males	Female	Male and female
Preschool (0–4)	Attention deficit hyperactivity disorder (ADHD) Dyslexia Specific language impairment Autistic spectrum disorders		Eating difficulties, such as fads and pica Sleeping difficulties Separation anxiety
Children (5–11)	Tourette's syndrome Nocturnal enuresis	Diurnal enuresis	Separation disorders Specific phobias Oppositional disorders Conduct disorders
Adolescents (12+)	Conduct disorders Completed suicide Schizophrenia	Depression Eating disorders Social phobia Panic Intentional self-injury Somatic disorders	Substance misuse Mania Bipolar disorder

UK studies have suggested prevalence rates are 3.62 per cent for boys and 0.85 per cent for girls for ADHD, and 1 per cent for hyperkinetic disorder (National Statistical Office 2005). Although generally thought of as a childhood disorder it is now viewed as a lifespan condition.

Diagnosis requires a minimum of six months chronicity and onset prior to 7 years. School reports and a school observation, by a CAMHS professional, are valuable. The assessment is usually supported using screening tools such as the Conners' Teacher's and Parent's Questionnaires (Conners 1973) and the Strength and Difficulties Questionnaire (Goodman 1997).

Guidelines support multi-modal treatment packages including medication, behaviour management, parent training programmes, psycho-education, classroom interventions and support (NICE 2008a). Parent training programmes, structured and informed by social learning theory, are the first line of treatment where there is a moderate impairment. Family support is crucial and parents need to adopt a consistent attitude with clear guidelines for acceptable behaviour.

Medication is not recommended as the first-line treatment, but reserved for severe symptoms and for those where parent training has either been refused or is not effective. Improvement in concentration and attention can increase academic performance leading to improved self-esteem and confidence. Modified release forms have provided some benefits. Common side-effects include reduced appetite, weight loss and difficulty in falling asleep. Normal growth can be affected and needs regular monitoring along with blood pressure.

Pervasive developmental disorders

Pervasive developmental disorders (PDD) are characterized by difficulties with social interaction, communication and behaviour that manifest before 3 years of age. PDDs include autism, Rett's disorder, childhood disintegrative disorder and Asperger's disorder. Prevalence rates vary but are generally estimated at 1 in 500.

Asperger's syndrome is a milder version of autism. These children are often aloof, distant and lack empathy. There is usually no delay in the development of vocabulary and grammar, though other aspects of language are abnormal.

Autism has a high genetic loading and an extended phenotype in families with subtle social and language defects, and circumscribed interests. It is associated with a number of medical conditions and there is strong evidence of pre-natal abnormality. The MMR vaccination as a causative agent has been ruled out by extensive research.

There are normally locally agreed, multi-agency pathways for recognition, referral and diagnosis. A comprehensive assessment is needed by a multi-disciplinary team involving a thorough neurological assessment and in-depth cognitive and language testing as well as observation of the child's behaviour and social communication skills.

Common abnormalities include resistance to change and stereotyped, narrow and repetitive patterns of play. Some children show intensive attachment to unusual objects or preoccupations and interests. Early signs of a lack of social interest may be missed but, by the second or third year of life, their social deficits become more noticeable. Some lose previously acquired skills.

Treatment aims to facilitate the normal development of cognition, language and socialization, decrease maladaptive behaviours and decrease the family's stress. Complete resolution of symptoms is generally not achieved. Benefit can come from a structured educational setting with behavioural programmes to reduce ritualistic behaviour, tantrums and aggressive behaviour while encouraging task-orientated work. Medication is sometimes used, particularly to manage anxiety, depression, hyperactivity and obsessive compulsive disorder (OCD). The prognosis is better in children with higher intelligence and those who acquire useful speech by the age of 5.

Tourette's syndrome

Tourette's syndrome affects 3–5 per 10,000 children. Prevalence is 10 times greater in children than in adults and the outcome for at least 50 per cent of children is favourable. The mean age of onset is 7 years and the essential features are the existence of multiple motor tics and at least one vocal tic. The most common symptoms involve eye-blinking and tics affecting the face, neck or head. Vocal tics usually occur later than motor tics. Coprolalia, the inappropriate and involuntary uttering of obscenities, is seen in about a third of patients. Anxiety, stress and fatigue can aggravate tics. Children with Tourette's syndrome are disproportionately likely to be obsessional. ADHD occurs in 25–50 per cent.

For the milder versions, explanation and reassurance to teacher, parents and the child has been shown to be helpful as well as self-help groups. Treatment is either medication or habit reversal (HR) based on social learning theory. Progressive Tourette's syndrome runs a lifelong course with symptoms waxing and waning over time.

Conduct disorders

Conduct disorders consist of repetitive and persistent patterns of behaviour which are age-inappropriate and violate social norms. These children often bully, intimidate or threaten others. Physical fights, cruelty to animals and people, serious violation of rules, such as damage to property, and involvement in the Youth Justice System are not uncommon. Disruptive behaviour in the classroom is common leading to repeated exclusion from school, poor interpersonal relationships and poor academic achievement. Oppositional defiant disorder is a sub-type of conduct disorder in younger children.

When assessing for conduct disorder alternatives need to be considered such as hearing problems, hyperkinetic disorder, chronic dental pain and specific learning difficulties. Co-morbid mental health problems are often present and it is important to be mindful of focusing solely on 'bad' behaviour.

The National Institute for Health and Clinical Excellence (NICE) is due to publish guidelines for conduct disorder in April 2013. Currently a technology appraisal for children aged 12 or under is available (NICE 2006a). This recommends parent training and group sessions based on social learning theory.

Treatment of children with conduct disorder can be complex and challenging, particularly as the young person can be uncooperative with a fear and distrust of adults.

Substance misuse in adolescence

A survey of British 15- to 16-year-olds found that almost half had tried illicit drugs at some time (Fergusson and Horwood 2000). While most children who experiment with illicit drugs do not go on to habitual abuse of drugs, the earlier the onset, the more persistent the habit becomes and some will become substance dependent as adults. When compared to adults, young people experience more rapid progression from first use to abuse and dependence, shorter time from first to second dependence diagnosis, and an increase in other mental health problems. Drug use is also a major risk in completed suicide.

NICE (2007) has issued guidance on community-based interventions to reduce misuse among vulnerable and disadvantaged children. While substance misuse is more likely to respond to early treatment in adolescence, motivation to accept treatment is generally poor. It is often the concern of others which leads to referral. Only 10 per cent of young people who would meet the criteria for treatment are actually referred to services (SAMHSA 2007). An assertive approach therefore needs to be adopted, usually involving other agencies. Drug and alcohol use is discussed in detail in Chapter 39.

Anxiety disorders

Anxiety disorders are associated with poor outcomes for children. Anxiety and depression are associated with immaturity, inattention and concentration problems, academic difficulties, poor peer relations, low self-esteem and low social competence as well as mental health problems in later life.

Separation anxiety arises in response to separation from parents and other attachment figures. When the intensity of anxiety is developmentally inappropriate and impacting significantly on the

child's life, separation anxiety disorder is diagnosed. Children with this condition are reluctant to let their parents out of their sight and complain of physical symptoms – for example, headaches and stomach ache – when separation is enforced (in the mornings before setting out for school).

Generalized anxiety disorders are present in roughly 3 per cent of children. They experience persistent anxieties and worries which are not related to a particular event or situation. Somatic complaints are common.

Specific phobias are common in early childhood. Anxiety leads to avoidance and distress. It is more common in girls. Cognitive behavioural therapy (CBT) has been shown to be helpful in the treatment of anxiety disorders, and is the first line of treatment, but there remain 20–60 per cent of children in research trials who do not show an improvement (Liber *et al.* 2008). In addition, family-based treatments, such as parent training programmes, group programmes and antidepressants are effective.

Obsessive compulsive disorder

While there are striking similarities between the phenomenology of OCD in children and adults, significant differences exist in terms of gender distribution, co-morbidity, familial contribution and developmental issues. Roughly a third of adults have their first symptoms before the age of 15. Although rare in young children, the rate increases towards adult rates at puberty.

Obsessions are recurrent, intrusive thoughts, ideas or images, or impulses that the person experiences as ego-dystonic and intensely distressing. A core characteristic of an obsession in adults is that they are resisted. Resistance to obsessions and compulsions in children is, however, not always present. Common obsessions in childhood focus on contamination, harm or death and symmetry. Compulsions are repetitive physical or mental acts that the person feels driven to perform in response to that obsession. The purpose of the compulsion is usually to reduce anxiety or magically prevent a dreaded event. Common examples are checking, touching, washing and repeating acts.

OCD is a chronic condition and needs long-term commitment to its management. CBT, including exposure and response prevention and involving the family is the first line of treatment (NICE 2005b). Medication, such as selective serotonin reuptake inhibitors (SSRIs), has been shown to be effective and is used when CBT has not had the desired effect. Good insight is related to better outcomes from treatment.

Disorders of social functioning
Selective mutism

This condition is characterized by a child's refusal to talk in certain situations while conversing normally in others. Generally, normal speech is present while in a minority there are problems of articulation and speech production. Milder forms present themselves at the start of school life and are usually transitory. High levels of social phobia have been found in children who are selectively mute. A speech and language assessment forms an important part of treatment. Treatment similar to that for anxiety has provided some success. There is also some evidence for psychopharmacology use.

Attachment disorders

The notion of attachment in infants was strongly influenced by the writings of John Bowlby (1980). According to these theories, a child needs to be attached to a protective figure. Children develop attachments to a relatively small number of figures. This relationship offers a secure base from which the child explores the world. Although all children develop attachments, their quality varies greatly. Children with attachment disorders have significantly more behavioural and psychosocial problems. Treatment requires establishing an attachment relationship when none exists and ameliorating disturbed attachments when they are evident. Coercive treatments are potentially dangerous and not recommended.

School refusal

Children with school attendance problems are sometimes referred to CAMHS. The school refusal may be linked to a conduct disorder, a school phobia or separation anxiety. With the latter the problem can present in a variety of ways including abdominal pain and headaches in the mornings before school. Onset may be abrupt, in which case a precipitating factor is likely to be found, or gradual, with the child increasingly reluctant to attend school. The child is often fearful of separating from the parent and leaving home. A lack of authority, on the part of the parents, to enforce attendance and parental illness can also play a part. Treatment involves dealing with the underlying condition and working with the parents to enable them to enforce school. Effective liaison with the school is essential to deal with issues such as bullying and to harness teachers' support. Change of schools rarely helps unless there are particular problems, for example, distance from school, or academic ability.

Elimination disorders
Enuresis

Primary enuresis is when bladder control has never been achieved and secondary enuresis is when bladder control is lost after a child has acquired it for at least six months. Once continence is achieved relapse occurs most commonly around the age of 5 or 6. Girls with enuresis are more likely to suffer from urinary tract infections. It is arguable whether enuresis is a mental health problem but it can be associated with stressful life events and separation. It is also thought culture has a role in prevalence, but in Europe the reported rate of nocturnal enuresis is 9–19 per cent at 5 years, 7–22 per cent at 7 years, 5–13 per cent at 9 years and 1–2 per cent at 16 years (Butler 1998). NICE (2011) details a comprehensive review of treatment options which include good bladder health, star charts, enuresis alarms, medication, training, education and support.

Encopresis

Encopresis or faecal soiling is the voiding of faeces in inappropriate places. At the age of 7, the prevalence in boys is 2.3 per cent and 0.7 per cent in girls. By the age of 11, less than 1 per cent of children soil once a month (Hersov 1994). Faecal soiling can occur for various reasons. Some children fail to achieve continence as they have never learned bowel control and this is usually found in the context of inconsistent or coercive toilet training practice. Treatment involves educating parents in proper toilet training methods. Fear of using the toilet can lead to some children soiling, for which cognitive behavioural techniques can help.

In some children encopresis occurs as a result of long-standing faecal retention. The original cause may be emotional or physical but it leads to constipation. Chronic constipation can lead to hard faeces acting as a plug. Liquid and semi-solid stools eventually leak past the plug causing soiling. A combination of family education, disimpaction and maintenance medications, a well-balanced diet and behaviour management is essential.

The provocative or aggressive soiler deliberately defecates onto furniture or smears faeces. There is an association with dysfunctional family systems based on social disorganization and coercive and abusive child-rearing practices. Management and treatment usually needs the coordinated input of several agencies including social services and education.

Depression

Young people can suffer from depression and depressive symptomology, starting before puberty and continuing into adolescence and adulthood. There are, however, some important developmental differences with children being relatively more reactive to their environment than adults. Depressed children are more likely to have parents with depression. Studies suggest a strong genetic loading while environmental factors play an important role. About 1–2 per cent of prepubertal children and about 3–8 per cent of adolescents have experienced a depressive episode before adulthood.

Young people will present with changes in mood, thinking and activity but may not have the emotional literacy to portray what they are experiencing. Instead they may describe somatic symptoms such as musculoskeletal pains and headaches. Poor concentration, low self-esteem and guilt are also common features. Depressed mood, hopelessness, misery and tearfulness are common and changes in the young person's experience of school and social life may often herald the onset of depression. The presence of behavioural problems is common in depressed children and may mask an underlying depression. Changes in appetite and weight loss are less common than in adults. Suicidal thoughts and behaviour may lead to referral by worried parents or teachers.

The onset of depression in adolescence may be acute or insidious. While brief periods of low moods are not uncommon in children, evidence of sustained low mood needs to be elicited for a diagnosis of depressive disorder. It is not uncommon for parents to be unaware of depression in their children.

NICE (2005a) has produced guidelines for depression in children and young people. Treatment aims at reducing depression, promoting social and emotional functioning and helping the family to understand and deal with their child's illness. Within three months 10 per cent will recover spontaneously and a further 40 per cent will within a year. Therefore a period of watchful waiting is recommended for mild depressions. CBT has been shown to be effective and programmes have been researched and validated that are computer-based as well as in manual form.

Antidepressant medication has been found to increase the risk of suicidal behaviour in adolescents and so should not be the first line of treatment. When it is offered it should be fluoxetine in the first instant, as this is the only one where the benefits have outweighed the risk of side-effects. Also, medication should be given in combination with a psychological therapy such as CBT unless the therapy has been declined. When taking the antidepressant the young person needs to be monitored for suicidal/self-injury behaviours and aggression.

Suicide and intentional self-injury

Suicide is the third leading cause of death in adolescence (Belfer 2008). Completed suicide is rare before puberty but its incidence increases during older adolescence. Suicidal behaviour and the meaning given to it are thought to be culturally specific and religion tends not to act as a protective factor, as it does in adults. The most consistent correlates of suicidal ideas are psychiatric disorders, child sexual abuse and maladaptive personality traits. Studies have rejected the idea that music genres cause suicide although it may be suggestive of a vulnerability.

Intentional self-injury behaviour peaks at adolescence and is generally low in childhood. Suicidal ideation is relatively common in adolescence with 10–20 per cent experiencing such thoughts over the past year. During early adolescence, self-injury rates are far higher in females than males, tending to start at around 12 years (Hawton and Harriss 2008). A history of sexual abuse or physical abuse and parental psychiatric disorder may be present.

All children who self-injure should have an assessment including a careful risk assessment, taking into account family history of mood disturbance and past attempts at self-injury. Children who do self-injure may be seen in emergency departments and be admitted to a paediatric ward as necessary. Some hospitals now have paediatric liaison nurses. Clear protocols need to be in place so that these children do not fall between medical and mental health services for children and those for adults. Factors indicating the suicide risk of children following an intentional self-injury are shown in Table 31.3. NICE (2004a) has published guidelines for the management of deliberate self-harm. Involvement of the family is beneficial. They should be encouraged to see self-harm as serious and play

Table 31.3 Suicide risk assessment in children following an intentional self-injury

	Low risk	High risk
Location	In public	Isolated
Timing	Intervention likely	Intervention unlikely
Precipitants	Impulsive	Extensive premeditation
Preparations for death	No suicide note	Suicide note
Attitude following overdose	Relieved about safe outcome	Still expressing suicidal intent
Re-evaluation of problems precipitating self-injury	Positive	Pessimistic outlook

a role in minimizing further risk. Dialectical behaviour therapy has good evidence of effectiveness with suicidal adolescents and those with emerging personality disorders.

Eating disorders

Eating disorders are conditions in which there is excessive preoccupation and concern with control of body weight and shape, with grossly restricted food intake or bingeing and vomiting. There are medical concerns particular to children with eating disorders due to the impact on their physical development. The term 'eating disorder' in young people covers a range of conditions where one or all of the psychological, social and physical areas of functioning is involved. It is important to note that eating disorders can arise secondary to other disorders such as depression and OCD (see Chapter 38).

Psychosomatic disorders

Developmental factors play an important role in the presentation of these disorders. Parental and cultural attitudes to 'illness behaviour' in children influence if and how children somatize. Very young children are less able to convey psychological distress based on their verbal competence and cognitive development. In the general population, 2–10 per cent of children have aches and pains, which are mostly unexplained, and 5–10 per cent of children and adolescents report distressing somatic symptoms or are regarded by their parents as 'sickly' (Garralda 2008).

The categories of somatic disorder differ based on the nature, chronicity and impact of unexplained somatic symptoms. There are certain factors associated with an increased reporting of physical symptoms. This may, in part, be related to the increase in symptom reporting associated with the onset of menarche.

Dissociative disorders

The most common symptom in young people is loss of motor function but loss of function in any modality may be reported. Complaints of sensory loss involving sight, hearing or consciousness are not uncommon. The symptoms can present as an 'epidemic' particularly involving girls where large numbers of children in a class report the same symptoms. Unlike the individual form, the disorder may arise in a number of individuals within a closed community. This variety of disorder is often described as 'epidemic hysteria'. Diagnosis of the condition is fraught with difficulties as a proportion of children diagnosed on follow-up have been shown to be suffering from an organic condition. Children who are referred usually have had extensive physical investigations. It is important to engage the family in exploring the psychological stressor without stigmatizing the patient as malingering. Individual and family work has been shown to be helpful.

Chronic fatigue syndrome

This is a condition in which severe disabling fatigue persists for over six months (three months in children) and is associated with a variety of other associated symptoms unexplained by primary physical or psychiatric causes. The most significant complaint on presentation is one of fatigue often preceded by a flu-like illness from which complete recovery has not been made. Associated low mood, mental fatigue and inability to concentrate are not uncommon. Girls are more affected than boys.

The aetiological model is complex and physical and psychological factors have been suggested. Low mood, anxiety and depression are not uncommon and, in up to a third of cases, depression may be present. While most cases remain ambulant, in very severe forms, children may be confined to a wheelchair. These children often present in paediatric clinics and may be resistant to transfer to CAMHS as they see the principle cause of the problems as organic. Individual work with the child in using behavioural and cognitive strategies in goal-setting and encouraging graded rehabilitation has been found to be beneficial.

Mania and bipolar affective disorder

Manic disorders are rare before puberty although a large-scale research study is currently investigating this further. In pre-pubertal children, symptoms of mania may be confused with ADHD. Manic patients present with irritability, euphoria or elated mood and insomnia. They tend to be hyperactive and may engage in reckless and impulsive behaviour. Mania may be part of a bipolar affective disorder with episodes of depression and mania. Onset is usually during adolescence or early adulthood. Neuroleptic drugs or lithium are commonly used to control acute episodes.

Psychosis

Although schizophrenia can occur in younger children, its onset before puberty is rare and it is usually preceded by a stage of behavioural and social difficulties, which may make early diagnosis difficult. Schizophrenia can have an onset in adolescence. Making a firm diagnosis is often difficult because of the limited verbal skills of the child and the confusion between vivid normal fantasy life and psychotic thinking. It can also be difficult to distinguish the prodromal stages of the illness from other disorders. Cannabis use has also been associated with the incidence of prodromal symptoms of psychosis.

Children with schizophrenia often present with earlier developmental delays and poor premorbid functioning. Developmental delays are particularly common in the areas of language development, reading and bladder control. A third of children also show difficulties in forming socio-emotional relationships. The onset of schizophrenia is usually insidious. There is usually a strong family history of psychosis.

Inpatient admission should be considered where there is serious risk to the safety of the young person or others. Lack of insight and poor compliance with treatment are other factors which need to be considered. Alternatively, the patient may be treated as a day patient or an outpatient.

The NICE (2006b) guideline for schizophrenia does not include children. Medication is the first line treatment and olanzapine and risperidone have been used with good effect. Psycho-education of parents and the patient about the illness, treatment and prognosis is an essential part of treatment, aiding their understanding of an illness which can be frightening and stigmatizing. Cognitive behavioural strategies and supportive counselling may be beneficial.

31.5 Principles of child and adolescent mental health treatment and care

Before an assessment or treatment it is important to seek consent from the patient and adults holding parental responsibility. Assessment of competence to give consent needs to be tailored to the young person's age and understanding of the purpose, nature and likely effects and risks. The Mental Capacity Act (MCA) (2005) is applicable to young people from the age of 16 although the Mental Health Act (MHA) (2007) does not have a lower age limit.

Once a comprehensive assessment has been completed, the child and parents need to be involved in drawing up a treatment plan. The success of this will often depend on the extent to which they feel their wishes, fears and anxieties have been addressed during the initial meetings. It is useful for goals to be set out for what will be seen as a successful outcome of treatment. A model, such as the Family Partnership Approach (Davis and Day 2010), can be used to facilitate this throughout the family's contact with the service.

Comprehensive CAMHS

The National Service Framework for Children, Young People and Maternity Services Standard 9 (DH/DfES 2004) sets out what CAMHS should look like. The underlying principles are that it is accessible, effectively commissioned, driven by a multi-agency assessment of needs and commissioned to meet the needs of the population safely, timely and effectively. For example, there should be appropriately trained staff for all 0–18-year-olds including those with a learning disability and 24-hour specialist CAMHS care should be available.

Safeguarding young people

Safeguarding children is the responsibility of everyone. Identifying and reporting suspected abuse, contributing to the child protection assessment and plan and treating the resultant emotional and behavioural problems are all roles the CAMHS nurse may have. Young people known to the service may be victims or perpetrators of abuse, or both.

Types of abuse include:

- physical abuse – non-accidental injury, burns, fractures, bruises;
- emotional abuse – threats, hostility, failure to protect;
- sexual abuse – penetrative, non-penetrative;
- neglect – lack of appropriate care and nurture, stimulation and supervision.

The primary aim is to prevent further abuse by safeguarding the child. A referral to the social care services is of utmost importance for an assessment and investigation. The second aim is to work, in partnership with the other agencies, to help meet the child's social, emotional and psychological needs while providing support to the family.

Multi-agency working

Mental health problems are not just the remit of CAMHS; commitment, input and investment are required from everyone involved in delivery of services to adolescents. Collaborative practices are now seen as the most efficient way of delivering high quality services and ensuring their effectiveness in being responsive to service user needs. Following the inquiry into the death of Victoria Climbié (Laming 2003) and *Every Child Matters* (DfES 2003) a number of measures to reform and improve children's care were proposed. The Common Assessment Framework (CAF) and the Team Around the Child (TAC) were introduced. The CAF is a standardized approach to conducting an assessment of a child's additional, rather than universal, needs. TAC meetings, where plans are decided, are attended by all relevant professionals, the child and parents or carers. A lead professional is allocated, who may be the CAMHS professional.

Youth justice

The current Youth Justice System was established by the Crime and Disorder Act 1998; its aim is to prevent offending by young people. There are youth offending teams (YOTs) in every area of England and Wales. Various agencies are represented including police, probation, social services, education and health. The Crime and Disorder Act 1998 stipulates YOTs should include 'a person nominated by a health authority any part of whose area lies within the local authority's area'; frequently this is a mental health nurse. This person is expected to ensure

young people are provided with 100 per cent access to health assessments.

As many as 23.7 per cent of offending young people report a prior suicide attempt (Howard *et al.* 2003). Prevalence studies suggest conduct disorders, suicide, depression, substance misuse, post-traumatic stress disorder (PTSD) and ADHD are more common. Young people at the interface of the Criminal Justice System and mental health services risk double jeopardy for social exclusion, alienation and stigmatization both from being involved in the Criminal Justice System and from having mental health problems (Bailey 1997). Affective disorders also play some role in youth violence and depression in adolescence can manifest itself as anger, which in turn is correlated with aggression (Bailey 2002). A substantial number of young people are not referred for treatment as the depression is misinterpreted as a conduct disorder.

Primary care

Although psychiatric disorders are relatively common in young people, only 1 in 10 of cases is seen in specialist CAMHS. Annually, around 2–5 per cent of children attending primary care present with emotional or behavioural disorders and they are more likely to be referred if they present with overt psychological problems. Recognition in primary care is an important factor in referral to specialist mental health services.

Many primary care practices employ counsellors, community psychiatric nurses and psychologists offering consultation and assessment. This has helped reduce referrals to increasingly long waiting lists for specialist child mental health services. They also have an input in enhancing GP skills in managing milder cases and making more appropriate referrals to specialist services.

Education

NICE has developed guidelines for social and emotional well-being in primary (2008b) and secondary (2009) education which detail both the role schools have in preventing mental health problems and the role of CAMHS in schools.

Prevention of childhood mental health problems

The mental health of young people and their vulnerability to physical, intellectual and emotional behaviour disorders, if untreated, has serious implications for adult life. Protective factors for young people include an adaptable temperament, a good relationship with a significant adult caretaker and engagement in pursuits in which the child has a good experience such as sports or school. Several studies have shown that a proportion of children exposed to gross deprivation and severe stress are resilient to developing psychiatric disorder, although the precise reasons why some children are resilient is not understood. The formation of secure attachments and the ability to be self-reflective are seen as protective factors.

 ## 31.6 The role of nurses in child and adolescent services

Nursing is a remarkably diverse discipline in CAMHS, with many identities, led by an increasingly well-qualified group of individuals who fulfil a wide range of responsibilities. As with all nursing posts, commitment to ongoing continuing professional development and lifelong learning is essential. The core nursing skills and competencies such as risk assessment and management, health promotion and education, physical health care and medication management, partnership working and relapse prevention can be valuably applied to the CAMHS setting, offering a unique perspective within the multidisciplinary team.

Nurses with specialist training in child and adolescent psychiatry are uniquely placed to work in all areas of the service including inpatient wards, community teams, schools, child health and primary care as generic CAMHS practitioners, advanced nurse practitioners, non-medical prescribers, modern matrons and consultant nurses. Nurses can also develop specialist training in a range of therapies, including CBT and family therapy. Nurses will continue to play a central role in the services for young people with first onset psychosis and ADHD.

Childhood, adolescence and parenting have different meanings to different people. Nurses working in CAMHS need to have an appreciation of the diversity of parenting approaches that are seen during the course of their work. This can vary not only between cultures but also between families. Keeping an open mind while having the safety and well-being of the child at the forefront of thinking can be challenging. However, with the focus on care and attending to all aspects of the patient, nurses are in a good position to engage and work with young people. The flexible and creative approaches that nurses develop are particularly helpful when working with those who may be reluctant to engage with services.

 ## 31.7 Conclusion

In summary, the key points of learning from this chapter are:

■ Compared to the high profile of adult mental health, the significance of the mental health needs of children has only recently been recognized. A National Service Framework for Children has been published setting out national standards for a comprehensive CAMHS.

■ Reported prevalence rates for mental health problems among children and adolescents vary. In this respect the use of mental health diagnoses for preschool children is highly contested.

■ Different patterns of mental health problems can be observed in young people, with typical age and gender patterns being noted for some disorders.

- Nurses may encounter mental distress and illness in young people in a wide variety of clinical and care settings.

- Multi-agency working is required to provide responsive, effective services with the allocation of a lead professional.

- Service users' views are important in guiding the future development of CAMHS. They have highlighted concerns with access to the service and waiting times, and the need for greater support of people in their parenting role.

Annotated bibliography

Rutter, M. and Taylor, E. (eds) (2008) *Child and Adolescent Psychiatry*, **5th edn. Oxford: Blackwell Publishing.**
The fifth edition is one of the most comprehensive textbooks in child and adolescent psychiatry and is highly recommended for readers wishing to research topics in depth.

McDougall, T. (2006) *Child and Adolescent Mental Health Nursing*. **Oxford Wiley-Blackwell Publishing.**
This book, written by a nurse consultant in CAMHS, offers further exploration of the nursing role within CAMHS.

www.rcpsych.ac.uk/mentalhealthinfoforall/youngpeople.aspx.
This is an excellent resource that is kept up to date, in line with the evidence base, by the Royal College of Psychiatrists. The site offers leaflets on matters relating to CAMHS, including information on specific diagnoses and what to expect when you are referred to CAMHS. There are specific resources for young people as well as resources for parents, teachers and health professionals. Leaflets can be downloaded and copied freely.

References

APA (American Psychiatric Association) (1994) *Diagnostic and Statistical Manual of Mental Disorders, DSM-IV*, 4th edn. Washington, DC: American Psychiatric Association.
Bailey, S. (1997) Adolescent offenders, *Current Opinion in Psychiatry*, 10: 445–53.
Bailey, S. (2002) Violent children: a framework for assessment, *Advances in Psychiatric Treatment*, 8: 97–106.
Bowlby, J. (1980) *Attachment and Loss: III. Loss, sadness and depression*.London: Basic Books.
Conners, C.K. (1973) Rating scales for use in drug studies with children, *Psychopharmacology Bulletin: Special issue on pharmacotherapy with children*, 9: 24–84.
Costello, E.J., Egger, H.L. and Angold, A. (2004) Developmental epidemiology of anxiety disorders, in T.H. Ollendick and J.S. March (eds) *Phobic and Anxiety Disorders in Children and Adolescents*. Oxford: Oxford University Press.
Davis, H. and Day, C. (2010) *Working in Partnership with Parents: The Family Partnership Model*, 2nd edn. London: Pearson.
DfES (Department for Education and Skills) (2003) *Every Child Matters*. Nottingham: DfES.
DH/DfES (Department of Health, Department for Education and Skills) (2004) *National Service Framework for Children, Young People and Maternity Services: The mental health and psychological well-being of children and young people*. London: DH/DfES.
Fergusson, D.M. and Horwood, L.J. (2000) Does cannabis use encourage other forms of illicit drug use? *Addiction*, 95: 505–20.
Garralda, E. (2008) Somatization and somatoform disorders, *Psychiatry*, 7(8): 353–6.
Goodman, R. (1997) The Strengths and Difficulties Questionnaire: a research note, *Journal of Child Psychology and Psychiatry*, 38: 581–6.
Hawton, K. and Harriss, L. (2008) The changing gender ratio in occurrence of deliberate self-harm across the life cycle, *Crisis* 29(1): 4–10.
Hersov, L. (1994) Faecal soiling, in M. Rutter, E. Taylor and L. Hersov (eds) *Child and Adolescent Psychiatry: Modern approaches*, 3rd edn. Oxford: Blackwell Science.
Howard, J., Lennings, C.J. and Copeland, J. (2003) Suicidal behaviour in a young offender population, *Crisis*, 24(3): 98–104.
Laming, H. (2003) *The Victoria Climbié Inquiry. Report of an inquiry by Lord Laming*. London: The Stationery Office.
Liber, J.M., Van Widenfelt, B.M., Utens, E.M.W.J. *et al.* (2008) No differences between group versus individual treatment of childhood anxiety disorders in a randomised clinical trial, *Journal of Child Psychology and Psychiatry and Allied Disciplines*, 49(8): 886–93.
National Statistical Office (2005) *UK 2005 – The Official Yearbook of the United Kingdom of Great Britain and Northern Ireland*. London: National Statistical Office.
NICE (National Institute for Health and Clinical Excellence) (2004a) *Self Harm*. London: NICE.
NICE (National Institute for Health and Clinical Excellence) (2004b) *Eating Disorders in Children and Adolescence*. London: NICE.
NICE (National Institute for Health and Clinical Excellence) (2005a) *Depression in Children and Young People*. London: NICE.
NICE (National Institute for Health and Clinical Excellence) (2005b) *Obsessive-Compulsive Disorder*. London: NICE.

NICE (National Institute for Health and Clinical Excellence) (2006) *Conduct Disorder in Children: Parent-training/education programmes*. London: NICE.

NICE (National Institute for Health and Clinical Excellence) (2007) *Community-based Interventions to Reduce Substance Misuse Among Vulnerable and Disadvantaged Children and Young People*. London: NICE.

NICE (National Institute for Health and Clinical Excellence) (2008a) *Attention Deficit and Hyperactivity Disorder*. London: NICE.

NICE (National Institute for Health and Clinical Excellence) (2008b) *Social and Emotional Well-being in Primary Schools*. London: NICE.

NICE (National Institute for Health and Clinical Excellence) (2009) *Social and Emotional Well-being in Secondary Schools*. London: NICE.

NICE (National Institute for Health and Clinical Excellence) (2011) *Nocturnal Enuresis: The management of bedwetting in children and young People*. London: NICE.

SAMHSA (Substance Abuse and Mental Health Services Administration) (2007) *Results from the 2006 National Survey on Drug Use and Health: National findings* (NSDUH Series H-28, DHHS Publication No. SMA 05–4062). Rockville, MD: Office of Applied Studies.

WHO (World Health Organization) (1996) *Mulitaxial Classification of Child and Adolescent Psychiatric Disorders: The ICD-10 Classification of Mental and Behavioral Disorders*. Geneva: WHO.

Chapter 32

Older People with Functional Mental Health Problems

Niall McCrae

I know the doctors and nurses care but I don't want to bother you; it's not like I'm sick.

(Mary – depression)

Since George passed away I just stay in most of the time, on my own. The brandy helps me sleep after another day of gloom.

(Alice – alcohol abuse)

It helped me to know something was wrong; the pills helped, but most of all I've got a lovely nurse who comes round and gives me strength.

(June – anxiety)

32.1 Introduction

In traditional societies, older people were venerated as an embodiment of family and social heritage and as a source of wisdom. In modern western culture family ties have loosened, and the skills and knowledge of older people have been undermined by technological progress and rapid cultural change. However, negative social attitudes towards senescence have been challenged by increasing numbers of older people leading healthy, active lives into their 70s and beyond. We live in an ageing society, and as life expectancy improves, people can look forward to three or four decades in retirement, ideally enjoying a healthy and active life. However, longevity is a double-edged sword, because there is strong correlation between age and morbidity. Although there is no evidence that older people overall are less happy, they have a disproportionately high frequency of depression and anxiety, as well as dementia. Older people have suffered from discrimination in service provision, with restricted access to therapeutic interventions, and reliance on institutional facilities often of poor quality. As demand grows, nurses are at the forefront of the mission to provide equitable and effective care for older people with mental health problems.

This chapter covers:

- issues and challenges of ageing that may impinge on mental health;
- mental health services for older people: policy and provision;
- four functional mental health problems of old age: depression, anxiety, delusional psychoses and substance misuse (organic mental disorders of old age are covered in Chapter 33).

32.2　The psychosocial challenges of ageing

In his book *Childhood and Society*, published in 1950, psychoanalyst Erik Erikson (1902–94) introduced his eight-stage theory of the human life cycle. Each stage presents a crisis, with conflict between a harmonious and a disruptive force, driving us to our next stage of development. Old age begins when the person senses his or her mortality, stimulating conflict between ego integrity and despair. Older people tend to review their life in terms of success or failure. If deriving satisfaction from accomplishments in life, the person will approach end of life in contentment and peace; someone reflecting only on difficulties and disappointments may feel that life was wasted or futile. In successful resolution, emotional and cognitive integration amounts to wisdom, which Erikson (1980) defined as an informed and detached view of life and death. The perspective of making a positive

contribution to future generations illustrates Erikson's humanitarian philosophy. Such theory lacks practical implications for nurses, but the emphasis on development as opposed to decline confers value both on older people and on the work of nurses with this age group.

Mental health problems in older people have tended to be neglected, partly due to a widespread belief that depression and cognitive decline are inevitable features of ageing. A negative attitude towards old age is strongest in western society, where status is determined by competence and capacity. The later years of life, particularly if tainted by mental impairment, are thus devalued. Such attitudes may contribute to an older person's sense of being a burden on others. To understand and to tackle mental health issues in older people, we must first consider the physical, psychological and social circumstances of ageing.

Physical changes

Ageing entails a gradual process of bodily change, which is apparent in all systems, influenced by both nature and nurture. Outward signs of deterioration include reduced elasticity of the skin, greying or loss of hair, decline in subcutaneous fat and changes in posture. The older person has lighter meals and reduced potential for physical exertion. Concentration and memory become less sharp. Older people are more prone to illness, with more likelihood of this becoming chronic. Mobility may be impaired by cardiovascular, endocrine, musculoskeletal or respiratory disorders, and there are tendencies for polymorbidity and polypharmacy as age advances. However, the number of older people retaining physical vitality into late age is growing.

Emotional and intellectual changes

A stereotypical characterization of an older person is inflexible with 'stuck in the mud' views, short-tempered, tardy and forgetful. However, an assumed intellectual decline of old age is refuted by cohort studies showing little decline in intelligence quotient scores after the peak reached in young adulthood.

Gradual loss of irreplaceable brain cells occurs in old age, and intracellular changes affect the process of neurotransmission, but the impact on mental functioning is debatable. Generally, intellectual deficits are insignificant in older people who maintain a positive, active lifestyle.

Emotional changes in older people may be reactive rather than an endogenous ageing process; bereavement and moving from the family home, for example, can lead to prolonged grief, insecurity and loneliness.

Social life

Social activity may increase after retirement, but networks tend to narrow in older age, or earlier if there are mobility, health or environmental constraints. In the 1950s gerontologists from the University of Chicago postulated the disengagement theory, whereby older people withdraw from social contact as a normal ageing process, but since then evidence has accumulated on the benefits of social activity. Surveys show that socially active older people have better physical and mental health, but the direction of causal relationship is reversible. Some people may take comfort in the warmth and familiarity of home, without detracting from their quality of life.

Sexuality

Society is in denial over the sexual activity of older people. Indeed the disparaging term 'dirty old man' demonstrates the revulsion of younger adults to such primal desires in advanced age. It is commonly assumed that older people are neither interested in, nor physically capable of, sexual intercourse. In the internet era, dating websites reveal a different picture, with the large number of single, divorced or bereaved older people generating a burgeoning social and sexual dynamic that challenges ageist assumptions.

Faith

A strong correlation has been found between religious practice and well-being in older people. However, it is not only the religious who ponder on the soul and spirituality in their later years. Instead of being overwhelmed by the challenges of ageing, lives can be enriched by a profound sense of purpose. Viktor Frankl (1963), who survived a Nazi death camp, professed that in dire circumstances people can find inner meaning. Drawing on Oriental philosophy, Lars Tornstam's (1996) theory of gerotranscendence describes a shift from a materialistic, pragmatic outlook to a sense of communion with a universal spirit or higher moral reality. Older people redefine life and death, meditating on their existence within a continuity of the past and future.

Gender

On average, women outlive men by four to five years (this gap has reduced since the Second World War, not only due to a period of relative peace but also to a decline in hazardous industrial labour). Husbands are typically older than their wives, ultimately lengthening the period of widowhood. Surveys show that more older women than older men suffer from disabling health conditions. As Nathanson (1977) commented, 'women get sick, but men die'. Retirement can be difficult for men whose job was a major determinant of identity, status and reward; while some enjoy freedom from the daily grind, others feel that life has lost its purpose. Such reactions may become more common in women, whose occupational activity has changed considerably in recent decades.

Poverty

A high percentage of older people live in poverty. Material deprivation is particularly common in women living alone, many of whom depend on a minimal state pension. A major factor for women is a discontinuous career due to child care, reducing the amount of occupational pension. Standard of living may also be impoverished if a spouse is or was a recipient of costly residential care. Although the government pays a heating allowance in the winter, older people often underheat their homes, potentially contributing to health problems.

Ethnicity

While the older population in the UK is predominantly white, the proportion from minority ethnic groups is increasing steadily. Compared to the host community, migrant groups tend to preserve social bonds between the generations, and this can be a substantial source of support. However, assumptions about family care in Asian communities, for example, may perpetuate disadvantage in access to services. Older people of minority ethnic groups may have language difficulties and may fear being placed in an environment with customs at odds to their own. Compared with older white people, black Caribbean and south Asian people are less inclined to consult general practitioners (GPs) for depression. Factors include limited awareness and pronounced stigma towards mental health problems; somatization of mental health problems is common in south Asian elders.

Quality of life

Well-being and quality of life defy precise definition, and the terms are often used synonymously. A survey of older people by Gabriel and Bowling (2004) revealed the following determinants of quality of life:

- good social relationships with family and friends;
- fulfilling social roles and participating in activities;
- good health and functional ability;
- pleasant home and neighbourhood;
- positive outlook and psychological well-being;
- adequate finance;
- independence.

However, quality of life is an inherently subjective matter. People judge life satisfaction emotionally rather than by a set of objective criteria. A key factor in well-being is psychological resilience, with some older people retaining a high level of satisfaction despite illness, loss or other adversities. Windle

et al. (2008) formulated resilience as a combination of self-esteem, competence and control.

32.3 Mental health services for older people

The *National Service Framework for Mental Health* (DH 1998) excluded the care of people aged over 65, who were covered instead by the *National Service Framework for Older People* (NSF-OP; DH 2001). The rationale for this division was the extent of overlap in the psychological, social and physical needs of older people. A key objective of the NSF-OP is 'to promote good mental health in older people and to treat and support those older people with dementia and depression' (p. 19), but there was a lack of specific targets and no extra resources were provided for the recommended service development. Services having evolved organically and inconsistently, the document *Everybody's Business* (Care Services Improvement Partnership 2005) presented a coherent model of a mental health service for older people, including social services and primary care. A single practitioner takes responsibility for each person's care, making appropriate use of statutory and voluntary services and other community resources, while building on the person's existing social support. The overarching aim of mental health services for older people is to provide prompt and effective care that enables patients to live as independently as possible in the community.

Assessment

In serving older people with overlapping health and social needs, there should be good collaboration between health and social services. The NSF-OP introduced the Single Assessment Process to avoid duplicate assessments and to ensure a more cohesive, holistic approach by health and social care agencies. The domains of the Single Assessment Process are as follows:

- user's perspective;
- clinical background;

- disease prevention;
- personal care and physical well-being;
- senses;
- mental health;
- relationships;
- safety;
- environment and resources.

Mental health should be covered in all assessments of older people. Practitioners should be looking for signs of mood disturbance, distorted perception or cognition, impaired insight, anxiety, speech abnormalities and substance misuse. Risk of self-harm or suicide should be examined by asking about recent thoughts and any past suicidal behaviour. Social factors impinging on mental health include domestic conditions, family support and dynamics, finance and other resources, and the wider social and physical environment.

Developing a therapeutic rapport

Assessment should be regarded as an ongoing process, alongside the nurturing of a therapeutic partnership. Nurses should clarify their role and how the service will work in each patient's situation; most first-time users will have limited knowledge of the complexities of mental health provision. The age and background of nurse and patient may be in stark contrast; acknowledging the older person's life experience can rebalance the power relationship. Attentive listening is crucial to assessment and rapport. Nurses should refrain from interrupting or raising their voice (not all older people are deaf). As verbal communication may be slower or impaired by sensory or cognitive deficits, the nurse should be receptive to non-verbal expression.

Mental health nursing should be holistic, rather than compartmentalizing a person's problems into a diagnosed condition. This is relevant to all age groups, but particularly so with older people, who often have overlapping health and social issues. Nursing interventions should be planned and agreed with the older person, with concise goals for

resolution, alleviation or adjustment to difficulties. Ideally the care plan will lead to discharge from professional input, but in every case the aim should be optimal independence and quality of life.

Working with family carers

After being overlooked or seen as a hindrance to health services in the past, the major role of family carers is now fully acknowledged in government policy. The *Carers Strategy* (DH 2008) emphasizes that services should regard carers not only as providers of informal care but also as people with needs of their own. Ultimately, a carer who is able to lead a fulfilling life is more likely to cope with the challenges of continually supporting a person with mental health problems. Carer stress is a major determinant of outcome for older people with mental health problems. Practical and supportive interventions for carers may prevent or delay institutionalization of the recipient of their care. These include support groups (which may require use of a sitting service), home care visits, welfare benefits and respite. The nurse can be of great value to carers by providing a listening ear for frustration and fears, responding with empathy, support and advice.

Cultural sensitivity

To prevent inequity in access and treatment, services must be culturally sensitive. The NSF-OP attributed inadequate detection of problems in minority ethnic elders to lack of cultural awareness in services. Iliffe and Manthorpe (2004) argued that application of broad categories such as 'black' and 'south Asian' ignores the heterogeneity within such groups. They explained that issues of language, culture and religion should be considered across the whole target population, rather than being restricted to an 'ethnic minority agenda'. The perspectives of smaller minority groups such as the Chinese and eastern Europeans have been overshadowed by a focus on the difficulties experienced by black and south Asian communities. Meanwhile, the literature has overlooked the asset of a culturally diverse mental health workforce.

32.4 Functional mental health problems in old age

Four disorders can present significant challenges to older people. Depression and anxiety are common conditions that can be extremely debilitating in old age. Delusional psychoses, which arise from various factors, are a leading cause of psychiatric admission of older people. Finally substance misuse is a growing problem that can compound mental and physical comorbidity.

Depression

Depression is the most common mental health problem in old age. In older people the condition

Malcolm

Malcolm, aged 68, is a retired civil servant with a reasonably good pension. Over the last year he has become inactive and socially withdrawn; he has gained weight and is breathless on minor exertion. Since retiring Malcolm has missed his regular social activity of meeting for drinks after work on Fridays. He was encouraged by one former colleague to play bowls, but lost interest. Recently Malcolm has been expressing negative thoughts about himself, seeing his life as devoid of purpose. Meanwhile his wife Judy, a retired nurse, maintains an active social life with her various groups of friends. Judy persuaded Malcolm to visit his GP, but when the prescribed antidepressants had no effect (although there were doubts over whether Malcolm was taking the tablets) a referral was made to the community mental health team (CMHT). Amy, a nurse from the team, assessed Malcolm at home. Completion of the Geriatric Depression Scale confirmed that he remained depressed. Discussing his past and recent history, Amy gradually built a rapport with Malcolm, who had been sceptical about input from the mental health service. Amy found little evidence of any mental distress in the past, except normal reactions to stressful events or bereavement. Malcolm's low mood seemed to be related to more recent experiences, particularly his response to retirement. Compounding the sense of loss, the office where he had worked for 20 years had been moved to another town. He was also upset by a newly-built block of apartments looming over his house, spoiling his enjoyment of the garden. Malcolm no longer read the newspaper because he thought that everything in the world was getting worse. Judy had been unable to console him. Amy assured them both that this was a treatable condition, and suggested a referral for cognitive behavioural therapy (CBT).

Thinking Space 32.1

Make a note of the features presented here that would indicate depression (feedback at end of chapter).

has tended to be under-detected, and consequently under-treated. To some extent depression has been regarded by health and social care workers as inherent to the inevitable mental, physical and social adversities of old age. A more positive response to depression among older people has been urged by government policy (DH 2001).

Risk factors

Risk of depression is increased by various factors including advanced old age, lack of a confiding relationship, bereavement and other distressing experiences, smoking and debilitating physical illness. Living alone does not necessarily add to the risk of depression. Incidence increases in men aged between 60 and 80, which may be attributed to loss of occupational and financial status. Depression sometimes arises when a person moves into residential care. A British study (McDougall *et al.* 2007) found a considerably higher prevalence in institutional settings: 27.1 per cent compared to 9.3 per cent of older people living in the community. Risk of depression in care homes is increased by a combination of physical disability and loss of autonomy. However, depression is poorly detected by nurses in care homes (Bagley *et al.* 2004).

Presentation and course

Depression often has a different clinical presentation in older people. Low mood may not be readily apparent; other signs include irritability, apathy, bodily complaints of dubious basis, and neglect of self-care. A severe form is sometimes found in older people, with delusions and a profound, nihilistic sense of physical and mental deterioration. Psychomotor retardation or agitation may be prominent features. While depression is normally a self-remitting condition, it is more likely to become chronic in old age if untreated. In a primary care study, Harris *et al.* (2006) found that 61 per cent of older patients who were depressed at baseline remained depressed two years later.

Suicide is disproportionately frequent in older people, although self-harm is less common than in younger adults. An attempted suicide is more likely to be completed by an older person, one factor being the ready availability of drugs for overdose. There are no clear predictors, but inquests show that a high proportion of older people who commit suicide were depressed at the time. Unlike with younger adults, most older people who commit suicide saw their health care providers during the month before death; this suggests opportunities for prevention.

Assessment

Older people tend not to complain when depressed. Somatization is common, partly because physical symptoms may have the greatest impact on the older person. As in younger adults, men report mental health problems less frequently than do women, but gender difference may be exacerbated by result of stoicism, denial and lack of emotional articulacy in men. There is difficulty in detecting depression in people who display cognitive impairment. Sometimes a depressive episode may be mistaken for dementia, and a pseudodementia syndrome may develop from severe depression. Fatigue, loss of appetite and sleep disturbance may be the result of physical illness or side-effects of medication rather than low mood. Diagnostic classification systems specify that symptoms suggestive of depression must be independent of other medical conditions. However, mental and physical health problems often overlap in older people, such that a person could have both depression and a physical illness contributing to impaired mood and volition. For this reason, generic screening instruments may be less useful in detecting depression in older people. The Geriatric Depression Scale (Yesavage and Brink 1983), a validated instrument that focuses more on thought patterns than on physical symptoms, is widely used.

A criticism of the use of standardized instruments is their limitations across cultural groups, but from their research on screening for depression in older people of African-Caribbean origin, Rait *et al.* (1999) argued that the important factor is the cultural sensitivity of the interviewer rather than the content of the instruments. On assessing older people, nurses should adapt terminology, where appropriate, to ensure mutual understanding. For example, it may be better to begin with terms such as 'sad' or 'feeling low' rather than 'depression'.

Treatment and care

For a full account of pharmacological treatment for depression see Chapter 26. In summary, the National Institute for Health and Clinical Excellence (NICE) recommends that prescription of antidepressants in older people should follow similar principles as in younger adults, but with special regard to tolerance and regular monitoring of side-effects.

While drugs are of limited value in severe depression, electro-convulsive therapy (ECT) appears to be as effective in older people as in younger adults, with a recovery rate of around 80 per cent. Its use is increasing, despite some concern about excessive use in older people (SCIE 2006). In the past, ECT was avoided in late-life depression due to cardiovascular risks, but there is now greater confidence in its tolerance by older people. Also, while there are cardiovascular and other contraindications, the balance of risk may be weighed in favour of ECT as a life-saving intervention. Short-term amnesia is common, and there should be a gap of at least three days between treatments to minimize cognitive dysfunction. Indications for ECT are similar across age groups, but in older people prominent factors may be delusional ideation and refusal of food.

Depression is more likely to be relieved if supportive interventions are provided by a practitioner such as a community nurse. This may take the form of a problem-solving approach, such as the 'skilled helper' model of Gerard Egan (1975). To overcome more fixed negative thinking, a structured therapy programme may be the best option. However, ageism continues to restrict access of older people to psychological therapies. This is partly due to myths as described by Laidlaw et al. (2003):

- you can't teach an old dog new tricks;
- getting old must be terrible: depression is inevitable;
- older people do not want psychotherapy and cannot deal with abstract formulations;
- poor cost-benefit ratio: therapeutic resources are best expended on younger people.

While considering life history in initial assessment, psychotherapeutic work with older people is orientated towards tackling current issues. Cognitive therapists explain depression as the result of distorted thought patterns, but a challenge is the tendency for older people to conflate thoughts and feelings. The person is encouraged to examine the evidence for negative thoughts, and to understand how automatic but irrational beliefs affect emotions and behaviour. The objective of CBT is to enable the person to recognize and overcome negative cognition, thus preventing recurrence of depression. Although there is evidence for CBT in treating depression in older adults, a Cochrane review recommended further research, due to the small scale of studies to date (Wilson et al. 2008).

Anxiety and obsessive compulsive disorder

Anxiety is a state of overwhelming apprehension, taking various forms (as described in detail in Chapter 37). Prevalence rates in older people vary considerably, with community estimates ranging from 1.2 to 15 per cent, suggesting conceptual and methodological inconsistency. While given less attention than depression and dementia, anxiety is a common disorder of old age, and it can have major impact on the quality of life of sufferers and their families.

Case Study

Maureen

Maureen, aged 80, is a widow whose husband died five years ago. Struggling with anxiety and sleep problems, she was referred by her GP to the mental health service for older people for assessment and treatment. John, a nurse from the CMHT, assessed Maureen at her home. Recently Maureen has been going out less and withdrawing from social contact; she has persistent nervousness with weight loss and insomnia. When she awakens at night she lies in bed worrying about being in difficult situations. She no longer goes into town to do her shopping, buying her food at inflated prices from a local convenience store. Her home is underheated and John had an impression of impoverishment. An antecedent to Maureen's distress was revealed in assessment. She had been accustomed to travelling everywhere in her husband's car, but after his death she began to use the bus. On one occasion she had a bad experience. On a crowded bus stuck at traffic lights, Maureen wanted desperately to use the toilet. She was suddenly overcome by a feeling of panic, and shouted 'let me off'. As she tried to get to the door, a young woman exclaimed 'she's mad'. Maureen was incontinent of urine in this debacle, and felt extremely embarrassed. Following the incident Maureen saw her GP who prescribed a benzodiazepine for short term only. Her anxiety has been worsening since she stopped taking this drug. She has a compulsion to use the toilet, and since she had been wetting the bed has resorted to using incontinence pads.

Thinking Space 32.2

Make a note of the main interventions that could be included in a care plan for Maureen (feedback at the end of chapter).

Risk factors

Anxiety is diagnosed twice as frequently in older women than in men. In some cases there is an obvious trigger of anxiety, but there may also be underlying issues or susceptibility. Precipitating factors include medical problems such as cardiac or respiratory disorders, social isolation, actual or anticipated adverse events (e.g. bereavement or loss of home), and drug side-effects or withdrawal. There is much overlap of anxiety and depression in older people.

Presentation and course

As well as general features such as restlessness, lack of concentration, irritability, tension and insomnia, older people with anxiety tend to worry more about their physical health than do younger people. There is much overlap with depressive symptoms. Older people are also more likely to somatize anxiety. Hypochondriasis, a preoccupation with bodily complaints of little or no factual basis, sometimes arises. Anxiety may become fixed on a rational concern. Agoraphobia is sometimes conflated with a reasoned fear of leaving the home. Older people are not more likely to be attacked, but they have more fear of crime, such insecurity reinforced by newspaper reports of muggings.

Obsessive compulsive disorder (OCD) is a type of anxiety with a disproprionately higher frequency in older women. Without treatment the condition may become increasingly disabling, as the person's life is dominated by persistent urges and rituals, which appear irrational to others but to the person are a necessity for maintaining control and reducing anxiety. In milder cases the obsessions and compulsions may be seen as an effective if irrational coping strategy. Common themes for OCD in older people are cleanliness, repetitive checking of taps and switches, and bodily functions (e.g. bowel movements).

Assessment

Like depression, anxiety is underdetected in older people. A limitation of screening tools for anxiety is the distinct cognitive and affective profiles of older people. A validated screening instrument specifically for older people is the General Anxiety Inventory (Pachana *et al.* 2007).

Treatment

For a full account of pharmacological treatments for anxiety see Chapter 26. Pharmacological treatment for the various forms of anxiety includes anxiolytic and antidepressant drugs. The evidence for pharmacological treatments is limited as few trials have evaluated treatments exclusively in older people.

There are two established psychological therapies for anxiety in older people. Anxiety management therapy is a structured approach including relaxation techniques to prevent and alleviate the symptoms of anxiety, but without tackling the underlying causes. There is modest evidence for CBT in treating anxiety in older people (NICE 2011). A priority for psychological treatment is for the person to recognize the thought processes contributing to anxiety and to be able to resume a sense of control.

Delusional psychoses

Persecutory delusions and paranoia

Unlike schizophrenia, paranoid delusional disorder often appears for the first time in later life. An older person might develop an unshakeable belief in being exploited or persecuted by a neighbour or family member. Predisposing factors include sensory or cognitive impairment, drug toxicity, premorbid personality and social isolation. There is also evidence of genetic and neuropathological factors. Paranoia can lead to irrational violence, but in many cases there is minimal constraint on everyday life. Behaviour that appears paranoid to a clinician may be a reaction to stressful events, environmental adversity or difficult relationships – for example, persecutory beliefs may be spurred by a genuinely conflictual relationship. Delusions may be comforting to some extent. However, paranoid or persecutory ideas can be distressing and detract from functioning and quality of life. Auditory hallucinations sometimes arise in paranoia; sometimes people imagine that the television or radio is conveying threatening messages. As hallucinations are also a feature of delirium, investigations may be necessary to check for urinary tract infection or other possible cause of acute mental disturbance. The nurse should build a rapport with the person to assess persecutory beliefs and possible causes. To confront such beliefs directly may be counterproductive, but rational explanations may be offered with due sensitivity to context. The nurse should also be aware that paranoia is often an early sign of Alzheimer's disease.

Antipsychotic drugs may be necessary for extreme agitation, hyperactivity, hallucinations and hostility. However, such drugs should be used with caution in older people due to anticholinergic effects, which include dry mouth, blurred vision, weight gain, sedation and postural hypotension. The dose should be started low and increased gradually, and reduced or stopped on mental state being stabilized. Tardive dyskinesia, a syndrome manifesting in involuntary and painful muscle contractions and abnormal body posture, is normally an effect of prolonged neuroleptic use, but it can occur after only a few weeks of treatment.

Schizophrenia

Schizophrenia is a chronic disorder that normally arises in younger adulthood. People under the care of mental health services for this condition will not necessarily transfer to the care of specialist services for older people on reaching the age of 65; there is debate about if and when such graduation should occur. People who have spent much of their adult lives in hospital or residential care may show lasting effects of institutionalization, although features such as stooped posture may also be the result of drug side-effects. Around 10 per cent of cases are diagnosed in old age, detection sometimes having been delayed by the person leading a reclusive life or being protected by family. Late-onset schizophrenia typically presents with paranoid thoughts (McClure *et al.* 1999). Development of cognitive impairment and other symptoms of dementia is disproportionately high in people with schizophrenia (Arnold and Trojanowski 1996).

Treatment entails antipsychotic medication, which is aimed primarily at positive symptoms (delusions, hallucinations and behavioural disturbance). For older patients with long-term use of such drugs, tardive dyskinesia is a common problem, but symptoms may be reduced by cholinergic drugs such as clonazepam. Important in the care of an older person with schizophrenia is promotion of exercise, which not only improves physical health but also channels energy into positive outlets, thus reducing the risk of aggression.

Substance misuse

Some older people develop habitual use of freely available, prescribed or illicit substances, including alcohol, painkillers, sedatives or cannabis. Alcohol and drug use may become a coping mechanism for loss, boredom, anxiety or depression. Addictive behaviour in older adults has tended to be overlooked, but there is now greater awareness of the extent of the problem. Alcohol use tends to decline as people get older, but there is a danger of a generational cohort continuing heavier social drinking habits into old age. A survey of British older people (Hajat *et al.* 2004) showed that 5 per cent of men and 2.5 per cent of women abuse alcohol. Dar (2006) presented three main factors for alcohol abuse in older people:

- emotional (e.g. bereavement);
- medical (e.g. pain);
- practical (e.g. poverty).

It should be acknowledged that alcohol is not harmful in moderation and a whisky or gin in the evening provides relaxing pleasure to many older people; indeed, in moderation it reduces the risk of cardiovascular disease. However, excessive drinking can have deleterious effects in old age. Due to slower metabolism, older people are more prone to toxic effects, raising the risk of cognitive impairment and delirium. There is danger of interaction with medication, particularly with central nervous system suppressants. Alcohol also reduces the effectiveness of hypoglycaemic and anticoagulant drugs. The older drinker is more at risk of injury from falls. Abstinence may be an appropriate goal for a person who has got into difficulties with alcohol dependency. Vitamin supplements may be required.

Although a potentially major factor in the mental health of older people, substance misuse may not be obvious to the mental health nurse in the community. As illicit drug use has increased over recent decades, the proportion of older substance misusers is growing. Some people use cannabis and opiates for the first time in old age, either to relieve discomfort or as a means of coping with emotional adversities. Another problem in older people is excessive use of painkillers and other 'over-the-counter' drugs. Prescribed medication such as sleeping tablets may be used inappropriately. Meanwhile the ready availability of drugs on the internet enables people to bypass the regulated system of medical prescription, potentially endangering users who have no guarantee that the drugs obtained are safe. Any use of substances with a stimulant or relaxant effect on the central nervous system is problematic, and may result in serious drug interaction, overdose or addiction.

In assessing substance misuse, it is important that the nurse develops a good rapport with the older person. A candid account of drinking or drug-taking habits should be encouraged, with assurance that the nurse will remain supportive, with a commitment to working in partnership with the person rather than simply encouraging abstinence. A constructive care plan will take account of the reasons for substance misuse, and deal with any underlying issues as a problem-solving approach.

32.5   Conclusion

This chapter has covered the psychosocial challenges of ageing and the common functional mental health problems. The main points of this chapter are:

- Prevalence of mental health problems increases with age.
- Physical, emotional and social adversities contribute to depression, anxiety and substance misuse.
- Functional psychoses may arise as a new episode but there are also growing numbers of people with schizophrenia who reach old age.
- Mental health services should confront ageism and present a positive attitude to care and treatment of mental disorders in older people.

Feedback to Thinking Spaces

1. In Malcolm's case the features which could indicate depression are:
   - inactivity and weight gain;
   - social withdrawal;
   - loss of interest;
   - negative thought patterns;
   - low self-esteem;
   - sense of helplessness.

2. On assessing Maureen, this is how John formulated a care plan.

   As a problem-solving, anxiety management approach, John encourages Maureen to think rationally about her fears, challenging her beliefs about what could happen in specific situations. He intends to work on these issues with Maureen over a series of visits. Maureen agrees to attend a relaxation class run by a voluntary organization, which arranges transport by minibus. John will review her progress. He will also discuss with the multi-disciplinary team the options for psychotherapeutic and pharmacological treatment. He will consult the social worker in his team on Maureen's inadequate heating and food, although only for advice at this stage, as these problems may be directly related to Maureen's anxiety. With Maureen's agreement, John may make a referral to the continence nurse if bedwetting problems persist.

Annotated bibliography

Stuart-Hamilton, I. (2006) *The Psychology of Ageing: An introduction,* **4th edn. London: Jessica Kingsley.**
An established and accessible text that covers the broader psychological issues of ageing, with a chapter on mental disorders.

Neno, R., Aveyard, B. and Heath, H. (2007) *Older People and Mental Health Nursing: A handbook of care.* **Oxford: Blackwell.**
A practical, evidence-based guide to nursing interventions in older people with mental health problems.

Yesavage, J.A. and Brink, T.L. (1983) Development and validation of a geriatric depression screening scale: a preliminary report, *Journal of Psychiatric Research,* **17: 37–49.**
The Geriatric Depression Scale is a validated 15-item scale widely used to detect depression in older people.

Pachana, N.A., Byrne, G.J., Siddle, H., Koloski, N., Harley, E. and Arnold, E. (2007) Development and validation of the Geriatric Anxiety Inventory, *International Psychogeriatrics,* **19: 103–14.**
This instrument has good psychometric properties for use in community and institutional settings.

References

Arnold, S.E. and Trojanowski, J.Q. (1996) Cognitive impairment in elderly schizophrenia: a dementia (still) lacking distinctive histopathology, *Schizophrenia Bulletin,* 22: 5–9.

Bagley, H., Cordingley, L., Burns, A. *et al.* (2000) Recognition of depression by staff in nursing and residential homes, *Journal of Clinical Nursing,* 9: 445–50.

Baldwin RC (2002): Depressive disorders. In *Psychiatry in the Elderly* (3rd edition) (eds R Jacoby, C Oppenheimer). Oxford: Oxford University Press. 627–626.

Baldwin R, Anderson D, Black S, Evans S, Jones R, Wilson K, Iliffe S (2003): Guidelines for the management of late-life depression in primary care. *International Journal of Geriatric Psychiatry,* 18: 829–838.

Benbow SB (1989): The role of electroconvulsive therapy in the treatment of depressive illness in old age. *British Journal of Psychiatry*, 155: 147–152.

Blow FC, Oslin DW (2003): Late-life addictions. *Geriatric Psychiatry*, 22: 111–143.

Butler RN, Lewis MI, Sunderland T (1998): *Aging and Mental Health: Positive Psychosocial and Biomedical Approaches* (5th edition). Needham Heights: Allyn & Bacon.

Conwell Y, Duberstein PR (2001): Suicide in elders. *Annals of the New York Academy of Science*, 932: 132–147.

Dar, K. (2006) Alcohol use disorders in elderly people: fact or fiction? *Advances in Psychiatric Treatment*, 12: 173–81.

Erikson, E.H. (1980) *Identity and the Life Cycle*. New York: W.W. Norton.

Frankl, V. (1963) *Man's Search for Meaning*. New York: Washington Square Press.

Gabriel, Z. and Bowling, A. (2004) Quality of life from the perspectives of older people, *Ageing & Society*, 24: 675–91.

Gilhooly MLM (2005): Reduced drinking with age: is it normal? *Addiction Research & Theory*, 13: 267–280.

Hajat, S., Haines, A., Bulpitt, C. and Fletcher, A. (2004) Patterns and determinants of alcohol consumption in people aged 75 years and older: results from the MRC trial of assessment and management of older people in the community, *Age & Ageing*, 33: 170–7.

Harris, T., Cook, D.G., Victor, C., DeWilde, S. and Beighton, C. (2006) Onset and persistence of depression in older people: results from a 2-year community follow-up study, *Age & Ageing*, 35: 25–32.

Harwood DMJ, Hawton K, Hope T, Jacoby R (2001): Suicide in older people: mode of death, demographic factors, and medical contact before death. *International Journal of Geriatric Psychiatry*, 15: 736–743.

Howard R, Rabins PV, Seeman MV, Jeste DV (2000): Late-onset schizophrenia and very-late-onset schizophrenia-like psychosis: an international consensus. *American Journal of Psychiatry*, 156: 172–176.

Laidlaw, K., Thompson, L.W., Dick-Siskin, L. and Gallagher-Thompson, D. (2003) *Cognitive Behaviour Therapy with Older People*. Chichester: John Wiley.

Levin CA, Wei W, Akincigil A, Lucas JA, Bilder S, Crystal S (2007): Prevalence and treatment of diagnosed depression among elderly nursing home residents in Ohio. *Journal of the American Medical Directors Association*, 8: 585–594.

Livingston G, Hawkins A, Graham N, Blizard B, Mann A (1990): The Gospel Oak study: prevalence rates of dementia, depression and activity limitation among elderly residents in inner London. *Psychological Medicine*, 20: 137–146.

McClure, F.S., Gladsjo, J.A. and Jeste, DV. (1999) Late-onset psychosis: clinical, research and ethical considerations, *American Journal of Psychiatry*, 156: 935–40.

McCrae N, Murray J, Banerjee S, Bhugra D, Tylee A, Huxley P (2005): 'They're all depressed, aren't they?' A qualitative study of social care workers and depression in older adults. *Aging & Mental Health*, 9: 508–516.

McDougall, F.A., Matthews, F.E., Kvaal, K., Dewey, M.E. and Brayne, C. (2007) Prevalence and symptomatology of depression in older people living in institutions in England and Wales, *Age & Ageing*, 36: 562–68.

Mirandi H (2007): Assessing older people with mental health issues. In *Older People & Mental Health Nursing: a Handbook of Care*. Oxford: Blackwell.

Nathanson, C.A. (1977) Sex, illness and medical care: a review of data, theory and method, *Social Science & Medicine*, 11: 13–25.

National Institute for Health & Clinical Excellence (2009): *Depression: the Treatment and Management of Depression in Adults (update)*. www.nice.org.uk/nicemedia/live/12329/45888/45888.pdf

NICE (National Institute for Health and Clinical Excellence) (2011): *Generalised Anxiety Disorder in Adults: Management in Primary, Secondary and Community Care*, available at: www.nice.org.uk/nicemedia/live/13314/52667/52667.pdf

Osborn PJ, Fletcher AE, Smeeth L, Stirling S, Bulpitt CJ, Breeze E, Ng ESW, Nunes M, Jones D, Tulloch A (2003): Factors associated with depression in a representative sample of 14217 people aged 75 and over in the United Kingdom: results from the MRC trial of assessment and management of older people in the community. *International Journal of Geriatric Psychiatry*, 18: 623–630.

Pachana, N.A., Byrne, G.J., Siddle, H., Koloski, N., Harley, E. and Arnold, E. (2007) Development and validation of the Geriatric Anxiety Inventory, *International Psychogeriatrics*, 19: 103–14.

Rait, G., Burns, A., Baldwin, R. *et al.* (1999) Screening for depression in African-Caribbean elders, *Family Practice*, 16: 591–5.

Sinoff G, Ore L, Zlotogorosky D, Tamir A (1999): Short anxiety screening test: a brief instrument for detecting anxiety in the elderly. *International Journal of Geriatric Psychiatry*, 14: 1062–1071.

SCIE (Social Care Institute for Excellence) (2006) *Practice Guide: Assessing the mental health needs of older people*, available at: www.scie.org.uk/publications/guides/guide03/index.asp.

Tornstam, L. (1996) Gerotranscendence – a theory about maturing in old age, *Journal of Aging & Identity*, 1: 37–50.

Wilson, K.C.M., Mottram, P.G. and Vassilas, C.A. (2008) Psychotherapeutic treatments for depressed older people, *Cochrane Library*, 1.

Windle, G., Marland, D.A. and Woods, B. (2008) Examination of a theoretical model of psychological resilience in older age, *Aging & Mental Health*, 12: 285–92.

Yesavage, J.A. and Brink, T.L. (1983) Development and validation of a geriatric depression screening scale: a preliminary report, *Journal of Psychiatric Research*, 17: 37–49.

Older People with Dementia

Niall McCrae

Don't let this illness own you. It doesn't have your soul, and it doesn't have your spirit.

(Hassan)

I like this group because everyone forgets here; in my house, I'm the only one.

(Beryl)

33.1 Introduction

Hardly a day passes without another report of research on a risk factor or putative treatment for dementia, with public interest guaranteed by the realization that as we live longer, more of us are likely to succumb to this disease. Dementia has become a clinical and sociopolitical priority, with increasing resources channelled into research on its prevention, care and treatment. Historically, care of people with 'senile dementia' was regarded as a backwater of mental health nursing, but it is now a rapidly developing and exciting area of practice.

Practitioners' attitudes have shifted from therapeutic nihilism to a more positive outlook. In the UK, nurses are at the forefront in implementing the National Dementia Strategy (DH 2009), which promotes 'living well with dementia'. This chapter covers:

- the nature of the disease;
- experiences of people with dementia and their families;
- principles and practice of person-centred care;
- specific therapeutic interventions;
- ethical considerations.

Case Study

Brian

Brian, aged 78, is a retired taxi driver diagnosed with dementia four years ago. The early signs of memory loss emerged years before diagnosis, but Brian had avoided medical consultation until his wife Joan insisted on this. Recent assessment has shown steady decline in his memory. Brian mostly sits in the lounge watching television; he tries to read the newspaper but cannot concentrate. He goes out every day walking the dog with Joan. He often misplaces items and has difficulty in initiating activities, but performs tasks well when prompted – for example, making a pot of tea. Brian enjoys visits by his sons and grandchildren but is unaware of when they are due. Joan manages his medication. She reports that Brian has good and bad days, but thinks that the donepezil 'must be doing something'. Brian went to a cognitive stimulation group once but did not enjoy it. He tends to become restless and irritable in the evenings and takes a long time to get to sleep. Alison, a community mental health nurse, has visited several times but Brian never remembers who she is. Alison is focusing on the evening restlessness and suggested that this may be related to Brian having worked late in the evenings before retirement. She has suggested more fulfilling daytime activity for Brian, including a gardening club run by a voluntary organization, and a weekly reminiscence group at a nearby church. When Joan asked about sleeping tablets for Brian, Alison explained the potential adverse effects. However, she has requested a medication review by the general practitioner (GP), and will discuss the situation with Brian and Joan on her next visit.

Throughout this chapter you will be invited to consider specific issues involving Brian. At each stage you can compare your judgements with those of the author by reading the feedback at the end of the chapter.

33.2 Epidemiology, course and symptoms

Historically, the term *dementia* literally meant loss of mind, in contrast to the congenital defect of *amentia*. Chronic confusional states common in older people became known as 'senile dementia'. Although a vascular cause was long suspected, it was a discovery by Alois Alzheimer (1864–1915) that undermined the notion of dementia as a normal ageing process. In 1901 Alzheimer began to observe a 51-year-old patient at the Frankfurt Asylum with unusual behavioural symptoms, including short-term memory loss. In 1906 she died and the brain was examined. Staining techniques revealed amyloid plaques and neurofibrillary tangles. Alzheimer presented the pathology and clinical symptoms of this case of pre-senile dementia, and Emil Kraepelin, founder of the modern classification of psychiatric disorders, referred to the condition as 'Alzheimer's disease'. Although not the only form of dementia, this is becoming an umbrella term in common parlance (e.g. the Alzheimer's Society in the UK is concerned with all types of dementia).

Types of dementia

The dementias (see Table 33.1) are a group of neurodegenerative syndromes of which the main feature is cognitive impairment, most prominently featuring memory loss and confusion.

Mild cognitive impairment (MCI) is a state not clearly distinguishable from the early stage of dementia. Apart from short-term memory problems,

Table 33.1 Common types of dementia

Type	Pathology	Symptoms
Alzheimer's	Amyloidal plaques and neurofibrillary tangles	Impairments in memory (particularly short-term), language and functional ability
Vascular	Impeded oxygen supply to brain caused by infarcts	Cognitive decline with reduced ability to concentrate and communicate Weakness in limbs Loss of coordination
Lewy body	Abnormal protein deposits in neurons	Hallucinations and disorientation Short-term memory loss Slowed movement
Frontotemporal (Pick's disease)	Degeneration of frontal and temporal lobes	Socially inappropriate behaviour, personality changes and obsessional behaviour
Korsakow's	General neurodegeneration	Impaired memory, judgement and social skills Loss of balance and coordination

cognitive function is normal, with no impairment of social or occupational functioning. Evidence suggests that MCI is prodromal, with dementia arising at a rate of 10–15 per cent annually, compared with 1–2 per cent of the general population (DeKosky and Marek 2003).

Prevalence and causes

Only 1 in 20 people will develop dementia, but the numbers are rising due to demographic trends. The *Dementia UK* report (tKnapp and Prince 2007)

estimated 700,000 existing cases, with a projected increase in 30 years to 1,400,000 (see Table 33.2).

The one indisputable risk factor for dementia is age, but researchers are investigating why some older people get dementia while others retain their mental faculties. According to the National Dementia Strategy (DH 2009), 'dementias affect all in society irrespective of gender, ethnicity and class'. There is no single cause of Alzheimer's disease, but evidence is accumulating on protective or predictive factors, both in nature and nurture.

Table 33.2 Estimated prevalence of dementia in the UK (Knapp and Prince 2007)

Age	Prevalence (%)
65–69	1.3
70–74	2.9
75–79	5.9
80–84	12.2
85–89	20.3
90–94	28.6
95 +	32.5

There is probabilistic evidence of genetic suscepti-bility, specifically involving a variant of the apoliproprotein gene. Risk increases for close rela-tives of a person with dementia, but familial pre-disposition may be influenced by shared environ-mental factors. Despite little difference in post-mortem neuropathology, dementia presents less frequently in more educated people, suggesting resilience. As well as regular intellectual activity, protective lifestyle factors include social engage-ment, physical exercise and a healthy diet. The psychosocial adversity of old age, with a decline in occupational and social activity, may be contribu-tory. A longitudinal study found that dementia was more likely to develop in people with depression at baseline assessment (Saczynski *et al.* 2010). Physical health factors correlating with Alzheimer's disease include midlife obesity, hypertension and diabetes mellitus.

Vascular dementia entails multiple, random infarcts producing areas of cortical damage. As these infarcts are caused by cerebrovascular occlu-sion, there is stronger aetiological evidence related to obesity, high fat diet, hypertension, smoking, dia-betes mellitus and stroke. Korsakow's dementia is firmly linked to chronic alcohol abuse.

Younger people with dementia

Knapp and Prince (2007) reported 15,034 cases of dementia in younger people (onset before the age of 65) in the UK, but as this was based on referrals it was likely to be an underestimate. While 2 per cent of the overall population of people with dementia are of early onset, this increases to 6 per cent in black and minority ethnic groups. Alzheimer's dis-ease accounts for only a third of the cases of dementia in younger people. Having a different social context, younger people may feel marginal-ized in generic service provision.

Course and symptoms

Dementia is normally a slow, progressive condition (see Table 33.3). Although the rate of onset and pro-gression varies widely, there are general patterns of deterioration in cognitive and behavioural function-ing. Cognitive symptoms are the cardinal feature, with deficits in memory, attention, executive func-tion, language and visuospatial awareness. Memory problems are the earliest sign of Alzheimer's disease, typically revealed by forgetting appointments, repeating questions or mislaying items. Longer-term memory is retained, but amnesia gradually becomes more extensive. Difficulty in dealing with competing demands on attention and slower decision-making occur early in the disease course. Deficits in execu-tive function include impaired planning and prob-lem-solving, most noticeably in tasks requiring con-current manipulation of information. Verbal and written language become simpler in structure and disorderly, with wrong words used or nonsensical

Table 33.3 Stages of dementia

Mild stage	Moderate stage	Severe stage
■ Recent memory loss ■ Difficulty in perform-ing complex tasks ■ Decline in language skills ■ Able to mask impair-ment by avoiding chal-lenging situations ■ Depression, apathy and social withdrawal common	■ Can no longer mask condition ■ Pervasive memory loss has increasing impact on daily life ■ Rambling, irrational speech ■ Disorientation to time and place ■ Affective and behavioural disturbance ■ Mobility and coordination problems ■ Need for reminders and assis-tance with daily activities	■ General confusion ■ Loss of recognition of familiar people and places ■ Severe loss of verbal skills ■ Marked behavioural distur-bances; hallucinations and delirium ■ Worsening mobility; dysphagia; incontinence ■ Need for total nursing care ■ Death often caused by infection

ordering. Reliance on speech is replaced by nonverbal expression in later stages of dementia; some people become mute. Visuospatial deficits manifest in disorientation, difficulties in performing complex motor tasks (apraxia), and inability to recognize objects and faces (agnosia).

Behavioural and psychological problems include agitation, apathy, disinhibition, irritability, mood disorder, psychosis and aberrant motor activity. Typically, psychological symptoms emerge in the early stage, followed by a period of relative stability before the advanced stage when agitation increases. Apathy is the most common non-cognitive symptom of dementia, appearing early in the course and tending to persist. Showing reduced initiation, indifference and blunted emotional response, the person is less able to perform activities of daily living than cognitive ability would suggest. Apathy causes carer distress, often being misinterpreted as laziness or stubbornness. Depression frequently coexists with dementia, exacerbating cognitive impairment. Anxiety is also common. People with dementia sometimes behave aggressively, which may be due to fear, humiliation or frustration; another cause is psychosis, which often occurs in the early stage. A review showed that delusions occur in 36 per cent and hallucinations in 18 per cent of people with Alzheimer's disease (Ropacki and Jeste 2005). Persecutory delusions (perceived theft, harm or intrusion) are most common. Hallucinations are a bad prognostic sign, correlating with rapid cognitive decline, early institutionalization and increased mortality. Cerebral damage often leads to socially inappropriate behaviour such as uncharacteristic profanity, rudeness, undressing in public, staring at strangers or inappropriate sexual advances. Disinhibition typically arises in the moderate stage of Alzheimer's disease, but may be an early presenting feature of frontotemporal dementia.

Terminal stage

Dysphagia is common in the late stage of dementia due to neurodegenerative suppression of the

> **Thinking Space 33.1**
>
> Where would you place Brian on this trajectory? Note that the three stages are not discrete, and that a person may be functioning well in some areas while deteriorating in others. A person apparently on the cusp of transition to the next stage may be said to be 'mild-to-moderate' or 'moderate-to-severe'.

swallowing reflex. A potential complication is aspiration pneumonia. The dysphagic person needs more frequent, lighter meals, with care taken to prevent food entering the airway. A common cause of death in dementia is pneumonia or gastrointestinal infection. Influenza is highly infectious, with 50 per cent higher mortality in people with dementia than expected by age group. Morbidity and mortality from respiratory infection is higher in care homes due to a generally frail population, excessive use of antibiotics and rapid transmission of pathogens. Isolation is not feasible, but resilience may be boosted by diet and exercise.

33.3　Assessment and diagnosis

Early diagnosis is a priority of the National Dementia Strategy, which urges radical change to conventional assessment practice. Asserting that 'diagnosis is the gateway for care', the strategy recommends specialist input from the outset. Benefits of early diagnosis are as follows:

- enables the person and family maximum time to adapt to changing circumstances and plan for the future;
- financial and legal matters can be managed while the person retains cognitive abilities;
- interventions in the early stage can prolong premorbid level of functioning;
- early engagement in support networks;

- building an effective partnership with health and social care agencies;
- opportunity to participate in clinical trials of treatments for dementia.

However, many people with cognitive impairment do not seek consultation until symptoms are pronounced. The person may be unaware of a gradual decline in ability, attribute memory problems to old age, or be in fear or denial. Carers have an important role: in our case study, Brian was coaxed by his wife to see the doctor. Some people living alone may not get help until a crisis. Dementia can also be missed by clinicians, partly because it varies considerably in initial presentation. Until recently dementia was normally diagnosed in primary care, but concern about under-detection, reluctance in disclosure by some GPs and inadequate post-diagnosis support led to policy in favour of specialist assessment and diagnosis.

Memory clinics provide comprehensive diagnostic assessment including cognitive and neuropsychiatric testing, brain imaging and physical examination, combined with a detailed history from the person and family. Although some memory clinics allow self-referral, diagnosis relies heavily on referral by primary care, usually following brief screening assessment and blood testing to exclude other conditions. The National Dementia Strategy has been criticized for disregarding the contribution of primary care, and for supporting a relatively expensive assessment process (Greaves and Jolley 2010). Benefits of memory clinics have been reported, but further evidence is awaited on the strengths and weaknesses of this model.

The 'three Ds'

The symptoms of dementia overlap considerably with those of two other common disorders of old age: depression and delirium. As well as low mood, apathy and social withdrawal, depression may present with delusional thought patterns and cognitive impairment (particularly memory loss). It may be difficult to differentiate depression from dementia, and the conditions often coexist: around half of people with dementia have depressive symptoms (see Chapter 32).

Confusion is a prominent feature of both dementia and delirium; respectively, these are chronic and acute confusional states. Delirium has rapid onset, with clouding of consciousness and fluctuating orientation. With prompt treatment, it is fully reversible. The range of possible causes of delirium is wide, but a leading factor is febrile disease, particularly urinary tract infection. Two-thirds of cases of delirium occur in people with dementia who may have increased neurological vulnerability. Often people with dementia fail to regain premorbid functioning following an episode of delirium. Outcomes are improved by prompt detection, which requires blood tests. Delirium is a medical emergency usually requiring hospitalization for treatment of the underlying cause, prevention of complications, nursing care and behaviour management. For further information, see the National Institute for Health and Clinical Excellence (NICE) 2010 guidelines on delirium.

Assessment process

Standardized assessment is now embedded in clinical practice. The most widely used screening instrument for dementia is the Mini Mental State Examination (MMSE; Folstein et al. 1975), which tests orientation, attention, language, short-term memory and task performance. A score of 21–26 indicates mild dementia, 11–20 moderate and 0–11 severe. Low education, poor literacy skills, cultural differences and sensory deficits are limitations to the validity of this test. Cognitive testing should contribute to comprehensive assessment: dementia should not be diagnosed by MMSE alone.

Imaging technology is a boon to diagnosis. Computerized tomography is a type of X-ray that produces high resolution cross-sectional images of the brain. Magnetic resonance imaging (MRI) works by aligning particles of the brain by magnetic force, then bombarding these with radio waves; the signal emitted differentiates the type of tissue. MRI can show shrinkage of structures in the inner brain (e.g. hippocampus, the earliest site of damage in Alzheimer's disease). Changes in brain metabolism correlating with cognitive impairment can be detected by functional MRI, which highlights areas of high oxygen and glucose consumption. Electroencephelography (EEG) shows electrical impulses typical of dementia, but is not definitive. The ultimate diagnostic test is post-mortem examination, which often reveals mixed Alzheimer's and vascular neuropathology.

Assessment serves not only diagnosis but also individualized care planning. A tool for assessing behavioural symptoms is the Neuropsychiatric Inventory (Cummings *et al.* 1994), which measures delusions, hallucinations, mood problems, anxiety, agitation, disinhibition, irritability, apathy, movement disorders, appetite and sleep problems. The Bristol Activities of Daily Living Scale (Bucks *et al.* 1996) is one of several instruments for assessing everyday skills in dementia (including mobility, feeding, dressing, bathing and using the toilet), rated by the primary carer. Life history is a major component of assessment. As well as providing important information for assessment, such enquiry ensures a focus on the person rather than the disease.

The manner of assessing is important: a person who feels depersonalized and disempowered may not display their optimal ability. He or she should be informed of what will happen during and after assessment. Careful consideration should be given to how information or questions are presented to a person with cognitive impairment, including sensitivity to cultural differences. Simple but effective communication is required, as well as patience in allowing time for comprehension and response.

Disclosure of diagnosis

Research has revealed inconsistent practice in disclosing a diagnosis of dementia (Bamford *et al.* 2004), with many physicians reluctant to inform patients due to likelihood of distress, or perceived inability to understand the diagnosis. Although some carers wish to withhold the diagnosis, most people

with dementia prefer to be told. Furthermore, patients have a right to this information. Emotional distress sometimes arises in response to diagnosis, which may manifest as shock, intense sadness, anger (often directed at self), fear about getting into difficult situations, a sense of loss of identity, and anxiety about the future. However, most people do not display extreme emotional reactions to diagnosis of dementia. Ideally diagnosis should be disclosed by a practitioner with whom the person will have ongoing contact, and should be regarded as a process rather than an event. Post-diagnosis support should include information (on the condition, care and treatment options, and community resources), advice on getting help with future living arrangements and financial affairs, and emotional support (through individual or group sessions). Family carers also face an emotional challenge in coping with a diagnosis of dementia, with Laakkonen *et al.* (2008) finding that 68 per cent developed depressive symptoms. Carers can respond positively by accepting the diagnosis, grieving the loss of lifestyle rather than the person, being realistic about the relationship, and preparing to communicate on a different level.

33.4 Experience of dementia

Until recently professional discourse on dementia was dominated by neuropathology and attribution of all aberrant cognition and behaviour to an underlying disease process. Pessimism was illustrated in book titles such as *Alzheimer's Disease: Coping with a living death* (Woods 1989), but since the seminal work of Tom Kitwood in the 1990s, a more positive approach has emerged. Kitwood's (1997) person-centred philosophy is now at the heart of policy, with acknowledgement that personal and social factors have much influence on the experience and course of dementia.

Impact of the social environment

Kitwood (1997) asserted that people with dementia have a right to meaningful relationships based on understanding, sharing, collaboration, equality, dignity, trust and respect. Social interactions and relationships have a significant impact on quality of life, but these may be tainted by negative attitudes towards dementia. Due to perceived lack of rational judgement and autonomy, the person may be stripped of roles and responsibilities regardless of retained abilities. Kitwood coined the term 'malignant social psychology', describing seventeen common attitudes and behaviours towards a person with dementia:

1. Treachery
2. Disempowerment
3. Infantalization
4. Intimidation
5. Labelling
6. Stigmatization
7. Outpacing
8. Invalidation
9. Banishment
10. Objectification
11. Ignoring
12. Imposition
13. Withholding
14. Accusation
15. Disruption
16. Mockery
17. Disparagement

Malignant social psychology detracts from personhood, which Kitwood (1997) defined as 'a standing or status that is bestowed upon one human being, by others in the context of relationship and social being'.

Coping with cognitive impairment

People with dementia face mounting challenges in sustaining their lifestyle prior to diagnosis. Ability to perform everyday tasks is hindered by failing memory, and the pace of life slows as activities require more thought and effort, and sense of time becomes less reliable. Communication skills deteriorate, both in expression and comprehension. Withdrawal from roles and responsibilities may be necessary, but this may reduce self-esteem. Opportunities for social interaction decline, with difficulties in attending events due to orientation problems. Friends may drift away. Feeling insecure and devalued, the person retreats to the psychological safety of home. It is understandable for people like Brian to stay in their 'comfort zone', but a life devoid of activity and social interaction ultimately contributes to decline in physical and mental functioning.

Negative feelings about having dementia are inevitable and understandable. The person may become self-reproachful for forgetfulness or failure to perform tasks, or perceive themselves as a burden to others. However, many people with dementia adapt positively. Clare (2002) categorized coping strategies as self-protective (denial, social withdrawal, minimization or normalization of memory problems) or self-adjusting (relinquishing old roles and developing new roles, accepting support, and preparing for future needs). Quality of life is subjective, and depends on various factors including personality, social circumstances and health. Ratings of people with dementia and their carers often diverge, with the latter tending towards more negative judgements. While judgement may be impaired by cognitive impairment, the perspective of the person with dementia should be respected.

Glen Campbell's story

Glen Campbell is one of the most popular country singers of all time, with worldwide hits including 'Wichita Lineman' and 'Rhinestone Cowboy'. Campbell has Alzheimer's disease, yet he continues to perform at large concert venues. His family revealed his condition in summer 2011, when Glen was aged 75. His wife Kim said:

When he goes on stage, it's just like a light switch turns on. It's really good for him to keep going. But we know at some point it's going to be time to stop . . . It's depressing to think about the future. We're not at a severe stage yet, but this thing always progresses . . . We savour every experience with him.

Asked about having dementia, Campbell says: 'I'm fine. I don't feel it. You just forget, and that's a blessing sometimes' (McCormack 2011). There is evidence that listening to music involves more areas of the brain than any other activity, and that connections to songs can be so strong that they endure in people with advanced Alzheimer's disease. Whatever the explanation, Glen Campbell shows that people with dementia can lead fulfilling lives – and continue to be themselves.

33.5 Person-centred care: from rhetoric to reality

Person-centred care emphasizes the uniqueness of the person and his or her life story, character, relationships and experience of dementia. While embraced in policy and professional training, the person-centred philosophy is not always applied in practice, where constraints include dominance of the biomedical model, risk-averse services, limited resources, routinized practice and an inadequately trained workforce.

Communication

Communication is essential to person-centred care at all stages of dementia, but services vary in this fundamental activity. Allowances must be made for cognitive impairment, but without disempowering the person. Useful tips for nurses are provided by the Alzheimer's Society (2010):

- approach the person from the front, making face-to-face contact;
- minimize distractions;
- use simple language, speaking slowly and clearly;
- repeat words if necessary, but do not shout;

- relate to the person as an adult and as a unique human being;
- allow extra time for the person to understand your message, and to respond;
- do not put pressure on the person to respond;
- use facial expressions as a supplement to verbal communication;
- do not contradict or argue with the person;
- if the patient has difficulty in remembering faces, use a familiar greeting to help with recognition;
- maintain eye contact: if the person is sitting drop to their eye level (standing over someone can be intimidating);
- a person with dementia can interpret non-verbal communication and this is a useful supplementary means of interaction;
- speak clearly and calmly, with short sentences, making one point at a time;
- do not ask questions requiring complicated answers or offering too many choices;
- processing information will take the person longer, so be patient, waiting for an answer and if necessary repeating the question;
- listen attentively;
- if the person has difficulty in finding the right words or finishing a sentence, suggest different ways of saying what was intended;
- do not let the person feel patronized.

Non-verbal expressions may be understood long after verbal communication failure. Some people retain intact and functional emotional capacity at the late stage of dementia; there is little correlation between cognitive and emotional functioning because these involve different parts of the brain. Affective signals (e.g. anger, tearfulness) may be understood by family carers or care staff as meaningful communication. Nurses should be aware of cultural differences in facial expressions, degree of eye contact, posture, proximity and touch.

Developing effective partnerships

Mike Nolan and his colleagues (2004) have argued that Kitwood's person-centred philosophy is too narrow. Their relationship-centred model prioritizes the person with dementia but also addresses the network of personal and caring relationships vital to the person's well-being and quality of life, and considers the needs of carers themselves. Services should support key relationships to promote an 'enriched environment of care'. Good relationships emerge when all parties are able to work together and appreciate each other's input. Nolan *et al.* devised the 'Six Senses Framework' as a guide for sustaining effective relationships:

- sense of security;
- sense of continuity;
- sense of belonging;
- sense of purpose;
- sense of achievement;
- sense of significance.

An excessive focus on the dyad of 'person with dementia and primary carer' neglects other family and social networks, and denies the wider impact of dementia. In a triadic relationship, people with dementia, their families and paid carers, contribute to combined expertise. Zarit *et al.* (1985) promoted a systemic approach whereby care within the family is acknowledged as a transactional process with mutual gratification. To be person-centred, care must also be relationship-centred.

Integrating physical and mental health

Kitwood's (1997) concept of personhood was based on an existential ontology that rejects mind/matter dualism. Holistic care does not mean considering physical, psychological and social needs in parallel, but regarding mind and body as *one*. Inextricably, a healthy mind serves a healthy body, and vice versa. As dementia progresses, physical health needs become more prominent, but this should not detract from person-centred care.

Diet, exercise and sleep are vital factors in health and well-being. Gradual weight loss is normal in old age, but may be marked in people with dementia due to restlessness and inadequate dietary intake. By contrast, some people with dementia become less active, and a sedentary lifestyle may lead to disability and disease. Regular exercise improves mood, self-esteem and cognitive function in people with dementia; it also prevents constipation. Disrupted sleep pattern may cause a vicious cycle, inhibiting daytime activity while causing safety risks at night. Sensory stimuli such as indoor lighting should be suppressed before and during bedtime. Sedatives may be used for acute insomnia, but may cause daytime drowsiness and confusion. People with dementia are more prone to falls and resulting hip fracture, partly due to increased sensitivity to anticholinergic drugs, which cause sedation and loss of balance. Medication should be reviewed regularly.

Thinking Space 33.2

If Brian is not interested in attending the groups or structured activities suggested by Alison, what else might he be encouraged to do to relieve his evening restlessness?

Sensory deficits exacerbate cognitive impairment. Eye care is often neglected in people with dementia (McKeefry and Bartlett 2010). Hearing loss may not be detected if lack of interaction is attributed to dementia. Spectacles and hearing aids are often not worn by people with dementia due to impairments in memory and manual dexterity. Care staff should remind and assist people to use their sensory aids, which are not only functional but also symbols of identity.

Care settings

Wherever dementia care occurs, practitioners should endeavour to nurture equitable and enabling partnerships; this requires an ethos of power-sharing, negotiation, cooperation, openness and respect.

Living at home

Two-thirds of people with dementia live at home. Policy promotes this, because it is generally preferred by the person with dementia and their family, while also reducing health and social care expenditure. Cohabitant carers play a major role: people with dementia living alone are 20 times more likely to move into residential care. Supporting the person at home entails adapting to changing needs, and a compromise between minimizing risk and maximizing independence.

People with dementia and their carers have informational, instrumental and emotional needs. The Care Needs Assessment Pack for Dementia (McWalter *et al.* 1998) is a tool for systematic assessment of people living at home, comprising seven domains:

1. Health and mobility
2. Self-care and toileting
3. Social interaction
4. Thinking and memory
5. Behaviour and mental state
6. Housework
7. Community living

Occupational therapists have expertise in assessing functional ability, and in fitting appropriate equipment including mobility and safety aids (e.g. hand rails, signs on doors, cooker safety switches), and assistive technology (e.g. electronic prompt for meals and medication). An infra-red beam emitter can detect movement at night, automatically switching lights on and alerting the family carer. The front door can be linked to a call centre, and tracking devices can locate the person if lost. Hints on assistive technology are provided in a guide for family carers by the Dementia Services Development Centre at the University of Stirling (2010). Such tools work best if they are reliable and unobtrusive, and the person with dementia and their carer are motivated to use them.

The Alzheimer's Society (2011) makes six policy recommendations for supporting people with dementia in the community:

1. Concerted effort to support people with dementia to live independently at home and avoid unnecessary admission to long-term care.
2. Commissioners to consider and engage a wide range of health and social care resources.
3. Better support for family carers.
4. Joint-working across health and social care to become the norm.
5. Standards of care to be raised by expanded sharing of good practice.
6. Support for home care workers in providing effective care in the community.

Hospital

Many people with dementia have physical comorbidity. In a survey by Sampson *et al.* (2009) of 617 older people admitted to general hospital, 42 per cent had dementia (of which only half were diagnosed prior to admission). Urinary tract infection and pneumonia are common causes of admission. Hospital can be disorientating and frightening for the person with dementia, whose behaviour may be difficult to manage. People with dementia have more likelihood of complications. Following reports of malnutrition and dehydration, additional training in dementia for nurses and health care assistants may be indicated, although the Care Quality Commission (CQC) (2011) saw lack of compassion as the main cause of neglect; this may reflect negative attitudes towards older people compounded by the stigma of dementia. Dementia is a strong factor in 'bed blocking' by older patients, potentially contributing to functional decline. Discharge planning should begin on admission, involving the person with dementia, family and care providers. Supporting people with dementia to leave hospitals one week earlier would save up to £80 million annually in the UK (Alzheimer's Society 2009).

Care homes

Knapp and Prince (2007) estimated there were 21,5000 people with dementia living in residential and nursing care homes in England, where they constitute a high proportion of residents: approximately 88 per cent in facilities for the elderly mentally ill and 74 per cent in other care homes (Macdonald and Cooper 2007). A steady shift from the state to private sector has continued since the 1980s, but many private homes have closed in recent years, creating a dilemma of increasing demand and reducing resource. Sadly, reports of unsatisfactory standards arise frequently in care homes, with degrading standards reinforced by poor management and low morale, in turn leading to behavioural problems and excessive use of antipsychotic medication.

Care homes are regulated by the Care Standards Act 2000, with a formal inspection regime. The NICE Quality Standards Programme promotes quality assurance, which encompasses the experience of care as well as structures, resources and procedures. As Gibson et al. (2010) have argued, the focus in long-term care settings should be on quality of life, for which indicators include social interaction among residents and between staff and residents, family involvement, and sustaining personal identities. The National Dementia Strategy gives explicit guidelines for improving standards in care homes:

- identification of a senior staff member to develop and implement a quality improvement strategy;
- reduced use of antipsychotic medication;
- commissioning of in-reach by community mental health teams and primary care;
- readily available guidance for staff on best practice in dementia care.

Respite care

Respite care can provide welcome relief for the primary carer. However, such provision has tended to neglect the perspective of the person with dementia, for whom temporary relocation may be upsetting, possibly exacerbating deterioration in functioning. Evidence for respite care is inconclusive, but brief, planned respite may contribute to sustaining a caring relationship, enabling the person with dementia to remain at home for longer.

Thinking Space 33.3

If Brian's wife began to suffer from stress caused by her caring situation, such that she was expressing doubts about Brian continuing to stay at home, would a period of respite care be appropriate? Consider the pros and cons for Brian and his wife.

33.6 Therapeutic interventions

Pharmacological treatments

Antidementia drugs arose from an observation that pharmacological suppression of the neurotransmitter acetylcholine causes confusion. A reduction in acetylcholine is observed in post-mortem brain examination in Alzheimer's disease, correlating with cognitive impairment. Treatment is aimed at acetylcholinesterase, an enzyme that breaks down acetylcholine in the cerebral cortex. Acetylcholinesterase inhibitors (donepezil, rivastigmine and galantamine) were introduced in the 1990s. Cholinergic depletion is not the only cause of cognitive impairment in Alzheimer's disease. Another treatment is memantine, which reduces the neurotoxic effects of excessive release of the neurotransmitter glutamate. Cholinergic deficits also appear in vascular and Lewy body dementias, but not in frontotemporal dementia.

Trials show a positive response to antidementia drugs in around 40 per cent of cases, but up to 80 per cent in clinical practice, possibly exaggerated by a placebo effect. Antidementia drugs are expensive, although costs may be mitigated by reduced demand on services and delayed institutionalization. In 2005, NICE recommended antidementia drugs for the moderate stage only, while awaiting more evidence of cost-effectiveness. Campaign groups expressed concern that people would not seek help if treatment was withheld. Responding to further evidence and public and professional pressure, NICE (2011) revised its guidance, recommending antidementia drugs for all stages, prescribed by a specialist following full neuropsychiatric assessment. Meanwhile, promising results have emerged from trials of concentrated vitamin B supplements, particularly in people with high blood levels of the amino acid homocysteine, a factor that may raise the risk of Alzheimer's disease fourfold. Compared to donepezil, vitamin B tablets appear at least as effective with minimal side-effects and low cost.

Antipsychotic drugs were until recently the standard treatment for agitation and aggression in dementia, despite limited evidence. Of the various conventional and atypical antipsychotic drugs, risperidone was found most effective, but with only modest benefits (Ballard and Howard 2006). Typically prescribed in care homes on a discretional *pro re nata* basis, antipsychotic medication has been described as a 'chemical cosh' (Bullock 2005), with side-effects including sedation, extrapyramidal symptoms and falls, and toxic drug interactions. Such medication is also likely to exacerbate cognitive decline. Due to increased risk of stroke, the UK Committee on Safety of Medicines (2004) decreed that risperidone and olanzapine should not be used for agitation in dementia. An independent review for the Department of Health (DH) (Banerjee and Wittenberg 2009) estimated 180,000 people with dementia taking antipsychotic drugs, to which was attributed a high incidence of cardiovascular problems and an excess of 1,800 deaths per year. Antipsychotic medication may be justifiable in preventing harm to self or others, but only as a short-term intervention following risk-benefit assessment.

Psychosocial therapies

Amidst concern about the effectiveness and toxicity of drug treatment, psychosocial therapies are recommended as front-line treatments for dementia (NICE/SCIE 2006). Claimed benefits for the wide range of psychosocial interventions include reduction in symptoms, improved mood, slower cognitive decline, sustained activities of daily living and better quality of life for the person with dementia and their carer.

Reality orientation aims to improve cognitive functioning by enhancing awareness of time, place and people. It is delivered as structured group sessions, and as ongoing reinforcement in care homes with a prominent orientation board showing information such as the date, weather and scheduled activities. Erroneous beliefs or memory lapses are corrected. It has been criticized for emphasizing impairment and unnecessary confrontation. A Cochrane review showed modest benefits (Spector *et al.* 2000).

Reminiscence therapy engages people in discussion about their past experiences. Typically conducted in a group setting, it uses prompts such as photographs, familiar items and music. A Cochrane review showed some evidence of improved cognition, mood, social engagement and well-being (Woods *et al.* 2005), however there is danger in raising unresolved emotional trauma from the past.

Validation therapy is a communicative strategy devised by Naomi Feil (1993) for people in the moderate to severe stage of disorientation. It focuses on the underlying meaning of verbal and emotional expression. In a group format, topics for discussion are chosen to share common feelings, such as a sense of loss. By verbalizing thoughts and having these acknowledged, members may feel better understood and accepted. A criticism is its concern with deeper meaning rather than the current situation. A Cochrane review indicated a reduction in behavioural and psychological symptoms, but studies were of small samples (Neal and Barton-Wright 2003).

Cognitive stimulation therapy (CST) entails various interventions, usually as group sessions, to improve memory and cognitive functioning. It draws on elements of reality orientation but with more flexibility and sensitivity. The NICE/SCIE guidelines on dementia care (2006) state that people with mild to moderate dementia should be offered a cognitive stimulation programme. Compared with usual care, recipients score significantly better in cognition, mood, behavioural disturbance and quality of life.

Behaviour therapy is useful in tackling stereotypical behaviours. For optimal effect, behavioural programmes require skilled assessment and consistent implementation. Antecedents, behaviour and consequences are assessed to determine triggers and reinforcements. Interventions should reinforce desired behaviour, taking account of the person's perspective.

Other therapeutic interventions with some evidence of cognitive or behavioural benefits include music therapy, art therapy activities such as dancing or walking groups, aromatherapy, sensory stimulation and doll therapy. As each therapeutic activity will suit some people more than others, a range of options should be available.

Limited evidence of efficacy for psychosocial interventions does not mean lack of efficacy. A problem in evaluation is inconsistent application: unlike drugs, psychosocial therapies cannot be fully standardized. As care workers are the instrument, training and resources are determinants of availability, process and outcome. Stronger support has emerged from qualitative research, showing facilitators and barriers to successful interventions:

Facilitators

- Intervention tuned to individual needs and preferences
- Reassurance and encouragement by staff
- Family involvement
- Flexibility with delivery (pace, complexity)

Barriers

- Lack of time/understaffing
- Prioritization of physical over psychological needs
- Staff dislike activity; not perceived as their job

Thinking Space 33.4

Brian has been offered psychosocial interventions. He declined to continue with a CST group, but are there other structured therapies that he might find helpful?

Interventions for carers

Despite a right to assessment under the Carers (Recognition & Services) Act 1995, two-thirds of family carers do not have their needs assessed (National Audit Office 2007). *Carers at the Heart of 21st Century Families and Communities* (DH 2008) urges services to support carers in maintaining a healthy and fulfilling lifestyle. A wide range of interventions has been devised for carers of people with dementia, including social support, advice and training to improve behaviour management and coping skills. Promoted by the National Dementia Strategy, there is a prima facie case for such activity, but evidence is fragmentary due to the diversity of interventions and outcome measures, and small-scale studies of limited generalizability. Meta-analysis by Thompson *et al.* (2007) produced tentative evidence that psycho-educational group interventions enhance carers' psychological well-being. Victor (2009) found that education improves knowledge but is less effective in changing carers' behaviour.

33.7 Ethical considerations

According to the Nuffield Council for Bioethics (2009), ethical problems arise frequently in the day-to-day care of people with dementia, and while policies and guidelines inform practice, critical judgement is necessary for decisions to be made in a flexible and compassionate way. While as a general principle practitioners should tell the truth, there are situations where this might detract from a person's well-being. It could be wrong to tell a partial truth in one situation but right in another similar situation, due to a difference in context. Without being prescriptive, the Nuffield report provides an ethical framework for the dilemmas in caring for a person with dementia. Ethical issues more generally are discussed in Chapter 11.

Safeguarding

Abuse is a major issue in dementia. It may be inflicted on the carer by the person with dementia, or vice versa; it could also be reciprocal. Abuse can take various forms: physical, sexual, emotional, financial or neglect. The person with dementia is also vulnerable to discrimination or teasing. Actions such as locking a person in a room indefinitely, violence or financial extortion are plainly wrong, if not criminal. However, there are many situations where the lack of capacity and behaviour of a person with dementia blur the boundaries of what is acceptable. For example, is it abusive for a loving husband of a woman with established dementia to persist with sexual intercourse? A general principle of consent may apply, but it cannot be assumed that a spouse is able to make a sound judgement. There is neither a legal right to sex, nor a liability to prove consent. Sometimes carers will act in ways that may seem harsh, but are doing so in the best interests of the person with dementia. The nurse should always be aware of the possibility of abuse in the domestic or institutional setting, being watchful of changes in behavior, appearance or mood, and enabling the person with dementia to express concern about his or her treatment. Detection of abuse is enhanced by good communication skills and the nurturing of a relationship based on trust. See the leaflet by Action on Elder Abuse (www.elderabuse.org.uk).

End of life care

Perhaps the most contentious ethical issue in dementia is about how and when to die. While many people with dementia would prefer to die in dignity at home, a high proportion of deaths occur in an impersonal, hospital environment. Admission to hospital in the terminal stage of illness should be avoided wherever possible. However, intensive nursing care is required for the person with marked weight loss, incontinence, constipation, lack of mobility and feeding difficulty, compounded by confusion. Pain may be inadequately detected and treated, particularly as standard pain assessment tools have limitations in advanced dementia. Good palliative care follows the principles of person-centred care, with the best possible quality of life maintained until death. This requires skill in managing discomfort and distress. Dementia practitioners have specialist expertise in communicating with people with advanced dementia and managing behavioural and psychological symptoms of the illness, but palliative care specialists should be consulted for instruction and support. The decision to replace active treatment with palliative care can be difficult and raises practical, ethical and emotional issues that necessitate an active dialogue between the care team and family carers. Early detection of deterioration of a person's condition can avert a crisis. If a decision is made for hospital admission, the person's beliefs and preferences should be documented; care home workers get to know the values, hopes and expectations of family carers over time, and will be in a good position to provide such information. Ideally a palliative care pathway should be implemented, with the agreement of the family, and in a flexible, sensitive manner. Cardiopulmonary resuscitation is rarely successful in severe dementia and may cause unnecessary trauma.

The person with dementia may have stated his or her preference for end of life care in an advance directive under the Mental Capacity Act (MCA), which care staff must follow (see Chapter 10). An advance directive cannot be made for life to be ended, or to refuse basic care. Refusal of life-sustaining treatment must be in writing, signed by a witness, and verified by a statement saying that it is to apply to the specified treatment even if life is at risk. If any practitioner is unwilling to comply with the terms of the advance directive, management of the patient's care should be transferred to another practitioner. A clinician does not incur liability for treating or not treating a patient, unless an advance directive is ignored. In the absence of an advanced directive, family carers can face difficult decisions in pressurized circumstances. Common decisions relate to the use of feeding tubes, catheters, antibiotics, investigative procedures and interventions, and whether to transfer the person to hospital in a terminal condition.

While assisted suicide and euthanasia are illegal in the UK (regardless of capacity), anyone may decide to end his or her life. Influential figures such as author Terry Pratchett and philosopher Peter Singer argue that people with dementia lack the means for suicide, and should therefore be offered a medically-assisted death. Medical ethicist Baroness Warnock has argued that dementia sufferers have a 'duty to die' as they are consuming resources for a hopeless condition (Doughty 2008). The notion of people with dementia being merely a burden provoked ire. However, society appears divided on this issue. Perhaps the focus should shift from the outcome to the process of terminal care. Hertogh et al. (2007) argued for better alleviation of suffering through improved palliative care: the aim is life without suffering, not life without dementia. People often make comments such as 'If I ever get dementia, please put me out of my misery', but research shows that people in the later stages of dementia continue to have enjoyment in their lives. A sense of self exists even in the advanced stage of dementia.

33.8 Conclusion

In summary, the main learning points from this chapter are:

- Dementia is a disease of slow progression.
- People with the condition may lead a fulfilling life by adapting to change in circumstances, with support from family and/or professional carers.
- Nurses should display a positive attitude to dementia, following the principles of person-centred care.
- The most important role of the practitioner is to build an effective therapeutic partnership with the person and his or her family, and to promote optimal autonomy and quality of life at every stage.
- Specific therapeutic interventions include medication and psychosocial therapies.
- Various ethical challenges arise in dementia care: nurses should understand and adhere to the legal framework, always acting in the person's best interests.

Feedback to Thinking Spaces

1. Brian appears to be graduating from the mild to moderate stage of dementia. His memory deficits have become more obvious, with adverse impact on his functioning. Behavioural disturbance and sleep problems have emerged, albeit manageable. However, Brian is able to prepare a pot of tea, which indicates that he retains cognitive capacity and coordination for complex tasks. There is no marked disorientation to time and place. With a regular routine and support from his wife and the community nurse, Brian may be able to function at around the current level for some time yet.

2. As Alison has observed, Brian was previously active in the evenings and he may be restless due to inadequate daytime activity. Like some other older people (particularly men) he may not appreciate therapeutic discussion groups. Practical activity such as a gardening group may be more suitable, but the company may not be to Brian's taste. He may prefer to be more active in his own environment, perhaps by resuming past hobbies or interests. Tending the garden at home, going for longer walks one or two days per week, or alternating the venue of family visits may be helpful. As always, choice should be emphasized, but encouragement and support may also be necessary.

3. While it may be possible to delay deterioration in Brian's functioning by maintaining a supportive environment, inevitably the dementia will worsen over time. Feeling appreciated for one's efforts is important, but eventually carers will need greater support from health and social services. Carers may be reassured that they will not become overwhelmed by the stress of their role. A period of respite may help to sustain the caring relationship, affording Joan a break from her ongoing responsibilities. She may make use of the time to engage with her social network, or simply to relax and enjoy a good rest. However, Brian may find the strange environment of the care home unsettling, and this may have adverse impact on his cognitive functioning. But he too may benefit from a brief interlude from the day-to-day stress at home, and on returning home he and Joan may be more appreciative of each other's company.

4. An important point about CST is that it is not a single, structured method but a range of interventions to maintain or enhance cognitive functioning. The purpose of CST should be explained to Brian and his wife, with various options considered. It may be possible to apply elements of CST in the home, as a regular activity with Joan's encouragement. Another potentially beneficial activity for Brian is life story work, whereby he would build a narrative of his life, with reflections aided by photographs, documents, souvenirs, music, etc.

Annotated bibliography

Downs, M. and Bowers, B. (2008) *Excellence in Dementia Care: Research into practice.* **Maidenhead: Open University Press.**
A comprehensive guide for dementia care, with a strong person-centred theme throughout chapters by experts in the field.

DH (Department of Health) (2009) *Living Well with Dementia: A national strategy*. **London: Department of Health.**
A positive approach to dementia, albeit selective in emphasis, with more on assessment and drug treatment than on nursing care. Freely available from the DH website.

Stuart-Hamilton, I. (2006) *The Psychology of Ageing: An Introduction*, **4th edn. London: Jessica Kingsley.**
An established and accessible text that covers the broader psychological issues of ageing, placing dementia and delirium in context.

References

Alzheimer's Society (2009) *Counting the Cost: Caring for people with dementia on hospital wards*, available at: www.alzheimers.org.uk.
Alzheimer's Society (2010) *Top Tips for Nurses: Communication*, available at: www.alzheimers.org.uk.
Alzheimer's Society (2011) *Support, Stay, Save: Care and support of people with dementia in their own homes*, available at: www.alzheimers.org.uk.
Ballard, C. and Howard, R. (2006) Neuroleptic drugs in dementia: benefits and harm, *Nature Reviews Neuroscience*, 7: 492–500.

Bamford, C., Lamont, S., Eccles, M., Robinson, L., May, C. and Bond, J. (2004) Disclosing a diagnosis of dementia: a systematic review, *International Journal of Geriatric Psychiatry*, 19: 151–69.

Banerjee, S. and Wittenberg, R. (2009) Clinical and cost effectiveness of services for early diagnosis and intervention in dementia, *International Journal of Geriatric Psychiatry*, 24: 748–54.

Bucks, R.S., Ashworth, D.L., Wilcock, G.K. and Siegfried, K. (1996) Assessment of activities of daily living in dementia: development of the Bristol Activities of Daily Living Scale, *Age & Ageing*, 25: 113–20.

Bullock, R. (2005) Drug treatment in dementia, in S. Curran and R. Bullock (eds) *Practical Old Age Psychopharmacology: A multi-professional approach*. Abingdon: Radcliffe.

Clare, L. (2002) We'll fight it as long as we can: coping with the onset of Alzheimer's disease, *Aging & Mental Health*, 6: 139–48.

Committee on Safety of Medicines (2004) *Atypical Antipsychotics and Stroke*, available at: www.mca.gov.uk.

CQC (Care Quality Commission) (2011) *Dignity and Nutrition for Older People*, available at: www.cqc.org.uk.

Cummings, J.L., Mega, M., Gray, K., Rosenberg-Thompson, S., Carusi, D.A. and Gornbein, J. (1994) The Neuropsychiatric Inventory: comprehensive assessment of psychopathology in dementia, *Neurology*, 44: 2308–14.

DeKosky, S.T. and Marek, K. (2003) Looking backward to move forward: early detection of neurodegenerative disorders, *Science*, 302: 830–4.

Dementia Services Development Centre (2010) *10 Helpful Hints for Dementia Design at Home: Practical design solutions for carers living at home with someone who has dementia*. Stirling: University of Stirling.

DH (Department of Health) (2008) *Carers at the Heart of the 21st Century Families and Communities: A caring system on your side, a life of your own*. London: DH.

DH (Department of Health) (2009) *Living Well with Dementia: A national strategy*. London: DH.

Doughty, S. (2008) Old people with dementia have a duty to die and should be pushed towards death says Baroness Warnock, *Daily Mail*, 20 September.

Feil, N. (1993) *The Validation Breakthrough: Simple techniques for communication with people with Alzheimer's-type dementia*. Baltimore, MD: Health Professions Press.

Folstein, M.F., Folstein, S.E. and McHugh, P.R. (1975) 'Mini-mental state': a practical method for grading the cognitive state of patients for the clinician, *Journal of Psychiatric Research*, 12: 189–98.

Gibson, M.C., Carter, M.W., Helmes, E. and Edberg, A-K. (2010) Principles of good care for long-term care facilities, *International Psychogeriatrics*, 22: 1072–83.

Greaves, I. and Jolley, D. (2010) National Dementia Strategy: well-intentioned – but how well founded and how well directed? *British Journal of General Practice*, 60: 193–8.

Hertogh, C.M.P.M., de Boer, M.E., Droes, E. and Eefsting, J.A. (2007) Would we rather lose ourselves than lose our self? Lessons from the Dutch debate on euthanasia for patients with dementia, *American Journal of Bioethics*, 7: 48–56.

Kitwood, T. (1997) *Dementia Reconsidered: The person comes first*. Buckingham: Open University Press.

Knapp, M. and Prince, N. (2007) *Dementia UK*. London: Alzheimer's Society.

Laakkonen, M.L., Raivio, M.M., Eloniemi-Sulkava, U. *et al.* (2008) How do elderly spouse care givers of people with Alzheimer's disease experience the disclosure of dementia diagnosis and subsequent care? *Journal of Medical Ethics*, 34: 427–30.

Macdonald, A. and Cooper, B. (2007) Long-term care and dementia services: an impending crisis, *Age & Ageing*, 36: 16–22.

McCormack, N. (2011) The quiet courage of Glen Campbell, *Daily Telegraph*, 20 October 2011.

McKeefry, D. and Bartlett, R. (2010) *Improving Vision and Eye Health Care to People with Dementia*, available at: www.pocklington-trust.org.uk.

McWalter, G., Toner, H., McWalter, A., Eastwood, J., Marshall, M. and Turvey, T. (1998) A community care needs assessment: the Care Needs Assessment Pack for Dementia (CareNAPD) – its development, reliability and validity, *International Journal of Geriatric Psychiatry*, 13: 16–22.

Neal, M. and Barton-Wright, P. (2003) Validation therapy for dementia, *Cochrane Database of Systematic Reviews*, 3. CD00(1394).

NICE (National Institute for Health and Clinical Excellence) (2010) *Delirium: diagnosis, prevention and management*, available at: www.nice.org.uk.

NICE (National Institute for Health and Clinical Excellence) (2011) *Alzheimer's Disease: Donepezil, galantamine, rivastigmine and memantine (review)*, available at: guidance.nice.org.uk.

NICE/SCIE (National Institute for Health and Clinical Excellence/Social Care Institute for Excellence) (2006) *Dementia: Supporting people with dementia and their carers in health & social care*, available at: www.scie.org.uk.

Nolan, M.R., Davies, S., Brown, J., Keady, J. and Nolan, J. (2004) Beyond 'person centred care': a new vision for gerontological nursing, *International Journal of Older People's Nursing*, 13: 45–53.

Nuffield Council for Bioethics (2009) *Dementia: Ethical issues*, available at: www.nuffieldbioethics.org.

Ropacki, S.A. and Jeste, D.V. (2005) Epidemiology of and risk factors for psychosis of Alzheimer's disease: a review of 55 studies published from 1990 to 2003, *American Journal of Psychiatry*, 162: 2022–30.

Saczynski, J.S., Beiser, A., Seshadri, S., Auerbach, S., Wolf, P.A. and Au, R. (2010) Depressive symptoms and risk of dementia, *Neurology*, 75: 35–41.

Sampson, E.L., Blanchard, M.R., Jones, L., Tookman, A. and King, M. (2009) Dementia in the acute hospital: prospective cohort study of prevalence and mortality, *British Journal of Psychiatry*, 195: 61–6.

Spector, A., Orrell, M., Davies, S. and Woods, N. (2000) *Reality Orientation for Dementia, Cochrane Library*, 4.????

Thompson, C.A., Spilsbury, K., Hall, J., Birks, Y., Barnes, C. and Adamson, J. (2007) Systematic review of information and support interventions for caregivers of people with dementia, *BMC Geriatrics*, 7: 18.

Victor, E. (2009) *A Systematic Review of Interventions for Carers in the UK: Outcomes and explanatory evidence.* Woodford Green: Princess Royal Trust for Carers.

Woods, B., Spector, A., Jones, C., Orrell, M. and Davies, S. (2005) Reminiscence therapy for dementia, *Cochrane Database of Systematic Reviews*, 18. CD00(1120).

Woods, R.T. (1989): *Alzheimer's Disease: Coping with a living death.* London: Souvenir Press.

Zarit, S.H., Orr, N.K. and Zarit, S.M. (1985) *The Hidden Victims of Alzheimer's Disease: Families under stress.* New York: New York University Press.

Chapter 34

The Person with a Diagnosis of Psychosis or Schizophrenia

Jacqueline Sin

Schizophrenia changed my life and that of my family. There's still no cure for it, the medication only helps to a certain extent with a lot of trade-off in side-effects. Over the years, I had to deal with a few breakdowns and learn to live with it even though I take the medication regularly. The hardest thing of all is to get on with my life as there's not much help out there for my recovery like finding something to do, making friends who won't shun me, other than for my symptoms to be sure I won't cause trouble for myself and others.

(A service user in his 30s)

 ## 34.1 Introduction

Schizophrenia is a major psychiatric disorder (or cluster of disorders), and the most common form of psychiatric disorder which alters a person's perception, thoughts and behaviour. Given its severity and multiple domains affected by the signs and symptoms, and that its onset tends to peak in late teenage or early adulthood – a significant developmental stage for most people (WHO 1992) – the implications and impact of the illness on the person with schizophrenia and his or her family can be far-reaching. This chapter explores schizophrenia through discussion of its prevalence, common presenting problems, aetiology and theories of causation. Discussion on care and treatments in a variety of mental health care settings across the course of the illness follows, together with a case study to illustrate the impact of the illness on a young man and his family. Throughout the chapter, the relevance and applications of assessment, formulation, care planning and treatment are drawn out with reference to the case study.

In summary, this chapter covers:

- medical classification and diagnostic criteria with reference to ICD-10;
- prevalence and incidence of schizophrenia;
- common signs and symptoms;
- prognosis and recovery;
- aetiology;
- Comprehensive assessment;
- treatments;
- nursing care.

34.2 Psychosis and schizophrenia within a broad spectrum of psychological experiences

This chapter is concerned with the understanding, assessment, treatment and nursing management of what is called schizophrenia, and related psychotic disorders. Although the precise terminology used for these disorders has been debated over the years, this chapter relates particularly to those identified by the tenth edition of the *International Statistical Classification of Diseases and Related Health Problems* (ICD-10) (WHO 1992). The National Institute for Health and Clinical Excellence (NICE), the powerhouse of evidence-based treatment for health conditions across England, Wales and Northern Ireland, has explicitly categorized schizophrenia with psychosis in its latest psychosis and schizophrenia guideline (NICE 2012). This grouping is due to the considerations of their shared commonalities in service-level interventions.

'Psychosis' could be regarded as a broad category of mental health conditions that have 'psychotic' symptoms as their hallmarks. Common psychotic symptoms include: delusional thoughts and ideas (i.e. false or ungrounded beliefs); having false sensations like hearing non-existent voices or sensing strange communications; and having disordered thoughts, sometimes described as one's thoughts being 'blocked' or 'inserted/controlled' by an external forces. While these psychotic symptoms may sound alien and strange, a small degree of such experiences, especially in a transient duration, is experienced by many people.

Thinking Space 34.1

Have you ever experienced the following:

- Feeling sick and anxious with worrying thoughts that never materialized?
- Having a little voice repeating your own worries or thoughts inside your head?
- Thinking and believing that some random coincidence was full of meaning to you, and just to you?
- Having telepathic or sixth sense and being proven correct?

While it is important for us to understand how to assess and treat psychosis and schizophrenia as a severe mental illness, it is also crucial to acknowledge that all of us lie somewhere on a spectrum between mental health and illness. Psychotic symptoms on their own do not make a diagnosis or label of mental illness. The key is to understand how such experiences impact on someone's emotions, functioning and identity, especially in such a prolonged and entrenched way that the negative impact of these experiences on the individual's mental health and overall life is maintained. To differentiate normal experiences from the symptoms and presentations indicative of a severe mental illness thus requires a comprehensive assessment and reference to medical classification and diagnostic systems.

34.3 Classification and diagnostic criteria

The ICD-10 (WHO 1992) provides the contemporary diagnostic framework for schizophrenia and its related disorders. Such disorders are grouped into F20 of the ICD-10 and within this group different presentations of the illness are named with specific features, as illustrated in Table 34.1.

NICE follows the ICD-10 definition, framework and terminology of schizophrenia and its cluster of disorders in its updated guidelines for schizophrenia (NICE 2010). However, its classification also includes schizoaffective disorder, schizophreniform disorder and delusional disorders, as well as those who are receiving treatment and support from Early Intervention in Psychosis Services (EIPS) for 'early onset psychosis' or 'first episode psychosis' (DH 2001).

The diagnosis of schizophrenia and its related disorders implies a major psychiatric disorder that alters an individual's perception, thought, affect and behaviour. Despite the variations across individual presentations, ICD-10 indicates that symptoms spanning multiple domains are required to diagnose schizophrenia, as summarized in Table 34.2.

To satisfy a diagnosis of schizophrenia, ICD-10 requires that at least one diagnostic symptom from one of the domains listed as A to D in Table 34.2 should be clearly present for at least one month. ICD-10 also confirms the diagnosis if at least two of the symptoms listed as E to H have been present in a less clear manner over the same time frame. However, the diagnosis of schizophrenia should not be made if prominent mood symptoms are present, such as depression or mania.

Another seminal diagnostic system, the *Diagnostic and Statistical Manual of Mental Disorders*

Table 34.1   Summary of ICD-10 codes and subtypes of schizophrenia cluster

ICD-10 code	Diagnosis	Specific and dominant features
F20.0	Paranoid schizophrenia	This is probably the most common form of schizophrenia in which stable delusions and auditory hallucinations are prominent
F 20.1	Hebephrenic schizophrenia	This form of schizophrenia usually starts with negative symptoms experienced in late teenage years and early adulthood and tends to have a poor prognosis
F 20.2	Catatonic schizophrenia	Disturbances of movement and strange or symbolic body postures are the main abnormality
F20.3	Undifferentiated schizophrenia	This category refers to illnesses meeting the criteria for schizophrenia, but not conforming to any one of the above subtypes, or showing the features of more than one subtype
F20.4	Post-schizophrenia depression	This signifies a probably prolonged depressive illness that arises after a schizophrenic illness with some of the psychotic symptoms still being present
F20.5	Residual schizophrenia	This is a chronic stage in the development of a schizophrenic illness in which there has been clear progression from an early stage, with acute symptoms, to a later stage, with long-term, negative symptoms
F20.6	Simple schizophrenia	This is an uncommon condition in which there is slowly worsening 'odd' conduct, an inability to cope, and a decline in good behaviour
F20.8	Other schizophrenia	This subtype includes cenesthopathic schizophrenia, the presentation of which is marked and dominated by abnormal bodily sensations and schizophreniform disorder NOS (not otherwise specified).
F20.9	Schizophrenia, unspecified	

Table 34.2   Symptoms categories according to ICD-10

A	Thought echo, thought insertion or withdrawal, and thought broadcasting
B	Delusions of control, influence or passivity, delusional perception
C	Hallucinatory voices
D	Persistent delusions of other kinds that are culturally inappropriate and completely impossible, such as religious or political identity, or superhuman powers and abilities
E	Persistent hallucinations in any modality, when accompanied either by fleeting or half-informed delusions without clear affective content, or by persistent over-valued ideas, or when occurring every day for weeks or months on end
F	Breaks or interpolations in the train of thought, resulting in incoherence or irrelevant speech, or neologisms
G	Catatonic behaviour, such as waxy flexibility and stupor
H	'Negative' symptoms such as marked apathy, paucity of speech and blunting or incongruity of emotional responses

(DSM-IV) (APA 1994), ICD-10's counterpart in North America, further stipulates that there should be evidence of ongoing symptoms persisting for at least six months. Each subtype of the disorder cluster has its specification to satisfy, usually in terms of unique and dominant signs and symptoms in addition to the general criteria outlined above. For instance, ICD-10 F20.2 (catatonic schizophrenia) has a specific requirement for stupor, waxy flexibility and rigidity as a dominant clinical presentation. A diagnosis of schizophrenia should not be made if the presentation of psychosis is a first episode, however the service-level comprehensive assessment and interventions detailed in this chapter should apply for all those who are affected by psychotic symptoms (NICE 2012). Further information related to diagnostic and classification terminology of psychotic disorders can be found in the ICD-10.

There are also wide variations in the presentation, course and outcomes of schizophrenia. People who develop schizophrenia will each have their own unique combination of symptoms and experiences, the precise pattern of which is believed to be influenced by their particular circumstances and cultural background. NICE (2010) recommends that in spite of the practical requirement for diagnostic categories, mental health professionals should exercise caution to avoid making simplistic prognoses for individual service users. Wide variations in individual experience continue to fuel the ongoing controversy about whether a diagnosis of schizophrenia really represents the presence of a single underlying disorder.

 34.4   Prevalence and incidence

Over a lifetime, about 1 per cent of the population will develop schizophrenia, averaging between 0.4 and 1.4 per cent (Cannon and Jones 1996). The UK National Survey of Psychiatric Morbidity found a population prevalence of 5 per 1,000 of psychiatric disorder in people aged 16–74 years (Singleton *et al.* 2000). These figures project schizophrenia as a relatively common illness and certainly the most common form of psychotic disorder. Average rates for men and women are similar, although there is a lower female rate in late adolescence and early adulthood onset. While the average peak onset age for men in the UK is estimated as 22 years, the mean age of onset in women is about five years older, with a second smaller peak in women after the menopause (NICE 2010). Across the UK, African-Caribbean people and south Asian people have been shown to have a higher incidence of schizophrenia (Kirkbride *et al.* 2006). No definitive explanation is available for this phenomenon thus far, but the NICE update on schizophrenia (2012) urges further research and development to pro-mote cultural competence in the mental health workforce and culturally sensitive treatment practices.

Case Study

Simon

Simon is 23 years old. He is the only child of Ghazala and Aamir who emigrated from Pakistan soon after their marriage, wanting to raise their young child in England to provide him with a better education and life prospect. Simon was a very quiet child throughout his childhood. While he was good academically, he found school life difficult as he had few friends throughout his school years. His secondary school years were even more difficult because he experienced bullying from age 15 onwards. He was constantly singled out and teased as a 'geek' or 'loner with no mates'. Simon was beaten up and on two occasions stripped of his clothes when the bullies made fun of him. Simon was so frightened that he isolated himself further and did not report the incidents for fear of worrying his parents and that the bullies would cause him more trouble. Simon was accepted at university to study accountancy. However, he found university life marked with adjustment difficulties as a result of being away from home for the first time. He struggled to cope with living in shared accommodation and did not like mixing with other student residents and his classmates. There was no bullying but he made no friends among the other students who were just getting on with their own lives. One year into his degree Simon started to feel tired all the time for no good reason. He did not like attending full lecture theatres but also found tutorials difficult because he became anxious at the prospect of small group discussion. Simon spent more and more time in his room and fell behind in his academic work and attendance at classes. Consultations with the university general practitioner (GP) led to no clear diagnosis, but a suspicion of depression and chronic fatigue syndrome. After another six months with hardly any progress Simon dropped out of university and his parents took him home.

The same pattern of lethargy, depressed mood and anxiety continued for another year at home. Simon's parents grew increasingly worried and frustrated which led them to seek help from their GP. The GP explained that he could not help unless Simon came to see him in person and that he could not force Simon to take any medication against his will, even if it might help him, particularly as he was not posing any risk to himself or others.

At age 21 when Simon would have graduated from his university, he started to experience delusional ideas along with auditory hallucinations. He believed that his computer was communicating special messages to him. He became convinced that his old school mates and others he did not know at all were plotting against him, to spread news about his failures and plan ways to make his life miserable. Simon believed that these people sent messages to each other via the TV, radio and internet. He also believed that his GP was part of the conspiracy, particularly because the GP asked him all sorts of questions about his failures and routines. The relationship between Simon and his parents became more and more strained. Frequent arguments broke out whenever they tried to reason with Simon about his worries and thoughts, or encourage him to return to his studies. Over the months and years, Simon's family became increasingly isolated from their extended family and friends because they felt embarrassed and were at a loss about how to explain Simon's situation. One night, Simon trashed his bedroom and broke all the electronic appliances including his computer and TV.

34.5 Symptoms and presentations

Schizophrenia is a major psychiatric disorder (or cluster of disorders) as its symptoms alter an individual's perception, thoughts, affect and behaviour, to an extent that their basic functions, sense of individuality and self-direction are disturbed.

The symptoms of schizophrenia are broadly categorized into 'positive' and 'negative' (WHO 1992). 'Positive' symptoms are those that broadly represent symptoms of excessive, 'out of the norm' thinking, beliefs and behaviour, commonly related to delusions (false beliefs) and hallucinations (false sensations), thought disorder and behavioural disturbances such as agitation and distress. Although the nature and presentation of the hallucinations, delusions and thought disorder can vary widely from one person to the next, there are some classic and signature presentations, such as:

- **Perception disturbances:** these can take a variety of forms, for example, one's most intimate thoughts, feelings and acts are often felt to be known or shared by others, colours or sounds may seem unduly vivid or altered in quality, and irrelevant features of ordinary things may appear more important than the whole object or situation (e.g. in Simon's experiences, the way the computer screen turned on and the idiosyncratic flickers the monitor made were full of special meaning to him, despite being nothing out of the ordinary for anyone else).

- **Hallucinations:** auditory hallucinations, in verbal or non-verbal form, such as whistling or humming, are the most common type. 'Voices', in the form of a second person (i.e. the voices 'talking' directly to the individual) and commentary and/or commanding voices (i.e. the voices comment on the individual's actions/behaviour/thoughts, and/or give commands and orders for the individual's behaviour/thoughts) are a cardinal feature of schizophrenia.

- **Delusions:** false beliefs or explanations, commonly reinforced by the perceptual and hallucinatory disturbances described above. Individuals frequently jump to a conclusive belief that everyday situations possess a special, usually sinister, meaning intended uniquely for them (i.e. delusion is marked by paranoia or persecutory content or themes). Very often, natural or supernatural forces are believed to be at work to influence the afflicted individual's thoughts and actions in ways that are often bizarre and pseudo-philosophical. This often leads to never-ending but futile rationalizations of firmly-held beliefs that are, nevertheless, false.

- **Thought disorders:** various mental activities, especially thinking, can become vague, elliptical and obscure and speech can become incomprehensible. Breaks and interpolations in the train of thought are frequent, and thoughts may seem to be controlled or withdrawn by some outside agency (i.e. thought block, thought withdrawal).

'Negative symptoms' refer to a deficit or poverty in normal mental activity and its consequences – for example, feelings and drive. Their definition and exact aetiology remain mysterious although the prominence of negative symptoms in presentation, especially at onset, has been correlated to poor outcome and prognosis in the long run (Murphy et al. 2008). Andreasen (1982) defined five groups of negative symptoms:

- blunted affect – a reduced range of intensity of emotional responses;
- alogia – poverty of thought;
- avolition – loss of motivation or drive;
- anhedonia – diminished capacity to experience pleasures;
- inattention – distractibility and difficulty focusing on tasks.

These negative symptoms can appear in the prodromal, acute phase as well as the recovery or remission phases, alongside the positive symptoms or on their own.

Compared to positive symptoms, which tend to be florid and acute, negative symptoms tend to remain for longer and are identified as the most distressing and burdensome by service users and carers. Negative symptoms are often misunderstood as part of the service user's behaviour and being within their control, for which the individual can be unfairly criticized or blamed. Despite their debilitating effects, negative symptoms receive comparatively less attention in terms of treatment and support (Sin 2000).

Common co-morbid health and social issues

As the symptoms and experiences associated with schizophrenia are often widespread and distressing, the effects of the disorder can be pervasive. Schizophrenia is also commonly associated with a number of co-morbidities and secondary ill-health issues. Depression, anxiety, higher risk of suicide, alcohol and substance misuse, and an increased risk of a wide range of physical health problems especially diabetes, obesity and cardiovascular diseases are the most commonly cited co-morbid problems (NICE 2010). A European study across six countries found that over 80 per cent of adults with this diagnosis had some persistent social functioning problems, with up to 80 per cent also remaining unemployed (Thornicroft et al. 2004).

In addition to recurrent episodes and/or continuing symptoms of schizophrenia that may explain the majority of impediments brought on by the illness, a number of other reasons for these impediments are well known. According to Sartorius (2002), 'stigma remains the main obstacle to a better life for the many hundreds of millions of people suffering from mental disorders'. People diagnosed with schizophrenia still encounter prejudice, difficulties and discrimination when finding employment and feel excluded from society. Moreover, unpleasant side-effects of medication treatment, social adversity and isolation also play a part.

The word schizophrenia still carries a lot of burden and stigma with it, I don't bring it up at all as you can see people being uncomfortable with it. Even people I've known for a long time, as I'd lost friends before because of the S word, they just suddenly grew scared of you.

(A service user in her 40s)

Case Study

Simon: *Commentary*

Simon's presentation and insidious onset over a period of three years illustrate the challenges in detecting and diagnosing early onset psychosis. Simon's experiences also illustrate the wide range of symptoms commonly experienced by individuals with psychosis and the impact of the illness on all aspects of life. His prodromal period seemed to be marked by negative symptoms and depression, which may be concurrent or secondary to the psychotic experiences. The manifestation of the positive symptoms was more acute with florid paranoid delusion and hallucinations which made it difficult for Simon to engage with others. Simon became suspicious of everyone including his own parents and GP, let alone any mental health workers from local community mental health services. Simon's behaviour, in response to the delusion and hallucinations, appeared irrational and could potentially put himself and others at risk, as he did not eat or sleep well at all for weeks, and he would appear aggressive and violent to his suspected persecutors. Following intervention by police and his GP after Simon trashed his room, he was admitted to hospital for assessment and then treatment under a section of the Mental Health Act (MHA) (see Chapter 11).

Thinking Space 34.2

Try to put yourself into Simon's shoes: how does he feel? Why does he behave as he does?

Feedback

Simon may feel confused and bewildered by his own experiences – they are all so bizarre but also so real. He is feeling extremely frightened. He may also experience shame and guilt, blaming himself for letting his study and independence go and for his own behaviour and responses to his thoughts; these took him by surprise as he was never an aggressive person. He feels that nobody, even his parents, understands him and he cannot trust anyone. Loss of sleep and lack of food, together with the constant fear and prolonged solitude, has further hampered Simon's rationality. Remember the reflective exercise at the start of the chapter on common psychotic experiences most of us may have experienced? In most cases, such experiences are transient in time and minor in degree of pervasiveness – most of us would shake our head, having our rational mind and the objective evidence kick in that would dispel minor and fleeting paranoid thoughts or psychotic beliefs. However, in Simon's case the psychotic experiences have become so entrenched, his body and mind so compromised and his social circumstances so impeded and isolated, that it is no longer easy to shake them off. Depression becomes intrinsic, both to the psychosis and to its impact and consequences. Both Simon and his parents feel embarrassed and stigmatized given the sectioning at their home. They worry a lot how their neighbours, extended families and others perceive them. They worry about whether others will understand that Simon is unwell and what they should say if people ask about him; and above all, what Simon's future may hold for them as a family.

34.6 Prognosis, course and recovery

It has been observed that the onset of most schizophrenias is preceded by a prodromal period which can be insidious over weeks and months, although onsets vary considerably across individuals (Murphy *et al.* 2008). Common initial, or so-called prodromal, symptoms and difficulties include: social withdrawal; unusual and uncharacteristic behaviour; disturbed communication and affect; bizarre ideas and perceptual experiences; and reduced interest in and motivation for doing day-to-day activities (those commonly described as 'negative' symptoms). Because the prodromal period and its symptoms can be insidious and subtle, confounded by the individuality of each presentation and onset, psychosis can often remain undetected and untreated. The average duration of untreated negative symptoms

(DUN), from when they first appear until they fall below diagnostic thresholds, is estimated to be just under 94 weeks (Murphy *et al.* 2008).

Such prodromal symptoms are usually exacerbated in an acute phase, which is marked by characteristic 'positive' symptoms of hallucinations, delusions and behavioural disturbances. The length of the acute phase, and indeed the various phases, varies widely from one person to the next. Some individuals experience no prodromal period at all. Some have brief acute phases that are effectively resolved with treatment. Others may live with residual psychotic symptoms for months or years.

Recent research suggests a more positive outlook on prognosis, with between 14 and 20 per cent of individuals estimated to have a full recovery following an episode of psychotic illness. The remaining three-quarters of people with schizophrenia will experience recurrent relapse and some continued disability. However, findings of longitudinal studies that follow up individuals diagnosed with schizophrenia over 20 to 40 years suggest that there is a moderately good long-term global outcome in over half of people with schizophrenia, with a smaller proportion having extended periods of remission of symptoms without further relapses (NICE 2010).

34.7 Aetiology of schizophrenia: theories of causation

The aetiology of schizophrenia has been debated for many years. While much of the research evidence is consistent with the longstanding 'stress-vulnerability model' (SVM) proposed by Zubin and Spring (1977), a number of mythical theories have been proposed that have shaped the public perception of the illness over the last century.

In the late nineteenth century, a German psychiatrist, Emil Kraepelin, popularized the term 'dementia praecox' (a premature dementia or precocious madness) to describe and discuss the psychotic disorder. Kraepelin's view of dementia praecox being a progressively deteriorating illness from which no one can recover, despite being disproven by the twentieth century, has always overshadowed the illness with pessimism (Porter and Berrioros 1995). A decade later a Swiss psychiatrist, Eugen Bleuler, first coined the term 'schizophrenia' which roughly translates as 'splitting of the mind'. This new terminology for the condition included a realization that some patients improve rather than deteriorate. However, the term's origin from its Greek root unintentionally led people to associate the condition with a 'split' or 'sheltered' mind and planted the myth of split/multiple/dissociated minds/personalities as the meaning or presentation of schizophrenia.

It used to be thought that schizophrenia was a 'functional' disorder, by which was meant that there was no sign of brain disease or brain damage, as there is in 'organic' disorders such as Alzheimer's disease and head injury cases. However, it is now well established with technological advances like computerized tomography (CT) scans and magnetic resonance imaging (MRI) scans, that abnormalities in the structure and function of the brain are present in most people who suffer from schizophrenia. Some psychoanalysts have suggested that certain patterns of parenting and upbringing could confuse children so much that they develop schizophrenia in later life (e.g. the double-bind theory of Bateson et al. 1956). There was really no empirical research or scientific basis for such theories. However, the stigma and blame that such mis-concepts brought to individuals suffering from schizophrenia and their families, and the damage to the mental health professional–carer relationship, should not be underestimated.

Since the 1970s, multiple contributory causes have been suggested, including genetics, biological factors (brain biochemistry and pathology) and psychological and social factors. While none of these can account independently for the causes of schizophrenia, the SVM proposed by Zubin and Spring (1977) successfully encompasses the complex interaction of them all. In addition to the varying individual levels of vulnerability due to the combination of the factors mentioned above, the SVM also emphasizes that life event stressors play a major role in the putative causes of onset, relapse and maintenance of schizophrenia, similar to other major physical and mental disorders. A life event stressor is an incident – such as bereavement, a broken relationship, migration or even promotion at work – that requires the adjustment or reorganization of a person's life. A list of vulnerability factors categorized into bio-psycho-social domains is presented in Table 34.3. While this list is extensive, it is not exhaustive.

Zubin and Spring's SVM and the interaction of its two dynamic ingredients are illustrated in Figure 34.1. This model hypothesizes the dynamic interaction between stressors and vulnerability in a way that, as long as the stress induced by the challenging life event stays below the threshold of vulnerability, the individual copes with the stressor using his or her usual repertoire of bio-psycho-social resources (that may include problem-solving by self, calling

Table 34.3   List of possible vulnerability factors

Main domain	Vulnerability factors
Biological domain	• Genetic factors (e.g. the greatest risk for developing schizophrenia is having a first-degree relative with the disease) • Brain biochemistry, especially the problems in regulation of the neurotransmitter dopamine in the prefrontal cortex • Brain pathology (e.g. structural changes as discussed earlier)
Psychological domain	• Basic cognitive functions such as learning, attention, memory or planning; and • Biases in emotional and reasoning processes. For instance, depression and anxiety are found to contribute to the symptoms of schizophrenia in research (e.g. Birchwood 2003)
Social and environmental domain	Known factors that increase vulnerability include: • urban birth and rearing • social adversity and trauma • heavy cannabis use • migration and stressful life events

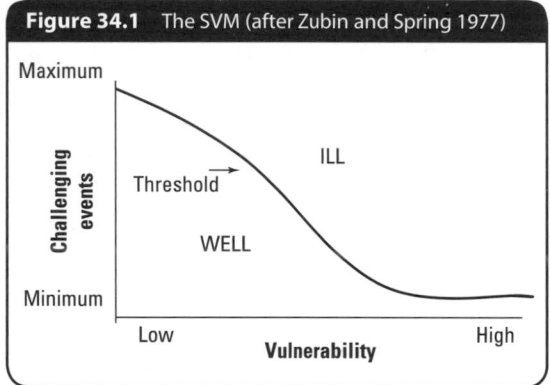

Figure 34.1   The SVM (after Zubin and Spring 1977)

on family/friends to help out, or putting in extra work and hours as required) and remains well within the limits of normality. When the stress exceeds the threshold (e.g. all the coping strategies mentioned above are exhausted and have failed to resolve the stress), the person is likely to develop a psychopathological episode of some sort. Moreover, the SVM postulates that the episode is time-limited. When the stress abates and sinks below the vulnerability threshold, the episode ends and the individual returns to a pre-episode level of adoption.

Thinking Space 34.3

Simon's background may shed some light on his vulnerability for developing psychosis. What vulnerability factors and stressors might be indicative in Simon's case?

Feedback

Around and before the onset of his illness Simon had to adjust to a new environment and pressure in study, while living away from home the first time. In terms of vulnerability factors, consider the various domains as outlined in Table 34.3. Biologically, prolonged poor sleep, diet and self-care may have compromised

Simon's brain function. Psychologically, Simon has a pre-morbid personality (being shy and asocial) that may have contributed to inadequate coping with adjustment to university and exacerbated difficulties in problem-solving. In the last domain of socio-environmental factors, Simon has higher than average vulnerability to psychosis due to being a second generation migrant with a southern Asian ethnic background and having suffered bullying in his developmental years.

34.8   Assessment

Given the complexity of schizophrenia and the high incidence rate of co-morbidity and social problems as a consequence, comprehensive and specialist assessment is always needed. The NICE guideline on schizophrenia (2010) states that people suspected of schizophrenia should receive comprehensive mental health assessment from a multi-disciplinary mental health team. The assessment should include a psychiatric, psychological and physical health evaluation and also address accommodation, culture and ethnicity, economic status, occupation and education (including employment and functional activity), prescribed and non-prescribed drug history, quality of life, responsibility for children, risk of harm to self and others, sexual health and social networks (NICE 2010). The principles and good practice of a systematic and comprehensive assessment are discussed in Chapter 14, and those focusing on the risk of self-harm and aggression in Chapters 17 and 18. These should be followed here, in addition to some further specific considerations focusing on psychosis and schizophrenia.

Mental health assessments with individuals showing signs and symptoms suggestive of psychosis are usually conducted for a number of reasons, including:

- to reach a diagnosis;
- to develop a psychological formulation;
- to identify strengths and needs;
- for screening purposes, including the detection of risk;
- to measure outcomes and evaluate progress.

For diagnosing the condition, as well as evaluating progress following a course of treatment, a comprehensive assessment that explores and investigates the various signs and symptoms discussed above is needed. Assessments are often conducted by psychiatrists and mental health nurses, over a period of time. While there is no definitive diagnostic test (e.g. blood test or MRI scan) available for schizophrenia, a number of psychiatric assessment measures or tools are commonly used for these purposes, including:

- Brief Psychiatric Rating Scale (BPRS – Overall and Gorham 1962);
- Positive and Negative Syndrome Scale (PANSS – Kay et al. 1989);
- Schedule for the Assessment of Positive Symptoms (SAPS) and Schedule for the Assessment of Negative Symptoms (SANS – Andreasen 1982).

These tools share a common characteristic in that they have multiple sections of semi-structured questions that explore positive and negative symptoms which are signatory of a psychotic disorder, by eliciting both experiential information from the individual and allowing for objective data collection through clinical observation and information-gathering from notes/records and families/carers. Skilful engagement and assessment incorporating interviewing and investigating skills are essential, in addition to knowledge and competence in using such tools.

Assessment of affect and mood is also important given that secondary or concurrent affective disturbances in schizophrenia are common (Birchwood 2003). While the comprehensive psychiatric assessment tools such as BPRS or PANSS will explore affective symptoms as part of a comprehensive overview, specific and discrete assessment focusing on depression and anxiety should be considered. Assessment of depression is particularly indicative in cases where a differentiation between depression and negative symptoms and/or risk of self-harm and suicide is highlighted. Anxiety is also commonly reported as a co-morbid condition as well as a common reaction to the psychotic signs and symptoms (e.g. paranoid ideations, auditory hallucinations of a derogatory nature), so its assessment is often indicated. Some useful assessment tools for consideration include:

- Beck Depression Inventory (BDI-II – Beck *et al.* 1996)
- Beck Anxiety Inventory (BAI – Beck *et al.* 1988)
- Hospital Anxiety and Depression Scale (HAD – Zigmond and Snaith 1983)
- Physical Health Questionnaire (PHQ 9 – Spitzer *et al.* 1999)

Most of these psychometric tests are self-administered questionnaires designed to elicit the individual's subjective feelings and emotions.

There are many tools to explore an individual's strengths and needs in terms of their overall quality of life and goals of recovery. Emerging research suggests that assessment tools that include the service user's views and which employ service-user rated measures are particularly relevant and meaningful. The Recovery Star (MacKeith and Burns 2008) and the Wellness Recovery Action Plan (WRAP – Copeland 1997) are regarded as popular tools for these reasons and both cover areas considered important by the individuals themselves, including identity and self-esteem, living skills, social networks, relationships, physical health and self-care, stressors and coping strategies. Specific assessment of the carers/families of individuals with schizophrenia in their own right for support, as well as in their pivotal role in supporting the service user's recovery, is also required. It is well documented that carers of individuals with schizophrenia have higher vulnerability to develop ill health, both physically

and mentally, due to the stress and burden of caring. Research evidence also identifies that individuals having close contacts with carers or families who exhibit critical, hostile or over-involved behaviour and attitudes towards them will encounter more relapses and have poorer outcomes (see Pharoah *et al.* 2010 for an overview). Each mental health service will have its specific carer assessment measures, but generally they serve the following purposes according to Department of Health (DH) guidance (DH 2002):

- determine what measures the carer feels would allow them to continue/start caring while maintaining their own health and well-being;
- determine whether the carer is eligible for support from/via social services;
- ensure a positive, outcome-focused engagement with carers;
- positively reduce the stigmas associated both with mental health problems and identification as a carer.

Chapter 25 discusses working with families and carers.

The wealth of information collated through systematic assessment helps to provide a comprehensive understanding of the individual's unique situation through a process called *case formulation*. Case formulation seeks to assemble and organize the assessment information to understand the stress-vulnerability interactions relevant to the individual, their unique vulnerability factors in various domains, their stressors, their coping capacity and strengths, their aspirations and motivations, in the onset and the maintenance and the prognosis of the illness episode(s). A collaborative case formulation between the mental health worker and the service user may be therapeutic in itself. It also serves as a springboard between assessment and care planning and treatment, with the aim of identifying evidence-based interventions targeting problems and needs, and drawing on resources from mental health workers and services, as well as from the service users and their families/carers, and the wider community.

Thinking Space 34.4

What strategies, principles and techniques are relevant to assessment and care planning with Simon and his parents?

Feedback

There are multiple challenges to engaging with Simon to undertake a comprehensive assessment given his paranoia and risk of self-neglect. You may wish to consider a collaborative approach incorporating some engagement strategies focusing on Simon's needs, motivation and aspiration, in addition to his symptoms and behaviour. Consider using the recommended tools in a sensitive manner to explore how Simon perceives the meaning behind his experiences and behavioural responses. Try to address his concerns and distress during the assessment and care planning process. Simon may not be forthcoming in talking about his psychotic symptoms for a number of reasons (e.g. embarrassment, shame, fear, or simply confusion). Instead, it may help if you show concern over Simon's worries. He may worry what the future may hold. He may wonder why the psychosis happened in the first place and what treatment is available. Simon's parents are well placed to provide detailed information and so should be involved in the assessment. They will also require support given the stress they have experienced in looking after Simon so far, and his need for their future support along his journey towards recovery.

34.9 Treatments to promote recovery

Treatment for people with schizophrenia should promote recovery, above and beyond symptom control or reduction. This requires new approaches by mental health workers to support people in settings of their own choosing, enabling access to community resources such as housing, education, work and friendships in whatever ways an individual sees as critical to their own recovery.

The concept of recovery (which is the focus of Chapter 5) has gathered momentum over recent decades and is now recognized as the ultimate goal and philosophy of treatment for severe mental illnesses. According to Anthony, 'Recovery . . . It's a way of living a satisfying, hopeful and contributing life even with limitations caused by illness' (1993: 13). The definition of recovery varies from one individual to another, nonetheless some common themes emerge across literature and policies in mental health service provision, including:

- pursuit of health and wellness;
- a shift of emphasis from pathology and morbidity to health and strengths;
- the importance of hope and belief in positive change;
- meaning and spiritual purpose;
- support received as mentoring not supervisory;
- identity explored as a cultural issue;
- social inclusion and empowerment through information, role change, self-care, awareness of positive language use;
- personal wisdom encouraged in professional practice;
- creative risk-taking (CSIP/RCPsych/SCIE 2007).

Research is ongoing to develop and identify specific evidence-based interventions that promote recovery. Nonetheless, it is widely believed that recovery-promoting relationships and work practices that promote care planning and treatment focusing on an individual's values and preferences, tapping into their strengths (e.g. the Strengths Model of Rapp and Goscha 2006) and striving towards personal goals are important.

Treatments for schizophrenia usually require a combination of medication, psychological and social interventions, considering the complex and multi-factorial nature of the predisposing factors associated with the development and maintenance of the illness. Planning and implementing treatment requires a collaborative partnership alongside an understanding of the SVM to inform the case formulation and subsequent interventions. The NICE guideline on schizophrenia recommends the following evidence-based treatments.

Pharmacological interventions

Antipsychotic medication has been the mainstay of treatment for schizophrenia for over half a century. There is well established evidence for its efficacy in both the treatment of acute psychotic episodes and for relapse prevention over time. However, considerable problems remain. A substantial proportion of service users, up to 40 per cent, have a poor response to conventional antipsychotic drugs and continue to show moderate to severe positive and negative psychotic symptoms. Moreover, despite the advances in the development of antipsychotic drugs, especially in recent decades with the manufacturing of 'atypical' or second-generation antipsychotics (SGAs like Olanzapine, risperidone, Aripiprazole), in addition to the conventional or 'typical' antipsychotics (FGAs, like chlorpromazine, haloperidol), antipsychotic medication as a whole is associated with a high incidence and broad range of unpleasant side-effects (NICE 2010). Therefore, although NICE recommends that oral antipsychotic medication should be prescribed to people who are newly diagnosed with schizophrenia, the initiation of antipsychotics should ideally be managed by a psychiatrist or an independent nurse prescriber, rather than in the primary care setting, and regarded as an individual

therapeutic trial (NICE 2010). Decisions about which antipsychotic to use should be made in partnership with service users and their carers, with service users' agreement, taking into account the potential of individual drugs to cause extrapyramidal side-effects (such as akathisia), metabolic side-effects (such as weight gain) and others (including unpleasant subjective experiences). Psycho-education on the indicators for a potential side-effects and a risk-benefit profile are an essential part of medication treatment. Once treatment starts, collaborative work to monitor tolerance, therapeutic effects and side-effects is crucial to optimize service users' understanding, commitment and self-management of their treatment regimes.

Combinations of antipsychotics should not normally be prescribed except for short periods – for example, when changing medication. Use of other psychotropic drugs (e.g. antidepressants) should be carefully considered within the context of a comprehensive treatment plan as well as the risk and disadvantages of side-effects caused by poly-pharmacy.

For people with schizophrenia who do not respond well to antipsychotic treatment, there is only one antipsychotic drug, clozapine, that has a specific licence for treatment with this treatment resistant group of people. Psychosocial interventions should also be considered and offered to these service users (NICE 2010). Detailed information on psychopharmacology inclusive of antipsychotic medication is available in Chapters 26 and 27. Specific interventions to optimize medication management are discussed in Chapter 28.

Psychological and psychosocial interventions

Compared to pharmacological treatment, the use of specific psychological and psychosocial interventions to help people with schizophrenia is relatively recent and increasingly recognized as crucial. The limitations of pharmacological treatment became more and more obvious when the deinstitutionalization of service users gained ground in the 1970s and resulted in people with schizophrenia being discharged from long-stay hospitals to live in the community. Often, they struggled to cope independently. The multiple impacts of the illness on the individual's life and their families/carers mean that adjustment and recovery over an array of life domains is essential. These lessons from deinstitutionalization in the 1970s and 1980s have informed the development of a number of psychosocial interventions.

Family intervention

Family intervention in the treatment of schizophrenia has evolved from studies of the family environment, especially a concept called 'expressed emotion' and its possible role in affecting the course of schizophrenia after an initial episode. It should be noted that in this context 'family' includes people who have a significant emotional connection to the service user, regardless of biological links, such as parents, siblings, partners and significant support networks like close friends and hostel support workers. Brown et al. (1962; Brown and Rutter 1966) developed a measure for the level of 'expressed emotion' within families and were able to show that the emotional environment within a family was an effective predictor of relapse in schizophrenia. The importance of this work lay in the realization that it was possible to design and develop family intervention (or 'family work' according to Kuipers et al. 2002) that could change the management of the illness by service users and their families, and influence the course of schizophrenia. Family intervention has been proven to be effective in preventing relapse in people with schizophrenia for a period at least 24 months following treatment, with a strong and corroborated evidence base from systematic reviews conducted by the Cochrane Collaboration (Pharoah et al. 2010) as well as NICE (2010).

Family intervention in schizophrenia derives from behavioural and systemic ideas, adapted to the needs of the families of those with psychosis. More recently, cognitive appraisals of the difficulties have been emphasized (NICE 2010). Family intervention models aim to help families/carers cope with their loved one's problems more effectively, provide support and education for the family, reduce levels of distress, and improve the ways in which the family communicates and negotiates problems and tries to prevent relapse by the service user. Family intervention is normally complex and lengthy, lasting for more than 10 sessions over a period of 3 to 12 months. It is delivered in a structured format with individual families, and includes the service user as much as possible. Multi-family group intervention, where carers and/or families of more than one service user receive the intervention in a group format, can be considered if the families/carers prefer a group format. Family intervention can be offered to the service user and their families/carers at any point in the course of their illness, ranging from the acute inpatient phase to sustaining recovery in the community.

Nurses, provided they have appropriate training and competencies in family intervention with reference to a well recognized treatment manual and access to regular clinical supervision, are ideally placed to work collaboratively with service users and their families/carers in family intervention. In line with all evidence-based interventions, a collaborative and comprehensive case formulation should inform the identification of goal(s) for treatment, which in turn should be evaluated using outcome measures and service users' and carers' feedback.

Cognitive behavioural therapy

By the late 1980s, cognitive behavioural therapy (CBT) approaches originally developed in the 1970s for depression were first applied to aid the reduction of distressing psychotic symptoms and then broadened to address emotional problems and functioning. CBT for psychosis (CBTp) has since evolved and now tends to be formulation-based. The overall aim of CBTp is to help the individual normalize and make sense of their psychotic experiences, and to reduce the associated distress and impact on functioning. NICE (2010) defines CBTp as a discrete psychological intervention where service users:

- establish links between their thoughts, feelings or actions with respect to the current or past symptoms, and/or functioning; and

- re-evaluate their perceptions, beliefs or reasoning in relation to the target symptoms.

It includes at least one of the following components:

- people monitoring their own thoughts, feelings or behaviours with respect to the symptom or recurrence of symptoms; and/or
- promotion of alternative ways of coping with the target symptoms; and/or
- reduction of distress; and/or
- improvement of functioning.

NICE further recommends that CBTp on a one-to-one basis over a course of at least 16 planned sessions should be offered to all people with schizophrenia. Such a recommendation is based on CBTp's efficacy in reducing rehospitalization (including the duration of an admission) and symptom severity, especially in respect of hallucinations and depression.

In recent years, mindfulness-based 'third-wave' CBT (Chadwick *et al.* 2009) and acceptance and commitment therapy (ACT) (Hayes *et al.* 2004, 2006), have gathered popularity in treating people with psychosis. Mindfulness-based CBT is relatively new in terms of being tested through trials with a study population of people with psychosis and it is not yet included in the NICE guideline (NICE 2010).

Again, similar to family intervention, training and relevant competencies in CBTp are essential for all those who provide the intervention, inclusive of mental health nurses. Access to regular clinical supervision is key for continuous professional development and for the quality assurance of such an intervention. Chapter 21 provides further information on generic CBT.

Arts therapies

The update guideline on schizophrenia (NICE 2010) introduced a new recommendation on arts therapies, which are particularly beneficial in alleviating negative symptoms. There are four modalities of arts therapies: art, music, drama and dance movement therapies. While the modalities prescribe different arts media and a variety of techniques, they share a common focus in the creation of a working therapeutic relationship between service users and therapists, in which strong emotion can be expressed and processed. The art form is also seen as a safe way to experiment with relating to others in a meaningful way when words can be difficult.

NICE (2010: 252) defines arts therapies as 'complex interventions that combine psychotherapeutic techniques with activities aimed at promoting creative expression. In all arts therapies, the aim is to enable the service user to experience him/herself differently and develop new ways of relating to others'. Arts therapies should be provided by a Health Professions Council registered arts therapist with experience of working with people with schizophrenia. Contrary to the one-to-one format favoured by family intervention and CBTp, groups are the preferred format for arts therapies.

While all the psychosocial interventions discussed above apply to all who suffer from schizophrenia, they are of particular importance for those who are identified as 'treatment-resistant' or whose illness has not responded adequately to drug treatment. Nurses should work collaboratively with the service user to review engagement and consider use of all recommended psychosocial interventions as outlined above. They should consider also other causes of non-response, such as co-morbid substance misuse, the concurrent use of other prescribed medication or physical illness.

Other approaches to promote physical health and recovery

While the NICE guideline on schizophrenia (2010) emphasizes promoting physical health and recovery in people with schizophrenia, it does not recommend specific interventions. As discussed, the evidence base on recovery approaches or interventions is evolving rapidly. Interventions to optimize physical health, well-being and recovery tend to span primary and secondary health care settings, as much as they span health care and societal boundaries to address complex issues (e.g. anti-stigma, employment and education, citizenship). This sets new challenges for research and the generation of a practice evidence base.

Thinking Space 34.5

Consider the relevance of various interventions and treatment approaches for Simon and his parents.

Feedback

Simon will need a comprehensive package of care including antipsychotic medication and psychological interventions, such as CBT, directed towards helping him make sense of his psychotic episode and develop more effective coping mechanisms for residual symptoms and relapse prevention. Family intervention for Simon and his parents is also indicated to help them all understand and support Simon's recovery. Simon's priority would focus around getting back on his own feet and back to his life. Recovering from the bizarre psychotic symptoms he has experienced will only be a beginning. In the future, Simon may need help in coming to terms with these experiences and any impediment they may have brought about (e.g. depression, social isolation). Social interventions using community resources may also be considered to help Simon resume his education and pursue other life aspirations, such as finding employment, making friends, and perhaps, in the longer term, moving out of his parents' home.

 ## 34.10 Nursing care

Contexts of care for people with schizophrenia rest mainly in secondary (specialist) mental health services. The inpatient services that admit people with schizophrenia comprise a range of statutory, independent and third-sector provision ranging in degree of restriction and cost from high (secure hospitals), to medium-secure units and low-secure units for mentally disordered offenders, through to intensive care, acute beds and rehabilitation units. In recent decades and in line with the recovery philosophy, most nursing care is community-based and spans a variety of community team models. Since the *National Service Framework for Mental Health* (DH 1999) placed emphasis on various alternatives to inpatient services to promote social inclusion and a seamless transition on to community services, an array of mental health services have been established, in addition to traditional community mental health services, such as community mental health teams (CMHTs) and psychiatric outpatient clinics. These relatively new community-based services include assertive outreach teams or 'community treatment', day hospitals or centres, crisis resolution services, home treatment services and respite services. EIPS have also been established across the UK to detect, assess and care for people who develop psychosis for the first time, to optimize their long-term trajectory and recovery from the illness (DH 2001). These community services, though still evolving, emphasize alternatives to inpatient admission, with treatments and interventions focused on the service user's usual environment and context.

Mental health nurses form the majority of the workforce in all these care contexts. Often, nurses act as the care coordinator for the service user in community services or the key nurse on an inpatient ward. In other words, nurses play a key role in all aspects of care and in the phases of treating schizophrenia discussed in this chapter. Nurses who work closely and collaboratively with service users and their carers, often over a substantial period of time, are well placed to undertake comprehensive assessments and plan care directed towards achieving the service user's goals and aspirations which incorporates access to evidence-based psychosocial interventions, identifies indications for treatment and makes referrals to and promotes engagement with interventions. Specialist mental health nurses with appropriate training and supervision can also provide specific interventions.

Another common feature of care involving people with schizophrenia is its relatively long duration due to the long-term nature of the illness and the involvement of multiple agents across care settings. It is quite common that while service users progress along the care pathway of schizophrenia over a duration of years or decade, they also have input from other health professionals across primary (e.g. GP, practice nurse), secondary (e.g. occupational therapist from CMHT; other general health care specialties like diabetic care) and even tertiary (e.g. specialist clinical psychologist within the local post-traumatic stress clinic) care settings. This will mean that the mental health nurse often acts as the agent who ensures continuity of care as well as being a central point of communication with various health and social agents (e.g. housing, job centre). To promote and optimize recovery, service users also need support in accessing employment, education and occupational activities to help integrate them into their usual social context and role and realize their aspirations. Mental health nurses should take a leading role in this process, working alongside service users to seek out opportunities beyond health care service settings.

 Conclusion

To conclude, the main points made in this chapter are:

- The scientific concepts and terminology of schizophrenia in the UK follow the ICD-10 diagnostic framework. Prevalence and incidence

of schizophrenia is estimated as 5 per 1,000 of psychiatric disorders in working-age adults, making schizophrenia the most common form of psychotic disorder.

- Schizophrenia implies a wide range of signs and both positive and negative symptoms that tend to impact upon multiple domains of the individuals' lives. The SVM that encompasses the complex interaction of biological, psychological and social factors in the understanding of the aetiology of schizophrenia has the best research evidence in explaining its onset, maintenance and prognosis.

- Comprehensive strengths and needs-based assessment conducted by a multi-disciplinary mental health team which incorporates validated scales is advocated for people suspected of developing psychosis.

- Treatments informed by a collaborative case formulation should aim to promote recovery. Combinations of medication, psychological and social interventions are often indicative to address the complex and multi-factorial nature of the illness and its impacts.

- Mental health nurses comprise the majority of the workforce in various mental health services across inpatient and community services within secondary and tertiary mental health care settings, so are well placed to work closely with individuals with schizophrenia and their families/carers, over a sustained period of time, along their journey towards recovery.

Annotated bibliography

Cockburn, P. and Cockburn, H. (2011) *Henry's Demons – Living with Schizophrenia: a father and son's story.* **London: Simon & Schuster.**
This book is written in a narrative style from both a service user's (Henry) and his father's (Patrick) perspectives. It tells a moving story about the son and father's experiences of living with schizophrenia since Henry's onset of psychosis in 2002. Henry's journey to a partial recovery also covers a wide range of care facilities, treatments, and the differing attitudes of health professionals as experienced by Henry and his family.

Gamble, C. and Brennan, G. (eds) (2006) *Working with Serious Mental Illness: A manual for clinical practice*, **2nd edn. Edinburgh: Elsevier.**
A manual for mental health professionals focusing on psychosis that provides detailed information elaborating on the various sections of this chapter, including explanatory models, signs and symptoms, assessment and formulation approaches, and various interventions.

NICE (National Institute for Health and Clinical Excellence) (2010) *Clinical Guideline 82: Schizophrenia – core interventions in the treatment and management of schizophrenia in adults in primary & secondary care*, updated edn. London: NICE.
This full version of the updated guideline combines a detailed review on various evidence-based interventions for people with schizophrenia as well as a comprehensive picture of contemporary mental health practices. The full guideline can be downloaded from NICE website (www.nice.org.uk). There is a further review of this guideline on psychosis and schizophrenia, just started from early 2012 with a view to update the recommendations and support implementation on evidence-based treatments.

References

Andreasen, N.C. (1982) Negative symptoms in schizophrenia, *Archives of General Psychiatry*, 39(7): 784–8.
Anthony, W.A. (1993) Recovery from mental illness – the guiding vision of the mental health services in the 1990s, *Psychosocial Rehabilitation Journal*, 16(4): 11–23.
APA (American Psychiatric Association) (1994) *Diagnostic and Statistical Manual of Mental Disorders*, 4th edn (DSM-IV). Washington, DC: APA.
Bateson, G., Jackson, D.D., Haley, J. and Weakland, J. (1956) Towards a theory of schizophrenia, *Behavioural Science*, 1: 251–64.
Beck, A.T., Epstein, N., Brown, G. and Steer, R.A. (1988) An inventory for measuring clinical anxiety: psychometric properties, *Journal of Consulting and Clinical Psychology*, 56(6): 893–7.
Beck, A.T., Steer, R.A. and Brown, G.K. (1996) *Manual for the Beck Depression Inventory – II*. San Antonio, TX: Psychological Corporation.
Birchwood, M. (2003) Pathways to emotional dysfunction in first-episode psychosis, *British Journal of Psychiatry*, 182: 272–5.
Brown, G.W. and Rutter, M. (1966) The measurement of family activities and relationships: a methodological study, *Human Relations*, 19: 241–63.
Brown, G.W., Monck, E., Carstairs, G.M. *et al.* (1962) Influence of family life on the course of schizophrenic illness, *British Journal of Preventive and Social Medicine*, 16: 55–68.
Cannon, M. and Jones, P. (1996) Schizophrenia, *Journal of Neurology, Neurosurgery and Psychiatry*, 60: 604–13.
Chadwick, P., Hughes, S., Russell, D., Russell, I. and Gagnan, D. (2009) Mindfulness groups for distressing voices and paranoia: a replication and randomised feasibility trial, *Behavioural and Cognitive Psychotherapy*, 37(4): 103–412.
Copeland, M.E. (1997) *Wellness Recovery Action Plan*. West Dummerston, VT: Peach Press.
CSIP/RCPsych/SCIE (Care Services Improvement Partnership/Royal College of Psychiatrists/Social Care Institute for Excellence) (2007) *A Common Purpose: Recovery in future mental health services*. London: SCIE.
DH (Department of Health) (1999) *National Service Framework for Mental Health: Modern standards and service models*. London: DH.
DH (Department of Health) (2001) *The Mental Health Policy Implementation Guide*. London: DH.
DH (Department of Health) (2002) *Guidance on Developing Services for Carers and Families*. London: DH.
Hayes, S.C., Masuda, A., Bassett, R., Luoma, J. and Guerrere, L.F. (2004) DBT, FAP & ACT: how empirically oriented are the new behavioural therapy technologies? *Behavioural Therapy*, 35(1): 35–54.
Hayes, S.C., Luoma, J.B., Bond, F.W., Masuda, A. and Lillis, J. (2006) ACT: model, processes and outcomes, *Behavioural Research & Therapy*, 44: 1–25.
Kay, S.R., Opler, L.A. and Lindermayer, J.P. (1989) The Positive and Negative Syndrome Scale (PANSS): rationale and standardization, *British Journal of Psychiatry*, 155 (suppl. 7): 59–65.
Kirkbride, J.B., Fearon, P., Morgan, C. *et al.* (2006) Heterogeneity in incidence rates of schizophrenia and other psychotic syndromes: findings from the 3-center AeSOP study, *Archives of General Psychiatry*, 63, 250–8.
Kuipers, E., Leff, J. and Lam, D. (2002) *Family Work for Schizophrenia: A practical guide*, 2nd edn. London: Gaskell.
MacKeith, J. and Burns, S. (2008) *Mental Health Recovery Star – Organisational Guide*. London: Mental Health Providers Forum.
Murphy, B., Stuart, A.H. and McGorry, P.D. (2008) Duration of untreated negative symptoms and duration of active negative symptoms: proof of concepts, *Early Intervention in Psychiatry*, 2: 27–33.
NICE (National Institute for Health and Clinical Excellence) (2010) *Clinical Guideline 82: Schizophrenia – core interventions in the treatment and management of schizophrenia in adults in primary & secondary care*, updated edn. London: NICE.
NICE (National Institute for Health and Clinical Excellence) (2012) *Psychosis and Schizophrenia (Update): Final Scope*, available at: http://guidance.nice.org.uk/CG/WaveR/113/Scoping/Scope/pdf/English, accessed 29 May 2012.
Overall, J.E. and Gorham, D.R. (1962) The Brief Psychiatric Rating Scale, *Psychological Report*, 10: 799–812.
Pharoah, F., Mari, J., Rathbone, J. and Wong, W. (2010) Family intervention for schizophrenia, *Cochrane Database of Systematic Reviews 2010*, Issue 12. Art. No.: CD000088. DOI: 10.1002/14651858. CD000088. pub3.
Porter, R. and Berrioros, G.E. (1995) *A History of Clinical Psychiatry: The origin and history of psychiatric disorders*. London: Athlone Press.
Rapp, C. and Goscha, R.J. (2006) *The Strengths Model: Case management with people with psychiatric disabilities*, 2nd edn. New York: Oxford University Press.
Sartorius, N. (2002) Iatrogenic stigma of mental illness, *British Medical Journal*, 324: 1470–1.
Sin, J. (2000) One step at a time, *Mental Health Care*, 41(31): 97–101.
Singleton, N., Bumpstead, R., O'Brien, M. *et al.* (2000) *Psychiatric Morbidity Among Adults Living in Private Households, 2000: Report of a survey carried out by the Social Survey Division of the Office for National Statistics on behalf of the Department of Health, the Scottish Executive and the National Assembly for Wales*. London: HMSO.

Spitzer, R., Kroenke, K. and Williams, J. (1999) Validation and utility of a self-report version of PRIME-MD: the PHQ primary care study, *Journal of the American Medical Association*, 282: 1737–44.

Thornicroft, G., Tansella, M., Becker, T. *et al.* (2004) The personal impact of schizophrenia in Europe, *Schizophrenia Research*, 69: 125–32.

WHO (World Health Organization) (1992) *International Statistical Classification of Diseases and Related Health Problems (ICD-10)*. Geneva: WHO.

Zigmond, A.S. and Snaith, R.P. (1983) The Hospital Anxiety and Depression Scale, *Acta Psychiatrica Scandinavica*, 67(6): 361–70.

Zubin, J. and Spring, B. (1977) Vulnerability – a new view of schizophrenia, *Journal of Abnormal Psychology*, 86: 103–26.

Chapter 35

The Person Who Experiences Depression

Sue Gurney

A lot of people don't realize that depression is an illness. I don't wish it on anyone, but if they would know how it feels, I swear they would think twice before they just shrug it.

Jonathan Davis

But if somebody dies, if something happens to you, there is a normal process of depression, it is part of being human, and some people view it as a learning experience etc.

Bob Geldof

35.1 Introduction

The term depression is a general expression used to describe a state of health characterized by low mood and/or loss of pleasure in most activities. Although the experience of depression is common for most people, particularly when experiencing adversity, it can be a life threatening condition. This chapter offers an overview of aspects of depression and provides information for consideration in application to mental health nursing practice. The chapter covers:

- what is depression?
- the causes of depression;
- screening, assessment and diagnosis;
- approaches to care and treatment;
- implications for mental health nursing practice.

35.2 What is depression?

Depression (low mood) is an umbrella term used to describe an experience that affects the whole person in terms of feelings, thoughts, judgements and behaviour. Depression presents a diverse picture, from mild to severe and lasting from a few weeks to a lifetime. Sometime it is obvious while in others it may be barely perceptible. Although depression is

Box 35.1 Signs and symptoms of depression (adapted from APA 1994)

Core (key) symptoms

- Persistent low mood or sadness
- Marked loss of interest or pleasure in activities or hobbies normally enjoyed

Other common symptoms

- Ability to think, concentrate, remember or make decisions is impaired, with even simple tasks seeming to be difficult
- Changes in appetite with under- or overeating and consequential weight loss or gain
- Changes in sleep patterns with either difficulties in sleeping or sleeping excessively
- Behaviour that is agitated or slowed down
- Fatigue, tiredness and decreased energy, aches or pains, headaches, cramps or digestive problems that do not ease even with treatment
- Thoughts of worthlessness, hopelessness, helplessness or excessive or inappropriate guilt
- Thoughts of death or suicide (with or without a specific plan), or attempt of suicide

Case Study

Brian

Brian is in his late 50s; he separated from wife and family about 10 months ago, moved into temporary accommodation and lost his job as a store manager when the firm went into receivership three months ago.

Brian visited his general practitioner (GP) as he felt he 'couldn't go on'. He'd lost a significant amount of weight, looked unkempt, wasn't sleeping and was exceedingly anxious and despondent about his future. Based on Brian's presentation the GP formulated that he was possibly suffering from moderate to severe depression combined with complex life problems.

common, it is a serious condition and is often characterized by some, or many, of the signs and symptoms outlined in Box 35.1.

If projections prove accurate, then by 2020, depression will become the second cause of the global disease burden. Already depression affects around 121 million people (WHO 2011), with almost half of the population of the western world experiencing at least an episode of depression during their lifetime. The resulting economic impact of depression is large – within England the annual

estimated cost of depression in 2007 was estimated between £20.2–23.8 billion a year (DH 2011a).

Thinking Space 35.1

List the possible problems that Brian is facing and the support he may need immediately and over the next 12 months. You will have an opportunity to review your ideas at the end of the chapter in relation to an account of Brian's care and treatment.

The causes of depression

There is a large volume of literature on the risk/causative factors associated with developing depression. Theories and evidence exist in supporting: psychosocial factors involving basic life experience; psychological attributes related to vulnerability and coping skills; changes in brain functioning; genetic predisposition; life events and stressors (particularly involving losses and major long-term difficulties); poor relationships; and social, cultural and environmental factors. In most cases the roots of depression are generally accepted as multi-dimensional.

Depression in children

An estimate of the prevalence of childhood and adolescent depression in the community ranges from 0.5 to 10 per cent (NICE 2005). Mood disorders can be difficult to identify and may be masked by developmental stages. Research has identified risk factors to include family discord, bullying, physical, sexual or emotional abuse, history of parental depression, ethnic and cultural factors, homelessness, refugee status and institutional living (NICE 2005).

Depression in women

Women experience depression almost twice as often as men. Research has often focused on the biological differences between the genders that possibly contribute to this increased rate. However, research on biological, psychological and sociopolitical explanations is offering a more integrated approach to informing the development of appropriate prevention/treatment approaches (Corey and Goodman 2006).

Depression in men

Men often experience depression differently than women. While women with depression are more likely to have feelings of sadness, worthlessness and guilt, men may be more likely to have feelings of tiredness, irritability and sleep disturbance. Although men are less likely to suffer depression than women the rate of suicide in men is three to four times that of women, although more women attempt it. While a wide range of explanation and risk factors are proposed, robust explanations for these gender differences have yet to be established.

Depression in the elderly

The incidence of depression and suicidal intent, in combination with physical symptoms, is higher in the elderly and is also one of the most frequently missed diagnoses with resulting negative effects on quality of life. Combined with increasing longevity, greater numbers of older people are experiencing depression. Research has identified risk factors to include poor social integration, loneliness, adverse life events, physical frailty/illness and lack of support from services.

Depression with coexisting conditions

People with depression often have other physical or mental conditions such as anxiety disorders, alcohol and/or substance abuse or dependence, heart disease, stroke, cancer, HIV/AIDS, diabetes, Parkinson's disease, etc. Mental health problems such as depression are also much more common in people with a physical illness. NICE (2009a, 2009b) suggests that people with three or more conditions are seven times more likely to have depression, and that having depression with a coexisting condition has been found to delay recovery (Mykletun et al. 2007), increase mortality by 50 per cent (NICE 2009a, 2009b) and doubles the risk of coronary heart disease in adults (Hemingway and Marmot 1999).

Cultural issues

Although the experience of depression is recognized across different cultures, the challenge is in identifying genuine differences without being misguided by ethnic stereotyping. This research arena is complex. In this era of increasing globalization it is proposed that individual differences are as great as ethnic ones with the headline message of treating the individual.

Box 35.2 NICE guidelines

Published NICE guidelines relevant to depression at the time of writing

- Common mental health disorders
- Depression
- Depression in adults
- Depression in children and young people
- Depression with a chronic physical health problem
- Pregnancy and complex social factors
- Medicines adherence
- Self-harm

Published technology appraisals at the time of writing

- Depression and anxiety – computerized cognitive behaviour therapy (CCBT)
- Electroconvulsive therapy (ECT)

Published pathway/s

- Depression

Published quality standards

- Depression in adults

The reader is referred to the NICE website (www.nice.org. uk) for the latest information.

35.3 Screening, assessment and diagnosis

Within the UK the National Institute for Health and Clinical Excellence (NICE) provides guidance and information on promoting health and treating ill health. The main recommendations related to depression are located in the form of published guidelines, technology appraisals, pathways and quality standards. Those available at the time of writing, that are relevant to depression, are summarized in Box 35.2. In addition the Map of Medicine offers a web based resource of evidence-based care maps for clinicians and includes depression pathways (Map of Medicine 2011).

Screening

People experiencing mood disorders may turn for help to numerous informal and formal sources. The type of help-seeking behaviour is generally influenced by the conceptual belief/model that the individual holds (e.g. a psychological model generally associated with self-help compared to a biological model with help-seeking behaviours). Occasionally, at-risk situations require people to be detained for assessment/treatment under the Mental Health Act (MHA).

All NICE depression guidelines recommend routine screening in primary care of at-risk groups, such as people with a history of depression, the experience of recent major life events etc. An initial two-part screening question is recommended (NICE 2009a):

During the last month, have you often been bothered by: been feeling down, depressed or hopeless? have little interest or pleasure in doing things?

If depression is potentially identified then a more comprehensive assessment by a mental health professional who is competent in mental health assessment is required.

Assessment

Best practice follows a person-centred, holistic approach in undertaking a comprehensive assessment informed by the *person's voice*. The reader is also referred to Chapters 14 on assessment, 17 on assessing and managing risk and 12 on engaging with clients in their care and treatment.

The following are key components of assessment for suspected depression:

- **physical assessment:** presentation, health history, current treatments and lifestyle related to physical well-being;
- **mental health assessment:** duration, severity and degree of functional impairment and/or disability associated with the possible depression and the duration of the episode; assessment of both past and current experience including thoughts, self-worth, self-esteem, risk, coping abilities, mental health history and lifestyle related to mental well-being;
- **social circumstances:** stressors in life, relationships, religious/spiritual needs, networks, employment, accommodation, finance, interests, potential support systems and identification of carers.

Risk

An element of the assessment process is the routine exploration of risk. Although there are many forms of risk, suicidal thoughts are common. It is also important to:

- identify the risks of self-neglect and self-harm and make sensitive enquiry about abuse from others (physical, sexual or emotional) and

actual and potential risk to others (e.g. identifying a need for safeguarding children);
- identify past and current use of prescribed/non-prescribed drugs.

Risk can be generally categorized into:

- **low risk:** no current/infrequent thoughts;
- **intermediate risk:** frequent current thoughts but no intention/plan;
- **high risk:** current thoughts/plans/preparations.

The reader is referred to Chapter 17 on assessing and managing risk of suicide and self-harm for further information.

Screening tools and assessment measures

In screening and reviewing progress, the routine use of validated measures in informing clinical decisions is recommended (NICE 2005, 2009a, 2009b). Many measures are available and the art lies in choosing the measure that best fits the practice setting. Regardless of the measures employed it is the interpretation of results that require validation with the individual that is most important. Some examples of frequently used measures are given in Table 35.1.

Medical classification of depression

A diagnosis of depression is determined by medical classification. The NICE (2009a) guideline has used DSM-IV. DSM-IV has specific criteria that classifies subcategories of depression and determines the type and severity of a depressive condition. This is dependent on symptoms, course, prevalence, pattern and differential diagnosis (which other types of depression can have similar symptoms). See Box 35.3 for more detail.

Diagnosis/classification also refers to a spectrum of depression conditions such as postnatal depression (low mood following childbirth), seasonal affective disorder (SAD) (low mood during winter) and dysthymia (persistent uncomfortable mood). The symptoms of depression may also

Table 35.1 Examples of screening and assessment measures

Measure	Source
General measures	
The Work and Social Adjustment Scale	Mundt *et al.* (2002)
General Health Questionnaire	Goldberg and Williams (1988)
Brief Psychiatric Rating Scale (BPRS)	Lukoff *et al.* (1986)
The Client Satisfaction Questionnaire	Attkisson and Zwick (1982)
Disorder-specific measures	
Patient Health Questionnaire (PHQ-9)	Spitzer *et al.* (1999)
Hospital Anxiety Depression Scale (HAD)	Zigmond and Snaith (1983)
Beck Depression Inventory (BDI-I)	Beck *et al.* (1961)
Beck Depression Inventory (BDI-II)	Steer *et al.* (2000)
Geriatric Depression Scale (GDS)	Sheikh and Yesavage (1986)
Edinburgh Postnatal Depression Scale (PDS)	Cox *et al.* (1987)
Beck Hopelessness Scale	Beck *et al.* (1993)
Case-specific measures	
Case specific measures are highly personal and simple to use (e.g. scoring an experience/view on a scale of 0 to 10). However, they cannot be used for screening purposes or in comparison with treatment groups.	

present in combination with other mental health medically classified conditions such as anxiety, bipolar affective disorder and other forms of psychoses and physical health problems.

Formulating a care plan

A comprehensive assessment will inform the formulation of an appropriate care plan which addresses the following broad themes:

- all possible physical causes such as hormonal conditions, medication side-effects, etc. have been excluded or been/being treated;
- the 'diagnosis', severity and impact of the 'experience' is ascertained;
- the level of risk is identified: low/medium/high;
- other relevant psychosocial factors are also considered.

The reader is also referred to Chapters 15 and 16 on care planning, admission and discharge planning.

 ## 35.4 Approaches to care and treatment

In common with care for people with other mental disorders described in this book, the overarching guiding principle relates to person-centred care, which is based on a collaborative approach, informed by the severity and complexity of the person's condition and their preferences. Clinical judgement is based on a comprehensive assessment, best evidence and available services. Good communication is essential, supported by evidence-based information, to allow people to reach informed decisions about their care. Both the Map of Medicine (www.mapofmedicine.com) and the NICE depression pathway (www.nice.org.uk) offer practitioners a web-based resource of evidence-based clinical pathways, to help inform clinical decision-making. Systematic monitoring and review are essential in deciding and delivering the most appropriate and effective care and treatment.

Box 35.3 Clinical features indicating different levels of depression severity (After NICE 2009a)

1. **Subthreshold depressive symptoms:** this is where you have less than the five symptoms needed to make a diagnosis of depression. So, it is not classed as depression but can cause distress and require treatment. If this condition persists for a period of over two years it is often called dysthymia.

2. **Mild depression:** few, if any, symptoms in excess of the five required to make the diagnosis, and symptoms result in only minor functional impairment characterized by having symptoms for two weeks or longer that do not meet full criteria for major depression.

3. **Moderate depression:** five or more symptoms or functional impairment between 'mild' and 'severe' is characterized by symptoms that may not be severe enough to disable a person but can prevent normal functioning or feeling well.

4. **Severe depression:** most symptoms are severe and the symptoms markedly interfere with functioning. It can occur with or without psychotic symptoms. It is characterized by a combination of symptoms that interfere with a person's ability to work, sleep, study, eat and enjoy once-pleasurable activities.

Note: some forms of depression are slightly different, or they may develop under unique circumstances. However, not everyone agrees on how to characterize and define these forms of depression.

Table 35.2 Stepped care model (after NICE 2009a)

Step	Who is responsible?	The focus	What they do
Step 5	Inpatient care, crisis teams	Risk to life, severe self-neglect	Medication, combined treatments, ECT
Step 4	Mental health specialists including crisis teams	Treatment-resistant, recurrent, atypical and psychotic depression and those at significant risk	Medication, complex psychological interventions, combined treatment, case management
Step 3	Primary care team, primary care mental health worker	Moderate or severe depression	Medication, psychological interventions, social support
Step 2	Primary care team, primary care mental health worker	Mild to moderate depression	Watchful waiting, guided self help, computerized CBT, exercise, brief psychological interventions
Step 1	GP, practice nurse	Recognition	Assessment

Stepped care

Stepped care is recommended for the management of a number of conditions including depression (NICE 2009a, 2009b). Stepped care is a model of care originating from the USA. The two principles of this approach are firstly in offering treatment likely to provide a significant health benefit, but which is the least intensive of those available. Secondly that any decision to 'step up' care is informed by the findings of systematic monitoring, indicating that the current treatment is not achieving the desired gain.

Table 35.2 illustrates some of the main care and treatment approaches at each of the steps based on current evidence. Many mental health nurses will work in specialist services with those at Steps 3 and 4. Recent health policy developments have invested and continue to invest in the Improving Access to Psychological Therapies (IAPT) programme. This national programme is developing primary care capacity, particularly at Steps 1 to 3, to deliver evidence-based interventions for depression and anxiety and other common mental health problems (DH 2011c).

Interventions

NICE (2009a, 2009b) recommends that interventions should be:

- delivered by competent practitioners who receive regular high-quality supervision;
- systematically monitored and reviewed, using outcome measures, to inform treatment efficacy (NICE 2009a, 2009b);
- engaging in monitoring and evaluation of treatment adherence and practitioner competence (NICE 2009a).

Improving and maintaining well-being

It is often very easy to overlook and neglect the importance of factors of well-being. The 'Five Ways' model (Box 35.4) recommended by the Foresight Report (Government Office for Science 2008) offers a simple framework of actions that individuals can adopt to improve and maintain their well-being and

recovery. The importance of these approaches is recommended by NICE in promoting techniques to manage depressive symptoms, such as structured exercise, activity scheduling, engaging in pleasurable and goal-directed activities, ensuring adequate diet and sleep, and seeking appropriate social support.

> ### Thinking Space 35.2
>
> How often do you apply the Five Ways model to yourself? Do you see it being applied in practice? If not why not?

Psychological approaches for depression

Psychological approaches, or talking therapy interventions, for the treatment of depression are wide ranging and include approaches such as CBT, interpersonal therapy, couples therapy, brief therapy, counselling, short-term psychodynamic psychotherapy, problem-solving, behavioural activation, education and self-help methods. CBT generally challenges negative styles of thinking and behaving associated with depression, whereas psychodynamic therapies are sometimes used to focus on resolving people's conflicting feelings. Although there are many forms of psychological intervention there is robust evidence for the efficacy of short-term CBT and interpersonal therapy in the treatment of depression.

Box 35.4 The Five Ways model (adapted from the Government Office for Science 2008)

Five ways to improve your well-being

- **Connect** – with the people around you, family, friends and neighbours
- **Be active** – go for a walk or a run, do the gardening, play a game
- **Take notice** – be curious and aware of the world around you
- **Keep learning** – learn a new recipe or a new language, set yourself a challenge
- **Give** – do something nice for someone else, volunteer, join a community group

For the treatment of mild to moderate depression, brief psychological approaches are recommended as a first-line treatment. This is usually in the form of around six to eight sessions over 6 to 12 weeks. Generally, as the severity of the depression increases the psychological intervention is extended over a longer period of time and may also involve other psychological approaches such as family therapy and include strategies for managing relapse. A range of computerized and web-based CBT and therapy-based programmes are also available.

Medication

Readers are referred to Chapters 26, 27 and 28 for detail on pharmacological interventions and medication for depression. NICE recommends the use of antidepressants, in conjunction with a high-intensity psychological intervention, in the treatment of moderate and severe depression. The first-line choice is from the selective serotonin reuptake inhibitor (SSRI) group, as these drugs are associated with fewer side-effects. Antidepressants take time to establish therapeutic levels and so generally need to be prescribed for a minimum of six weeks, or more, before being considered ineffective. Antidepressants are not considered for routine use to treat mild depression as the benefit ratio is low.

Augmentation of medication may be required in treating combinations of depression with anxiety, psychosis and other conditions. Specific arrangements need to be made for careful monitoring of progress, side-effects and adverse drug reactions with prescribed and un-prescribed drugs and when switching antidepressants. Generally, treatment is continued for at least six months after an episode but this depends on symptoms, support and current/potential stressors. People who have had two or more depressive episodes in the recent past and who experience significant functional impairment are usually advised to continue medication for at least two years. Discontinuation should be gradual.

Alternative and complementary therapies

A vast array of alternative or complementary therapies exist such as light therapy, transcranial magnetic stimulation, vagus nerve stimulation, herbalism, aromatherapy, massage, Traditional Chinese Medicine, hypnosis, folate, St John's wort, meditation, acupuncture, self-help and web and online sources. The extent of usage of these interventions in primary and secondary care is currently constrained, as evidence to support their efficacy remains limited. Because a number of people use such approaches as their main health care system, or in supplementing conventional treatments, it is important for mental health nurses to have awareness and knowledge of these approaches. The reader is referred to Chapters 19 and 29 for further information on self-management and complementary and alternative therapies.

Electroconvulsive therapy

Electroconvulsive therapy (ECT) has been in use since the 1930s and how it works is still not fully understood. NICE guidance on the use of ECT is published, at the time of writing, as *Technology Appraisal 59* (NICE 2003). The Royal College of Psychiatrists (RCPsych 2005) has also produced guidance and developed an accreditation scheme related to ECT administration (RCPsych 2009).

Although the use of ECT in the UK is declining it is still administered to a substantial number of people. NICE (2003) recommends ECT to be used as a treatment for people suffering from a severe depressive illness, prolonged or severe mania, or catatonia, and that it must be used only for conditions which are life-threatening and unresponsive to existing treatment and after all other treatment options have failed. ECT is not used as maintenance therapy.

ECT is undertaken under general anaesthetic and so general preparation and guidance for pre- and post-general anaesthetic care applies. While under anaesthesia electrodes are placed at precise locations on the head to deliver electrical impulses. The electrical stimulation causes a brief (about 30-second) seizure within the brain. The choice of electrode placement and stimulus dose related to seizure threshold should balance efficacy against the risk of cognitive impairment. Bilateral ECT is more effective than unilateral ECT but may cause more cognitive impairment; similarly with unilateral ECT a higher stimulus dose is associated with greater efficacy, but also increased cognitive impairment. To achieve full therapeutic benefit it is recommended that several sessions of ECT be given each week over a three- to six-week period. Memory loss is the most frequently reported side-effect following ECT.

The decision to use ECT needs to be made, as far as possible, jointly with the person. The decision needs to take into account, where applicable, the requirements of both the Mental Capacity Act (MCA) and the MHA. Also be aware that valid informed consent should be obtained (if the person has the capacity to grant or refuse consent) without the pressure or coercion that might occur as a result of the circumstances and clinical setting. The decision is also based on the outcome of a full cost-benefit analysis taking into account such issues as advanced directives, advocacy, the risk of anaesthesia, current health and co-morbidities, adverse events such as potential cognitive impairment, age, risk of not receiving treatment and perceived benefits.

ECT remains a controversial treatment because of its uncertain theoretical basis and its practical application. One service user, Caroline Hearst, sums up her attitude towards ECT as follows:

> On Mind's website a psychologist compares ECT to the 'assumption a broken television could be mended as readily with a sledgehammer as with a screwdriver: you might jog the right bit'. Well, if you don't have a screwdriver and you need the television, using the sledgehammer might be better than nothing. I feel I needed that sledgehammer, but I also needed to know all the risks involved in its use.

(Hearst 2007: 21)

Relapse prevention

Along with advice on managing depressive symptoms, people with depression, who are considered to be at significant risk of relapse, should be offered specific psychological interventions such as CBT or mindfulness-based CBT. For people with recurrent severe depression or depression with psychotic symptoms and for those who have been treated under the MHA, it is recommended that collaborative development of advanced decisions and advance statements should be considered, to influence future care delivery.

 35.5 ## Mental health nursing: caring for people with mood disorders

Context of mental health nursing

The emphasis of mental health nursing care is on providing care through meaningful therapeutic engagement and supporting people through their distressing symptoms. The national policy emphasis is on services working collaboratively together to address all that is implied in the *No Health Without Mental Health* strategy (DH 2011a). This policy context includes a vision of a seamless and connected care system which is consumer focused and recovery oriented. The context of mental health nursing in England remains set within the recommendations of the *Review of Mental Health Nursing* (DH 2006). The review sets the direction of travel for mental health nursing in moving from a traditional medical model to a psychosocial approach. However, Gallop and Reynolds (2004) suggest that the biological, psychological and sociological models have operated as distinct entities, and while we may refer to 'holistic care' the reality is limited in practice and even more so in research.

Mental health problems are common and although most people experiencing depression are seen in primary care, they may or may not be offered effective treatments. Mental health nurses

(MHNs) are the largest professional group providing both care to those with high severity/complex needs, or in supporting other workers in caring for those with less complex needs. This places MHNs in a unique position to fully comprehend the needs and views of people who use our services, thus enabling MHNs to influence change in improving care and advancing practice.

For most people in contact with specialist mental health services, treatment and care is delivered through the Care Programme Approach (CPA) process (DH 2008) with an emphasis on care delivery set within a philosophy of a recovery, as mentioned previously. Each situation will be influenced by the needs of the individual, the care group, the care setting and the availability of appropriate treatments/interventions. This will mean working with individuals in a range of ways that improve the social aspects of their lives, such as social skills, self-esteem, encouraging engagement with other groups in society and helping to identify further training or work opportunities.

The following sections explore some emergent themes from the mental health nursing literature in caring for people experiencing depression.

Mental health nursing and stigma

A study of mental health nursing students' attitudes towards people with depression found that they were similar to those held by the general public – that people with depression have some control of and responsibility for their experience. As the students progressed through their learning this attitude lessened and the students displayed increasing attitudes of help and pity. Although the desire to help is consistent with choosing a nursing career, feelings of pity, although viewed positively, can be viewed negatively as condescending and exclusionary.

In caring for vulnerable people whose reality may be very different to the majority in the community, nurses may be at risk of developing despair and pity. Some care settings are also challenging in attempting to meet all individuals' needs and remaining continuously empathic and understand-

ing. Within this context MHNs may develop coping strategies that adopt a symptom/task approach to care with a resulting disassociation with the person. There is also evidence that MHNs hold positive views towards the 'good, unproblematic, trusting patient' and negative views to all others (Lilja *et al.* 2004: 552).

Fundamental nursing practice

Mental health nursing has championed an interpersonal context at its core (see Chapter 3) and so the concept of inspiring hope is also central to mental health nursing practice. However, inspiring hope generally appears to be achieved by the presence of certain aptitudes and traits in MHNs rather than technical skills alone. Although the interpersonal context is central to mental health nursing, the nurse–person relationship may not always be a positive and enabling one.

Advanced nursing practice

Current research into the efficacy of treatments for depression supports, in the main, pharmacological and psychological approaches. MHNs may now prescribe and are routinely involved in the administration and monitoring of medication. However, there are reports that MHNs are often ill prepared for this aspect of practice (Gray *et al.* 2010) and also that they are not adequately trained to provide psychological support (Crowe and Luty 2005). Having time to spend caring, and delivering psychotherapeutic care, are two different things. However, CBT and brief-term psychological therapies have proven efficacy and MHNs are well placed to incorporate these within their practice.

The true expert

Acknowledging the negative impact of the experience of depression and contact with mental health services, it is proposed that for some people this experience reinforces a 'sick role' and hinders recovery. MHNs can gain invaluable learning from listening to the experiences of people who use mental health services. Gallop and Reynolds (2004: 64) suggest that 'When we [nurses] are able to hear all voices then nurses will be able to frame research and practice in ways that can profoundly impact on clients' lives'.

An understanding of the complexity of mood disorders

An understanding of cultural expectations and their relation to mental distress provides a reference for understanding the meaning of behaviours that may be regarded as mental disorders. Aware that 'depression' is experienced by nearly all of us, we might conclude that this human commonality informs mental health nursing practice; but this may not be so according to the following personal story:

> I do not believe that depression is instructive in many ways. It does not necessarily help you to understand others better, and it does not in my view, make you a better nurse. The danger with having a particular 'experience' is always that we can believe that other people's experiences may be the same: they may or may not be. It does occasionally allow you to see things from two different perspectives: the health-care professionals' and the consumers'. And sometimes these are very different. I can still remember the sister in the psychiatric outpatient clinic who said: 'Oh you are a psychiatric nurse! Are they going to keep you on in your job?' At a time when I felt it difficult to carry on with very much at all, this was of little comfort. Recently, in asking me to recount my symptoms, a doctor asked me: 'Do you feel worthless?' I replied that, as a diagnostic question, I thought it was terrible.

(Burnard 2006: 245)

 35.6 Conclusion

This chapter has provided an overview of depression. It has described briefly what it is, possible causes, screening, assessment, diagnosis, common care and treatment approaches and some points for consideration for mental health nursing practice. In the main these areas have been discussed in relation to the current NICE recommendations and the current context and strategic direction for mental health nursing. Within this context the nature, the art and science, and future, of mental health nursing will evolve.

In summary the main points from this chapter are:

- Depression is an umbrella term describing a spectrum of low mood experience.

- Mood disorders are multi-faceted, complex phenomena.

- Medical diagnosis acts as a frame of reference with MHNs adopting an integrated approach.

- The art and science of nursing: the core being of mental health nursing lies in an enabling therapeutic alliance/relationship with people. However, care and treatments need to be delivered that are competency- and evidence-based.

- There are challenges for MHNs in particular care settings in providing holistic, individualized person-centred care.

- A more standardized, cohesive and evolving approach to effective care and treatments is being recommended by NICE.

- Achieving holistic integrated person-centred care is beset with challenges and opportunities.

- Good communication is essential, supported by evidence-based information, to allow people to reach informed decisions about their care.

- There is a shift of focus from mental illness to mental wellness and well-being.

- The person's voice guides practice in offering person-centred care.

Feedback to Thinking Space 35.1

In line with NICE guidance, Brian's GP made a referral to the specialist crisis and home treatment service. Brian was assessed later that day at home by two members of the team. The MHN leading the assessment took a skilled and empathic approach to engaging with and understanding Brian's situation – as Allan and Dixon (2009: 866) point out: 'When mental health nurses work in partnership with the patient, the patient's story becomes the focus of the therapeutic relationship'.

The initial assessment, which was subsequently confirmed, was that self-neglect was a major risk. It was decided that the team would work with Brian at home, although this decision would be reviewed on each visit and if the situation deteriorated. Although a number of team members would be working with Brian, the MHN was the named worker. The team initially visited Brian twice a day. Once a general physical examination was completed, including blood tests, to exclude any underlying medical conditions, Brian commenced medication in an attempt to alleviate his depressive symptoms and help him develop a regular sleep pattern. The MHN made contact with Brian's brother who met with the team and became involved in supporting Brian, and an appointment was made with a debt adviser to begin to develop a strategy of clarifying and planning the management of Brian's financial problems. The team worked with Brian for six weeks and their input was lessened as his symptoms became less severe.

In view of the severity of Brian's symptoms and the nature of his ongoing stressors it was decided that ongoing support would be required from the community mental health team (CMHT). The CMHT MHN liaised with the crisis intervention team and began working with Brian as the crisis team withdrew.

The CMHT MHN worked with Brian as his care coordinator for the next 10 months. During this time Brian had further input from a psychiatrist, social worker, support worker and psychological therapist. Key elements of activity included: monitoring and review of medication adherence; access to high-intensity psychological therapy; practical assistance and support in managing benefits and debt; support to make lifestyle choices; coping and relapse strategies; and support to develop a vision and goals for the future.

Annotated bibliography

NICE (www.nice.org.uk).
Familiarize yourself with this website which includes mental health clinical guidelines, technology appraisals, quality standards, pathways and public health initiatives, along with the NHS Evidence in Depression Update (April 2012). This work summarizes new evidence relevant to NICE *Clinical Guideline 90: The treatment and management of depression in adults* (2009).

Stahl, S.M. (2009) *Stahl's Illustrated Antidepressants.* New York: Cambridge University Press.
This publication, as with many of the 'Stahl range', where a picture is 'worth a thousand words', presents a complex subject in an enjoyable format.

Royal College of Psychiatry (www.rcpsych.ac.uk).
The mental health information pages of this website have a range of information and although aimed at the general public they are a useful resource.

Living life to the full (www.llttf.com) and **Mood Gym (www. moodgym.anu.edu.au)** are two free quality CBT web-based self-help programmes – have ago.

Map of Medicine (www.mapofmedicine.com).
This resource creates and offers evidence-based informed care maps for clinicians. Familiarize yourself with the depression pathways.

References

Allan, J. and Dixon, A. (2009) Older women's experiences of depression: a hermeneutic phenomenological study, *Journal of Psychiatric and Mental Health Nursing*, 16(10): 865–73.

APA (American Psychological Association) (1994) *Diagnostic and Statistical Manual for Mental Disorders*, 4th revision. Washington: American Psychiatric Association.

Attkisson, C. and Zwick, R. (1982) The client satisfaction questionnaire: psychometric properties and correlations with service utilization and psychotherapy outcome, *Evaluation Program Planning*, 5: 233–7.

Beck, A., Ward, C., Mendelson, M. *et al.* (1961) An inventory for measuring depression, *Archives of General Psychiatry*, 4: 561–71.

Beck, A., Steer, R., Beck, J. and Newman, C. (1993) Hopelessness, depression, suicidal ideation and clinical diagnosis of depression, *Suicide and Life-Threatening Behaviour*, 2: 139–45.

Burnard, P. (2006) Sisyphus happy: the experience of depression, *Journal of Psychiatric and Mental Health Nursing*, 13: 242–6.

Corey, L. and Goodman, S. (eds) (2006) *Women and Depression*. New York: Cambridge University Press.

Cox, J., Holden, J. and Sagovsky, R. (1987) Detection of postnatal depression: development of the 10-item Edinburgh Postnatal Depression Scale, *British Journal of Psychiatry*, 150: 782–876.

Crowe, M. and Luty, S. (2005) Interpersonal psychotherapy: an effective psychotherapeutic intervention for mental health nursing practice, *International Journal of Mental Health Nursing*, 14: 126–33.

DH (Department of Health) (2006) *From Values to Action: The Chief Nursing Officer's review of mental health nursing*. London: DH.

DH (Department of Health) (2008) *Refocusing the Care Programme Approach*. London: DH, available at: www.dh.gov.uk.

DH (Department of Health) (2011a) *No Health Without Mental Health: A cross-government mental health outcomes strategy for people of all age*s. London: DH, available at: www.dh.gov.uk.

DH (Department of Health) (2011b) *No Health Without Mental Health: A cross-government mental health outcomes strategy for people of all age*s, supporting document: the economic case for improving efficiency and quality in mental health. London: DH, available at: www.dh.gov.uk.

DH (Department of Health) (2011c) *Talking Therapies: A four-year plan of action – a supporting document to No Health Without Mental Health: A cross-government mental health outcomes strategy for people of all ages*. London: DH, available at: www.dh.gov.uk.

Gallop, R. and Reynolds, W. (2004) Putting it all together: dealing with complexity in the understanding of the human condition, *Journal of Psychiatric and Mental Health Nursing*, 11: 357–64.

Goldberg, D. and Williams, P. (1988) *A User's Guide to the General Health Questionnaire*. Windsor: NFER-Nelson.

Government Office for Science (2008) *Mental Capital and Wellbeing: Making the most of ourselves in the 21st century – final project report*, available at: http://tinyurl.com/ ForesightReportMentalcapital.

Gray, R., White J., Schulz, M. and Abderhalden, C. (2010) Enhancing medication adherence in people with schizophrenia: an international programme of research, *International Journal of Mental Health Nursing*, 19(1): 36–44.

Hearst, C. (2007) Blasted into the present, *Openmind*, 144: 20–1.

Hemingway, H. and Marmot, M. (1999) Evidence-based cardiology: psychosocial factors in the aetiology and prognosis of coronary heart disease – systematic review of prospective cohort studies, *British Medical Journal*, 318: 1460–7.

Lilja, L., Ordell, M., Dahl, A. and Hellzen, O. (2004) Judging the other: psychiatric nurses' attitudes towards inpatients as measured by the semantic differential technique, *Journal of Psychiatric and Mental Health Nursing*, 11: 546–53.

Lukoff, D., Neuchterlein, K. and Ventura, J. (1986) Manual for the Expanded Brief Psychiatric Rating Scale (BPRS), *Schizophrenia Bulletin*, 12: 594–602.

Map of Medicine (2011) Available at: www.mapofmedicine.com.

Mundt, J., Marks, I., Shear, M. and Greist, J. (2002) The work and social adjustment scale: a simple measure of impairment of functioning, *British Journal of Psychiatry*, 180: 461–4.

Mykletun, A., Bjerkeset, O., Dewey, M., Prince, M., Overland, S. and Stewart, S. (2007) Anxiety, depression and cause-specific mortality: the HUNT study, *Psychosomatic Medicine*, 69(4): 323–31.

NICE (National Institute for Health and Clinical Excellence) (2003) *Technology Appraisal 59: Guidance on the use of electroconvulsive therapy*, available at: www.nice.org.uk.

NICE (National Institute for Health and Clinical Excellence) (2005) *Clinical Guideline 28: Depression in children and young people*, available at: www.nice.org.uk.

NICE (National Institute for Health and Clinical Excellence) (2009a) *Clinical Guideline 90: Depression: treatment and management of depression in adults* (updated edition), available at: www.nice.org.uk.

NICE (National Institute for Health and Clinical Excellence) (2009b) *Clinical Guideline 91: Depression in adults with a chronic physical health problem – treatment and management*, available at: www.nice.org.uk.

RCPsych (Royal College of Psychiatrists) (2005) *The ECT Handbook*, 2nd edn. London: Royal College of Psychiatrists.

RCPsych (Royal College of Psychiatrists) (2009) The ECT Accreditation Service, available at: www.rcpsych.ac.uk/quality/ qualityandaccreditation/ectclinics/ectas.aspx.

Sheikh, J. and Yesavage, J. (1986) Geriatric Depression Scale (GDS): recent evidence and development of a shorter version, in T.C. Brink (ed.) *Clinical Gerontology: A guide to assessment and intervention*. New York: Hayworth Press.

Spitzer, R., Kroenke, K. and Williams, J. (1999) Validation and utility of a self-report version of PRIME-MD the PHQ Primary Care Study, *Journal of the American Medical Association* 282: 1737–44.

Steer, R., Rissmiller, D. and Beck, A. (2000) Use of the Beck Depression Inventory-II with depressed geriatric patients, *Behaviour Research and Therapy*, 38(3): 311–18.

WHO (World Health Organization) (2011) *Disorders Management: Mental health*, available at: www.who.int/mental_health/ management/depression/definition/en/.

Zigmond, A. and Snaith, R. (1983) The Hospital Anxiety Depression Scale, *Acta Psychiatrica*, 67: 361–70.

Chapter 36

The Person with a Bipolar Affective Disorder

Sue Gurney

I went to a doctor and told him I felt normal on acid, that I was a light bulb in a world of moths. That is what the manic state is like.

Carrie Fisher

Manic intentions are always good; manic consequences, almost never.

Terri Cheney 2009

36.1 Introduction

The term bipolar disorder, also known as bipolar affective disorder or manic depression, is used to describe a state of health commonly associated with episodes of severe mood swings (highs and lows). Far from being a discrete diagnostic entity there is increasing recognition of a spectrum of bipolar disorders that range from very severe (potentially life threatening) to milder mood variations, which can become difficult to distinguish from the normal ups and downs that most of us experience. This chapter offers an overview of bipolar disorder and provides information to inform mental health nursing practice.

The chapter covers:

- what is bipolar disorder?
- diagnosis and assessment;
- approaches to care and treatment;
- implications for mental health nursing practice.

What is bipolar disorder?

The term bipolar disorder is an umbrella term which refers to the experience of opposite states of mood, whereby low mood/depression alternates with the experience of elevated mood/mania. These cyclic mood changes may be gradual or rapid and dramatic; with occasionally mania (elated mood and

> ## Box 36.1 Everyone's experience of bipolar disorder is different (Bipolar UK 2011)
>
> - Some people are more affected by depression with just the occasional period of mania.
>
> - Some people experience extreme mood swings only occasionally, with long periods of stability in between. Others experience up to five or six episodes a year or more, sometimes called 'rapid cycling', while some may even experience several mood swings in one day.
>
> - For some people mood swings seem to be triggered by stressful events in their lives, for others they appear to come out of the blue.
>
> - For some people, the highs and lows are relatively short, and for others they may last many months.
>
> - Some people have just one or two mood swings in their life, others have mood swings for many years, but these often become less severe with increasing age.

behavior) or hypomania (elevated mood) occurring on its own. Although an abnormally elevated mood and disturbed behaviour changes are the defining characteristics of bipolar disorder, most people spend more time experiencing low mood/episodes of depression. However, everyone's experience of bipolar disorder is highly individual (see Box 36.1).

NICE (2006) reports that the lifetime prevalence of bipolar disorder is estimated at around 1 per cent of the population, although studies report higher rates when including a wider range of the spectrum of bipolar disorder presentations. The peak age of onset is in late adolescence or early adulthood with a further small increase in incidence in mid to late life. The WHO (2008) reports psychosis, which includes bipolar 1 disorder, as one of the top 20 leading causes of disability worldwide. In the UK the annual cost of bipolar disorder, to society, is estimated at about £2 billion (NICE 2006). However, this might be an underestimate as bipolar disorder may remain unrecognized or misdiagnosed as unipolar depression. As a consequence the resulting suboptimal treatment, in non-detection, could contribute to an increase in the health care cost.

Although the onset of bipolar disorder is often triggered by stressful or life-changing events, the research agenda has a focus on susceptibility factors. There is strong evidence of genetic linkage demonstrated through twin and familial studies and the neuroanatomic and neurodevelopmental areas associated with this related to susceptibility.

Medical classification, signs and symptoms

The medical classification systems DSM-IV (APA 1994) and ICD-10 (WHO 1992) have diagnostic criteria for bipolar disorder (see Boxes 36.2 and 36.3). However, there are crucial differences between the two systems, focusing on the number of 'manic' episode(s) required for a diagnosis and a distinction between bipolar I and II disorders in DSM-IV. DSM-IV requires one single episode of mania/hypomania plus a single major depressive episode for a diagnosis of bipolar disorder, whereas ICD-10 requires at least *two* episodes (one of which must be mania/hypomania). Apart from significant mood alterations, both systems require that the person's behaviour/levels of activity are significantly disturbed (NICE 2006). A DSM-IV diagnosis of bipolar II disorder requires the experience of at least one major depressive episode and at least one hypomanic episode. Any history of manic or mixed episodes rules out a diagnosis of bipolar II disorder (NICE 2006). For further distinctions between the two diagnostic classification systems, readers are referred to NICE (2006).

Manic, and less severe hypomanic episodes usually begin abruptly and last on average around four months; depressive episodes usually last longer, around six months. Recovery may or may not occur between mood episodes. Generally the longer bipolar symptoms are experienced the greater the increase in depressive episodes; an early age of

Box 36.2 DSM-IV diagnostic criteria for a manic episode

A. distinct period of abnormally and persistently elevated, expansive or irritable mood, lasting at least one week.

B. During the period of mood disturbance, three (or more) of the following symptoms have persisted (four if the mood is only irritable) and have been present to a significant degree:

1. Inflated self-esteem or grandiosity

2. Decreased need for sleep (e.g., feels rested after only three hours of sleep)

3. More talkative than usual or pressure to keep talking

4. Flight of ideas or subjective experience that thoughts are racing

5. Distractibility (i.e., attention too easily drawn to unimportant or irrelevant external stimuli)

6. Increase in goal-directed activity (either socially, at work or school, or sexually) or psychomotor agitation

7. Excessive involvement in pleasurable activities that have a high potential for painful consequences (e.g. engaging in unrestrained buying sprees, sexual indiscretions or foolish business investments).

Box 36.3 ICD-10 diagnostic criteria for bipolar disorder

A diagnosis of bipolar disorder requires the experience of at least two mood episodes, one of which must be manic or hypomanic (unlike DSM-IV).

A. A distinct period of abnormally and persistently elevated, expansive or irritable mood, lasting at least one week

B. During the period of mood disturbance, three (or more) of the following symptoms have persisted (four if the mood is only irritable) and have been present to a significant degree:

1. Inflated self-esteem or grandiosity

2. Decreased need for sleep (e.g. feels rested after only three hours of sleep)

3. More talkative than usual or pressure to keep talking

4. Flight of ideas or subjective experience that thoughts are racing

5. Distractibility (i.e. attention too easily drawn to unimportant or irrelevant external stimuli)

6. Increase in goal-directed activity (either socially, at work or school, or sexually) or psychomotor agitation

7. Excessive involvement in pleasurable activities that have a high potential for painful consequences (e.g. engaging in unrestrained buying sprees, sexual indiscretions, or foolish business investments).

onset also tends to indicate greater depressive symptom burden.

 ## 36.2 Differential diagnosis

An accurate diagnosis of bipolar disorder requires time, sometimes years, because presentations can be so wide ranging. Careful consideration also needs to be given to differential diagnoses. This is because the manic/hypomanic stage can often resemble other conditions and may also coexist with them. For example, the presentation may be the symptom of an underlying cerebral condition such as epilepsy, encephalitis, dementia, demyelinating white matter lesions, such as those seen in multiple sclerosis and HIV infection, and space-occupying lesions; metabolic conditions such as hypothyroidism, Cushing's disease, Addison's disease, vitamin B12 deficiency and effects of dialysis; psychotic symptoms can be mistaken for schizophrenia; substance and alcohol misuse can induce manic-like symptoms as can some prescribed medications such as corticosteroids, stimulants and antidepressants (NICE 2006).

Case Study

Stephen

Stephen was in his late twenties, he had relationship difficulties, held a high pressured job, had some ongoing physical health problems and had recently moved house. At the request of his family he was referred to the crisis team by his general practitioner (GP). Stephen was seen and admitted to hospital for assessment under the Mental Health Act (MHA).

At school Stephen had mood swings but this was attributed to 'growing up'. Over recent years he had experienced several periods of depression for which he had seen a therapist and found it helpful. Over recent months he had become increasingly busy, then really busy and multi-tasking big time. He remortgaged the house and started recklessly spending and running up debt into tens of thousands of pounds. He had also started spending business funds. Stephen felt great, he had loads of energy and ideas, he hardly slept and ate and was becoming sexually promiscuous and disinhibited.

When Stephen arrived on the ward he was eccentrically and inappropriately dressed. He was restless, agitated, angry, frightened and talked so excessively fast that his speech was slurred. He had also lost a significant amount of weight. Following a thorough physical and mental health assessment a diagnosis of mania was made and medication suggested. Stephen was angry, and viewed the diagnosis as incorrect.

Stephen's named nurse approached him to explore his 'world' and spent some time over the following week providing information and talking it through. Finally Stephen was willing to 'give it a try'; he accepted the medication and 30 days later was discharged from hospital to the care of the community mental health team (CMHT).

The community team and the nurse, along with his Care Programme Approach (CPA) care coordinator, supported Stephen's care and treatment which in the main was medication, a psycho-education package that included cognitive behavioural therapy (CBT) and membership of a support group. Stephen's life had changed; the experience resulted in the loss of a relationship, home and job. On discharge from hospital his spirits lifted but his life seemed empty as if in a vacuum.

Eighteen months down the line and life is beginning to rebuild. Stephen has moved out of his parents' home into a small flat and is planning to move from voluntary work to commence a course in graphic design.

Stephen self-monitors his mood with a mood diary and mood calendar and holds ambivalent views about his family for the life-changing event that brought him into contact with mental health services.

Thinking Space 36.1

1. What communication approaches might nurses adopt in their time spent with Stephen?

2. What other aspects of support might Stephen require to assist his recovery journey?

Jot down your thoughts. Feedback is given at the end of the chapter.

36.3   Assessment

Within the UK the National Institute for Health and Clinical Excellence (NICE) provides guidance and information on promoting health and treating ill health. At the time of writing the NICE bipolar recommendations are published as *Clinical Guideline 38* (NICE 2006). In addition the Map of Medicine offers an evidence-based web resource of care maps for practitioners which includes bipolar care pathways (Map of Medicine 2011).

People experiencing mood disorders may turn for help to numerous informal and formal sources. The type of help-seeking behaviour is generally influenced by the conceptual belief/model that the individual holds (e.g. a psychological model generally associated with self-help compared to a biological model with help-seeking behaviours) (Goldstein and Rosselli 2003). Occasionally, in-risk situations require people to be detained for assessment/treatment under the MHA.

Best practice follows a holistic, person-centred approach to assessment with clinical judgement informed by the 'person's voice' and current best practice. The reader is referred to Chapters 14 on assessment, 17 on assessing and managing risk and 12 on engaging clients in their care and treatment.

In screening, assessing and reviewing progress, NICE (2006) recommends the routine use of valid measures to inform clinical decisions. Regardless of the measures employed it is the interpretation of results that require validation with the individual

Table 36.1   Examples of screening and assessment measures

Disorder-specific measures	
Measure	**Source**
Mood Disorder Questionnaire	Hirschfeld *et al.* (2001)
Bipolar Spectrum Diagnostic Scale (BSDS)	Ghaemi *et al.* (2005)
Mania Scale	Bech *et al.* (1979)
Case-specific measures	
Case-specific measures are highly personal and simple to use (e.g. scoring an experience/view on a scale of 0 to 10). However, they cannot be used for screening purposes or in comparison to treatment groups.	

that is most important. Some examples of valid measures for bipolar disorder are given in Table 36.1. Examples of measures for depression can be found in Chapter 35.

The following outlines the core principles and key components of assessment:

- effective communication skills in building, maintaining and closing person-centred relationships;

- holistic assessment with the involvement of family and carers as appropriate;

- taking full account of the voice and views of what is important to the person, families and carers and all those involved in the delivery of care; and

- acknowledging strengths and working with these.

The key components of assessment include:

- **thorough physical assessment:** presentation, health history, current treatments and lifestyle related to physical well-being;

- **mental health assessment:** duration and severity of the current experience including the symptom profile: thoughts, self-worth, self-esteem, risk, coping abilities, mental health history (full history including family history, previous episodes and symptoms between episodes), co-morbidities including alcohol and/or drug misuse and lifestyle related to mental well-being;

- **social circumstances:** stressors in life, triggers, relationships, social and personal functioning, religious/spiritual needs, networks, employment, accommodation, finance, interests, potential support systems and identification of carers and obtaining, if possible within the bounds of confidentiality, a corroborative history from a family member or carer.

Risk assessment

It is also important to identify the risks of:

- **self-neglect and self-harm:** people with bipolar disorder have a very high risk of suicide which usually occurs early in the onset of the disorder; the completion rate is 1 in 3 compared to 1 in 30 in the general community (Van Meter *et al.* 2011)
- **abuse from others:** physical, sexual or emotional;
- **actual and potential risk to others:** for example, identifying a need for safeguarding children; and
- **past and current use of prescribed/non-prescribed drugs.**

Risk can be generally categorized into:

- **low risk:** no current/infrequent thoughts;
- **intermediate risk:** frequent current thought but no intention/plan;
- **high risk:** current thoughts/plans/preparations.

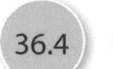 ## 36.4 Care planning

A comprehensive assessment will inform the formulation of an appropriate care plan which addresses the following broad themes:

- all possible physical causes such as organic brain and metabolic conditions, medication

side-effects, etc. have been excluded or have been/are being treated;

- the 'diagnosis' and severity of the 'experience' is established;
- the level of risk is identified: low/medium/high;
- other relevant psychosocial factors are considered.

For most people in contact with specialist mental health services, treatment and care is delivered through the CPA process (DH 2008). This will be influenced by the needs of the individual, the care group, the care setting and the availability of appropriate treatments/interventions. The reader is referred to Chapters 15 and 16 on care planning, admission and discharge planning.

 ## 36.5 Approaches to care and treatment

The overarching guiding principle for care and treatment relates to person-centred care, which is based on a collaborative approach, informed by the severity and complexity of the person's condition and their preferences. Clinical judgement should be based on a comprehensive assessment, best evidence and available services. Good communication is essential, supported by evidence-based information, to allow people to reach informed decisions about their care. Both the Map of Medicine (www.mapofmedicine.com.) and the NICE depression pathway (www.nice.org.uk) offer practitioners a web based resource, of evidence based clinical pathways, to help inform clinical decision-making. Systematic monitoring and review are essential in deciding and delivering the most appropriate and effective care and treatment (NICE 2006).

Primary care

NICE (2006) recommends that any new or suspected presentations of bipolar disorder in primary care are referred for specialist assessment. As more people access and receive treatments in primary care it is imperative that primary care practitioners become more skilled at both recognition and interventions for bipolar disorder. Generally, shared care, between specialist services and primary care, or transfer back from specialist services to primary care is recommended once the condition/situation is stable.

Specialist services

Specialist mental health teams can offer a range of services including early intervention, crisis and home treatment, inpatient care, intensive care units and other specialties. Admission to an inpatient unit is usually considered for people presenting with significant risk of harm. Specialist services should provide expertise in diagnosis, pharmacological and psychosocial interventions.

Pharmacotherapy

The treatment of bipolar disorder, both acute and long term, is primarily based on psychotropic medication (mainly mood stabilizers such as lithium and anticonvulsants). Medication is employed to reduce the severity of symptoms, stabilize mood and prevent relapse. Individual variation in response to medication will often determine the choice of drug, as will the side-effects and potential harms associated with each drug (NICE 2006). Much is unknown about how the medications used to manage bipolar disorders act, but they act on neurotransmitter chemical imbalances. The major neurotransmitters that seem to be involved in bipolar disorder are dopamine, norepinephrine, serotonin and gamma-aminobutyric acid (GABA). Inadequate release or faulty storage mechanisms may cause the imbalance (Murphy 2006).

NICE (2006) does not use the term 'mood stabilizer', as there is no agreed definition. Instead it applies the term 'antimanic drugs' (or medication) to a range of preparations that can be used to treat bipolar disorder. These include antipsychotics (olanzapine and risperidone, quetiapine) lithium and some anticonvulsant drugs (carbamazepine, semisodium valproate and lamotrogine). These medications may be used alone or in combination (Pandya 2010).

Women of childbearing age

It is important to note increasing evidence, and confirmation for valproate, that foetal exposure to antimanic preparations may raise the risk of congenital malformations and neurodevelopmental delays (Galbally et al. 2010). Consequently, prescribing for women of childbearing age requires a careful, flexible approach that is responsive to the needs of clients and their families. Prescribing decisions need to be balanced with the risk of relapse, poor pregnancy and potential child outcomes with the untreated maternal bipolar disorder (Galbally et al. 2010). What also needs to be flagged is the experience of side-effects of medication such as nausea, vomiting, constipation and weight gain, which can mask the classic signs and symptoms of pregnancy and indirectly facilitate the occurrence of pregnancy complications, foetal and neonatal problems (Gentile 2011).

Readers are referred to Chapter 26 for information on medication for bipolar disorder.

Management of an acute episode

Medication is the primary treatment approach and in an acute episode this will consist of:

1. The rapid control of hyperactivity, sleeplessness, irritability, and possible psychotic features with atypical antipsychotics.
2. The selection of an antimanic preparation which should not be delayed beyond the point at which the client is willing to accept oral medication. The choice of the antimanic preparation needs to be based on decisions about future prophylactic treatment, likely side-effects and whether the client is a woman of childbearing age.

If the client exhibits seriously disturbed behaviour, or is at risk of doing so, then they require care delivery in the least stimulating, most supportive environment available, with a constant review of their safety and health needs and the possible employment of distraction techniques. The care setting should seek to provide an emotionally warm, safe, culturally sensitive and supportive environment, with high levels of positive engagement between staff and clients and access to a psychiatric intensive care unit if required (NICE 2006). Pharmacological management of severe behavioural disturbance may be required and the reader is referred to NICE *Clinical Guideline 25* (2005) and Chapters 17 and 18 on assessing and managing risk.

Management and treatment of an episode of depression

If a person is taking antidepressants at the acute onset of mania they are generally stopped or titrated off. Current practice raises the need for caution in prescribing antidepressants for low mood episodes in case it triggers a switch to mania. If antidepressants are prescribed NICE (2006) recommends that an adjunctive antimanic preparation is also prescribed. Few studies provide guidance on the management of acute bipolar depression and it remains unclear whether or not antidepressants provide any additional benefit to ongoing antimanic medication (El-Mallakh *et al.* 2010).

Care of rapid-cycling bipolar disorder and acute mixed episodes

The recommended approach to both these situations is to consider treating the client as if they had an acute manic episode, avoid prescribing antidepressants and monitor closely, particularly for suicide risk (NICE 2006).

Long-term maintenance: management

The least studied phase of bipolar disorder is the maintenance phase (El-Mallakh *et al.* 2010). Generally treatment with antimania medication lasts around two years after the first episode and up to five years if the person has risk factors such as a history of frequent relapse and ongoing stressors (NICE 2006). Once again arrangements need to be made for careful monitoring of progress. Particular awareness needs to be given to the toxicity of some of these preparations and when switching from one medication to another, titrating doses and discontinuing

(NICE 2006). Despite the many advances in the pharmacotherapy of bipolar disorders, the overall prognosis does not appear to have changed; bipolar disorder remains a severe illness often leading to impaired functioning and disability (Slaney *et al.* 2011).

The use of ECT in severe mania and depressive episodes

Electroconvulsive therapy (ECT) is considered only for rapid and short-term improvement of severe symptoms after other treatments have proved ineffective or if the condition is life threatening (NICE 2006). The decision to use ECT as an intervention will be based on cost-benefit analysis of risks associated with the anaesthetic, current comorbidities and anticipated adverse events, particularly cognitive impairment, against the perceived benefits and risks of not having treatment. If ECT is used to treat bipolar disorder then consideration is given to stopping or reducing any antimanic medication, monitoring the length of fits, particularly if the client is taking anticonvulsants, and close monitoring of mental state for evidence of switching to the opposite pole. The reader is referred to Chapter 35 for details on ECT in treating depression.

Psychosocial interventions

Although pharmacology plays a significant part in the treatment of bipolar disorder, full functional recovery is not achieved for many clients. In response, a range of psychosocial interventions have been developed or adapted as an adjunct to medication (NICE 2006). Examples of interventions include: individual therapy such as CBT; psycho-education; promoting a healthy lifestyle; communication skills, problem-solving skills; medication adherence; mood monitoring; detection of early warning signs and development of coping strategies; acceptance of the illness; and family therapy. NICE (2006) also includes advice about techniques such as structured exercise, activity scheduling, engaging in pleasurable and goal-directed activities, ensuring adequate diet and sleep and seeking appropriate social support.

Jung and Newton's (2009) systematic review of Cochrane reviews of non-psychosocial interventions for psychosis identified six studies related to bipolar disorder interventions. These studies focused on prodromals (early warning signs and symptoms), self-help treatments and psychological approaches used to teach people to both recognize and manage early warning signs and therefore better manage their conditions. The main outcomes of the interventions were positive in reducing symptoms, hospitalization and cost.

Monitoring physical health

The available evidence suggests that bipolar disorder is associated with increased premature mortality, secondary to general medical illnesses (NICE 2006) NICE guidance for the monitoring of physical health is outlined in Box 36.4.

Complementary medicine

Jarman *et al.* (2010) propose that motivations for using complementary and alternative medicines or therapies in people with serious mental illness may vary by population and condition. This view challenges previous work which has tended to suggest that people who are dissatisfied with treatment for medical conditions are more likely to use complementary therapies and medicines. A review of com-

plementary medicine applied in combination with conventional antimanic medications in the treatment of bipolar disorder has highlighted some favourable findings relating to supplements (zinc or omega-3) and possibly acupuncture (Sarris *et al.* 2011). Complementary therapies are discussed in Chapter 29.

 ## 36.6 Implications for mental health nursing practice

This section explores some of the emergent themes from the literature related to the mental health nursing care of a person with bipolar disorder; each theme concludes with a point for practice consideration. Similarly, themes relating to mental health nursing for people with depression are given in Chapter 35.

Nurse competency, caring and trustworthiness

There is strong evidence to support that a core element that aids the recovery of clients with severe mental illness, which includes bipolar disorder, is the development of positive trusting relationships with practitioners. Green *et al.* (2008) found that

---

Box 36.4 Monitoring physical health in bipolar disorder (after NICE 2006)

People with bipolar disorder should have an annual physical health review, normally in primary care, to ensure that the following are assessed each year:

- lipid levels, including cholesterol in all clients aged over 40 even if there is no other indication of risk;
- plasma glucose levels;
- weight;
- smoking status and alcohol use;
- blood pressure.

The results of the annual review should be given to the person, and to health care professionals in primary and secondary care (including whether the person refused any tests). A clear agreement should be made about responsibility for treating any problems.

Note: Appendix D of the NICE guideline includes a list of the physical monitoring required.

what is valued most by clients is healthy, collaborative, mutually trusting relationships with competent, trustworthy, caring practitioners 'who treat encounters "like friendships", increase willingness to seek help and continue care when treatments were not effective and support "normal" rather than "mentally ill" identity' (Green *et al.* 2008: 9). These elements provide a healthy framework for dialogues between practitioners and clients, increasing the likelihood that health care will be planned and carried out in ways that promote, rather than endanger, recovery.

In a Swedish study exploring how nurses' attitudes influence the time nurses spend with clients, Hellzén *et al.* (2005) found that the attitude of empathy may be difficult for mental health nurses (MHNs) to portray in certain situations. Their research suggests that when clients exhibit disturbed behaviour or if they are very cognitively impaired, then it is very difficult for nurses to empathically 'place themselves in their client's shoes' as the experience is so 'foreign'. However, the research does indicate that in these circumstances the desire to care in nurses seemed to be 'triggered' by visual perception and moral concern to care raised by curiosity. The researchers propose that this has important implications for practice – i.e. does lack of curiosity, in these circumstances, relate to a neglect in caring? Although this raises further questions it does highlight the importance of supervision, education and reflective practice for MHNs, discussed further in Chapter 7.

Mental health nursing

The delivery of mental health nursing care should ideally be based and built on evidence-based practice. However, the ideal and reality often differ.

The review by Goossens *et al.* (2007) of nursing literature on care for people with bipolar disorder concludes that although mental health nurses are involved in the provision of care for this client group, there are no agreed nursing standards assuring quality and more research is needed to provide a knowledge base for integrated evidence-based nursing care. The reviewers pose a range of questions to investigate the daily practices of nurses working with bipolar disorder clients, which are listed in Box 36.5. A later study by this research team (Goossens *et al.* 2008) explored the practice of Dutch community MHNs in their care for people with bipolar disorder. They found that although the nurses' daily practice covered relevant issues in caring for people with bipolar disorder there was a lack of specific, systematic, structured bipolar nursing assessment and the formulation of nursing care plans.

Goossens *et al.* (2007: 176) identify what they refer to as the most promising nursing processes for the care of a client with bipolar disorder, which they suggest should be carried out as part of a multidisciplinary approach to care and treatment. These nursing processes are:

- a specific bipolar disorder nursing assessment;
- concrete formulation of both care and crisis plans;

Box 36.5 What do MHNs do in caring for people with bipolar disorder? (Goossens *et al.* 2007)

- Which interventions do they use and when?
- What goals do they set when nursing clients with bipolar disorder?
- What are the critical decision points during the nursing process?
- What information do nurses use to make these decisions, and how do they obtain this information?
- And how do nurses evaluate the outcomes of their decisions with respect to client with a bipolar disorder?

Table 36.2 Psychological interventions applied in nursing practice to the care of people with bipolar disorder and their potential benefits (adapted from Crowe *et al.* 2010)

Psychological intervention	Main benefits
Psycho-eduction	Positive outcomes were achieved in reducing relapse
Family interventions (mostly psycho-education)	Indications of enhanced medication adherence and reduction of symptoms of depression
CBT	The approaches were adapted to include psycho-education, management of stress, recognition of early warning symptoms/signs, developing coping strategies, healthy living techniques, etc.
Interpersonal social rhythm therapy	This approach combined interpersonal therapy with a social rhythm matrix to promote routine to the lifestyle. The focus was on mood and symptoms, importance of daily routine, social relationships and techniques to manage disruption of routine
Systematic/chronic care models	These approaches were very case management based and included general support, psycho-education and some group work over a period of several years
Intensive therapies	A range of different individual therapies were used

- protection;
- psycho-education measures;
- other measures aimed to enhance self-management and treatment compliance;
- support for the client, caregivers, family and friends;
- observation of treatment effectiveness and any side-effects of medication;
- easy access to nurse as case manager.

Psychosocial interventions are recommended in the NICE guidelines for schizophrenia and bipolar disorder. Although education and training initiatives have evolved over the last few decades to help equip the mental health workforce, serious problems remain in implementing such interventions into routine practice (Sin and Scully 2008).

Crowe *et al.* (2010) propose that mental health nurses are well positioned to implement and develop psychosocial work for people with bipolar disorder. Their review of the mental health nursing literature between 1990 and 2009 identified 35 nurse-led psychological interventions applied in nursing practice to the care of people with bipolar disorder (see Table 36.2), although they conclude that research in this field is in its infancy.

General mental health context

In exploring a National Health Service (NHS) NHS trust's adherence to the NICE (2006) bipolar guidelines, Kumar and Rao (2010) discovered omissions in discussing pharmacological options with clients to help them make informed choices, and a deficit in offering psychosocial interventions and lifestyle advice.

A retrospective national benchmarking audit of lithium monitoring against recommended standards collected from 3,373 client clinical records, from 38 NHS trusts found that for clients commencing lithium therapy there were documented baseline measures of renal function in 84 per cent of cases and thyroid function in 82 per cent of cases. For clients prescribed lithium for a year or more, the NICE standards for monitoring lithium serum levels and renal and thyroid function were met in lithium serum levels completed for 30 per cent of cases, in renal function tests for 55 per cent and in thyroid function for 50 per cent. Since these finding fell short of the NICE (2006) recommended standards, they, along with reports of harm received by the National Patient Safety Agency (NPSA), prompted a patient safety alert mandating primary care, mental health and acute trusts, and laboratory staff to work together to ensure systems are in place to support recommended lithium monitoring (Collins *et al.* 2010).

Physical health

It is now widely accepted that there are higher levels of physical morbidity and mortality in people with serious mental illness, which includes bipolar disorder, than in the general population (see Chapter 30). The available evidence indicates that this increased physical morbidity and premature mortality is secondary to general medical illnesses, unhealthy lifestyle, biological factors, adverse pharmacologic effects and disparities in health care. In light of this evidence NICE (2006) recommends a schedule for the physical monitoring of clients with bipolar disorder. However, Nayrouz *et al.* (2011) identify weaknesses in monitoring activities, responsibilities and information-sharing between primary and secondary care and recommend closer working relationships which not only guide improved health screening but also improved selection of antipsychotic prescribing and psychosocial interventions.

36.7 Conclusion

This chapter has described the presentation of bipolar disorder, possible causes, assessment, diagnosis, key care and treatment approaches and some points for consideration for mental health nursing practice. In the main these areas have been discussed in relation to the current NICE guidance and the current context of mental health nursing practice. Within this context the art and science, and future, of mental health nursing practice will evolve.

In summary the main points from this chapter are:

- Bipolar disorder is an umbrella term describing a spectrum of high and low mood experiences.
- A more standardized and cohesive approach to effective care and treatments is being provided by NICE and the Map of Medicine.
- Medical diagnosis acts as a frame of reference, however the essence of mental health nursing involves working with the person and their distress.
- Pharmacology remains the primary intervention for both acute and long-term maintenance of bipolar disorder.
- MHNs play a key role in monitoring and reviewing the efficacy and adherence issues of prescribed medication for bipolar disorder.
- A range of psychosocial interventions are available as an adjunct to medication for people with bipolar disorder. MHNs are well placed to deliver and implement these.
- It is well established that people with bipolar disorder have poor physical health and higher morbidity. MHNs are well placed to influence practice to change this situation.
- The person's voice guides practice in offering person-centred care, preferences and choice.
- Better understanding of bipolar disorder and improved diagnosis and management by both primary and secondary care providers has the potential to dramatically improve clients' and their families' ability to function in society.

Feedback to Thinking Space 36.1

1. Along with the givens of dignity, respect and empathy, communication approaches will be influenced by Stephen's behaviour and degree of concentration and understanding. As this is

generally reduced in both manic and depressive episodes communication needs to be delivered in clear, simple and 'appropriate concentration tailored' amounts. The communication may also require repetition and revisiting in gaining clarification of understanding. Consideration should be given to the need and appropriateness of communicating with his family and other relevant relationships.

2. Other areas might include: managing mental health including relapse prevention, a crisis plan and an advanced directive; building identity, self-esteem and confidence; meeting carers' needs and support requirements; ensuring good self-care (e.g. diet and cooking skills and physical health) is promoted; support with living skills (e.g. welfare, accommodation needs; addressing relationship needs; developing relationship skills and social networks; addressing addictive behaviours; undertaking meaningful activities, work and employment).

Annotated bibliography

Reavley, D. (2008) The work of a clinical nurse specialist in bipolar disorder is examined, *Nursing Standard*, 22(27): 24–5.
This article describes the role and contribution of a bipolar clinical nurse specialist.

Biploar UK (www.bipolar.org.uk). Bipolar UK is the national charity dedicated to supporting individuals with the condition of bipolar disorder, their families and carers.
This website has a range of resources and information.

NICE (www.nice.org.uk).
Familiarize yourself with the range of bipolar guidelines.

Map of Medicine (www.mapofmedicine.com).
Familiarize yourself with the bipolar and associated care pathways.

NHS Choices (www.nhs.uk) is the online 'front door' to the NHS. It is the country's biggest health website and has information on bipolar disorder.

References

APA (American Psychological Association) (1994) *Diagnostic and Statistical Manual for Mental Disorders*, 4th revision. Washington: American Psychiatric Association.

Bech, P., Bowlig, T., Kramp, P. and Rafaelson, O. (1979) The Bech-Rafaelson Mania Scale and the Hamilton Depression Scale, *Acta Psychiatrica Scandinavica*, 49: 248–56.

Bipolar UK (2011) Available at www.bipolar.org.uk.

Collins, N., Barnes, T.R., Shingleton-Smith, A., Gerrett, D. and Paton, C. (2010) Standards of lithium monitoring in mental health Trusts in the UK, *BMC Psychiatry*, 10(80): 1471–244x.

Crowe, M., Whitehead, L., Wilson, L. *et al.* (2010) Disorder-specific psychosocial interventions for bipolar disorder: a systematic review of the evidence for mental health nursing practice, *International Journal of Nursing Studies*, 47(7): 896–908.

DH (Department of Health) (2008) *Refocusing the Care Programme Approach*. London: DH.

El-Mallakh, R.S., Elmaadawi, A.Z., Loganathan, M., Lohano, K. and Gao, Y. (2010) Bipolar disorder: an update, *Postgraduate Medicine*, 122(4): 24–31.

Galbally, M., Roberts, M. and Buist, A. (2010) Mood stabilizers in pregnancy: a systematic review, *Australian & New Zealand Journal of Psychiatry*, 44(11): 967–77.

Gentile, S. (2011) Drug treatment for mood disorders in pregnancy, *Current Opinion in Psychiatry*, 24(1): 34–40.

Ghaemi, S.N., Millar, C., Berv, D.A., Klugman, J., Rosenquist, K. and Pies, R.W. (2005) Sensitivity and specificity of a new bipolar spectrum diagnostic scale, *Journal of Affective Disorders*, 84: 273–7.

Goldstein, B. and Rosselli, F. (2003) Etiological paradigms of depression: the relationship between perceived causes, empowerment, treatment, preferences and stigma, *Journal of Mental Health*, 12(6): 551–63.

Goossens, P.J., van Achterberg, T., van der Klein, T. and Knoppert, E.A.M (2007) Nursing processes used in the treatment of patients with bipolar disorder, *International Journal of Mental Health Nursing*, 16(3): 168–77.

Goossens, P.J., Beentjes,T.A.A., de Leeuw, J.A.M., Knoppert-van der Klein, E.A.M. and van Achterberg, T. (2008) The Nursing of Outpatients with a Bipolar Disorder: What Nurses Actually Do? *Archives of Psychiatric Nursing* 22(1): 3–11.

Green, C.A., Polen, M.R., Janoff, S.L. *et al.* (2008) Understanding how clinician-client relationships and relational continuity of care affect recovery from serious mental illness: STARS study results, *Psychiatric Rehabilitation Journal*, 32(1): 9–22.

Hellzén, M., Ingbritt, L., Annika, D. and Hellzén, O. (2005) Psychiatric nurses' attitudes towards identified inpatients as measured by the semantic differential technique, *Scandinavian Journal of Caring Science*, 19: 12–19.

Hirschfeld, R.M.A., Williams, B.W.J., Spitzer, R.L. *et al.* (2000) Development and validation of a screening instrument for bipolar spectrum disorder: the mood disorder questionnaire, *American Journal of Psychiatry*, 157(11): 1873–5.

Jarman, C., Perron, B., Kilbourne, A. and Farmer, C. (2010) Perceived treatment effectiveness, medication compliance and complementary and alternative medicine use amongst veterans with Biopolar Disorder. *The Journal of alternative and Complementary Medicine* 16(3): 251–5.

Jung, X.T. and Newton, R. (2009) Cochrane Reviews of non-medication-based psychotherapeutic and other interventions for schizophrenia, psychosis, and bipolar disorder: a systematic literature review, *International Journal of Mental Health Nursing*, 18(4): 239–49.

Kumar, A. and Rao, K.P. (2010) Local adherence to national guidelines in the management of bipolar affective disorders, *European Psychiatry*, 25: 0924–9338.

Map of Medicine (2011) Available at: www.mapofmedicine.com.

Murphy, K. (2006) Managing the ups and downs of bipolar disorder, *Nursing*, 36(10): 58–64.

Nayrouz, S., Ploumaki, S., Farooq, R., Stock, D. and Lim, H. (2011) Physical health problems in patients with severe mental illness: relationship between antipsychotic treatment and physical health, *European Neuropsychopharmacology*, 21: S480–1.

NICE (National Institute for Health and Clinical Excellence) (2005) *Clinical Guideline 25: Violence: the short-term management of disturbed/violent behaviour in psychiatric inpatient settings and emergency departments*, London: NICE, available at: www.nice.org.uk.

NICE (National Institute for Health and Clinical Excellence) (2006) *Clinical Guideline 38: Bipolar disorder – the management of bipolar disorder in adults, children and adolescents, in primary and secondary care*, London: NICE, available at: www.nice.org.uk.

Pandya, S. (2010) Mood stabilizers: use, actions and prescribing rationale, *Nurse Prescribing*, 8(10): 492–6.

Sarris, J., Lake, J. and Hoenders, R. (2011) Bipolar disorder and complementary medicine: current evidence, safety issues, and clinical considerations, *Journal of Alternative & Complementary Medicine*, 17(10): 881–90.

Sin, J. and Scully, E. (2008) An evaluation of education and implementation of psychosocial interventions within one UK mental healthcare trust, *Journal of Psychiatric & Mental Health Nursing*, 15(2): 161–9.

Slaney, C., Garnham, J., Manchia, M. and Donovan, C. (2011) Outcome measures in a bipolar disorder, *International Clinical Psychopharmacology*, 26: e19.

Van Meter, A., Freeman, A., Holdaway, A. and Youngstrom, E. (2011) Temperament as a predictor of suicidality, *International Clinical Psychopharmacology*, 26: e30–1.

WHO (World Health Organization) (2008) *Global Burden of Disease: 2004 update*. Geneva: WHO.

WHO (1992) *International Classification of Disease* (10th edn). Geneva, WHO.

Chapter 37

The Person with an Anxiety Disorder

Sally Askey-Jones and Ryan Askey-Jones

'I am going to pass out', 'I will have a heart attack', 'I will choke to death', 'I will act foolishly', 'I will not be able to control myself', 'I am going to die', 'I am going to suffocate.'

(Typical utterances from someone with an anxiety disorder)

37.1   Introduction

Anxiety disorders are some of the most common and debilitating mental disorders. They can often be chronic and result in impairments across personal and occupational domains. This chapter examines the prevalence of anxiety disorders and how they affect people, and considers assessment tools and interventions that nurses can use in hospitals and in the community.

The chapter explores the different aetiological theories for anxiety, focusing in particular on biological and cognitive-behavioural explanations. The skills required for accurate screening and assessment of the different anxiety disorders are considered and potential treatments reviewed, including both pharmacological and psychological

interventions. The chapter concludes with a discussion of the nursing role for a person with an anxiety disorder. The chapter covers:

- definitions of anxiety disorders;
- aetiology of anxiety disorders;
- screening of anxiety disorders;
- assessment of anxiety disorders;
- psychological treatments;
- pharmacological treatments;
- the role of the mental health nurse.

37.2   What is anxiety?

Fear is a normal emotional reaction that occurs in response to external threatening events in the here and now. It is understood to be an evolutionary mechanism designed to avoid threat and enhance survival, and consists of behavioural, cognitive and physiological reactions.

Anxiety, conversely, is an emotion similar to fear, but occurs in the absence of a threatening situation and can be in response to a perceived future threat to either internal or external stimuli. Anxiety is maintained by the intolerance of uncertainty.

The distinction between anxiety symptoms and anxiety disorders is important as while fear is a normal response to a threatening situation, persistent anxiety interferes with daily functioning and negatively affects people's quality of life.

Anxiety disorders are diagnosed when anxiety is excessive and causes a variety of different cognitive, emotional, behavioural and physiological responses. They are diagnosed according to their intensity and the duration of the anxiety response.

Physiological symptoms

- **Cardiovascular:** palpitations, heart racing, increased blood pressure, faintness.
- **Respiratory:** rapid breathing, shortness of breath, shallow breathing, choking.
- **Neuromuscular:** increased reflexes, muscle spasms, tremors, rigidity, fidgeting, wobbly legs.
- **Gastrointestinal:** abdominal discomfort, nausea, vomiting.
- **Urinary tract:** frequency of urination.
- **Skin:** flushed face, sweating, hot and cold spells.

Behavioural symptoms

People who experience anxiety can find that they freeze, become inhibited, are avoidant of situations, feel restless, may hyperventilate or may have speech difficulties. Furthermore, many patients will describe safety-seeking behaviours that keep the person safe in stressful situations. For example, drinking alcohol before engaging in social activities or leaving a situation if you believe you may embarrass yourself.

Cognitive symptoms

People, who experience anxiety may display particular cognitive styles. Many people with anxiety have selective attention, in which they focus primarily on sources of danger or safety. Furthermore, many may describe erroneous thinking styles such as fortune-telling, catastrophizing, personalizing, mind reading and black and white thinking. People may experience repetitive negative thinking in the style of worry and rumination and some may also have positive and negative beliefs about worry (known as meta-cognitive beliefs). People with anxiety may also describe poor memory, forgetfulness and reduced ability to concentrate.

Prevalence

Anxiety disorders affect around 6 million people in the UK and while they are some of the most common mental disorders, less than 30 per cent of individuals seek treatment and can often remain undiagnosed by health professionals. As a consequence it is estimated that only around 10 per cent are adequately treated (McManus *et al.* 2007). This untreated common mental health problem costs around £26 billion a year in sickness and absence from work (Sainsbury Centre for Mental Health 2007). The costs to the government in paid benefits and lost tax revenues are around £7 billon per year (Layard *et al.* 2006).

The prevalence of anxiety disorders can be difficult to establish due to disagreements about thresholds, changes in diagnostic criteria and the use of different interview rating scales or the methods used within research. However, current evidence focusing on the prevalence of anxiety worldwide suggests that 16.6 per cent of people have a lifetime risk of developing an anxiety disorder and there is a one-year prevalence of approximately 10.6 per cent (Somers *et al.* 2006), with the US National Co-Morbidity Survey suggesting lifetime prevalence of 31.2 per cent and 12-month prevalence rates of 19.1 per cent (Kessler 2007). On average, anxiety rates are twice as high for females than males. Table 37.1 describes the

Table 37.1 Lifetime and 12-month prevalence rates of anxiety disorders

Disorder	Lifetime prevalence (%)	12-month prevalence (%)
Generalized anxiety disorder	5.7	4.4
Panic disorder	4.7	2.7
Agoraphobia	1.3	1.0
Post traumatic stress disorder	6.8	3.0–3.6
Phobia	12.5	1.4–9.1
Obsessive compulsive disorder	2.3	1.2
Social phobia	12.1	7.1

lifetime and 12-month prevalence for the different anxiety disorders.

Anxiety disorders create high individual and social burdens, have a tendency to be chronic, and can be debilitating for the person and their family. Furthermore, they can also arise co-morbidly with another condition. For example, anxiety can often be co-morbid with depression, with co-morbidity being the rule in these conditions, rather than the exception. NICE (2011) suggests that more than half of people who meet criteria for one mental health disorder will experience co-morbid anxiety and depressive disorders.

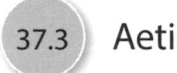

37.3 Aetiology

Alternative explanations for anxiety disorders are underpinned by different theoretical perspectives including cognitive-behavioural, learning, biological, developmental and psychodynamic.

Cognitive theories suggest that people with anxiety have a tendency to overestimate danger and that it is this misperception that creates anxiety. Furthermore, not only do people overestimate the threat, but they also underestimate their ability to cope with the threat and the potential rescue factors. Anxiety is then maintained by processes such as selective attention, selective memory, thinking errors, recurrent thinking and avoidance and safety seeking behaviours that aim to reduce anxiety, but

in the long term increase the preoccupation with the threat and maintain the anxiety.

In contrast, biological theories of anxiety focus on neurotransmitters or neurophysiology. Neurochemical theories suggest there is an imbalance in certain neurotransmitters. The neurotransmitters implicated in the genesis of anxiety are gamma-aminobutryic acid (GABA), serotonin (5HT) and noradrenaline (NA). For anxiety, it is suggested that there are reduced levels of GABA and 5HT and increased levels of NA. Further reading that provides an overview of alternative theories of anxiety is provided in the annotated bibliography at the end of this chapter.

Specific anxiety disorders

The term 'anxiety disorders' defines several conditions in which anxiety is the predominant feature. They are classified according to the American Psychiatric Association's (APA) *Diagnostic and Statistical Manual of Mental Disorders* (DSM-IV) (APA 2000) or the World Health Organization's (WHO) *International Statistical Classification of Diseases and Related Health Problems* (ICD-10) (WHO 1992). These systems provide clear criteria on which diagnoses can be made. This chapter draws on DSM-IV criteria.

Generalized anxiety disorder (GAD)

GAD can be a debilitating condition that can greatly reduce a person's quality of life. GAD is characterized by persistent and excessive anxiety and worry. People

Box 37.1 DSM-IV criteria for GAD

- Excessive anxiety, worry and apprehension about a number of events
- Present for at least six months
- The worry is difficult to control
- Three (or more) of the following six symptoms: restlessness, easily fatigued, difficulty concentrating, irritability, muscle tension, sleep disturbance (difficulty falling or staying asleep, or restless unsatisfying sleep)
- Significant distress or impairment in social, occupational or other important areas of functioning
- The symptoms are not due to the effects of substances, medications or a medical condition (e.g. hyperthyroidism)

may worry about their family, their house, their financial security, their health, and these worries may be unrealistic or inappropriate. As a result of these worries, they may feel apprehensive the majority of the time and experience motor tension, apprehension and hypervigilance. Worry is a key component of GAD, and as such GAD should be conceptualized as a disorder about worry (see Box 37.1). People with GAD find it difficult to identify their sources of worry and may complain of physical symptoms such as muscle aches, fatigue and difficulties with controlling the worrying thoughts. Furthermore, even if a particular worrying thought is resolved, it is often replaced by another concern. The course of GAD is often chronic, but fluctuates and worsens during periods of acute stress. Diagnosing GAD can be challenging, and it has the lowest diagnostic reliability of all anxiety disorders.

There is a strong overlap between the physical symptoms of GAD and other anxiety disorders, and the only physical symptom that does not exist in other anxiety disorders is that of muscle tension. However, it is difficult to diagnose a disorder based on muscle tension alone, and therefore it is important to assess the nature and impact of the worry.

GAD can commonly present with other disorders such as depression or substance misuse, or other anxiety disorders. Moreover, cultural context can influence symptoms; in some cultures, somatic symptoms may predominate, whereas in other cultures cognitive symptoms may be dominant.

Panic disorder

Panic disorder is characterized by patterns of recurring, unforeseen panic attacks and persistent worry about experiencing another panic attack in the future (see Box 37.2). People who experience panic attacks also experience physical symptoms such as palpitations, chest pain, shortness of breath, dizziness and sweating, and patients often misinterpret these symptoms as life-threatening. Panic attacks also affect behaviour – for example, people may stop shopping if previous attacks have occurred at shopping centres. Panic attacks can occur unexpectedly and may not be provoked by any external stimulus. Up to 65 per cent of people with panic disorder can also develop agoraphobia, which is a fear of being in places from which escape might prove difficult in the event of a panic attack. In more severe cases, people may not leave their homes.

Diagnosis of panic attacks requires at least four of the following symptoms that develop abruptly and reach a peak within 10 minutes and occur in the absence of real danger: palpitations, sweating, trembling or shaking, shortness of breath, choking, chest pain or discomfort, nausea or abdominal distress, feeling dizzy, lightheaded or faint, derealization (feelings of unreality) or depersonalization (being detached from oneself), fear of losing control, fear of dying, paresthesias (numbness or tingling sensations) and chills or hot flushes.

Box 37.2 DSM-IV criteria for panic disorder without agoraphobia

At least one of the attacks has been followed by one month (or more) of one (or more) of the following:

- Frequent worry about having new attacks
- Concerns about the consequence of another attack, such as 'having a heart attack', 'dying', 'going mad'
- A significant change in behaviour related to the attacks
- Agoraphobia is not present
- The attacks are not due to effects of a substance (e.g., a drug of abuse, a medication) or a general medical condition (e.g. hyperthyroidism)
- the attacks are not better accounted for by another mental disorder, such as social phobia, specific phobia, obsessive-compulsive disorder, posttraumatic stress disorder, or separation anxiety disorder

Panic attacks can vary in their frequency. Some people may experience them periodically, whereas others can experience them on a daily basis. Some people can also experience panic attacks at night, with attacks occurring in the first three hours of sleep. People may develop fears and avoidance around panic attacks – for example, some people may start to fear sleep. These panic attacks could lead to sleep deprivation, which can lead in turn to an increase in anxiety symptoms.

Phobias

Fears of specific events are a common occurrence among the general population, and can serve as a useful safety mechanism in the appropriate environment. For example, fear of snakes may seem excessive in the UK where most snakes are not poisonous; however in other countries, this fear would be a realistic and rational response. When fears interfere with a person's daily life they can become a phobia.

Phobias, according to ICD-10, are defined as:

A group of disorders in which anxiety is evoked only, or predominantly, in certain well-defined situations that are not currently dangerous. As a result these situations are characteristically avoided or endured with dread. The patient's concern may be focused on individual symptoms like palpitations or feeling faint and is often associated with secondary fears of dying, losing control, or going mad. Contemplating entry to the phobic situation usually generates anticipatory anxiety.

(WHO 2010)

Specific phobias

People with a specific phobia experience anxiety about a particular object or situation (see Box 37.3). There are a wide range of phobias that people can experience – for example, people can develop fears about animals, bridges, injections, blood, vomit, dentists and heights. When people are exposed to the object, they become very anxious and may experience symptoms similar to a panic attack. This can result in people needing to leave the situation or avoid it. Some may also endure it but experience severe distress. In people who develop animal phobia, distress is experienced in the form of fear, whereas people who have blood injury phobia experience distress in the form of disgust and repulsion. It is thought that phobias can develop in childhood or

Box 37.3 DSM-IV criteria for specific phobias

- Persistent, excessive fear that occurs in the presence or anticipation of an object or situation (e.g. storms, lifts, enclosed spaces, heights, animals, vomit, blood)
- Exposure to the phobic stimulus leads to an anxiety response, which may take the form of a panic attack
- The person is aware that the fear is excessive or unreasonable
- The object/situations is/are avoided or endured with intense anxiety or distress
- The avoidance, anticipation or distress causes significant disruption of the person's life, functioning, relationships or social activities
- The anxiety is not better accounted for by other anxiety disorders

adolescence but decline in older age and are almost twice as common in females as in males.

Having a specific phobia can lead to a reduced quality of life and a restricted one. For example, avoidance of crowded places can lead to a curtailment of social activities. Phobias can develop following trauma such as being attacked by a dog, observing others being fearful of a particular animal and by transmission of information – for example, parents or the media communicating to children the dangers of certain animals or information about plane crashes. The majority of feared objects tend to involve something that represents a threat or has been a threat over the course of human evolution.

Agoraphobia

Agoraphobia is a contentious category as DSM-IV suggests that it is not a codable disorder, but is only diagnosed in the context of panic disorder (see Box 37.4). However, some studies suggest that it can occur independently of panic attacks and therefore should be considered as a separate disorder.

Agoraphobia is defined as the fear of crowds, public places, travelling alone or travelling away from home. The person experiencing agoraphobia will experience anxiety in the feared situation and will have several autonomic arousal symptoms. They will also experience significant distress and be aware that their response is excessive. The person will only experience symptoms when in the feared situation(s) or when thinking about them.

Social phobia

Social phobia is characterized by fear of negative appraisal, which the person anticipates will occur due to poor performance. The anxiety may not just occur in performance situations, but can occur in everyday tasks in which the person is under examination, such as eating in public or speaking to a stranger or a group. The person with social phobia believes that they will act in a way which is unacceptable and will lead to rejection or loss of self-worth. For example, a person eating in public may worry that they will be seen shaking, or a person speaking in public may worry that they are blushing excessively.

For the diagnosis to be made, the person must experience anxiety when they are exposed to the situation. The person with social phobia will also avoid the situation or will endure it with significant distress (see Box 37.5). Some people may experience panic attacks either prior to, or within, the situation. Individuals with social phobia almost always experience symptoms of anxiety (e.g. palpitations, tremors, sweating, gastrointestinal discomfort, diarrhoea, muscle tension, blushing, confusion) in the feared social situations, and, in severe cases, these symptoms may meet the criteria for a panic attack.

A further diagnostic criterion for social phobia is that it must cause significant interference with the person's routine, occupational or academic functioning, or social activities or relationships, or the person must experience marked distress about having the phobia.

Box 37.4 DSM-IV criteria for agoraphobia

- Agoraphobia is not a codable disorder and should be coded as panic disorder with agoraphobia or agoraphobia without history of panic disorder
- People with agoraphobia will be anxious in places or situations in which escape might be difficult or help not available in the event of having an unexpected panic attack or panic-like symptoms
- Situations might include: being outside the home alone; being in a crowd or standing in a line; being on a bridge; and travelling in a bus, train or car
- People with the disorder will avoid the situation or endure it with significant distress

Box 37.5 DSM-IV criteria for social phobia

- Persistent fear of social or performance situations in which the person is exposed to new people or to potential scrutiny by others. The individual worries that they will act in a way that will be humiliating or embarrassing
- Exposure to the feared social situation provokes anxiety that is similar to a panic attack
- The person is aware that the fear is excessive or unreasonable
- The feared social or performance situations are avoided or endured with intense distress
- The avoidance, anticipatory anxiety or distress causes significant interference in the person's occupational, social and routine functioning

People who have social phobia may also be oversensitive to criticism, negative evaluation or rejection; they may have difficulties with acting assertively and may also have low self-esteem.

Obsessive compulsive disorder

Obsessive compulsive disorder (OCD) is characterized by obsessions and compulsions that interfere with the functioning of the person and cause considerable emotional distress (see Box 37.6). Obsessions are defined as intrusive and recurrent thoughts, impulses or images that are distressing and lead the person to engage in compulsive mental or physical behaviours in order to reduce their discomfort. As the obsessions are often intrusive and inappropriate, they are known as 'ego-dystonic'. This suggests that the content of the obsession is alien, and not within the individual's control. The person with the obsession is able to recognize that they are products of their own mind and not from elsewhere, as in thought insertion. The person who experiences obsessions will attempt to ignore or suppress such thoughts or impulses or to neutralize them with some other thought or action (i.e. a compulsion).

The compulsions can be overt behaviours such as people washing their hands, checking taps or cleaning things, or mental actions such as counting, praying and reassuring themselves; all these rituals aim to reduce the person's discomfort. Patients will continue doing the ritual until the discomfort has subsided, and while some can delay them, they find it difficult to stop doing them. Furthermore, the rituals are aimed at preventing some harm from occurring and are always excessive in comparison to the actual threat. OCD is diagnosed when functioning becomes affected, and rituals are lasting longer than one hour a day.

Box 37.6 DSM-IV criteria for OCD

Obsessions defined as

- Recurrent and persistent thoughts, impulses or images that are experienced, at some time during the disturbance, as intrusive and inappropriate and that cause marked anxiety or distress
- The thoughts, impulses or images are not simply excessive worries about real-life problems
- The person attempts to ignore or suppress such thoughts, impulses or images, or to neutralize them with some other thought or action
- The person recognizes that the obsessional thoughts, impulses or images are a product of their own mind (not imposed from without as in thought insertion)

Compulsions defined as

- Repetitive behaviours or mental acts that the person feels must be performed in response to the obsession
- The behaviours (physical or mental) are aimed at preventing or reducing distress or some dreaded event
- The person recognizes that the obsessions or compulsions are excessive
- The obsessions or compulsions cause distress, are time consuming (for one hour a day or more) and cause interference with functioning

OCD symptoms can be classified according to the following subtypes:

- harming, religious, sexual obsessions with mental/checking rituals;
- contamination obsessions with washing/cleaning rituals;
- obsessions about certainty with ordering rituals;
- counting/repeating/checking compulsions;
- hoarding (Y-BOCS scale) (Goodman *et al.* 1989).

Many patients will have more than one obsession and compulsion, so the subtypes may not translate into types of patient.

 37.4 Screening

For screening NICE (2011) recommend the GAD-7 (Spitzer *et al.* 2006), a brief measure designed to identify probable cases of GAD. The GAD-7 comprises seven items and is short and easy to administer, with good psychometric properties. Scores of 1–5 indicate mild anxiety, 6–10 indicate moderate anxiety, 11–15 moderately severe anxiety and 16–21 severe anxiety.

The NICE guidelines (2011) suggest that primary and secondary care clinicians should collaborate to create local care pathways that promote access to mental health services. The guidelines propose that all clinicians should be alert to the possibility of a person presenting with anxiety, especially if that person has a history of anxiety or has recently experienced a traumatic event. The guidelines recommend that clinicians initially ask two questions from the GAD-7 (Spitzer *et al.* 2006). These are:

1. Over the past two weeks, how often have you been bothered by feeling nervous, anxious or on edge?

2. Over the past two weeks, how often have you been bothered by not being able to stop or control worrying?

Answers are scored as 0 = not at all, 1 = several days, 2 = more than half the days, 3 = nearly every day.

If the person scores more than 3 on these questions, then a more thorough assessment is required. If they score less than 3 on the questions, but the clinician still suspects an anxiety disorder, then the person should be asked:

Do you find yourself avoiding places or activities and does this cause you problems?

If the person answers yes to this, then a more thorough assessment is required.

NICE (2011) also recommends the Hospital Anxiety and Depression Scale (HADS-A, HADS-D) (Zigmond and Snaith 2003) as a measure of psychological distress within the population. The scale was designed to measure anxiety and depression in populations with physical health problems. It comprises 14 items, with two subscales for depression and anxiety. A score over 8 indicates possible depression or anxiety, and 10 indicates a problem.

If a person has been screened and identified as requiring further assessment, they should be assessed by a competent clinician who should consider the nature, severity and duration of the disorder, symptom severity and the impact on daily functioning, and then identify appropriate treatment pathways.

 37.5 Assessment

Richards and Whyte (2008) advocate patient-centred interviewing as a way of identifying the patient's

symptoms and of acknowledging the patient as a unique person. The interviewer's aim is to use the patient's own experience to guide the assessment. The assessment techniques mentioned in Chapter 14 can help facilitate the assessment and build the therapeutic relationship, however there are also specific standardized instruments that can be used (see Table 37.2).

Stepped care

There are NICE guidelines available for the treatment of GAD and panic disorder (with or without agoraphobia) (NICE 2011), OCD and body dysmorphic disorder (NICE 2005), and PTSD (NICE 2005). No guideline currently exists for social anxiety disorder, although this is currently in development. NICE (2011) recommends the use of a stepped care model (see Figure 37.1) to organize the provision of services and to ensure people with GAD receive treatment appropriate to their needs. Stepped care is designed to provide the patient with the least intrusive intervention initially, and if that does not work the person can be escalated to more intensive interventions. Decisions to 'step up' care are based on patient progress and whether there is any significant gain being made with the current level of health care provision. Progress can be measured utilizing standardized instruments.

In Step 1, clinicians assess and diagnose anxiety and provide psycho-education about the disorder. People assessed as having mild to moderate anxiety can be moved to Step 2 in which they receive low

Table 37.2 Standardized instruments for anxiety assessment

Anxiety disorder	Standardized Instrument and description
GAD	Penn State Worry Questionnaire (Meyer *et al.* 1990) This is a 16-item questionnaire that measures trait symptoms, frequency and intensity of worry on a five-point scale. The questionnaire can be used prior to treatment, during treatment and at the end of treatment
Panic disorder	Panic Disorder Severity Scale (Shear *et al.* 1997) This is a 7-item questionnaire that measures severity of panic attacks on a scale from 0–4 with 0 indicating no panic and 4 indicating extreme panic and disability. Shear *et al.* (2001) suggest a cut off score of 8 to indicate someone with symptoms that require further assessment and possible treatment

(Continued)

Table 37.2 Standardized instruments for anxiety assessment *(Continued)*

Anxiety disorder	Standardized Instrument and description
Specific phobias	The Fear Questionnaire (Marks and Mathews 1979)
	This is a well validated measure that assesses severity of phobias. The items are rated on 0–8 Likert scales with 0 indicating no problem and 8 indicating severe problems. The item ratings can be added up to provide subscale scores or a total phobic avoidance score with a range of 0 to 120. The Fear Questionnaire can be completed on a weekly basis.
	Fear of Vomiting Questionnaire (Veale and Lambrou 2006)
	This is a very comprehensive self-report questionnaire that clinicians can use to assess beliefs, safety behaviours, potential consequences of vomiting, avoidance behaviours and effects on daily living that fear of vomiting induces in the person
	Fear of Spiders Questionnaire (Szymanski and O'Donohue 1995)
	This is an 18-item self-report questionnaire that assesses the severity of spider phobia. It is quick to administer and takes approximately five minutes
Agoraphobia	The Mobility Inventory for Agoraphobia (Chambless *et al.* 1985)
	This is a 27-item questionnaire that measures agoraphobic avoidance behaviour and panic attack frequency. The questionnaire can be completed prior to treatment, during treatment and at the end of treatment
	Agoraphobic Cognitions Questionnaire (ACQ) (Chambless *et al.* 1984)
	The ACQ has 14 items which can either be scored as a total scale, or according to its subscales: Loss of Control and Physical Concerns. Both subscales have 7 items. The questionnaire can be completed on a weekly basis
Social phobia	Social Phobia Inventory (SPIN) (Connor *et al.* 2000)
	This is a 17-item questionnaire that measures symptoms of fear, avoidance and physiological arousal in social phobia. It is easy to administer and scores range from 0–68. Caseness for social phobia is defined as a score over 19. A score over 40 indicates severe social anxiety
OCD	Obsessive Compulsive Inventory (Foa *et al.* 1998)
	This measures frequency of obsessions and compulsions over the last month and distress caused. There are 42 items distributed in seven subscales: washing, checking, doubting, ordering, obsessions, hoarding and neutralizing. The distress scores range from 0–168 with a score of 40 or more suggestive of OCD
	The Yale Brown Obsessive-Compulsive Scale (Y-BOCS) (Goodman *et al.* 1989)
	The Y-BOCS is designed to be used by highly trained clinicians. It measures the severity of the symptoms and is a 10-item scale with scores ranging from 0–40. A score above 8 is considered clinically significant and should warrant treatment
Post-traumatic stress disorder (PTSD)	Impact of Event Scale (Horowitz *et al.* 1979)
	This is a 15-item questionnaire that measures intrusive thoughts and avoidance after a traumatic event
Health anxiety	Health Anxiety Inventory (Salkovskis *et al.* 2002)
	This measures health anxiety symptoms and has two sections. The first section considers symptoms of health anxiety and the second considers how a person would act if they were to develop a severe illness

Figure 37.1 Stepped care model for GAD (NICE 2011)

Focus of the intervention	Nature of the intervention
STEP 4: Complex treatment-refractory GAD and very marked functional impairment, such as self-neglect or a high risk of self-harm	Highly specialist treatment, such as complex drug and/or psychological treatment regimens; input from multi-agency teams, crisis services, day hospitals, or inpatient care
STEP 3: GAD with an inadequate response to step-2 interventions or marked functional impairment	Choice of a high-intensity psychological intervention (cognitive behavioural therapy/applied relaxation) or a drug treatment
STEP 2: Diagnosed GAD that has not improved after education and active monitoring in primary care	Low-intensity psychological interventions: non-facilitated self-help,* guided self-help, and psycho-educational groups
STEP 1: All known and suspected presentations of GAD	Identification and assessment; education about GAD and treatment options; active montioring (see Table 1)

intensity interventions for their anxiety from psychological wellbeing practitioners. These include interventions such as guided self-help and computerized cognitive behavioural therapy (cCBT) or group sessions. If the patient does not improve or if they have a moderate to severe episode of anxiety, they can be escalated to Step 3, in which they receive high intensity interventions such as face-to-face CBT or other appropriate interventions such as applied relaxation (for GAD) or eye movement desensitization and reprocessing (EMDR) from a specially trained therapist if they have PTSD. People at this level may also be assessed as appropriate for pharmacological treatment and these can be prescribed by their general practitioner (GP). Those who do not respond to these treatments can be moved to Step 4 and offered intensive treatment with a community mental health team (CMHT) or inpatient service.

The IAPT programme

In the UK, the Improving Access to Psychological Therapies (IAPT) programme has been developed to support the implementation of the NICE guidelines for depression and anxiety, as it was recognized that a lack of access to CBT practitioners was preventing routine National Health Service (NHS) delivery of the guidelines. This led to a training programme of mental health professionals, including mental health nurses, to become CBT therapists. CBT was found to be as effective as medication in helping people with depression and/or anxiety, and better at preventing relapse, and this led to an economic case for the development of the IAPT programme (DH 2011). Furthermore, it was argued that if these interventions were combined with employment support, then it would enable people to return to work and reduce reliance on benefits. IAPT provides the stepped care model for several anxiety disorders and depression.

37.6 Psychological treatments

Psychological treatments for people diagnosed with an anxiety disorder are usually categorized as low intensity and high intensity interventions.

Low intensity interventions

According to Bennett-Levy (2010), low intensity interventions represent a new paradigm in which the traditional delivery of CBT has been altered. Low intensity refers to low usage of therapist time in which more people are able to access effective, evidence-based mental health resources. This can include self-help approaches such as cCBT or self-help books, brief therapies and group treatments.

Low Intensity interventions aim to provide the key CBT principles in accessible ways and in flexible formats. The practitioner's role is to support the use of these materials, but they must also understand the principles of CBT so that they can provide advice, should the patient require it.

There are several low intensity interventions that can be used with people who have anxiety disorders, however prior to that the patient can be provided with information. This information can include details about the anxiety disorder they are experiencing, and details of potential pharmacological and psychological treatments. It is also important to signpost patients to services in the community that could be of benefit to them. Further details about other forms of support can also be provided if appropriate.

Low intensity Interventions that can be used for people with anxiety include guided self-help, exposure therapy, problem solving, cognitive restructuring and sleep hygiene.

Guided self-help

This is a structured treatment that utilizes a CBT or problem-solving approach and is usually based on health technologies such as cCBT, freely available websites or written materials. The patient is encouraged to develop goals to work towards, to work through the self-help materials and is provided with limited support from a health care professional over a limited period of time. This support can be face to face, over the telephone, by email or by Skype.

Exposure therapy

When people experience anxiety, they will often avoid the situations they fear. While this avoidance is beneficial in the short term as it reduces anxiety, in the long term it maintains the anxiety and creates longer-term difficulties. Exposure is the planned confrontation of a feared situation. It is effective for anxiety disorders such as panic, specific phobias, agoraphobia, social phobia and OCD.

Exposure works through a process known as 'habituation'. There is a natural reduction in physiological arousal when a person allows themselves to remain with the feared object over a period of time. In contrast, when a person avoids a feared object, the arousal quickly reduces but only when the person escapes the situation. When the person is in the feared situation again, their arousal levels will spike. Through habituation, less anxiety will occur on each subsequent session of exposure.

The main guidelines for exposure suggest that it should be graduated, repeated and prolonged, and tasks should be clearly specified in advance (Hawton et al. 1989).

Problem solving

This can be used with patients who have anxiety over specific problems that they need to deal with but which appear too big to manage. There is some evidence that people who experience worry are slower to use problem solving, possibly because the worry acts as an avoidance strategy – therefore, learning problem solving may help them to overcome these difficulties. Problem solving consists of a series of steps, described by Richards and Whyte (2008).

Sleep hygiene

Sleep problems are common in people with anxiety. Through interview the clinician can establish how difficult it is to get off to sleep, whether the person can stay asleep, whether they wake early and can't get back to sleep or whether they wake up and don't feel refreshed. Patients can be asked to keep sleep diaries to gather information about their sleep patterns.

Patients are provided with information about sleep and encouraged to develop a regular sleep routine. They should also be informed that sleeping during the day will create disruption in their evening routine.

Cognitive restructuring

Cognitive restructuring is a way of altering unhelpful thoughts by identifying, examining and challenging them. Cognitive theory suggests that it is not the situation per se that causes emotional distress, but the thoughts about the situation.

High intensity interventions

High intensity interventions are delivered by specially trained cognitive therapists from different professional groups such as nurses, psychologists and counsellors. They consist of interventions that are delivered face to face over a certain period of time. Depending on the evidence, people can receive up to 20 sessions of CBT (e.g. for example, the NICE 2011 guidelines recommend 12–15 weekly sessions of CBT for someone with GAD).

There are different treatment models for anxiety disorders. For example, there is a specific model of panic developed by David Clark (1986), and models for the treatment of GAD (Ladouceur *et al.* 2000), OCD (Salkovskis 1985) and social phobia (Clark and Wells 1995).

Many therapists follow a transdiagnostic approach to treatment and treat according to the specific formulation of each individual person's problem, focusing on the key processes that maintain the disorder. Therapists will work with people to develop their formulation, will identify their erroneous cognitions and develop behavioural experiments in which the person can test out the validity of their beliefs.

Mindfulness and acceptance-based interventions

Mindfulness and acceptance-based interventions aim to decrease emotional distress through a process of developing awareness of the present with compassion and acceptance, rather than through avoidance or suppression. Williams (2010) suggests that mindfulness teaches participants to observe objects and their reactions to them, and particularly to notice how they have a tendency to want positive states to continue, to want negative states to end and to want neutral states to be less boring. The main aim of these strategies is not to alter the thoughts themselves, as in CBT, but to alter the *relationship* with the thoughts that the person has. As anxiety and worry are often future-focused, training in mindfulness may enable the person to develop an alternative and more flexible response to the worrisome thoughts. Mindfulness and acceptance are developed through a series of exercises in which the person attends to the present moment in a non-judgemental manner.

In a systematic review and meta-analysis completed by Vøllestad *et al.* (2011), results from studies utilizing mindfulness-based interventions revealed significant reductions in people diagnosed with several different anxiety disorders. While many of these studies were uncontrolled, there were several controlled trials that still revealed significant results against waiting list controls.

More research is needed to establish the value of mindfulness-based interventions in the treatment of anxiety disorders. However, practitioners of mindfulness-based stress reduction (MBSR) interventions and mindfulness-based cognitive therapy (MBCT) are required to practise mindfulness themselves in order to be able to deliver it to others (Kabat-Zinn 2003). Therefore nurses who are interested in delivering these interventions need to be cultivating their own practice before commencing work with patients.

 ## 37.7 Pharmacological treatments

NICE guidelines for OCD, GAD and panic disorder (NICE 2005, 2011) recommend that pharmacological treatment be provided when the person has a marked impairment that is impacting on their daily functioning or when their symptoms have not improved with low intensity interventions. The person can choose between a high intensity face-to-face CBT intervention and pharmacological treatment. For all anxiety disorders except PTSD, NICE recommends initiating treatment with a selective serotonin reuptake inhibitor (SSRI). For a full account of the pharmacological treatment of anxiety disorders see Chapter 26.

Sarah

Sarah is a 25-year-old married mother of one child. She has been to see her GP due to chest pains and concerns that she is developing coronary heart disease. She describes the pain as occurring suddenly and she notes that she experiences palpitations and shortly afterwards develops chest pain. She is worried that she is having a heart attack.

Her GP has completed medical tests but these are normal and she has referred her to see the IAPT team. Upon assessment, it is established that the chest pains occur on a frequent basis and are accompanied by other symptoms such as palpitations, sweating, wobbly legs, dizziness and a sense of unreality. Sarah describes experiencing these sensations on a regular basis, at least two or three times a week. The sensations are very intense for her and can last for approximately 10 minutes. In order to cope with these sensations, she leaves the situation she is in and finds a place to sit down and tightens the muscles in her legs until she feels that the sensations have passed by. She also tries to control her breathing by slowing it down and taking deep, slow breaths. She has now been observed to be avoiding shops or places that are unfamiliar to her because she fears that if she collapses no one will rescue her.

Thinking Space 37.1

1. What do you think would be Sarah's diagnosis?

2. As a nurse, how would you support Sarah?

3. Sarah is avoiding shops or places that are unfamiliar to her. As her nurse, how will you encourage her to reduce her avoidance? What strategies could you use?

Feedback is provided at the end of the chapter.

37.8 The role of the nurse

In the 1990s, a review of community psychiatric nursing (CPN) highlighted that the average caseload of CPNs contained only 27 per cent of clients with schizophrenia (White 1990). In response to this, it was suggested that specific training for nurses in the use of psychosocial interventions for people with severe mental illness was required so that nurses could focus their care on people with severe mental illness as opposed to those with depression and anxiety. As a result of this, clients with common mental health problems such as anxiety were neglected (Gournay 2005). Due to this lack of provision for clients affected by anxiety disorders, graduate mental health workers were recruited to meet the needs of this population while mental health nurses focused on the needs of clients with severe and enduring mental health problems. At present, the responsibility of working with people with anxiety and depression is based in primary care.

The majority of people with anxiety will be treated in primary care by IAPT services or other primary care practitioners; however there will also be around 50 per cent of people with severe mental illness who will experience anxiety and this can often go undetected. Furthermore, nurses may meet people with long-term conditions or physical health problems in either primary or secondary care who may also be experiencing anxiety, and therefore it is imperative that all nurses regardless of their background should be able to screen for anxiety disorders and know who to refer to should they suspect that someone is experiencing excessive anxiety.

Mental health nurses (MHNs) need to be able to recognize, detect and differentiate the different anxiety disorders that people can experience. They need to have a working knowledge of assessment methods and rating scales that can be used to help detect anxiety disorders. They should also be aware of local stepped care provision and understand how their role fits in with this.

It is important that MHNs can provide psychoeducation to patients and their families about anxiety disorders and are able to help patients to problem-solve any current difficulties they may be experiencing. MHNs also need to know the different treatment methods appropriate for anxiety – for example, delivering low intensity interventions to people with anxiety disorders and having knowledge regarding guided self-help, sleep hygiene, cCBT and relaxation techniques. Some will have the opportunity to work in IAPT as high intensity therapists and will be able to deliver face-to-face therapy to people with moderate to severe anxiety.

There are several barriers that need to be addressed in order for nurses to carry out low intensity interventions with clients affected by anxiety disorders. Regular allocated time is required for nurses to review their interventions with a trained supervisor in order that they adhere to evidence-based low intensity interventions. Nurses also need to be given the opportunity to train and be supported in updating their knowledge base. They need to be given protected time to deliver such interventions rather than this being viewed as an ad hoc activity. Lack of vision and perceived lack of efficacy in low intensity interventions need to be challenged at a senior level in order for these interventions to be embedded within the general culture of nursing care.

37.9 Conclusion

This chapter has provided the reader with an overview of anxiety disorders. It has also discussed the co-morbidity of anxiety with other mental health problems and the importance of being able to screen and detect anxiety disorders adequately. Mental health nurses need to be aware of different treatment methods and be able to deliver low intensity interventions to their client groups.

In summary, the key points of learning from this chapter are:

- Anxiety disorders are common in the general population and present co-morbidly with severe mental illness.
- Nurses need to be aware of the possible presence of anxiety disorders and be be able to assess them accurately.
- The stepped care model will ensure that people with mild to moderate and moderate to severe episodes of anxiety are treated in IAPT services and that those with more protracted and severe episodes receive treatment in secondary care services.
- Patients with anxiety may be treated with pharmacological agents, with psychological treatments such as CBT and in severe cases with both.
- Through the provision of low or high intensity interventions, nurses will be involved in the care and treatment of people with anxiety disorders and it is essential that they are trained adequately to fulfil this role.

Feedback to Thinking Space 37.1

1. Sarah would likely be diagnosed with panic disorder.
2. The nurse worked with Sarah to develop a formulation using Clark's (1986) model of panic disorder. Once the formulation was developed, the nurse checked that Sarah did not have any medical

conditions that could explain the panic attacks. There were no medical conditions such as hyperthyroidism that explained the attacks and Sarah was informed that it was possible that she had panic disorder. She was provided with psycho-education about this. The nurse and Sarah practised interoceptive exposure, in which both the nurse and Sarah hyperventilated in the session for at least five minutes and the nurse clarified what Sarah was noticing and whether she was doing anything to keep herself safe. She became aware that Sarah was not pushing herself and was tightening her legs and leaning against the wall. After discovering these safety-seeking behaviours, they developed behavioural experiments to test out Sarah's predictions that she would collapse of a heart attack and die.

3. Eventually experiments were taken outside the office, into the shops where the nurse feigned a collapse and Sarah was asked to observe this and see what would happen. People came to the nurse's rescue very quickly and this led to Sarah repeating this experiment herself and eventually to her slowly increasing her activities outside through the use of a graded programme. She discovered that nothing catastrophic happened to her.

Annotated bibliography

Andrews, G. et al. (2010) Generalized worry disorder: a review of DSM-IV generalized anxiety disorder and options for DSM-V, *Depression and Anxiety*, 0: 1–14.
This is an interesting paper that questions the future of GAD and reconceptualizes it as generalized worry disorder. The authors make recommendations for the forthcoming DSM-V and therefore this paper is extremely topical.

Wells, A. (1997) *Cognitive Therapy of Anxiety Disorders: A practice manual and conceptual guide.*
An excellent manual on the use of cognitive therapy for anxiety disorders. It considers cognitive conceptualizations of different anxiety disorders and how they can be treated.

Bennett-Levy, J. (2010) *Oxford Guide to Low Intensity CBT Interventions*. Oxford: Oxford University Press.
A useful guide designed to help clinicians understand low intensity interventions and how they can be delivered to people with anxiety and depression. It is extremely useful for nurses looking to enhance their care of people with anxiety.

Richards, D. and Whyte, M. (2008) *Reach Out: National programme educator materials to support the delivery of training for psychological wellbeing practitioners delivering low intensity interventions*, 2nd edn. ?????: Rethink, available at: www.iapt.nhs.uk/silo/files/reach-out-educator-manual.pdf.
A useful guide designed to help educators deliver low intensity training to psychological wellbeing practitioners.

NICE (National Institute for Health and Clinical Excellence) (2011) www.nice.org.uk/nicemedia/live/13314/52599/52599.pdf.
The NICE guidelines for GAD and panic disorder were amended in 2011 to reflect current changes in the evidence base and are important for nurses to be familiar with as many patients will present with pure GAD or it will be present in comorbid conditions.

Self-help resources

Websites

www.bemindful.co.uk. A useful website that provides information on mindfulness and a short four-week online course for people to begin to develop skills in mindfulness.

www.livinglifetothefull.com. An excellent resource for patients and professionals that provides modules on anxiety, depression, low self-esteem, assertiveness, healthy living skills, sleeping skills and problem solving.

www.moodjuice.scot.nhs.uk. An excellent resource for patients and professionals that provides resource guides for managing difficulties such as anxiety, anger, sleep problems and depression.

References

APA (American Psychiatric Association) (2000) *Diagnostic and Statistical Manual of Mental Disorders*, 4th edn. Washington, DC. APA.

APA (American Psychiatric Association) (1994) *Diagnostic and Statistical Manual of Mental Disorders*, 4th edn (DSM-IV). Washington, DC: APA.

Bennett-Levy, J. (2010). *Oxford Guide to Low Intensity CBT Interventions*. Oxford: Oxford University Press.

Chambless, D.L., Caputo, C.G., Bright, P. and Gallagher, R. (1984) Assessment for fear of fear in agoraphobics: the Body Sensations Questionnaire and the Agoraphobic Cognitions Questionnaire, *Journal of Consulting and Clinical Psychology*, 52: 1090-7.

Chambless, D.L., Caputo, C.G., Jasin, S.E., Gracely, E.J. and Williams, C. (1985) The Mobility Inventory for Agoraphobia, *Behavioural Research & Therapy*, 23: 35-44.

Clark, D.M. (1986) A cognitive approach to panic, *Behaviour Research and Therapy*, 24: 461-70.

Clark, D.M. and Wells, A. (1995) A cognitive model of social phobia, in R.G. Heimberg, M. Liebowitz, D. Hope and F. Scheier (eds) *Social Phobia: Diagnosis, assessment, and treatment*. New York: Guilford Press.

Connor, K.M., Davidson, J.R.D., Churchill, L.E., Sherwood, A., Foa, E. and Wesler, R.H. (2000) Psychometric properties of the Social Phobia Inventory (SPIN), *British Journal of Psychiatry*, 176: 379-86.

DH (Department of Health) (2011) *Talking Therapies: A four-year plan of action*. London: DH.

Foa, E.B., Kozak, M.J., Salkovskis, P.M., Coles, M.E. and Amir, N. (1998) The validation of a new obsessive compulsive disorder scale: the Obsessive Compulsive Inventory (OCI), *Psychological Assessment*, 10: 206-14.

Goodman, W.K., Price, L.H., Rasmussen, S.A. *et al.* (1989) The Yale-Brown Obsessive-Compulsive Scale, I: development, use, and reliability, *Archives of General Psychiatry*, 46: 1006-11.

Gournay, K. (2005) The changing face of psychiatric nursing: revisiting . . . mental health nursing, *Advances in Psychiatric Treatment*, 11: 6-11.

Hawton, K., Salkovskis, P.M., Kirk, J. and Clark, D.M. (1989) *Cognitive Behaviour Therapy for Psychiatric Problems: A practical guide*. Oxford: Oxford University Press.

Horowitz, M., Wilner, N. and Alvarez, W. (1979) Impact of Event Scale: a measure of subjective stress, *Psychosomatic Medicine*, 41: 209-18.

Kabat-Zinn, J. (2003) Mindfulness-based interventions in context: past, present, and future, *Clinical Psychology: Research and Practice*, 10: 144-56.

Kessler, R.C. (2007) The global burden of anxiety and mood disorders: putting the European Study of the Epidemiology of Mental Disorders (ESEMeD) findings into perspective, *Journal of Clinical Psychiatry*, 68(suppl. 2): 10-19.

Ladouceur, R., Gosselin, P. and Dugas, M.J. (2000) Experimental manipulation of intolerance of uncertainty: a study of a theoretical model of worry, *Behaviour Research and Therapy*, 38: 933-41.

Layard, R., Clark, D., Bell, S. *et al.* (2006) *The Depression Report: A new deal for depression and anxiety disorders*. London: The Centre for Economic Performance's Mental Health Policy Group, LSE.

McManus, S., Meltzer, H., Brugha, T., Bebbington, P. and Jenkins, R. (2007) Adult psychiatric morbidity in England, 2007 results of a household survey, appendices and glossary, *The NHS Information Centre for Health and Social Care*, 9(6379).

Meyer, T.J., Miller, M.L., Metzger, R.L. and Borkovec, T.D. (1990) Development and validation of the Penn State Worry Questionnaire, *Behaviour Research and Therapy*, 28(6): 487-95.

NICE (National Institute for Health and Clinical Excellence) (2005) *Obsessive-compulsive Disorder: Core interventions in the treatment of obsessive-compulsive disorder and body dysmorphic disorders*. London: NICE.

NICE (National Institute for Health and Clinical Excellence) (2011) *Common Mental Health Disorders: Identification and pathways to care*. London: NICE.

Richards, D. and Whyte, M. (2008) *Reach Out: National programme educator materials to support the delivery of training for psychological wellbeing practitioners delivering low intensity interventions*, 2nd edn. ?????: Rethink, available at: www.iapt.nhs.uk/silo/files/reach-out-educator-manual.pdf.

Sainsbury Centre for Mental Health (2007) *Mental Health at Work: Developing the business case*, policy paper 8. London: Sainsbury Centre for Mental Health.

Salkovskis, P.M. (1985) Obsessive-compulsive problems: a cognitive-behavioural analysis, *Behaviour Research and Therapy*, 23: 571-83.

Salkovskis, P.M., Rimes, K.A., Warwick, H.M.C. and Clark, D.M. (2002) The Health Anxiety Inventory: development and validation of scales for the measurement of health anxiety and hypochondriasis, *Psychological Medicine*, 32: 843-53.

Shear, M.K., Brown, T.A., Barlow, D.H. *et al.* (1997) Multicenter collaborative Panic Disorder Severity Scale, *American Journal of Psychiatry*, 154: 1571-5.

Somers, J.M., Goldner, E.M., Waraich, P. and Hsu, L. (2006) Prevalence and incidence studies of anxiety disorders: a systematic review of the literature, *Canadian Journal of Psychiatry*, 51(2): 100-13.

Spitzer, R.L., Kroenke, K., Williams, J.B. *et al.* (2006) A brief measure for assessing generalised anxiety disorder: the GAD-7, *Archives of Internal Medicine*, 166: 1092-7.

Szymanski, J. and O'Donohue, W. (1995) Fear of Spiders Questionnaire, *Journal of Behaviour Therapy and Experimental Psychiatry*, 26(1): 31-4.

Veale, D. and Lambrou, C. (2006) The psychopathology of vomit phobia, *Behavioural and Cognitive Psychotherapy*, 34(2): 139-50.

Vøllestad, J., Birkeland Nielsen, M. and Høstmark Nielsen, G. (2011) Mindfulness and accetance-based interventions for anxiety disorders: a systematic review and meta-analysis, *British Journal of Clinical Psychology*, DOI: 10.1111/j.2044-8260.2011.02024.

White, E. (1990) *A Quinquennial Survey of Community Psychiatric Nursing.* Manchester: University of Manchester, Department of Nursing.

Williams, J.M.G. (2010) Mindfulness and psychological process, *Emotion*, 10: 1–7, doi:10.1037/a0018360.

WHO (World Health Organization) (1992) *International Statistical Classification of Diseases and Related Health Problems* (ICD-10). Geneva: WHO.

Zigmond, A.S. and Snaith, R.P. (1983) The hospital anxiety and depression scale, *Acta Psychiatry Scandinavia*, 67(6): 361–70.

Chapter 38

The Person with an Eating Disorder

David Morning and Anthony Ross

She thought she was in control of her eating and she felt a thrill of being in control of something for once. She had never felt the importance of being in control before, of being the boss, but she wasn't in control of anything. Anorexia was the boss and in control of everything.

(Taken from a story written by a 15-year-old girl about her experience of being under the influence of anorexia nervosa)

I was not even aware of lads having anorexia... It might be awkward for them to come forward as they think it's a girl's illness.

(Mother of a 16-year-old boy whose referral into treatment was delayed due to a lack of awareness by professionals)

I've got my son back.

(The same mother after her son had improved following care and treatment)

 ## 38.1 Introduction

In 1689 English physician Richard Morton described the 'sad and anxious' cases of young women who were 'wasting away'. Morton also described two other cases, one of which was an 18-year-old male

and it is thought that this is the first description of what would be termed today as anorexia nervosa (Brumberg 1988).

In the nineteenth century, Lasegue (Paris) and Gull (London) both independently published papers in 1873 outlining cases of young women suffering from a condition which Gull himself termed as 'anorexia nervosa'. Initially Gull had named the condition 'anorexia hystericus', believing that it was unique to female gender types. This reflected the Victorian belief at the time that the womb had a significant role to play in females' psychological and emotional problems. Realizing that it could also manifest itself in males, he changed the term to anorexia nervosa. The translation of this is 'a nervous loss of appetite', which can be misleading as sufferers of the condition often report having a voracious appetite and their main objective is to control and suppress this. Gull (1873: 26) recommended that the treatment required is: 'obviously that which is fitted for persons of unsound mind. The patients should be fed at regular intervals and surrounded by persons who have moral control over them; relations and friends being generally the worst attendants'. While recognizing the Victorian context, this still remains a challenge for today's mental health nurse – feeding an individual who for many perceived reasons does not want to be fed.

This chapter focuses specifically on anorexia nervosa and bulimia nervosa, and provides a brief overview of eating disorders not otherwise specified (EDNOS). This does not negate the fact that there are other disordered patterns of eating, but it reflects the current 'trans-diagnostic' perspective. This model of care proposes that all types of eating disorder can benefit from the same treatment approaches and that they should not necessarily be viewed as separate conditions (Van der linden *et al.* 2007; Fairburn 2008). The chapter covers:

- diagnosis of eating disorders;
- prevalence and incidence;
- the causes and aetiology of eating disorders;
- screening and assessment;
- contemporary treatments;
- recovery from eating disorders.

The case of Alison, a 16-year-old girl with an eating disorder, is used to illustrate some of the content in this chapter and her case study is integral to the screening, assessment, treatment and recovery sections.

38.2 Diagnosis of eating disorders

Whereas the diagnosis of anorexia nervosa is over 140 years old, bulimia nervosa is a much more recent term, Russell (1979) first referring to the condition as a separate entity. The following diagnostic criteria for anorexia, bulimia nervosa and EDNOS have been adapted from the *Diagnostic Statistical Manual of Mental Disorders* (DSM-IV) (APA 2000) and the *International Statistical Classification of Diseases and Related Health Problems* (ICD-10) (WHO 2010).

Anorexia nervosa

Key diagnosis criteria are:

- A refusal to maintain body weight at or above a minimally normal weight for age and height, being maintained at least 15 per cent below that expected. Pre-pubertal individuals may show failure to make expected weight gain during period of growth.
- Amenorrhoea (at least three consecutive cycles) in postmenarchal girls and women.
- If onset is pre-pubertal, the sequence of pubertal events is delayed or even arrested (growth ceases; in girls the breasts do not develop and there is a primary amenorrhoea; in boys the genitals remain juvenile).
- Weight loss is self-induced by avoidance of 'fattening foods'. One or more may be present:
  - self-induced vomiting;
  - self-induced purging;
  - excessive exercise;
  - use of appetite suppressants and/or diuretics.
- Body-image distortion where there is an intense fear of gaining weight or becoming fat, even though underweight.

Bulimia nervosa

Key diagnostic criteria are:

- A persistent preoccupation with eating, and an irresistible craving for food; the individual succumbs to episodes of overeating in which large amounts of food are consumed in short periods of time.
- A sense of lack of control over eating during the episode, characterized by a feeling that the individual cannot stop eating or control what or how much they are eating.
- Dread of 'fatness'.
- Recurrent inappropriate compensatory behaviour to counteract the 'fattening' effects of food, including:
  - self-induced vomiting;
  - misuse of laxatives, diuretics, enemas or other medications;
  - alternating periods of starvation/fasting;
  - excessive exercise.

EDNOS

- For female patients, all of the criteria for anorexia nervosa are met except that the patient has regular menses.
- All of the criteria for anorexia nervosa are met except that, despite significant weight loss, the patient's current weight is in the normal range.
- All of the criteria for bulimia nervosa are met except that the binge eating and inappropriate compensatory mechanisms occur less than twice a week or for less than three months.
- The patient has normal body weight and regularly uses inappropriate compensatory behaviour after eating small amounts of food.
- Repeatedly chewing and spitting out, but not swallowing, large amounts of food.
- Binge-eating disorder is recurrent episodes of binge eating in the absence of regular inappropriate compensatory behaviour characteristic of bulimia nervosa.

38.3 Prevalence and incidence

Around 1 in 250 women and 1 in 2,000 men will experience anorexia nervosa at some point in their lives. It is estimated that bulimia is around five times more common than anorexia nervosa with 90 per cent of people with bulimia being female. Anorexia nervosa usually develops during adolescence around the age of 16 or 17, though it can occur earlier (Fairburn and Harrison 2003). The onset of bulimia nervosa is slightly later than anorexia nervosa, generally around 18 years. EDNOS, which incorporate binge eating, usually affect males and females equally though this generally occurs later in life, between the ages of 30 and 40.

Fairburn and Brownell (2002) report that at any one time 39 per cent of females and 21 per cent of male adults are currently trying to lose weight in western countries. Over a one-year period 55 per cent of females and 29 per cent of males had dieted to lose weight. Furthermore it was noted that between 25 and 33 per cent of adolescent females were also trying to lose weight. This may well reflect the cultural pressure and influences which link thinness to being attractive.

This process of defining self-image by weight (or lack of it) has the potential to become problematic (Stice 2001). Information from the National Eating Disorders Association (NEDA) indicated that more than one in three 'normal dieters' progresses to pathological dieting. Accepting this, eating disorders are complex phenomena that involve more than the restriction or consumption of food. The behaviour is generally an indicator of underlying distress and has specific meaning to the person (Shisslak et al. 1995).

38.4 What causes eating disorders?

The onset of an eating disorder is multi-factorial. Consequently, care and treatment has to both recognize and assess the individual from differing and sometimes complementary angles.

Control

An eating disorder can envelop the individual, becoming so important and significant that, paradoxically, it can be their reason for living. Compounding this fixation with the pursuit of thinness are health ramifications of self-starvation, which in turn make the person even more vulnerable to the slow process of literally becoming less of an individual, in a physical sense, especially if they are suffering from anorexia nervosa. These physical changes are accompanied by changes that are psychological and emotional – feelings of inadequacy and sometimes a perceived lack of control. Ogden (2010) describes the belief that the body is a controllable object and food is used as a statement of self-control. This theme of self-control and the maintenance of control appear to permeate the differing types of eating disorder. In adolescents it can be used to delay the onset of puberty and accordingly arrest normal development into adulthood. It can also be a way of coping with emotional distress and for some it may be the only way they have of expressing their true emotions.

Giordano (2005) refers to the addictive element of an eating disorder and postulates that treatment could benefit from some facets of treatment developed for those with addictions – for example, motivational interviewing. There can also be an interpersonal element involved in the development of an eating disorder. This can reflect troubled relationships within the family or with friends and peers, including emotional and sexual abuse. There could be a history of ridicule and bullying associated with the individual's weight and shape. Duker and Slade (2003) remind us that when an individual is undernourished, feelings and emotions can become blunted. The pursuit of starvation 'creates a sense of detachment, of being anesthetised, removed far from the rest of the world' (p.23).

Developmental issues

Crisp (1980) proposed a developmental model, with the origins of anorexia nervosa arising from biological and psychological experiences associated with the attainment of adult weight. This con-

flict arises as a consequence of reaching physical and psychological maturity. In an attempt to arrest and prevent these, individuals with anorexia use dieting and the associated self-induced starvation as a way to regress back to their pre-pubescent size, hormonal stages and general life experience. Crisp (1995, preface) develops this further:

> anorexia nervosa [is] a distorted biological solution to an existential problem for an adolescent and their family and is a crippling condition. Experienced as adaptive in the face of an otherwise imminent crisis, it results, through its massive and abortive effect on physical, psychological and social development, in increasingly destructive isolation for the individual as the years go by.

This reflects the external perspective of others around the individual, the frustration and hopelessness that can be experienced when family members feel helpless to effect any positive change.

Genetics

Keel and Klump (2003) report a chromosomal link to self-induced vomiting in bulimia nervosa and an evolutionary perspective is put forward by Gatward (2007), who links dietary restrictions to a perceived threat of being excluded from the 'group', which once would have been dangerous for the individual. As the weight loss associated with the restrictions continues, it dips below a certain level and an 'old adaptive response to the threat of famine is triggered thus enabling the weight loss to continue' (p.10). Gatward postulates that this could be why individuals can function at a low weight and why the disorder is often viewed in a positive way by the person.

The reviews of genetic studies on twins and families by Scherag et al. (2010) suggest a substantial genetic influence for anorexia and bulimia nervosa. Recognizing the multiple aetiological factors involved in the development of eating disorders they write about the interplay between genetics and the environment, citing for example high risk areas such as figure-skating and fashion modelling where a person predisposed genetically to develop the condition could become even more vulnerable to it as a result of being in these environments.

Culture

From a societal perspective there are cultures that present images of women (and men) in certain ways. The 'celebration' of thinness and the 'perfect body' can be significant in the development of anorexia and bulimia nervosa and the media can reinforce the role that the family and peers can have in pressuring the individual into becoming thin. Prestwood (2004) highlights that societal pressure to be thin can become internalized and consequent body dissatisfaction can lead to an eating disorder. This pursuit of thinness can become 'pathological' from a medical perspective and develop into, for example, anorexia nervosa.

Although originally thought to be the domain of western cultures, Simpson (2002) refers to the 'globalization' of fat phobia and the ongoing permeation of western images in other cultures, and an associated increase in the presentation of anorexia nervosa. Levine and Smolak (2010) report that, Antarctica aside, eating disorders have been found in all continents.

Case Study

Alison

Alison, aged 16, lives at home with her mother. Her parents separated two years ago due to arguments relating to her mother's alcohol consumption. Alison still sees her father regularly and has a 'good' relationship with him.

She describes her relationship with her mother as difficult. She is currently attending a local secondary school and is due to sit her A level exams. Alison has always done well academically, though finds studying difficult at the moment.

Alison is a popular pupil with a number of friends and a couple of 'best friends', however she has been reducing her contact with them and recently they have been arguing. She recently collapsed at school and was taken to the accident and emergency (A&E) department where her physical health observation indicated some abnormalities in her blood chemistry. She was followed up by her general practitioner (GP) and was referred to the local childrens' and adolescents' mental health team (CAMHS) for assessment.

Alison did not know why she was accessing mental health services – as far as she was concerned there was nothing wrong with her. Discussing her weight loss Alison identified that she has always been mindful of her weight and two years ago would be described as plump. Due to a family holiday she went on a diet so she would look good in a bikini and comments were made about how well she looked. Following her holiday she continued to diet and over the past year has lost approximately 12kgs. She restricts her calorie intake, her parents have found bags of what appear to be vomit in her room and she has also increased her visits to the gymnasium.

At the initial appointment her height was 1.57 m and her weight was 35kgs.

38.5   Screening and assessment

Screening

A questionnaire can be undertaken with clients to screen for the possibility of an eating disorder. One brief tool is the SCOFF, (Morgan *et al.* 1999), which comprises five items:

1. Do you make yourself **S**ick because you feel uncomfortably full?
2. Do you worry you have lost **C**ontrol over how much you eat?

3. Have you recently lost more than **O**ne stone in a three-month period?

4. Do you believe yourself to be **F**at when others say you are too thin?

5. Would you say that **F**ood dominates your life?

A positive response to two or more questions indicates that a more detailed assessment is required. Alternative screening questionnaires include the Eating Disorder Inventory (Garner *et al.* 1983) and The Eating Disorder Examination (Cooper and Fairburn 1987).

Assessment

Due to the potential impact of an eating disorder upon a client's physiology, a physical health assessment should be a priority, recognizing some of the complications of starvation. Irrespective of the type of eating disorder, good practice would require determining body mass index (BMI). The formula for calculating BMI is weight in kilograms divided by height in metres squared, and web-based tools are available to perform the calculation.

In children and adolescents the same calculation is used but is interpreted differently using BMI-for-age growth charts which allow translation of a BMI number into a percentile for a child's sex and age. A BMI of less than 14 would be of concern, a BMI of less than 12 is potentially life threatening. A low BMI alone is not necessarily an indicator of an eating disorder but used alongside a full assessment can inform the diagnosis (Bryant-Waugh 2006).

> ### Thinking Space 38.1
>
> Refer back to Alison's case study. Does Alison's body weight raise concerns about her physical well-being? Feedback is provided at the end of the chapter.

Physical assessment

Baseline health checks such as blood pressure (sitting and standing), pulse and temperature are indicated. Eating disorders can create physiological imbalances, therefore blood screenings should be done in order to obtain indicators of liver and kidney function. Electrolytes should be monitored as bulimic and anorexic behaviours can create electrolyte imbalances which may result in life-threatening cardiac arrhythmias or arrest. An electrocardiograph (ECG) would also be indicated to assess cardiac function, which can be compromised by an eating disorder, in particular bradycardia with anorexia. Low body weight can produce amenorrhoea in females so it is helpful when working with female clients to determine when they had their last period, which may give an indication of the duration of the eating disorder.

In anorexia nervosa the person may have fine downy hair known as laguno. This is produced naturally to prevent heat loss and maintain body temperature when there is loss of body fat. In the case of bulimia the patient may appear to have puffy cheeks; this is due to enlargement of the salivary glands which may be an indicator of vomiting.

Psychological assessment

Low self-esteem, poor self-image, perfectionist tendencies and setting high standards are all thought to potentially contribute to the development of eating disorders. Other psychological variables which can be present include depression, anxiety, anger and feelings of emptiness or loneliness. Approximately 50 per cent of people with eating disorders suffer obsessive compulsive spectrum disorders and/or have obsessive compulsive personality traits including an extreme concern with shape and weight, sometimes characterized as a fear of fatness or a drive for thinness. Some of the following cognitions could be present, such as a fear of gaining weight, of becoming fat, accompanied by fears of failure and perfectionism. This may be characterized by dichotomous or 'all-or-nothing' thinking where clients may perceive things in extremes.

Depressive and anxiety disorders associated with eating disorders have been reported (Brewerton *et al.* 1995) and low mood and poor cognitive functioning may be associated with a reduction in calorific intake and subsequent weight loss (Duker and Slade 2003) which may be alleviated as weight increases. The assessment of mood and any related suicidal ideation or intent is important because there is an increased mortality rate for people with eating disorders with approximately 1 in 5 people with anorexia nervosa committing suicide (Arcelus *et al.* 2011).

Thinking Space 38.2

Refer back to Alison's case study.

1. What issues are being highlighted that you would want to explore in more depth with Alison?
2. What issues would you make a priority?

Feedback is provided at the end of the chapter.

Behavioural assessment

When working with adolescent clients it is advisable to ask the client for consent and then ask the parents about any associated behaviour as they may provide an alternative history or extra, useful detail about time frame of behaviour. Obtaining this time frame for the development of any eating disorder and related behavioural changes can determine whether the condition had an acute onset or is more indicative of a severe and enduring eating disorder (SEED) (Robinson 2009). This information will help to gauge the level of risk when collated within the full asessment. The following questions could be explored:

- Are there any indications of binge eating?
- Is there any evidence of compensatory behaviours such as purging through vomiting?
- Does Alison visit the toilet straight after meals?
- Does Alison make excessive use of laxatives?
- Is Alison using slimming tablets or illicit stimulants?
- Are there any changes in Alison's eating habits such as omitting meals, avoiding eating in company or becoming isolated?
- Is there any evidence of excessive exercise?

Once the assessments have been carried out and a plan of care indentified there are a number of care and treatment options available.

 ## 38.6   Contemporary treatments

Psychological treatments

The National Institute for Health and Clinical Excellence (NICE) (2004) guidelines recommends that the following therapies should be considered for the psychological treatment of eating disorders:

- cognitive analytic therapy (CAT);
- cognitive behavioural therapy (CBT);
- interpersonal psychotherapy (IPT),
- psychodynamic therapy and family interventions which focus specifically on the eating disorder.

NICE guidelines reviewed in 2008 reported that CBT may reduce the risk of relapse for adults once they have had their weight restored; however, the efficacy of the approach in the underweight stage of anorexia nervosa is unknown. A Cochrane systematic review (Fisher *et al.* 2010) reports that there is evidence that family therapy could be effective in the care and treatment of many clients. However, the evidence base is weak, founded upon a number of small case studies and these researchers recommend larger trials for future research.

In another Cochrane review, Hay *et al.* (2007, revised 2009) evaluated the efficacy of CBT and other psychotherapies in the treatment of adults with bulimia nervosa or related syndromes of recurrent binge eating. They found that CBT was more effective than other psychotherapeutic approaches (and no treatment) in reducing binge eating. However, other psychotherapies were identified as useful, in particular IPT in the longer term. Self-help approaches that used structured CBT treatment manuals were also considered to be of promising therapeutic value.

A review by Perkins *et al.* (2006) compared pure self-help (PSH) and guided self-help (GSH) to psychological, pharmacological or control treatments and waiting lists. The review included bulimia but also anorexia nervosa, binge eating disorder and EDNOS. Perkins found some evidence that self-help and the use of manuals could reduce eating disorders and other symptoms.

CBT might be used to help identify thoughts and how these relate to feelings and behaviour. Its premise would suggest that in many cases emotions and associated behaviour are based upon cognitive appraisal of the situation and that there is an interactive relationship between these elements. By helping your clients gain an understanding of the relationship between these three elements, some of the core beliefs can be challenged, especially if they are not an accurate appraisal of the situation. This potential for change may then facilitate a reduction in emotional distress and unhelpful behaviours. CBT was developed more specifically for bulimia nervosa (CBT BN) by Fairburn (1981). Fairburn (2008) proposes a transdiagnostic view of eating disorders, not viewing them as separate conditions but proposing that patients can move between 'diagnoses', and has designed a model of CBT applicable to all eating disorders. This is known as enhanced cognitive behavioural therapy (CBTE). CBTE addresses four key maintenance factors that support and maintain eating disorders:

- clinical perfectionism;
- low self-esteem;
- mood intolerance;
- interpersonal difficulties.

Van der Linden (2008) provides a caveat in relation to the use of CBT. He reports that some individuals with an eating disorder still appear to be unable to adapt their thinking, despite the use of evidenced-based CBT approaches. So it is important to evaluate the associated research and treatment approaches as some individuals need different and/or concurrent treatment methodologies. We refer the reader to the specific chapters in this volume to learn more about these psychological approaches to treatment.

Family approaches

Even if they live alone, clients don't live in isolation and as such family members, including siblings, should normally be included in treatment – especially for children and adolescents with eating disorders (NICE 2004). Family therapy can make an important contribution to recovery through helping family members gain a better understanding of the complex nature of the eating disorder. It aims to improve communication skills with one another and teach strategies for coping with stress and negative feelings. A number of family therapy techniques could be applied. Milan systemic family therapy (Cecchin 1987), a long established approach, assumes that an eating disorder performs a function within the family system. In this approach the facilitator typically adopts a position of expertise and power and would prescribe tasks and homework for the client and the family in order to 'fix' the system. A more recent approach is the Maudsley Model of Family Therapy (Lock *et al.* 2001), which in contrast would enlist the family as a central player in the client's nutritional recovery, and would typically adopt three distinct phases to treatment:

- weight restoration;
- returning control over eating to the adolescent; and
- establishing a healthy adolescent identity.

Within this family therapy approach the parents would take charge of planning and supervising all meals and snacks. As recovery progresses, the client would gradually take on more personal responsibility for determining when and how much to eat. Finally, if the approach is to be successful, they would begin to develop their own 'healthy' identity. The New Maudsley Method (Treasure *et al.* 2010) highlights the importance of working collaboratively with the family, engaging families as part of the solution rather than part of the problem. The techniques adopted fit well with a nursing approach based upon a position of warmth, genuiness, a willingness to understand and a willingness to provide support and information. The New Maudsley Method draws on the lived experiences of families and fosters their willingness to share their experience to create stories of hope and optimism, so providing an antidote to the despair and the stigma associated with eating disorders.

A further development of family therapy for eating disorders is narrative therapy (White and Epston 1990) which is based upon a respectful, non-blaming approach. This could be particularly relevant in situations where the client may be held responsible and blamed for their eating behaviours and/or the parents may feel guilty for allowing such behaviours to develop. Lack of understanding can reinforce negative views of self and strengthen the position that someone is responsible for the problem. Narrative therapy takes the position that the person is not the problem; the problem is the problem – which allows the family to be united against the eating disorder and reduce blame and guilt within the family.

A potential challenge for nurses working with clients who present with eating disorders may be an apparent lack of motivation and ambivalence to change. This can create frustration and resistance within the relationship and compromise the development of any therapeutic alliance required to address the eating disorder. Motivational interviewing (Miller and Rollnick 2002) combined with reflective listening, open-ended questions and reflective paraphrasing may be used to empower clients, helping them to gain understanding of their motivations, and affirm and validate them as a person, while reducing arguments and resistance.

Pharmacological approaches

Claudino *et al.'s* (2006) review of seven studies did not draw definite conclusions about the benefits of antidepressants in acute anorexia nervosa. Bacaltchuk and Hay's (2003) review of 19 trials comparing antidepressants with placebos for people diagnosed with bulimia nervosa found that antidepressants were clinically effective but no particular antidepressant was preferred in terms of efficacy and tolerability.

Kruger and Kennedy (2000) recommend that outcomes for medication trials for individuals with eating disorders should focus upon the underlying biological disturbances and associated clinical symptoms. These include: the remission of core symptoms; prevention of relapse in the recovery phase; and the protection of biologically vulnerable individuals (longer term).

Similarly to Claudino *et al.* (2006) they report that medication had little effect in the treatment of anorexia nervosa, whereas selective serotonin reuptake inhibitors (SSRIs) are beneficial in the control of binge urges in bulimia nervosa. While the benefits of medication for anorexia nervosa are uncertain, some clients may benefit from medication for associated conditions which may include depression and/or anxiety.

 ## 38.7   Recovery

The underlying philosophy of recovery (see Chapter 5) is particularly apt when applied to clients presenting with eating disorders. Patching and Lawler (2009) discovered that recovery occurred when individuals re-engaged with their lives, developing necessary coping skills and thus rediscovering their sense of self. In essence their findings pointed to seeing the eating disorder as a search for self-identity. Some clients may have adopted anorexia nervosa as a way of achieving this, and associated behaviours could be gradually relinquished as clients realize that they are self-defeating.

Linked to this process, Duker and Slade (2003) point to an eating disorder as an attempt by an individual with little sense of self to gain some control over their life. They write: 'where every other action is fraught with the possibility of failure, where the rule is that failure and personal inadequacy are not allowed, where the demand is that the individual must be independent and strong, then food control comes into its own' (p. 141).

Van der Linden *et al.* (2007) investigated the views of patients and therapists about the 'necessary ingredients' for recovery from an eating disorder. For those with anorexia nervosa in particular, family therapy was seen by both groups as the treatment of choice. Also important were increasing self-esteem and learning problem-solving skills. In effect the views of patients and therapists supported the transdiagnostic model suggesting that all types of eating disorder can benefit from the same treatment approaches.

Williams and Reid (2010) offer a different perspective on recovery, exploring the perceived ambivalence that some sufferers have about recovering from anorexia nervosa. Using a phenomenological approach they explored the views held by those who use pro-anorexia ('pro-ana') websites. Their study found ambivalence about whether the condition gave them control or controlled them. This dichotomy led to ambivalence and uncertainty about whether they wished to recover or maintain the associated behaviours. Thus clients may perceive positive benefits from the condition, perceiving it as a friend or even a guardian. Pragmatically, mental health nurses need to recognize this especially when establishing a therapeutic relationship. Nurses need to be able to empathize with clients, which may be challenging when they want to starve themselves and as a consequence suffer emotional, psychological and physical complications.

Thinking Space 38.3

Refer back to the case study. Recognizing the importance of the eating disorder to Alison's sense of self-identity, consider the challenges of arresting the process of self-starvation.

Feedback is provided at the end of the chapter.

A particular challenge to mental health nurses working with people like Alison is alexithymia (difficulties in identifying and also describing emotions), which will make it difficult for Alison to share her feelings and associated thoughts. The nurse should also be aware that Alison may have been accessing some of the 'pro-ana' sites for support.

'Pro-ana' sites

Pro-ana websites first appeared in the early years of the century. 'Prettythin' proclaims itself as 'the world's largest community for individuals with eating disorders'. 'Prothinspo' offers a variety of ways to lose weight and numerous images of celebrities and others who have lost weight. 'The House of Thin' declares that 'there is no shame in being eating disordered'. These sites are not necessarily about 'recovery' but offer a 'safe' forum for individuals to talk and share their respective experiences. While some of these sites have a controversial mission, some researchers have recognized pragmatically that they may have a role to play.

Clarke (2008) discusses the notion of social capital in relation to 'pro-ana' websites. This theory recognizes the benefits of membership of a network and the sharing of common values. Csipke and Horne (2007) highlight the dangers that the sites pose for their respective visitors. Gauging the opinions of those accessing these sites, they refer to improvement in emotional well-being, especially when participation is active, whereas individuals who passively engaged with them found it fostered maintenance of their eating disorder. These findings point to some of the perceived benefits of active participation. Seeking friendship and support of other visitors had a positive effect on mental well-being. However, passive participants who access pro-ana sites, endeavouring to become 'better' at an eating disorder, fail to improve their feelings of isolation.

38.8 Conclusion

This chapter has highlighted the complexities involved in the development and maintenance of an eating disorder, and in an individual's recovery from the condition. In summary, the key points of learning from this chapter are:

- While anorexia nervosa as a diagnosis was first made over 140 years ago, bulimia nervosa is a more recent term, dating from 1979.

- Diagnostic criteria for anorexia, bulimia nervosa and EDNOS are contained in the *Diagnostic and Statistical Manual of Mental Disorders* (DSM-IV) and the *International Statistical Classification of Diseases and Related Health Problems* (ICD-10).

- Around 1 in 250 women and 1 in 2,000 men will experience anorexia nervosa at some point in their lives, with bulimia estimated to be around five times more common than anorexia nervosa.

- Anorexia nervosa usually develops during adolescence around the age of 16 or 17 with the onset of bulimia nervosa being slightly later at around 18 years. EDNOS usually affect males and females equally though this generally occurs later in life, between the ages of 30 and 40.

- Eating disorders arise from a complex interplay of factors that can include an individual's desire to exert self-control, developmental conflicts as an individual matures to adulthood, probable genetic influences and ever-present societal pressures that align thinness with beauty.

- A number of screening instruments are available to provide an indication of whether an individual has an eating disorder, such as the SCOFF.

- Comprehensive biopsychosocial assessments should be conducted: physical assessment is a priority due to the potential effects of an eating disorder on physiology and biological functioning; psychological assessments should explore an individual's self-image, any experiences of anxiety and/or depression, and any obsessive/compulsive beliefs and/or behaviours; social assessments should involve the individual's family whenever possible and appropriate to provide an additional perspective on the person's condition.

- A number of psychological and family-based interventions are effective in supporting the care and recovery of people with an eating disorder. Pharmacological interventions, such as antidepressants to treat underlying conditions, have a less certain evidence base.

Feedback to Thinking Spaces

Engaging clients in their care and treatment is the first step. You need to adopt a non-judgemental, open and honest approach, which can be difficult when faced with the reluctance and resistance that anorexia can bring into the relationship. By working collaboratively and actively listening to experiences, the foundations of a therapeutic relationship can be established.

In this instance, Alison's motivations may appear initially to be externally driven, reflecting her parents' concerns. Questions and dialogue can be used to develop internal motivation. It may be helpful to adopt a position of curiosity and by the use of circular questioning explore Alison's understanding of why people may be concerned about her.

- If we were to ask your parents and about your eating what might they say?
- What are they most concerned about?
- How do they describe how anorexia has changed their relationship with you?

The associated family dynamics should be explored in some depth. This is a priority especially if family members are to become integral to Alison's future recovery. It would also be helpful to gain an understanding of the relationship that anorexia has with your client. You might ask questions such as:

- What promises does anorexia make to you that allows it to have such an influence in your life?
- In offering these promises what has anorexia stolen from you?
- How has it influenced the relationship with your family/friends?
- If you were free from the constraints of anorexia what plans would you be able to make for your life?

Motivational interviewing techniques may be used to explore ambivalence about anorexia and weigh up its positive and negative aspects. If Alison can share what she views as the benefits of having the condition, this can be helpful as previously the conversations may have focused on the negatives; thus a more balanced picture may emerge. This in turn creates an opportunity for you to understand Alison's beliefs which can increase your understanding of her problems and also identify what support may be helpful. For example, if she says that anorexia reduces her anxiety, then alternative strategies to deal with anxious thoughts and feelings could be explored. This could also begin to create dissonance and help her move toward making a decision to change aspects of her behaviour. In effect you can help Alison to adopt more positive coping strategies than self-starvation and by exploring alternatives this can have an empowering effect and demonstrate empathy.

A female who is 1.57 m in height should normally weigh about 50kgs. Alison's weight is 35kgs and this is approximately 18 per cent lower than her average expected body weight (AEBW). This is cause for concern, not only may there be physical complications, she may be 'closing down' emotionally and there may be temporary cognitive impairment which could affect her ability to engage on a therapeutic level. Facilitating conversations with Alison and her family and providing education about the physical risks associated with anorexia may increase Alison's understanding of her parents' concerns and reinforce the need for monitoring her weight and her physical health. Due to the weight loss a goal for Alison should be to increase weight by a gradual amount of 0.5kgs per week to improve her physical health and minimize the potential for refeeding syndrome. You need to be mindful that while monitoring an increase in Alison's weight may feel very positive for you, paradoxically it may feel very negative for Alison. Indeed, negative feelings such as guilt, shame and failure may be associated with weight gain. This can provide an opportunity to explore the cognitions and emotional aspects of the condition, which might influence Alison's likelihood of relapse.

It would be helpful to negotiate involvement of Alison's family and to hand over control of eating to them temporarily, with an agreed weight gain target, which will then start a process of handing control back to Alison. Weekly weighing should be carried out within the outpatient department with the same pair of scales and clothes each week to minimize opportunities for Alison to question the validity of the monitoring. Given Alison's age it would be helpful for her GP and paediatric consultant to monitor her physical condition because weighing alone should not be the definitive marker for physical wellbeing.

The involvement of Alison's school should also be considered, perhaps to provide a work schedule that can be followed at home, and/or a phased return to school when Alison's energy levels have improved. This reduces the potential for anorexia to impact upon Alison's educational and future career prospects. Alison could be given the option of inviting her friends into a session to increase their understanding of what she is experiencing and to draw on them for support.

Individual work using a CBT approach supported with family work should be offered to address the individual and systemic issues that may be supporting the maintenance of anorexia.

Annotated bibliography

Agras, W.S. (ed.) (2010) *The Oxford Handbook of Eating Disorders.* **Oxford: Oxford University Press.**
This is a comprehensive text providing the reader with multiple perspectives on eating disorders, including the phenomenology, epidemiology, assessment and approaches to understanding the condition.

Beat Eating Disorders at: www.b-eat.co.uk.
Beat began life as the Eating Disorder Association and is now the UK's only nationwide organization supporting people affected by eating disorders, their family members and friends. The site has many useful links including one to the *European Eating Disorders Review* journal.

Crisp, A.H. (1995) *Anorexia Nervosa – Let me Be.* **Hove: Laurence Erlbaum Associates.**
This book has become a seminal text capturing the developmental aspects of anorexia and views the condition as the avoidance of normal adult weight. It provides the reader with insightful perspectives, especially in relation to empowerment of the individual and the family, leading towards recovery.

Miller, W.R. and Rollnick, S. (2002) *Motivational Interviewing: Preparing people to change addictive behaviour.* **New York: Guilford Press.**
This text presents the principles of motivational interviewing and uses case examples to illustrate the key points that underpin the approach. This is of particular benefit when we reflect upon the perceived ambivalence associated with eating disorders. It is identified within the literature that engagement is paramount and this book provides the concepts, skills and strategies required to engage and motivate people to change.

NICE (National Institute for Health and Clinical Excellence) (2004) *Clinical Guideline 9: Eating disorders – core interventions in the treatment and management of anorexia nervosa, bulimia nervosa and related eating disorders.* **London: NICE.**
Provides the reader with up-to-date evidenced-based information on eating disorders. It is regularly reviewed to accommodate the latest developments in the field.

References

APA (American Psychiatric Association) (2000) *Diagnostic and Statistical Manual of Mental Disorders*, revised 4th edn. Washington, DC: APA.

Arcelus, J. Mitchell, A., Wales, J. and Nielsen,S. (2011) Mortality Rates in patients with anorexia nervosa and other eating disorders a meta-analysis of 36 studies, *Arch Gen Psychiatr*, 68(7): 724–31.

Bacaltchuk, J. and Hay, P.P.J. (2003) Antidepressants versus placebo for people with bulimia nervosa, *Cochrane Database of Systematic Reviews*, Issue 4. Art. No.: CD003391. DOI: 10.1002/14651858. CD003391.

Brewerton, T.D., Lydiard, B.R., Herzog, D.B., Brotman, A.W., O'Neil, P.M. and Balenger, J.C. (1995) Comorbidity of Axis I psychiatric disorders in bulimia nervosa, *Journal of Clinical Psychiatry*, 56: 77–80.

Brumberg, J.J. (1988) *Fasting Girls: The history of anorexia nervosa.* New York: Penguin Books.

Bryant-Waugh, R. (2006) Recent developments in anorexia nervosa, *Child and Adolescent Mental Health*, 11(2): 76–81.

Cecchin, G. (1987) Hypothesizing, circularity, and neutrality revisited: an invitation to curiosity, *Family Process*, 26: 405–13.

Clarke, C. (2008) Creating communities in cyberspace: pro-anorexia web sites and social capital, *Journal of Psychiatric and Mental Health Nursing*, 15: 340–3.

Claudino, A.M., Silva de Lima, M., Hay, P.P.J, Bacaltchuk, J., Schmidt, U.U.S and Treasure, J. (2006) Antidepressants for anorexia nervosa, *Cochrane Database of Systematic Reviews*, Issue 1. Art. No.: CD004365. DOI: 10.1002/14651858. CD004365. pub2.

Cooper, Z. and Fairburn, C.G. (1987) The Eating Disorder Examination: a semi-structured interview for the assessment of the specific psychopathology of eating disorders, *International Journal of Eating Disorders*, 6: 1–8.

Crisp, A.H. (1980) *Anorexia Nervosa – Let me be.* London: Academic Press.

Crisp, A.H. (1995) *Anorexia Nervosa – Let me be new edn?.* Hove: Laurence Erlbaum Associates.

Csipke, E. and Horne, O. (2007) Pro-eating disorder websites: users' opinions, *European Eating Disorders Review*, 15: 196–206.

Duker, M. and Slade, R. (2003) *Anorexia Nervosa and Bulimia: How to help.* Buckingham: Open University Press.

Fairburn, C.G. (1981) A cognitive behavioural approach to the management of bulimia, *Psychological Medicine*, 11, 707–11.

Fairburn, C.G. (2008) *Cognitive Behaviour Therapy and Eating Disorders.* New York: Guilford Press.

Fairburn, C.G. and Brownell, K.D. (2002) *Eating Disorders and Obesity: A comprehensive handbook*, 2nd edn. New York: Guilford Press.

Fairburn, C.G. and Harrison, P.J. (2003) Eating disorders, *The Lancet*, 361(9355): 407–16.

Fisher, C.A., Hetrick, S.E. and Rushford, N. (2010) Family therapy for anorexia nervosa, *Cochrane Database of Systematic Reviews*, Issue 4. Art. No.: CD004780. DOI: 10.1002/14651858. D004780. pub2.

Garner, D.M., Olmstead, M.P. and Polivy, J. (1983) Development and validation of a multidimensional eating disorder inventory for anorexia nervosa and bulimia, *International Journal of Eating Disorders*, 2: 15–34.

Gatward, N. (2007) Anorexia nervosa: an evolutionary puzzle, *European Eating Disorders Review*, 15, 1–12.

Giordano, S. (2005) *Understanding Eating Disorders.* Oxford: Clarendon Press.

Gull, W.W. (1873) Anorexia nervosa (apepsia hysterica, anorexia hysterica), *The Lancet*, 22–8.

Hay, P.P.J., Bacaltchuk, J., Stefano, S. and Kashyap, P.(2009) Psychological treatments for bulimia nervosa and binging, *Cochrane Database of Systematic Reviews*, Issue 4. Art. No.: CD000562. DOI: 10.1002/14651858. CD000562. pub3.

Keel, P.K. and Klump, K.L. (2003) Are eating disorders culture-bound syndromes? Implications for conceptualizing their aetiology, *Psychological Bulletin*, 129: 747–69.

Kruger, S. and Kennedy, S.H. (2000) Psychopharmacotherapy of anorexia nervosa, bulimia nervosa and binge-eating disorder, *Journal of Psychiatry & Neuroscience*, 25(5): 497–509.

Levine, P. and Smolak, L. (2010) Cultural influences on body image and eating disorders, in W.S. Agras (ed.) *The Oxford Handbook of Eating Disorders*. Oxford: Oxford University Press.

Lock, J., Le Grange, D., Agras, W. and Dare, C. (2001) *Treatment Manual for Anorexia Nervosa: A family-based approach*. London: Guilford Press.

Miller, W.R. and Rollnick, S. (2002) *Motivational Interviewing: Preparing people to change addictive behaviour*. New York: Guilford Press.

Morgan, J.F., Reid, F. and Lacey, J.H. (1999) The SCOFF questionnaire: assessment of a new screening tool for eating disorders, *British Medical Journal*, 319: 1467–8.

NICE (National Institute for Clinical Excellence) (2004) *Clinical Guideline 9: Eating disorders – core interventions in the treatment and management of anorexia nervosa, bulimia nervosa and related eating disorders*. London: NICE.

Ogden, J. (2010) *The Psychology of Eating from Healthy to Disordered Behaviour*, 2nd edn. West Sussex: Blackwell Publishing.

Patching, J. and Lawler, J. (2009) Understanding women's experiences of developing an eating disorder and recovering: a life-history approach, *Nursing Inquiry*, 16(1): 10–21.

Perkins, S.S.J., Murphy, R.R.M., Schmidt, U.U.S. and Williams, C. (2006) Self-help and guided self-help for eating disorders, *Cochrane Database of Systematic Reviews*, Issue 3. Art. No.: CD004191. DOI: 10.1002/14651858. CD00419.

Prestwood, C. (2004) The person with an eating disorder, in I. Norman and I. Ryrie (eds) *The Art and Science of Mental Health Nursing*. Maidenhead: Open University Press.

Robinson, P. (2009) *Severe & Enduring Eating Disorder (SEED): Management of complex presentations of anorexia and bulimia nervosa*. Chichester: Wiley/Backwell.

Russell, G.F.M. (1979) Bulimia nervosa: an ominous variant of anorexia nervosa nervosa? *Psychological Medicine*, 9: 429–48.

Scherag, S., Hebebrand, S. and Hinney, A. (2010) Eating disorders: the current status of molecular genetic research, *European Child and Adolescent Psychiatry*, 19: 211–26.

Shisslak, C.M., Crago, M. and Estes, L.S. (1995) The spectrum of eating disturbances, *International Journal of Eating Disorders*, 18: 209–19.

Simpson, K.J. (2002) Anorexia nervosa and culture, *Journal of Psychiatric and Mental Health Nursing*, 9: 65–71.

Stice, E. (2001) A prospective test of the dual pathway model of bulimic pathology: mediating effects of dieting and negative affect, *Journal of Abnormal Psychology*, 110: 1–12.

Treasure, J., Schmidt, U. and Macdonald, P. (2010) *The Clinicians Guide to Collaborative Caring in Eating Disorders: The New Maudsley Method*. East Sussex: Routledge FALMER?.

Van der Linden, J. (2008) Many roads lead to Rome: why does cognitive behavioural therapy remain unsuccessful for many eating disorder patients? *European Eating Disorders Review*, 16: 329–33.

Van der Linden, J., Buis, H., Pieters, G. and Probst, M. (2007) Which elements in the treatment of eating disorders are necessary 'ingredients' in the recovery process? A comparison between the patient's and therapist's view, *European Eating Disorders Review*, 15: 357–65.

White, M. and Epston, D. (1990) *Narrative Means to Therapeutic Ends*. New York: Norton.

Williams, S. and Reid, M. (2010) Understanding the experience of ambivalence in anorexia nervosa: the maintainer's perspective, *Psychology and Health*, 25(5): 551–67.

WHO (World Health Organization) (2010) *International Statistical Classification of Diseases and Related Health Problems (ICD-10)*, 10th revision, available at: http://apps.who.int/classifications/icd10/browse/2010/en#/F50 Accessed 24/11/11.

Chapter 39

The Person with Co-existing Mental Illness and Substance Use Problems ('Dual Diagnosis')

Cheryl Kipping

The danger is that if [substance use and mental disorder] get separated, things can get missed. There are a lot of advantages of looking at the total picture to avoid people making assumptions that are incorrect about you. Sometimes there might not be a link but I know in my case that there was a link. I wouldn't have been able to stop drinking without having my mental health problems treated.

Anonymous service user; Rethink Dual Diagnosis Research Group (2004)

39.1 Introduction

Although dual diagnosis has been identified as one of the most challenging clinical problems facing mental health services, provision for dual diagnosis should be central to modern mental health care, and mental health nurses in all settings should be able to respond to the needs of this group (DH 2006). Many combinations of mental and substance misuse disorders occur and, while it is important that the needs of each individual are at the centre of assessment and care/treatment, some general principles can inform practice and help support people with dual diagnosis to achieve their recovery goals. This chapter covers:

■ introduction and overview of dual diagnosis and substance mis/use;

- foundations for working with people with a dual diagnosis;
- assessment, treatment and nursing care.

39.2 Concepts and terminology

'Substance use' is a broad concept. Use in itself may not be problematic. Many people experiment with, or use, substances on a recreational basis. However, adverse physical, psychological, psychiatric, interpersonal, social or legal consequences may be experienced, particularly with regular use. The 'problem', however, may not be perceived as such by users. 'Substance misuse' is use that is not socially or medically approved, or which is illegal. What is socially acceptable, medically approved or illegal in one culture, at one point in time, may not be in another or at another time. Although a distinction is made between drugs and alcohol, alcohol is a drug that happens to be legal. Other legal drugs include tobacco and caffeine – while caffeine is socially acceptable, tobacco is becoming less so.

'Dependence' indicates a compulsion to continue taking a substance on a regular, repetitive basis. Physical dependence occurs when the body adapts to repeated doses. Withholding it will result in withdrawal symptoms. Some substances do not create physical dependence but do create psychological dependence.

'Dual diagnosis' has been adopted as a convenient term for coexisting mental health and substance misuse problems. Some people think it is unhelpful because it is underpinned by the medical model, focuses on diagnoses, and suggests that people have just two problems. People with a 'dual diagnosis' may have more than two diagnoses and often have multiple needs – for example, physical health problems, housing, financial and legal difficulties. 'Complex needs' is sometimes used as an alternative. This shifts the focus away from the medical model and points to the wider range of needs and challenges experienced by service users, carers and service providers. Despite its limitations, given its widespread usage, 'dual diagnosis' is used in this chapter.

39.3 Overview of dual diagnosis

The range of people that might be considered to have a dual diagnosis is wide. Figure 39.1 illustrates this. Each person can be located on the figure by taking account of the severity of their mental illness (horizontal continuum) and the severity of their substance misuse (vertical continuum). Personality disorder is conceptualized as a separate dimension that can coexist with mental illness, a substance misuse problem, or both.

Complexity is added when the relationship(s) between mental illness and substance misuse are considered:

- substance use or withdrawal can produce psychiatric symptoms or illness;
- dependence, intoxication or withdrawal can produce psychological symptoms;
- psychiatric disorder can lead to a substance misuse disorder;
- substance misuse may exacerbate a pre-existing psychiatric disorder (Crome 1999).

In practice it can be difficult to identify which of these mechanisms is operating. To understand a person's presentation and disentangle which aspects may be due to substances, which mental disorder, and which may be a combination, a good understanding of substances, and the signs and symptoms of use, intoxication and withdrawal is required. Several websites provide such information including: FRANK (www.talk-tofrank.com) and Drugscope (www.drugscope.org.uk/resources/drugsearch). The Depertment of Health (DH) (2011) has also produced a publication on the harms associated with drugs (and alcohol). This includes details of acute and chronic, physical and psychological effects, and information about dependence, withdrawal and tolerance.

Figure 39.1 Scope of coexistent psychiatric and substance misuse disorder (After DH 2002)

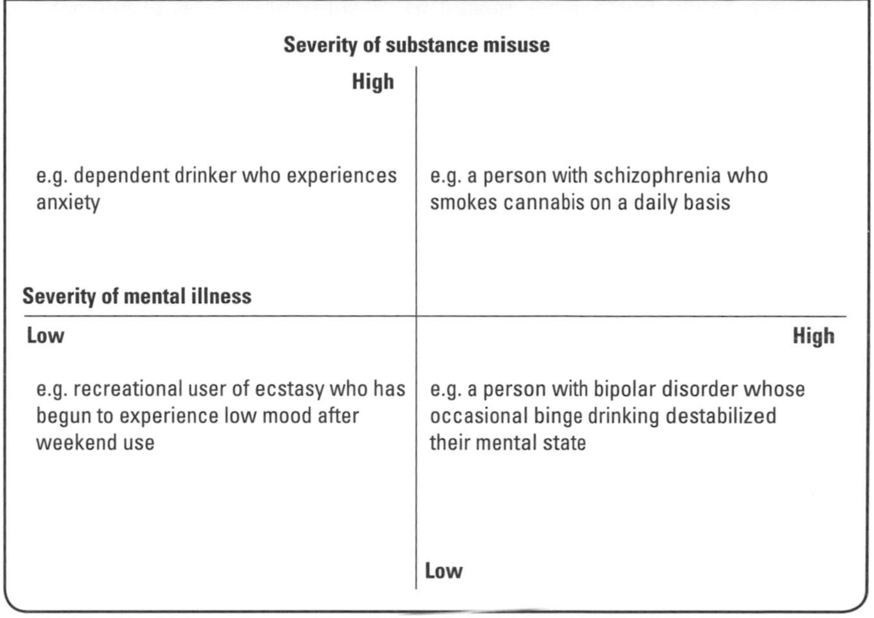

Severity of substance misuse

High

e.g. dependent drinker who experiences anxiety

e.g. a person with schizophrenia who smokes cannabis on a daily basis

Severity of mental illness

Low   High

e.g. recreational user of ecstasy who has begun to experience low mood after weekend use

e.g. a person with bipolar disorder whose occasional binge drinking destabilized their mental state

Low

Thinking Space 39.1

Think of two or three people with a 'dual diagnosis' that you have worked with (include people with different diagnoses and using different substances).

Where on Figure 39.1 would you locate them?

Now think about the difficulties these people experience as a consequence of having mental health and substance misuse problems: think about their mental state, physical health, relationships with family/carers/neighbours, accommodation, education/employment, finances, legal situation, prescribed medication and risks (self-harm, suicide, violence, accidents, self-neglect, abuse and exploitation, impact on children). In light of these do you think 'dual diagnosis' is a useful term, or is 'complex needs' move helpful?

Prevalence

Prevalence studies of dual diagnosis vary in their definitions of mental illness and substance misuse, sample selection, measurement tools and time frames. It is generally accepted that 30–50 per cent of people with a severe mental illness also have substance misuse problems and at least 70 per cent of people accessing substance misuse services have co-existing mental health problems. The diagnoses in this latter group tend to be anxiety and mood disorders.

Reasons for substance use and aetiological theories

People have many reasons for using substances. These include: dealing with negative feelings/situations (e.g. stress, anger, anxiety, boredom, poor sleep, blocking out past painful experiences); promoting positive feelings (e.g. the 'buzz', relaxation, confidence); and responding to social pressures (e.g. it is the norm within the peer group).

'Self-medication' has received particular attention in relation to people with mental health problems. Evidence of use to self-medicate negative symptoms, mood problems, anxiety and insomnia has been found but findings related to managing positive symptoms and medication side-effects are inconsistent.

Several models have been proposed to explain the high prevalence of co-morbid substance misuse and mental health problems. These include:

- common factor – a common vulnerability factor increases the risk of mental illness and substance misuse (e.g. genetic, childhood sexual abuse);

- secondary substance misuse – mental illness is a vulnerability factor for substance misuse;

- secondary psychiatric illness – mental illness develops as a consequence of substance misuse;

- bi-directional – both disorders are present and likely to interact.

While these models provide a conceptual framework for understanding co-morbidity, evidence to support them is equivocal.

39.4 Foundations for working with people with a dual diagnosis

As well as having a good understanding of substances and their effects, work with people with a dual diagnosis needs to be underpinned by four foundational components. The first is:

1. *An approach based on engagement, motivational enhancement and recovery principles*

The National Institute for Health and Clinical Excellence (NICE) (2011a) emphasizes the importance of engagement and building respectful, trusting, non-judgemental relationships in an atmosphere of hope and optimism. Working collaboratively and respecting service users' autonomy is essential if change is to be achieved. The principles set out in Chapters 5 ('Recovery and social inclusion') and 23 ('Motivational interviewing') are fundamental.

People with a dual diagnosis can be challenging. They can be difficult to engage and not view their substance use as problematic despite its negative consequences. This can result in staff feeling pessimistic. Maintaining belief in the possibility of change is important: people with a dual diagnosis do change and lead meaningful lives. Reflecting on one's views of substance use and people that misuse substances can be important as negative attitudes can be a barrier to working effectively with this group.

The second component for working with people with a dual diagnosis is:

2. *An integration of principles from the mental health and substance misuse fields*

Because mental health/illness and substance misuse impact on each other, addressing one in isolation from the other is unlikely to be effective. Consideration should be given to each *and* account taken of how they may interrelate. Treatment planning needs to consider the relative severity of each condition at a particular time (NICE 2011a).

Closing the Gap, the dual diagnosis capability framework (Hughes 2006), identifies the capabilities required to deliver effective nursing care to this group. It draws from mental health and substance misuse competency frameworks.

Capabilities are identified in three areas:

- values;
- utilizing knowledge and skills;
- practice development.

Within each there are three levels. All mental health nurses should have Level 2 capabilities. Those taking a leading role in dual diagnosis (e.g. dual diagnosis link workers/champions) should be aspiring to attain Level 3 capabilities.

The third component for working with people with a dual diagnosis is:

3. *Clarity regarding care pathways and which service(s) should provide care for different groups of people with a dual diagnosis*

Three service models have been identified for working with people with a dual diagnosis:

■ **Serial:** mental health and substance misuse disorders are treated consecutively by different services. Each expects the person to deal with the other problem first. This frequently results in people falling between services and is generally seen as poor practice.

■ **Parallel:** mental health and substance misuse interventions are provided concurrently by two services; mental health working on mental health problems and substance misuse services on substance misuse. Although this is an improvement on the serial model, the service user needs to attend two services and there is a risk that services may not work together or communicate effectively.

■ **Integrated:** mental health and substance misuse interventions are provided at the same time, in one setting, by one team.

Although robust research in support of the integrated model is limited, it is widely advocated. The service leading/coordinating care has responsibility for addressing needs associated with *both* disorders.

In recognition of the challenges this can present, when mental health services are coordinating care, substance misuse services should offer advice and support. Similarly, when substance misuse services are coordinating care, mental health services should offer advice and support (DH 2002; NICE 2011a).

The integrated model is the only realistic way forward for people with mental health problems who do not view their substance use as problematic: they would be very unlikely to engage with a substance misuse service. When the person is ready to make changes to their use and could benefit from specialist alcohol/drug treatment, joint work (in line with the parallel model) can be a constructive way forward (NICE 2011a).

Figure 39.1 provides an indication of the service best placed to lead/coordinate the care of someone with a dual diagnosis, in line with the integrated treatment model. People with severe mental illness (in the right hand quadrants) should usually have both their mental health and substance misuse problems addressed within mental health services. Those in the top left quadrant (severe substance misuse, low severity mental illness) should have both addressed within substance misuse services. People falling in the bottom left quadrant are unlikely to have any contact with services. If they do, the most appropriate would be primary care.

The fourth component for working with people with a dual diagnosis is:

Thinking Space 39.2

Identify which quadrant from Figure 39.1 each of the following cases falls into and, on the basis of this, which service should lead/coordinate care in line with the integrated treatment model.

1. Leroy has a diagnosis of schizophrenia. He uses cannabis and alcohol most days and crack two or three times each week. He does not think his substance use causes any problems for him.

2. Sandra has been dependent on heroin for many years. She also experiences persistent episodes of low mood and anxiety.

3. Ahmed has a diagnosis of bipolar disorder. He sometimes binges on alcohol and this can have an impact on his mental state.

4. Tony regularly uses alcohol and cocaine at weekends, and occasionally during the week. Sometimes he experiences episodes of anxiety and low mood following use.

Make a note of your thoughts. *Feedback is provided at the end of the chapter.*

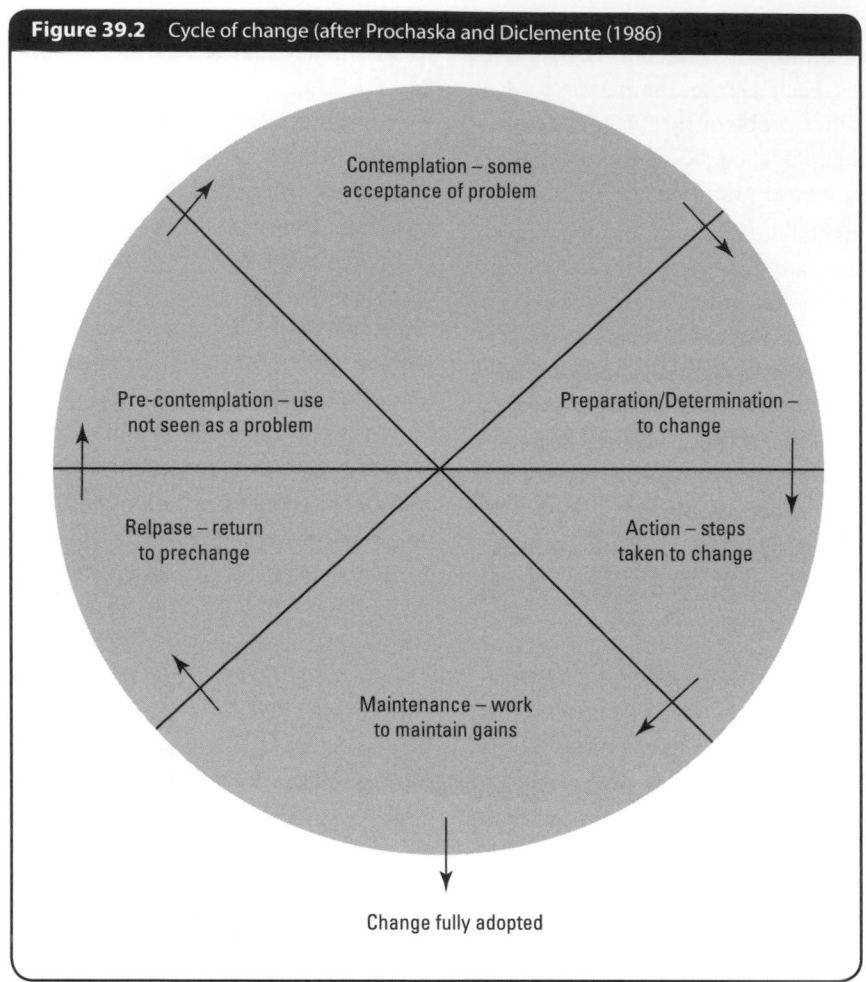

Figure 39.2 Cycle of change (after Prochaska and Diclemente (1986)

Contemplation – some
acceptance of problem

Pre-contemplation – use
not seen as a problem

Preparation/Determination –
to change

Relpase – return
to prechange

Action – steps
taken to change

Maintenance – work
to maintain gains

Change fully adopted

4. *An understanding of Prochaska and DiClemente's (1986) transtheoretical model of change and Osher and Kofoed's (1989) staged treatment model*

Together these models provide a framework to inform interventions. Prochaska and DiClemente (1986) view change as a process where the person moves from *precontemplation*, where their behaviour is not seen as problematic and change is therefore not considered, through *contemplation*, where there is some acknowledgement of difficulties and the possibility of change, on to *preparation/determination* where plans for change are made, and then *action* when change is made. *Maintenance* concerns sus-

taining long-term change. People are often unable to maintain change and *relapse* (see Figure 39.2). Because both mental illness and substance misuse are chronic relapsing conditions people are likely to move backwards and forwards round the cycle several times before change is sustained. A long-term perspective, often several years, is therefore needed.

Osher and Kofoed's (1989) staged treatment model comprises four stages: engagement, building motivation (persuasion), active treatment and relapse prevention. These map onto Prochaska and DiClemente's stages of change and it is by bringing these together that a framework for identifying appropriate interventions is produced (see Figure 39.3).

Figure 39.3 Stages of change, treatment stage and possible treatment approaches/interventions

Stage of change (Prochaska and DiClemente 1986)	Treatment stage (Osher and Kofoed 1989)	Possible treatment approches/interventions
Precontemplation	Engagement	Building relationships Assertive outreach Flexible working practices Identifying needs Address practical issues, e.g. housing, benefits Motivational interviewing Harm minimization Brief interventions Offering information and advice Pharmacotherapy–for stabilization of psychiatric symptoms Assessment of carer's needs Obtain initial information to begin building comprehensive assessment
Contemplation	Building motivation	Continue building realtionship Motivational interviewing Comprehensive assessment Decision metrices Readiness rules Diaries Pharmacotheraphy–for psychatric symptoms
Action	Active treatment	Motivational interviewing Goal setting and planning Solution focused approach Diaries Development of new skills and lifestyle changes, e.g. budgeting, building social networks, enhancing social skills, developing leisure interests, developing vocational skills Activity scheduling Pharmacotherapy–for psychiatric symptoms– for detox from substances: inpatient or community reduction Adjunctive therapy to address specific problems, e.g. bereavement issues, childhood sexual abuse Self-help groups, e.g. AA, NA, SMART Recovery
Maintenance	Relapse prevention	Motivational interviewing Pharmacotherapy–for psychiatric symptoms– for substance misuse relapse prevention Relapse prevention mental health and substance misuse Day programmes, residential programmes Consolidation of skills and lifestyle changes Self-help groups, e.g. AA, NA, SMART Recovery

39.5 Assessment, treatment and nursing care

Assessment

Assessment should not be thought of as separate from treatment. It is important for engaging the person, building a therapeutic relationship, enhancing motivation and offering information and advice. Assessment of substance use should be integral to mental health assessment. Failure to identify use can result in misdiagnosis and inappropriate treatment.

Key components of a comprehensive assessment are:

- current and recent use;
- past use;
- physical health (including sexual health);
- mental health;
- prescribed medication;
- social situation (including accommodation, relationships, family circumstances – especially children, employment, finances);
- legal situation;
- personal and family history;
- risk;
- client's perception of situation, reasons for using and motivation for change;
- strengths and supports;
- family/carer needs.

The remainder of this section focuses on the components of particular relevance to substance use: current and recent use; past use; and the client's perception, reasons for using and readiness for change.

Obtaining information about the impact of substance use on other assessment domains (e.g. physical, mental, social and legal circumstances) is important. Risk assessment is especially important. Substance use increases a range of risks potentially resulting in the person posing a risk to others and/or being vulnerable to risks themselves.

Consideration should be given to:

- Risks specifically associated with substances (e.g. withdrawal seizures, delirium tremens, blood-borne viruses, accidental overdose).
- The impact of substances on other risks (e.g. suicide, violence, self-neglect, exploitation, accidental injury).
- The potential interaction of substances and prescribed medication.
- Safeguarding issues. Substance misuse and mental illness frequently impact on children, whose needs are paramount. People with a dual diagnosis may also be very vulnerable themselves. Safeguarding procedures (children and/or vulnerable adult) should be followed where appropriate.

The DH (2011) publication on the health harms of drugs (including alcohol) is helpful for identifying risks.

Current and recent use

Information about which substances are being used (alcohol and drugs – illicit, over-the-counter and prescribed), the quantity, frequency and pattern of use, route of administration and length of time use has been at the current level should be obtained. Prompting for specific substances and further questioning to gain clarification (e.g. type/strength of beer, whether prescribed medication is taken as directed) may be necessary. Information about when the person last used each substance is important both for identifying risks and making sense of the person's current presentation. If the person is injecting, sites should be inspected and information about whether equipment is being shared obtained.

An assessment of dependency is also required (NICE 2011a). This may be achieved by further questioning or use of standardized tools. A history of the past five to seven days' use, starting with 'today' and working back, can indicate whether the person is dependent, and whether use is stable or fluctuating. A more detailed picture of use on a typical day may also be helpful. Other factors influencing use should be explored – for example, the person may use one substance to counteract another, or use heavily after benefit payments and then have several days of abstinence.

Details of withdrawal symptoms (from alcohol, benzodiazepines, opiates and GHB/GBL) are needed to establish whether the person is physically dependent and ensure that any life threatening withdrawal symptoms (e.g. alcohol withdrawal seizures and delirium tremens) are identified.

Observation is essential. Factors to observe include: signs of intoxication or withdrawal, injuries, jaundice, whether the person appears underweight, unkempt, agitated or anxious. Objective tests can provide further information (e.g. urinalysis, breathalyser readings and blood tests).

Throughout assessment opportunities for offering information about the potential impact of alcohol and drug use on physical and mental health, and how these harms might be reduced, should be taken.

Past use

A substance misuse history should establish when the person began taking each substance they have used, what prompted use, how it developed, its impact on the person's life (e.g. education, employment, relationships, finances, physical and mental health, contact with the criminal justice system), whether abstinence has been achieved and, if so, how, and details of any substance misuse treatment (what was provided, what was helpful and the outcome).

Client's perception of situation, reasons for use and readiness to change

With sensitive questioning and active listening this information is likely to emerge during assessment. Confirmation may be achieved by asking the person directly, in a non-judgemental way, whether they think their use is causing them difficulties and whether (or not) they want to make changes. On the basis of this information, the person's position on Prochaska and DiClementi's cycle of change can be identified.

Standardized tools

Standardized tools can complement the assessment process. Many have been developed for drugs and alcohol but few specifically for dual diagnosis. Caution is needed when using drug and alcohol assessment tools with the dual diagnosis population as they may not be sufficiently sensitive to detect problem use. For some people with mental health problems use is low and their scores may not meet threshold criteria, but even low level use can have serious consequences.

AUDIT (Alcohol Use Disorders Identification Test) (Babor *et al.* 1989) is a screening tool that assesses use over the past 12 months. It is recommended for all populations including people with mental health problems. The score indicates whether the person is drinking at 'lower', 'increasing' or 'higher' risk levels, or is 'possibly dependent'. Appropriate interventions have been identified for each (NICE 2010a). AUDIT is therefore a clinical decision tool too. It can also be used as an outcome measure (NICE 2011b).

A score in the 'possibly dependent' range indicates that the SADQ (Severity of Alcohol Dependence Questionnaire) (Stockwell *et al.* 1983) should be completed (NICE 2011b). As its name suggests, this measures how severely dependent the person is and provides an indication of whether an assisted alcohol withdrawal is needed. The score also indicates the appropriate dose of chlordiazepoxide from which to start a detoxification regimen (NICE 2010b).

NICE (2011b) recommends the LDQ (Leeds Dependence Questionnaire) (Raistrick *et al.* 1994) as an alternative measure of dependence. This can be used for alcohol or drug use and is valid for people with a severe mental illness.

For dependent drinkers admitted to hospital/residential care the CIWA-Ar (Clinical Institute Withdrawal Assessment for Alcohol – Revised) (Sullivan *et al.* 1989) is recommended for the assessment of alcohol withdrawal symptoms. This allows pharmacological treatment to be tailored to individual need as dosing is symptom triggered (NICE 2010c, 2011b).

NICE has not recommended any standardized screening tools for drug use. Several assessment tools have been developed specifically for dual diagnosis but none have been widely adopted into UK practice. The Drug Use Scale – Revised, and Alcohol Use Scale – Revised (Mueser *et al.* 2003) assess drug/alcohol use in people with severe mental illness. The Substance Abuse Treatment Scale (SATS) (McHugo *et al.* 1995) assesses the person's treatment stage (closely relating to Osher and Kofoed's 1989 staged treatment model). Both could be useful outcome measures.

Case Study

Leroy

Leroy has a diagnosis of schizophrenia and uses cannabis, alcohol and crack. His care is provided under the Care Programme Approach (CPA). Leroy lives with his parents and has a sister who lives locally. His grandmother, with whom he had a close relationship, also lived nearby. However, she died recently and since then Leroy's substance use has increased and his mental state deteriorated. His parents have found his behaviour increasingly difficult. He has become argumentative, is borrowing money and not repaying it, and is abusive towards a neighbour, who he believes is watching and talking about him. He stopped going to a music group he had been attending and missed appointments with his community psychiatric nurse (CPN).

Although always a bit inconsistent in taking his medication, as his substance use increased Leroy stopped taking it altogether. He became increasingly paranoid and talked about killing the neighbour. Given a history of violence in the context of increased substance use and paranoia he was admitted to hospital.

A nurse Leroy knew from previous admissions conducted the admission procedures. She reminded him of the boundaries regarding not using alcohol and drugs on the ward, asked if he had brought any substances in with him, and searched him and his possessions.

The admission assessment revealed an AUDIT score indicating 'possible dependence'. Over the past week Leroy had been drinking six to eight cans of strong lager (9 per cent alcohol by volume) and smoking six to eight cannabis joints daily, and shared three or four rocks of crack cocaine on three days. A urine drug screen provided confirmatory evidence of his use. Liver function tests showed some abnormalities likely to be a consequence of his drinking.

The CIWA-Ar was used to monitor his alcohol withdrawal symptoms and an alcohol detoxification regimen, using chlordiazepoxide, was commenced. He was also prescribed intra-muscular pabrinex (thiamine/vitamin B supplement) to prevent Wernicke's encephalopathy.

Thinking Space 39.3

A care plan was negotiated with Leroy that included:

- *interventions* to ensure that Leroy's alcohol detoxification was completed safely;
- offering *opportunities* to discuss his substance use and its effects;
- *strategies* to ensure that he remained abstinent from drugs and alcohol while on the ward.

What interventions, opportunities and strategies could be included within Leroy's care plan? Jot down your ideas. Feedback is provided at the end of the chapter.

Figure 39.4 Drink diary

Day	How much and what type of alcohol	Times drinking started and ended	Who with	Where drinking took place	Number of units	Thoughts, feelings and consequences	Cost (£s)
Monday							
Tuesday							
Wednesday							
Thursday							
Friday							
Saturday							
Sunday							

Further assessment tools

Assessment is an ongoing process. Building a detailed picture of the person's use, the way it developed over time, the role substances play in the person's life and their impact takes time. Following initial assessment further tools can be used to help the clinician and service user develop a fuller understanding of the person's substance use. These include:

- diaries;
- decision matrices;
- time lines;
- exploring a typical day;
- readiness rulers.

Diaries are useful for obtaining baseline information about use, and providing insights into reasons for, and influences on, use (see Figure 39.4). Formats can be adapted to meet individual need. For example, simplifying if the person's literacy skills are limited, adding columns to monitor psychiatric symptoms (e.g. mood). Diaries can also monitor progress over time. If gains are made they can provide encouragement and boost confidence in the person's ability to make further changes.

Decision matrices (see Figure 39.5) enable the person to explore the good and not so good things about their substance use (pros/cons, advantages/ disadvantages), and the potentially good and not so good things about stopping or reducing use. Although Figure 39.5 illustrates a 2 x 2 cell format, for people with severe mental illness a simpler two-cell format may be more appropriate (Martino and Moyers 2008).

Working with the service user to construct a chronological 'time line' of life events, mental health and substance misuse can provide insights into the interrelationship(s) between these, and a more detailed understanding of the person's history.

Exploring a typical day can provide further detail about the person's use and insights into other aspects of their life, and how substances fit with these. For example, how they spend their time, which people they have contact with, and whether these are likely to be positive or negative influences.

The readiness ruler can be useful in determining whether the person is ready for change. The person is asked to rate (on a scale of 0–10) how important change is and then how confident they feel about making the change. High scores on both suggest that the person is ready.

Although these tools have been included in the assessment section, using them in a collaborative manner with the service user can be an intervention as well, and help support the person to change.

Figure 39.5 Example of decision matrix (see case study)

Continuing to drink alcohol

Advantages/pros	Disadvantages/cons
Like being drunk	Having a bad effect on health (abnormal liver tests)
Like drinking with friends	Spending more than I can afford
Stops me feeling down about death of Gran	Arguments with parents
	Sister stops me going round and seeing children
	Got in mess, stopped taking medication and ended up in hospital

Reducing alcohol

Disadvantages/cons	Advantages/pros
Feelings about death of Gran will be strong	Improve health, will be fitter for playing football
Will feel left out when mates are drinking	Better relationships with family – won't owe parents money, sister will let me go round and see children
	May get to start computer course

Substance use varies over time so regular review is needed. For people under the CPA, this should be part of review meetings.

Treatment

Osher and Kofoed's (1989) staged treatment model provides the framework for this section. In practice, flexibility is required. Movement between stages is fluid and aspects of the various interventions will be used at each stage (see Figure 39.3). The emphasis here is on substance misuse interventions but these cannot be seen in isolation from mental health interventions. Many aspects of treatment are essential regardless of whether the person has mental health, substance misuse or co-morbid problems – for example, provision of safe accom-

modation, development of daytime activity, building support networks.

Engagement

This stage focuses on developing a therapeutic alliance. While some people acknowledge that they have mental health problems, others do not. Similarly, some recognize that their alcohol and/or drug use is problematic, others do not. People may therefore be difficult to engage. A motivational approach, with an emphasis on the spirit of motivational interviewing (being collaborative, compassionate, accepting including respecting the person's autonomy, and eliciting the person's own strengths and perspectives – evocation), is required, along with flexibility – seeing people at times and locations convenient to them. Support to resolve practical issues (e.g. benefit payments, accommodation difficulties) can also promote contact and relationship development. Focusing on substance use, and in particular reducing use, is not the aim at this stage. The emphasis is on reducing harm. Harm reduction is concerned with reducing health, social and economic harms to individuals, communities and societies (UK Harm Reduction Alliance 2007). It derives from the substance misuse field, where the emphasis has been on reducing injecting related harms, but the principles are applicable to other substances and broader issues associated with mental health (e.g. homelessness, physical health, exposure to violence).

Offering people information (verbal and written) about the effects of substances on physical and mental health, and strategies they could employ to use in less harmful ways is important as it enables people to make informed choices about their use.

Long-term engagement and treatment are required for many people with a dual diagnosis. However, there will be some people in contact with mental health services who use substances at a low level and this may not appear to be causing difficulties, at least currently. Nurses have a responsibility to address this too: early intervention may prevent more substantial problems at a later stage.

Brief interventions, or extended brief interventions, should be offered to 'increasing' or 'higher risk' drinkers (as identified by AUDIT) (NICE 2010a). These are short, motivationally based sessions where advice on reducing use is provided. The acronym FRAMES summarizes the elements of brief interventions (Bien *et al.* 1993):

F – *feedback* of current status and risk

R – emphasis on the client having *responsibility* for change

A – *advice* to change

M – a *menu* of change options

E – an *empathic* manner

S – reinforcing the client's *self-efficacy*

Building motivation (persuasion)

Once a positive relationship has been developed and regular contact established, attention can focus on building motivation for change. This stage maps to the contemplation stage of the cycle of change. Ambivalence – being in two minds – is characteristic. The person will have some reasons for changing and some for not doing so. Taking a motivational approach to help strengthen the person's readiness for change is the goal (see Chapter 23). The decision matrix tool can be useful for developing discrepancy between where the person is, and where they want to be, hopefully enabling them to make a decision for change. It can also highlight areas requiring attention if the person is to achieve change. For example, if a substance is used to help the person relax, attention may need to be given to finding alternative relaxation methods.

When there are indications that the person is at the preparation/determination stage of the cycle of change the readiness ruler can be useful for confirming this. If ratings of importance and confidence are high then change plans can be made. If not, further work is required to boost the dimension where ratings are low.

Active treatment

In this stage goals are identified and plans made and implemented. While abstinence is likely to be the ideal, many people will be unwilling or unable to achieve this. Health and social gains can be made by reducing the harms associated with use. Goals must be realistic and those of the service user. Ambitious goals (e.g. wanting a job) need to be broken down into smaller parts. Achieving small goals can be encouraging, build confidence and provide a platform upon which future change can be built. Not achieving can create a sense of failure and trigger a return to precontemplation or contemplation. Service users' suggestions about how to attain their goals should be elicited and consideration given to difficulties that may be encountered. Individuals and other services that can provide support should be identified. The person can then make an informed decision about which option(s) to pursue.

Strategies for cutting down or stopping use will be central. Some people can reduce use themselves, others need pharmacological interventions (e.g. detoxification, substitute prescribing). Advice from substance misuse services may enable alcohol/drug treatment to be delivered within a mental health service (in line with the integrated model) but some people will need to engage with specialist substance misuse services (parallel model).

Guidance on alcohol detoxification is provided by NICE (2010b, 2010c, 2011b). It includes criteria for inpatient and community detoxification (people with 'significant psychiatric co-morbidity' require inpatient detoxification), dosing regimens and thiamine prescribing (to prevent Wernicke-Korsakoff syndrome). Alcohol detoxification is achieved by prescribing a reducing regimen of a long-acting benzodiazepine (usually chlordiazepoxide) over about a week. Close monitoring is required because of the risks if the person drinks alcohol while taking benzodiazepines, and because of the severe complications that can be associated with withdrawal (e.g. seizures).

Detoxification from opiates is usually undertaken by prescribing methadone or buprenorphine (both opioids). Lofexidine may be considered in some cases. NICE has published guidance on opioid detoxification (NICE 2007a). Practical guidance on the clinical management of drug misuse and dependence is also available in DH England and the Devolved Administrations (2007).

Pharmacological interventions must be accompanied by psychosocial interventions (NICE 2007b). Attention needs to be given to behavioural, cognitive and lifestyle changes. These might include: learning new skills (e.g. social skills, vocational skills, coping with cravings, budgeting, drug refusal skills, relaxation techniques); structuring time (e.g. taking up a hobby, developing new social networks, going to college, becoming a volunteer); and addressing underlying issues (e.g. past sexual abuse, bereavement issues). Mutual aid/self-help groups, such as Alcoholics Anonymous, Narcotic Anonymous, Dual Recovery Anonymous and SMART Recovery (Self-management and Recovery Training) can be useful adjuncts to treatment (all have websites). Information about these should be offered to all service users.

Relapse prevention

Once use has been reduced or abstinence achieved, interventions should address preventing relapse. Substance misuse and mental illness relapse are often interrelated.

An approach for preventing and managing substance misuse relapse has been developed by Marlatt and his colleagues (Marlatt and Gordon 1985; Marlatt and Donovan 2005). A cognitive behavioural framework is used to identify high-risk situations and triggers for use, and the development of strategies for coping with them. Effective coping enhances the person's sense of self-control. If substance use does occur this is seen as a lapse or 'slip-up' that can be overcome, and from which learning can take place. In terms of Prochaska and DiClemente's (1986) model, the person returns to active treatment rather than precontemplation, or contemplation. This perspective contrasts with the sense of failure and hopelessness which can be engendered if drinking or using drugs is seen as a relapse, putting the person 'back to square one'.

Situations/triggers for relapse will be varied and include: negative emotional states (e.g. anger, anxiety, depression, boredom); positive emotional states (e.g. celebrations); interpersonal conflicts (e.g. with partner, family members, employer); social pressures (e.g. at a party); and associations with particular places, people, times/dates or situations. Diaries, decision matrices and reflecting on a typical day can help to identify triggers. Exploring the chain of events which led to past (re)lapses can also highlight triggers as well as points at which the person could have acted differently. Strategies for managing relapse risks will require new coping skills and lifestyle changes. Like all new skills they will require practice.

Family and friends can be a source of support. For example, inviting the person to a social outing to help structure their time, being available to provide a listening ear at times of low mood or craving, or giving the person a lift to an Alcoholics Anonymous meeting.

Planning to prevent psychiatric relapse is also essential. A process for identifying a 'relapse signature', the pattern of early warning signs likely to indicate impending relapse, and development of a 'relapse drill', the coping strategies to manage emergence of these indicators, has been described by Birchwood *et al.* (2000). Use of substances may be part of a person's relapse signature. Together the approaches of Marlatt and Birchwood provide a comprehensive approach to relapse prevention in people with a dual diagnosis.

Ongoing pharmacological management of psychiatric symptoms is important for preventing substance misuse relapse as substances may be used to manage symptoms. Pharmacological interventions can also play a direct part in preventing substance misuse relapse. People with opiate problems may find naltrexone helpful as it blocks the effects of opiates (NICE 2007c). Acamprosate or naltrexone may be beneficial for problem drinkers as they can reduce craving (NICE 2011b). Disulfiram (antabuse) acts as a deterrent to drinking as adverse consequences follow if alcohol is consumed (NICE 2011b).

Families and carers

Carers and family members can be important partners in supporting the person's recovery. They may contribute information to the assessment, as well as playing a role in helping the person make and sustain change. The mental health team needs to negotiate with the service user and his or her carer/family confidentiality and information sharing agreements.

Carers and family members also have needs which nurses have a role in addressing. They often bear the brunt of the distress and difficult behaviour of the person with a dual diagnosis – for example, being the victim of aggression, being coerced into handing over money for substances. Carers may also feel frustrated with services – for example, because they think their relative is being 'bounced' between mental health and substance misuse services; because they feel excluded from decisions when the service user does not consent to information being shared with them.

Although usually keen to support their relative, carer and family behaviour can have a negative impact. Arguing can increase resistance and service users' distress and may contribute to relapse. Enabling behaviours such as buying drink or drugs for the person and helping them pay bills can inhibit change. Developing an approach consistent with the stages of change model and motivational interviewing style can enable family members to be more effective in helping their relative (Barrowclough *et al.* 2001).

Carers and family members need information. Even if service users do not consent to their involvement in treatment, information can be provided, for example, about substances, their effects and complications, mental illnesses and their signs and symptoms, the impact of substance use on mental illness, the nature of care and treatment, and what to do and who to contact in a crisis. Information about family and carer support groups, such as Al-Anon, Al-Ateen and Families Anonymous should be offered.

Case Study

Leroy

Having been re-commenced on olanzapine, Leroy's mental state settled. His key nurse took a collaborative approach to working with him and made it clear that decisions about his use of alcohol and drugs were his. She used the decision matrix framework to explore with Leroy the good and not so good things about each of the substances he was taking (see Figure 39.5 for alcohol) and offered him verbal and written information about alcohol, cannabis and crack, and their potential effects on physical and mental health, drawing on his recent experiences to highlight some of the risks. Leroy acknowledged that, at times, he had been spending more than he could afford and his use had created arguments with his parents and sister, who had stopped him visiting because she did not want him near her children when he was intoxicated. He felt guilty about the money he owed to his parents and was worried that he had started building up debts to a drug dealer. The abnormal liver function tests were a shock and, although alcohol helped to numb the pain he felt from the loss of his grandmother he decided that he should set some limits to his use once he was discharged.

Leroy had always maintained that his substance use did not affect his mental health, however, following work on a time line that looked back at his mental health and substance use, he noted that it did appear that when his crack use escalated his mental health deteriorated, and that when his drinking and drug using were high he was more likely to stop taking his medication and this resulted in a relapse in his mental health and hospital admissions.

He decided that he would try to stop using crack and would cut down on drinking so that it was more 'social'. He found it difficult to identify a specific target but did think he would try and have at least two days each week when he was abstinent. Leroy was adamant that he did not want to stop using cannabis but did think he would try to cut that down too.

The nurse offered Leroy information about local substance misuse services but he wasn't interested in accessing them. His care coordinator visited him on the ward, and agreed that, following discharge, she would work with him to attain his goals.

Some of the things he thought may be useful in helping him to do this included: spending time away from his crack using friends; resuming the music group; starting a football group – he thought getting fit would be an additional incentive to reducing use; arranging to visit his sister and her children every week; drinking lower strength lager; and talking through his feelings about the loss of his grandmother with his parents and care coordinator. He agreed to try to keep a drink and drug diary to monitor his use.

Information was offered to Leroy's family on the support groups available for the family and friends of alcohol and drug users (Al-Anon, Families Anonymous) and his mother decided she would contact them. Leroy's family and care coordinator attended his discharge CPA meeting so that they could all be involved in planning how they could best support him on discharge.

39.6 Conclusion

This chapter has provided an overview of the assessment, care and treatment of people with co-morbid mental health and substance misuse problems. In summary, the main points of learning are:

- Substance misuse is common in people with mental health problems and all mental health professionals need knowledge and skills in this area.
- Dual diagnosis is a broad concept which encompasses a wide range of people with varying types and levels of mental illness and substance use.

- The relationship between mental illness and substance misuse is complex.
- Physical, psychiatric, interpersonal, social and legal complications can be associated with substance misuse.
- A variety of risks are associated with dual diagnosis.
- Assessment of substance use should be integral to mental health assessment.
- An integration of mental health and substance misuse interventions is needed for working with people with a dual diagnosis.
- A client's readiness to change should guide treatment interventions.

- Working with people with a dual diagnosis requires optimism, flexibility and a long-term perspective.
- The needs of families and carers require attention.

- The various services in contact with people with a dual diagnosis need to work collaboratively so that the person's experience is of seamless care provision.

Feedback to Thinking Space 39.2

1. Leroy would be located in the top right quadrant. He has a severe mental illness (schizophrenia) and is using alcohol and drugs most days of the week, suggesting that he has a severe substance misuse problem too. The mental health team should lead/coordinate care using the CPA. As Leroy does not think his substance use causes him any problems the mental health team must address needs associated with both his mental health and substance misuse. To support them in this they may seek advice from the substance misuse team. If, in the future, Leroy recognizes that his use is problematic and he could benefit from the interventions provided by the substance misuse team, it would be appropriate to make a referral. The mental health team would continue to lead/coordinate care under the CPA.

2. Sandra would be located in the top-left quadrant. She has a severe drug problem (dependent on heroin for many years) and a 'low' severity mental illness (low mood and anxiety). The substance misuse team should lead/coordinate care and ensure that both her substance misuse and mental health needs are addressed. Some substance misuse teams have psychologists that can deliver interventions for depression and anxiety. For those that do not, access for such treatment should be negotiated through primary care and would probably involve IAPT (Increasing Access to Psychological Therapies) services. A positive practice guide on working with drug and alcohol users has been produced for IAPT services (www.iapt.nhs.uk/silo/files/iaptdrugandalcoholpositivepracticeguide.pdf).

3. Ahmed would be located in the bottom-right quadrant. He has a severe mental illness (bipolar disorder) and although his drinking can impact on his mental state his use is not regular ('sometimes binges on alcohol'). His substance misuse is therefore not severe. The mental health team should lead/coordinate care using the CPA and address needs associated with both his mental health and substance misuse. They may want to seek advice from the substance misuse team.

4. Tony would be located in the bottom-left quadrant. Neither his mental health nor substance use are severe. It is unlikely that he would access any services in relation to his mental health or substance use. If he happened to see his general practitioner (GP) for other health issues his use and its consequences may be identified as part of an assessment. The GP may then offer him information about the possible consequences of his use on his health.

Feedback to Thinking Space 39.3

Interventions to promote safe alcohol detoxification

- Ensure chlordiazepoxide administered in line with detoxification regime
- Regular observations/monitoring of withdrawal symptoms

- Encourage fluids and diet when Leroy feels able to eat
- Offer space to discuss how he is feeling
- No baths or unescorted leave due to risk of withdrawal seizures

Opportunities to discuss substance use and effects

- Take a collaborative approach recognizing that Leroy needs to make his own decisions about future use
- Explore Leroy's perceptions of the good and not so good things about his use (using a decision matrix – see Figure 39.5)
- Offer him verbal and written information about alcohol, cannabis and crack and their possible effects on physical and mental health – also make him aware of websites that have further information
- Encourage him to attend any ward-based groups that may provide opportunities for him to reflect further on his use
- Work with Leroy to construct a time line to explore the relationship between his substance use and mental health

Strategies to promote abstinence on the ward

- Remind Leroy about the prohibition of alcohol and drug use on the ward
- Discuss with him strategies to help cope with cravings
- Ensure that he has opportunities to engage in ward-based activities (so that he is not bored)
- Once he has leave, plan this with him, including how he might manage any opportunities for drinking and using drugs – if use on leave appears inevitable, negotiate limits on this so that he does not return to the ward intoxicated
- As Leroy had used drugs on the ward in the past, make him aware that: he, and his room, may be searched if there is suspicion of use; drug detection dogs are used to search the ward from time to time; he will be searched on return from leave; a request to provide urine for drug screening or be breathalysed may be made at any time

Annotated bibliography

Turning Point/Rethink (2004) *Dual Diagnosis Toolkit*. **London: Rethink and Turning Point.**
This is an introductory text for working with people with a dual diagnosis. It can be downloaded from www.rethink.org/dualdiagnosis/toolkit.html.

Graham, H.L., Copello, A., Birchwood, M.J. and Mueser, K.T. (2003) *Substance Misuse in Psychosis: Approaches to treatment and service delivery*. **Chichester: Wiley.**
This volume is useful for those wanting a more in-depth understanding of dual diagnosis.

Graham, H.L. (2004) *Cognitive-Behavioural Integrated Treatment (C-BIT): A treatment manual for substance misuse in people with severe mental health problems*. **Chichester: Wiley.**
This manual provides a framework for delivering integrated treatment to people with severe mental illness and substance misuse problems. Guidance on how to deliver interventions appropriate to the person's stage of change is provided and case material included for illustration.

National Collaborating Centre for Mental Health (2011) *Psychosis with Co-existing Substance Misuse: The NICE guideline on assessment and management in adults and young people (National Clinical Guideline 120).* **Leicester/London: The British Psychological Society and The Royal College of Psychiatrists, available at: www.nice. org.uk/nicemedia/live/13414/53691/53691.pdf.**
This full version of the NICE guideline is a publication to dip into rather than read from start to finish. The 'Experiences of Care' chapter provides illuminating service user and carer accounts. The rigorous processes undertaken to develop the guidance are explained, summaries of the studies considered are provided and the recommendations identified.

Useful websites

www.talktofrank.com
www.drugscope.org.uk
www.alcohollearningcentre.org.uk
www.drugscience.org.uk
www.dualdiagnosis.co.uk

References

Babor, T., de la Fuente, J., Saunders, J. and Grant, M. (1989) *AUDIT, The Alcohol Use Disorders Identification Test: Guidelines for use in primary care.* Geneva: World Health Organization.
Barrowclough, C., Haddock, G., Tarrier, N. *et al.* (2001) Randomised control trial of motivational interviewing, cognitive behaviour therapy, and family interventions for patients with co-morbid schizophrenia and substance use disorders, *American Journal of Psychiatry,* 158 (10): 1706–13.
Bien, T.H., Miller, W.R. and Tonigan, J.S. (1993) Brief interventions for alcohol problems: a review, *Addiction,* 88(3): 315–35.
Birchwood, M., Spencer, E. and McGovern, D. (2000) Schizophrenia: early warning signs, *Advances in Psychiatric Treatment,* 6: 93–101.
Crome, I. (1999) Substance misuse and psychiatric co-morbidity: towards improved service provision, *Drugs: Education, Prevention and Policy,* 6: 151–74.
DH (Department of Health) (2002) *Mental Health Policy Implementation Guide: Dual diagnosis good practice guide.* London: DH.
DH (Department of Health) (2006) *From Values to Action: The Chief Nursing Officer's review of mental health nursing.* London: DH.
DH (Department of Health) (2011) *A Summary of the Health Harms of Drugs.* London: DH.
DH (Department of Health) England and the Devolved Administrations (2007) *Drug Misuse and Dependence: UK guidelines on clinical management.* London: DH, the Scottish Government, Welsh Assembly Government and Northern Ireland Executive.
Hughes, L. (2006) *Closing The Gap: A capability framework for working effectively with combined mental health and substance use problems (dual diagnosis).* Lincoln: Mansfield Centre for Clinical and Workforce Innovation, University of Lincoln.
Marlatt, G.A. and Donovan, D.M. (2005) *Relapse Prevention: Maintenance strategies in the treatment of addictive behaviours,* 2nd edn. New York: Guilford Press.
Marlatt, G.A. and Gordon, J.R. (1985) *Relapse Prevention: Maintenance strategies in the treatment of addictive behaviours.* New York: Guilford Press.
Martino, S. and Moyers, T. (2008) Motivational interviewing with dually diagnosed patients, in H. Arkowitz, H.A. Weston, W.R. Miller and S. Rollnick (eds) *Motivational Interviewing in the Treatment of Psychological Problems.* New York: Guilford Press.
McHugo, G., Drake, R., Burton, H. and Akerson, T. (1995) A scale for assessing the stage of substance abuse treatment in persons with severe mental illness, *Journal of Nervous and Mental Disease,* 183: 762–7.
Mueser, K.T., Noordsy, D.L., Drake, R.E. and Fox, L. (2003) *Integrated Treatment for Dual Disorders: A guide to effective practice.* New York: Guilford Press.
NICE (National Institute for Health and Clinical Excellence) (2007a) *Clinical Guideline 52: Drug misuse – opiate detoxification.* London: NICE.
NICE (National Institute for Health and Clinical Excellence) (2007b) *Clinical Guideline 51: Drug misuse – psychosocial interventions.* London: NICE.
NICE (National Institute for Health and Clinical Excellence) (2007c) *Technology Appraisal 115: Naltrexone for the management of opioid dependence.* London: NICE.
NICE (National Institute for Health and Clinical Excellence) (2010a) *Public Health Guidance 24: Alcohol use disorders – preventing harmful drinking.* London: NICE.
NICE (National Institute for Health and Clinical Excellence) (2010b) *Alcohol Use Disorders: Sample chlordiazepoxide dosing regimens for use in managing alcohol withdrawal.* London: NICE.
NICE (National Institute for Health and Clinical Excellence) (2010c) *Clinical Guideline 100: Alcohol use disorders: diagnosis and clinical management of alcohol-related physical complications.* London: NICE.

NICE (National Institute for Health and Clinical Excellence) (2011a) *Clinical Guideline 120: Psychosis with co-existing substance misuse*. London: NICE.

NICE (National Institute for Health and Clinical Excellence) (2011b) *Clinical Guideline 115: Alcohol use disorders – diagnosis, assessment and management of harmful drinking and alcohol dependence*. London: NICE.

Osher, F. and Kofoed, L. (1989) Treatment of patients with psychiatric and psychoactive substance abuse disorders, *Hospital and Community Psychiatry*, 40: 1025–30.

Prochaska, J. and DiClemente, C. (1986) Towards a comprehensive model of change, in W. Miller and N. Heather (eds) *Treating Addictive Behaviours: Processes of Change*. New York: Plenum.

Raistrick, D., Bradshaw, J., Tober, G. *et al.* (1994) Development of the Leeds Dependency Questionnaire (LDQ): a questionnaire to measure alcohol and opiate dependence in the context of a treatment evaluation package, *Addiction*, 89: 563–72.

Rethink Dual Diagnosis Research Group (2004) *Living with severe mental health and substance use problems*. Kingston-upon. Thames, UK Rethink.

Stockwell, T., Murphy, D. and Hodgson, R. (1983) The Severity of Alcohol Dependence Questionnaire: its use, reliability and validity, *British Journal of Addiction*, 78: 145–55.

Sullivan, J., Sykora, K., Schneiderman, J. *et al.* (1989) Assessment of alcohol withdrawal: the revised Clinical Institute Withdrawal Assessment for Alcohol Scale (CIWA-Ar), *British Journal of Addiction*, 84: 1353–7.

UK Harm Reduction Alliance (2007) www.ukhra.org.harm_reduction_definition.html.

Chapter 40

The Person with a Personality Disorder

Ian P.S. Noonan

When I was diagnosed [with borderline personality disorder], I felt a sense of relief. Now I could understand my symptoms. It felt like a weight had been lifted. I was offered treatment on [a] dialectical behaviour therapy (DBT) programme ... Although therapy helps, there is no cure for BPD (as I was told in writing by my psychiatrist) and this is something I will have to try and manage for the rest of my life.

Agata Cardoso

 ## 40.1 Introduction

Personality disorder is a powerful label that can evoke strong responses in clients, carers and clinicians. There are myths and misunderstandings about what the diagnosis means, what may lead to and maintain personality disorders and, importantly, what can treat and help someone live with a personality disorder. This chapter aims to address and dispel some of those myths by considering the impact of a personality disorder on the life of the person with the diagnosis, their carers and significant others and the mental health practitioners involved in providing their care.

Personality disorders are relatively common, but not all people with a personality disorder will come into contact with mental health services. According to the Office for National Statistics (ONS), 5.4 per cent of men and 3.4 per cent of women living at home have a personality disorder (Singleton *et al.* 2002). The numbers vary according to the type of personality disorder (more men are diagnosed with antisocial personality disorder and more women with borderline personality disorder), and the setting. Moran *et al.* (2000) report that 24 per cent of people attending primary care services have a personality disorder meeting the diagnostic criteria of DSM-IV (APA 2000), and in their systematic review Fazel and Danesh (2002) found that 65 per cent of male and 42 per cent of female prisoners has a personality disorder. This chapter will focus predominantly on 'Cluster B' type personality disorders (including borderline and antisocial) as people with these types of personality disorder are more likely to come into contact with mental health services.

A model of personality disorder which considers the balance of the aspects of an individual's personality as disordered, rather than only the total aspect or the person themselves, will be used to challenge the historical idea that personality disorders are untreatable. The chapter will provide definitions and diagnostic criteria for personality disorder, an overview of the symptoms experienced by someone with this diagnosis and a model for assessment that considers how to assess personality as well as how to assess personality disorder. The National Institute for Health and Clinical Excellence (NICE) guidelines for antisocial (2009a) and borderline (2009b) personality disorder will be used to highlight recommended nursing interventions in both general and specialist mental health settings.

The chapter covers:

- what is a personality disorder?
- diagnosis and clustering;
- aetiology of personality disorders;
- treatment and nursing care.

40.2 What is a personality disorder?

Traditionally psychiatric textbooks have regarded personality as something that is fixed by mid-adolescence and which remains the same in a wide range of different circumstances. However, if we accept that personality is fixed, it could lead us to the wrong assumption that personality disorder is fixed and therefore untreatable.

MIND offers a more flexible definition of personality:

The word 'personality' refers to the pattern of thoughts, feelings and behaviour that makes each of us the individuals that we are. Generally speaking, personality doesn't change very much, but it does develop as we go through different experiences in life, and as our circumstances change. We mature with time, and our thinking, feelings and behaviour all change depending on our circumstances. We are usually flexible enough to learn from past experiences and to change our behaviour to cope with life more effectively.

(Mind 2012)

This definition explicitly values individuality and suggests that differences in personality are a positive thing. While acknowledging that these patterns of response do not change very much, it suggests that we have the potential to learn and develop, to change and adapt. This adaptation is particularly difficult for people with personality disorder – they have to work much harder to achieve it, but it is our first indicator as to what we, as mental health nurses, should be helping our clients with: their ability to recognize experience, learn, change and try out alternative ways of thinking, feeling and behaving in various circumstances.

The nomenclature used to describe different types of personality disorder is complex: there are two main diagnostic guides and each uses slightly different terms. According to DSM-IV (APA 2000) a personality disorder is: 'An enduring pattern of inner experience and behaviour that deviates markedly from the expectations of the individual's culture, is pervasive and inflexible, has an onset in adolescence or early adulthood, is stable over time, and leads to distress or impairment'. The *International Statistical Classification of Diseases and Related Health Problems* (ICD-10) (WHO 2010) describes it as: 'a severe disturbance in the characterological condition and behavioural tendencies of the individual, usually

---

Thinking Space 40.1

Think about how you would describe the different aspects of your personality. To do this you might like to list your:

- character
- attitudes and beliefs

- relationships
- leisure activities
- prevailing mood
- habits

If you identify an aspect of one domain of your personality that could be viewed as a problem, think how this is balanced by other aspects.

Feedback to Thinking Space 40.1

For example, someone who has an anxious prevailing mood might manage this by the habit of planning things in advance, have a fairly shy character, enjoy routines and have a relatively low-risk lifestyle. We are able to balance the various aspects of our personalities as we have learned what we can tolerate, what overwhelms us and what we need to do to mediate our responses to our experiences. One way to understand the experience of a person with a personality disorder is to imagine what it would be like if we couldn't balance that anxious mood – if that were the aspect of ourselves that dominated every interaction and experience. How then might your behaviour and character appear to someone else?

involving several areas of the personality, and nearly always associated with considerable personal and social disruption'.

40.3 Diagnosis and clustering of personality disorders

There are many types of personality disorder which are labelled differently in the two diagnostic manuals. The symptoms and experiences that make up different types of personality disorder overlap to some degree, so a cluster system is used. Figure 40.1

shows the division of types according to the three clusters: odd or eccentric; dramatic, emotional or erratic; anxious or fearful.

The treatment section below will focus on Cluster B type personality disorders, as people in this group make the most use of mental health services.

Cluster A

Cluster A includes a range of thoughts and behaviours that might make someone appear eccentric. People with a paranoid personality disorder may

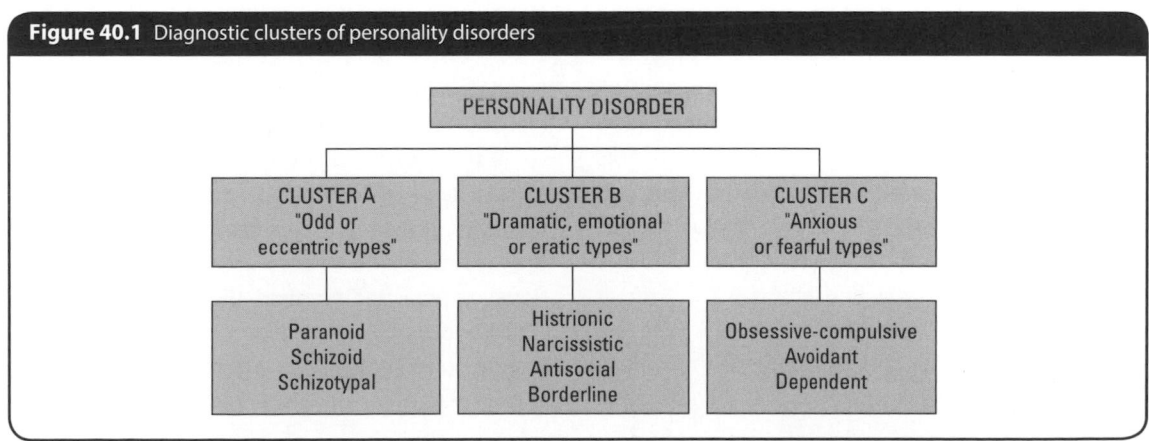

Figure 40.1 Diagnostic clusters of personality disorders

PERSONALITY DISORDER

CLUSTER A "Odd or eccentric types"	CLUSTER B "Dramatic, emotional or eratic types"	CLUSTER C "Anxious or fearful types"
Paranoid Schizoid Schizotypal	Histrionic Narcissistic Antisocial Borderline	Obsessive-compulsive Avoidant Dependent

appear suspicious, sensitive, mistrustful, argumentative, stubborn and self-important. The schizoid personality disorder diagnosis is used to describe someone who is emotionally cold, detached, aloof, humourless and introspective; and the term 'schizotypal' is used for people who are socially anxious, have an inability to make close friends, display eccentric behaviour, oddities of speech and an inappropriate affect, and experience ideas of reference and unusual perceptual experiences.

People with these types of personality disorder may not come in to contact with mental health services. However, typically, after a loss event – such as the loss of a home or threatened eviction – someone with a schizotypal personality disorder may come to the attention of their general practitioner (GP) or other primary care services. Their eccentric lifestyle, 'magical' thinking and unusual behaviour will raise concern and the person may be admitted for assessment. On admission their symptoms may be mistaken for schizophrenia. But, someone with schizotypal personality disorder will not be upset or concerned by their inability to make friends or maintain relationships – they will want to be alone and usually will not be troubled by their unusual vocal tics, neologisms or mannerisms, and preoccupied thoughts and behaviours. If anything, these seem to be comforting and the disruption to their usual routine caused by the admission and the invasion of privacy caused by the questions in our assessments will cause the most distress.

It is unlikely that someone with a Cluster A type personality disorder will want to accept treatment. Moreover, there is insufficient evidence to support any particular intervention. Supportive psychotherapy and social skills training may be helpful and the person may benefit from antipsychotic medication in an acute phase or crisis, but the disorder is chronic and enduring in its nature. The individual therapeutic relationship will be key to any psychological and social support offered. Someone with this type of personality disorder will find group work difficult and unhelpful. Hayward (2007) suggests that the nursing profession has yet to engage with working with this client group and argues that the empathic interpersonal communication skills on which we normally rely may not serve clients who do not respond appropriately to affective cues. He suggests maintaining a 'therapeutic distance' to enable the client to discover the value of the therapeutic relationship on their own terms rather than attempting to use it to challenge the client's point of view.

Cluster C

Avoidant personality disorder is characterized by social inhibition, feelings of inadequacy, extreme sensitivity to negative evaluation and avoidance of social interaction. It may at first appear that this is the opposite of a dependent personality disorder where someone has a pervasive psychological dependence on other people. Obsessive compulsive personality disorder (not the same as obsessive compulsive disorder) is characterized by rigid conformity to rules, moral codes and excessive orderliness.

People with Cluster C personality disorders recognize that there is a problem and may actively seek out help because of their anxious and fearful patterns of behaviour, the impact on their intrapersonal well-being and interpersonal relationships, and the state of depression, fear and panic that this leaves them in.

There may be people with undiagnosed Cluster C personality disorders attending primary care and community mental health teams (CMHTs) for repeated short-term treatments of their anxiety and low mood. Short-term psychotherapeutic interventions such as self-help, brief solution-focused therapy and cognitive behavioural therapy (CBT) are less likely to be effective with this group than longer-term treatments because of difficulties maintaining treatment effect. Eskedel and Demetri (2006) conclude that these 'defects in self-maintenance are reflected in the inability to self-soothe, experience self as real, develop self-esteem, and experience a sense of personal identity'. Psychodynamic and cognitive psychotherapies, delivered individually or in groups, have the greatest clinical effect with adaptations to traditional approaches required (Eskedel and Demetri 2006) and significant changes in symptom distress, interpersonal problems and personality functioning at two-year follow-up (Svartberg et al. 2004).

Cluster B

People with Cluster B personality disorders, particularly those with borderline type, are likely to have regular contact with health, social and criminal justice services, particularly when experiencing crises. This group includes the histrionic, narcissistic, borderline and antisocial personality disorders.

Someone with a histrionic personality disorder may appear to be outwardly confident, lively, sociable and emotionally responsive. However they may also be vain and self-centred, have short-lived enthusiasms, be acting a part, be self-deceiving and may demonstrate unrestrained emotional display. The term 'narcissistic personality disorder' is used to diagnose someone with a grandiose sense of self-importance, who may be preoccupied with fantasies of unlimited success, power and intellectual brilliance. Narcissists crave attention from others but are not warm towards other people; they exploit others without returning the favour and there is a very strong overlap with histrionic, borderline and antisocial personality disorders.

Borderline personality disorder

The DSM-IV(TR) (APA 2000) diagnostic criteria for borderline personality disorder cite a series of symptoms evident from early adulthood. When considering the criteria for frantic efforts to avoid real or imagined abandonment, and impulsivity in at least two self-damaging areas, suicidal behaviour should not be included as that is assessed as a separate criterion. Borderline personality disorder is:

A pervasive pattern of instability of interpersonal relationships, self-image and affects, as well as marked impulsivity, beginning by early adulthood and present in a variety of contexts, as indicated by five (or more) of the following:

■ Frantic efforts to avoid real or imagined abandonment.

■ A pattern of unstable and intense interpersonal relationships characterized by alternating between extremes of idealization and devaluation.

■ Identity disturbance: markedly and persistently unstable self-image or sense of self.

■ Impulsivity in at least two areas that are potentially self-damaging (e.g., promiscuous sex, excessive spending, eating disorders, binge eating, substance abuse, reckless driving).

■ Recurrent suicidal behaviour, gestures, threats or self-injuring behaviour such as cutting, interfering with the healing of scars or picking at oneself (excoriation).

■ Affective instability due to a marked reactivity of mood (e.g., intense episodic dysphoria, irritability or anxiety usually lasting a few hours and only rarely more than a few days).

■ Chronic feelings of emptiness.

■ Inappropriate anger or difficulty controlling anger (e.g., frequent displays of temper, constant anger, recurrent physical fights).

■ Transient, stress-related paranoid ideation, delusions or severe dissociative symptoms.

(APA 2000)

This list spells out the criteria, but it may lead to a better understanding of the experience of someone with a borderline personality disorder to use a model proposed by Moskovitz (2001) who groups the symptoms of borderline personality disorder into the four overlapping categories of disturbance experienced by the client: disturbed identity, perception, behaviour and mood (see Figure 40.2).

1. **Disturbed identity:**
   ● Self-image or sense of self persistently and markedly disturbed, distorted or unstable; chronic feelings of emptiness, frantic efforts to avoid real or imagined abandonment.

2. **Disturbed perception:**
   ● Transient, stress-related paranoid ideation, or severe dissociative symptoms.

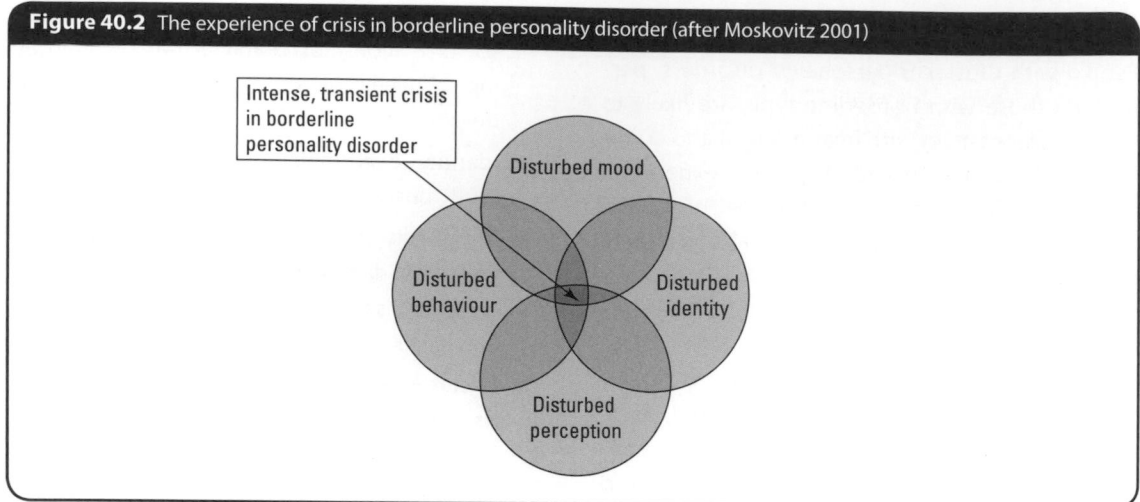

Figure 40.2 The experience of crisis in borderline personality disorder (after Moskovitz 2001)

3. **Disturbed behaviour:**

- Impulsiveness in at least two areas that are potentially self-damaging; spending, sex, substance-abuse, reckless driving, and binge eating.

- Recurrent suicidal behaviour, gestures, or threats, and/or self-harming behaviour.

4. **Disturbed mood:**

- Affective instability due to a marked reactivity of mood.

- Intense, episodic dysphoria, irritability or anxiety, usually lasting a few hours and only rarely more than a few days.

- A pattern of unstable and intense interpersonal relationships characterized by alternating between extremes of idealization and devaluation.

- Inappropriate, intense anger or lack of control of anger; frequent displays of temper, constant anger, recurrent physical fights.

Thinking Space 40.2

Review the following case study and identify how Judy experiences disturbed mood, identity, perception and behaviour.

Case Study

Judy

Judy is a member of a support group for people who self-harm. She is 24 years old and has a diagnosis of borderline personality disorder, which was made four years ago after a series of crisis admissions to an acute mental health ward. Judy has been able to reflect on both her views of her illness and what happens during a crisis. Here are three brief extracts from some autobiography work carried out in the group. She has given her permission for her story to be used and her name and other identifying details have been changed to protect her identity.

At university (aged 19)

'At university, things just fell apart. It was like one disaster after another. On one occasion, I couldn't log on to my college email and I thought, "That's it, I've been thrown off the course." I started to think what a fool I had been to even think that I could do it. For a split second I knew what was happening as what started as a thought then became something I could hear, inside my head: a voice telling me I was an idiot, that they only let me in because they felt sorry for me, that I was an embarrassment. I felt over- whelmingly angry and panicked, I figured, they couldn't throw me off the course if I was dead – I would show them all. I remembered that my lecturers and other students looked at me in funny ways in class and wondered if they wanted me dead, but just didn't care. I drank a half bottle of vodka, took some paracetamol and feminax [naproxen] and slit my wrist. It was as if, in a split second, every- thing had come to an end: I wanted to die, to stop feeling, to shut off the rushing sounds in my head, for someone to know how much I hurt and yet for no one to know. It is like feeling everything at once. I felt strong and decisive and then terrified and embarrassed. I called the ambulance, but people assume that shows I didn't mean it: as if I could mean anything when I feel like that.'

Now (aged 24)

'When I told Jack I was pregnant, I knew he would leave. He thought I only got pregnant to make him stay. I felt everything all at once; that I hated him, loved him, wanted him, wanted to kill him, wanted to kill myself. I thought if I got an abortion he would stay because it would prove that I wasn't trying to trap him, then I thought, if I killed myself, he would be free forever. I'm not sure if I really believed any of this, but I just couldn't slow my thoughts down enough to work out what I felt, what I wanted, or even who I was. I knew that if I cut myself, I would feel calm, and my breasts were feeling like they didn't belong to me. I cut them and watched the blood flow down across my belly and thought – well at least that is real.'

Thinking Space 40.3

Judy gives clear accounts here of some key moments relating to her self-harm. In the group, the purpose of writing autobiographical accounts is to slow participants' thoughts down enough for them to be able to discuss them and consider whether there were alternative options. Referring back to Moskovitz's (2001) model above, identify examples of Judy's disturbed mood, behaviour, perception and think when she might have been able to choose a different behaviour from her self-harm to manage these intense feelings, thoughts and perceptions.

Antiscial personality disorder

Antisocial personality disorder (DSM-IV(TR)) or disso- cial personality disorder (ICD-10) is a type of person- ality disorder that used to be referred to as 'psychopa- thy' or 'sociopathy' and which includes a marked 'dis- regard for' and 'violation of' the rights of others. Paris (2003) suggests that although diagnosis is not usually made until early adulthood, there is a strong correla- tion between conduct disorders in childhood and antisocial personality disorder in adulthood.

The NICE guidelines describe antisocial personality disorder as a combination of:

impulsivity, high negative emotionality, low conscientiousness and associated behaviours including irresponsible and exploitative behaviour, recklessness and deceitfulness. This is manifest in unstable interpersonal relationships, disregard for the consequences of one's behaviour, a failure to learn from experience, egocentricity and a disregard for the feelings of others. The condition is associated with a wide range of interpersonal and social disturbance.

(NICE 2009a)

The lack of regard for others may mean that someone with antisocial personality disorder is unlikely to see the need for treatment. However, the MIND (2012) definition cited above reminds us of the impact on carers and family and we may have an extended role in supporting them. Table 40.1 summarizes the diagnostic criteria in DSM-IV(TR) and ICD-10.

 ## 40.4 Aetiology of personality disorders

The causes of personality disorder are complex: there is no one thing that results in personality disorder; rather it seems to be a combination of predisposing factors that put someone at risk, and experiences that decrease their resilience to these risk factors. There are also different theories exploring the biological and environmental factors that variously contribute to the development of different types of personality disorder.

Krawitz and Watson (2003) identify the following possible causes:

Table 40.1 Diagnostic criteria for antisocial and dissocial personality disorders

Antisocial personality disorder (DSM-IV(TR))	Dissocial personality disorder (ICD10)
There is a pervasive pattern of disregard for and violation of the rights of others occurring since age 15 years, as indicated by three or more of the following: ■ Failure to conform to social norms with respect to lawful behaviours as indicated by repeatedly performing acts that are grounds for arrest ■ Deception, as indicated by repeatedly lying, use of aliases or conning others for personal profit or pleasure ■ Impulsiveness or failure to plan ahead ■ Irritability and aggressiveness, as indicated by repeated physical fights or assaults ■ Reckless disregard for safety of self or others ■ Consistent irresponsibility, as indicated by repeated failure to sustain consistent work behaviour or honour financial obligations ■ Lack of remorse, as indicated by being indifferent to or rationalizing having hurt, mistreated or stolen from another ■ The individual is at least age 18 years ■ There is evidence of conduct disorder with onset before age 15 years ■ The occurrence of antisocial behaviour is not exclusively during the course of schizophrenia or a manic episode	At least three of the following: ■ Callous unconcern for the feelings of others ■ Gross and persistent attitude of irresponsibility and disregard for social norms, rules, and obligations ■ Incapacity to maintain enduring relationships, though having no difficulty in establishing them ■ Very low tolerance to frustration and a low threshold for discharge of aggression, including violence ■ Incapacity to experience guilt or to profit from experience, particularly punishment ■ Markedly prone to blame others or to offer plausible rationalizations for the behaviour that has brought the person into conflict with society ■ Persistent irritability may also be a feature of the condition

- childhood experience of physical abuse, sexual abuse, neglect or trauma;
- decreased serotonin activity linked with impulsivity, irritability, anger, low mood and suicidality;
- dysregulation of the noradrenergic system response to stress;
- increased incidence of brain trauma, childhood attention deficit and hyperactivity disorder, neurocognitive impairment and learning disability;
- temperament characterized by high emotional pain, impulsivity and limited affect regulation;
- genetics.

However, the evidence to support any one theory is equivocal. There are people, for example, with no history of abuse who develop personality disorders, and survivors of abuse who do not go on to develop a personality disorder. One way to conceptualize the aetiology of personality disorders as a whole is to consider the interaction of predisposing and resilience-decreasing factors over time.

Genetic, neurotransmitter and neurocognitive predisposing factors combine with environmental factors which decrease an individual's resilience. These influence, and to some degree reinforce, each other, in turn leading to schema that risk forming personality disorders in adolescence. Diagnosis then occurs in adulthood when the impact of these schemas on relationships, work, housing, health, etc. leads to referral to or contact with services. The aetiology of personality disorders is illustrated in Figure 40.3.

Thinking Space 40.4

Review Judy's autobiographical writing exercise above and answer the following questions:

1. What predisposing and resilience decreasing factors can you identify?
2. What schemata has she formed, or how does she view herself in the world?
3. What impact is her self-harm likely to have on her referral to/contact with services now?

40.5 Treatment and nursing care

This section outlines treatment recommendations from the NICE guidelines for antisocial borderline and personality disorder (NICE 2009a, 2009b) and evidence for other types of treatment and the service characteristics required to optimize treatment efficacy. Nursing care should not be seen as something that is separate from the overall treatment plan. A multi-disciplinary approach is required as well as team supervision for working with this client group.

Personality disorders are not untreatable. They require a combination of psychological treatments reinforced by drug therapy at critical times. According to Bateman and Tyrer (2002) the following principles should apply to all therapeutic approaches with this client group. Treatment needs to:

- be well structured;
- devote effort to achieving adherence;
- have a clear focus;
- be theoretically coherent to both therapist and patient;
- be relatively long-term;
- be well integrated with other services;
- have a clear treatment alliance (with the client, carers and all agencies involved).

These principles usually underpin specialist mental health services for personality disorder such as therapeutic communities, CBT and cognitive-analytic therapy (CAT), dialectical behaviour therapy (DBT),

Figure 40.3 The aetiology of personality disorders (after Paris 2003; Krawitz and Watson 2003)

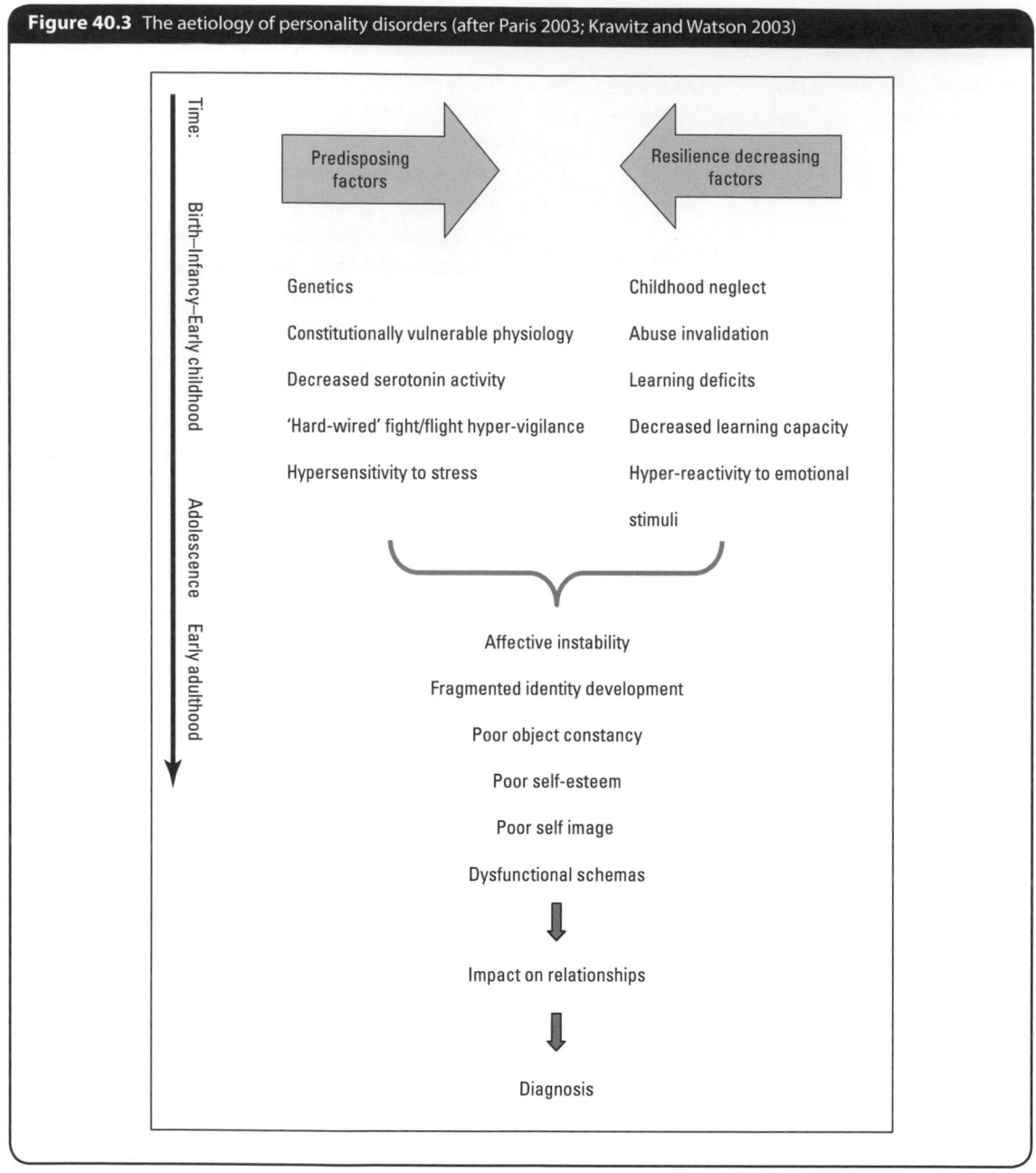

dynamic psychotherapy, sex offender treatment programmes and interventions to promote intentional awareness and reduce impulsivity such as thinking skills training, mentalization and mindfulness.

However, in reality people with personality disorders access care in a range of non-specialist services such as primary care, emergency departments, through social and criminal justice services, and in crisis admissions to acute mental health wards. The key to getting treatment right is to be clear about its goal. Is it to treat the underlying personality disorder or to manage the current crisis? The former requires evidence-based long-term psychotherapeutic treatment in specialist services, the latter employs core nursing skills with a tertiary health promoting approach – to prevent the crisis from worsening, manage risk and offer a positive engagement with a view to later referral for specialist treatment.

Borderline personality disorder

Core recommendations for the management and treatment of borderline personality disorder from NICE (2009b) are summarized in Box 40.1.

NICE guidelines emphasize that person-centred care must underpin the management and treatment of clients with borderline personality disorder, outlining the importance of good communication with the client and choice of their preferred treatment. This includes having written information about their treatment and, with their consent, making this available to their carers and relatives.

There are two significant areas where conflicts may occur in the management and treatment of borderline personality disorder. These relate to managing crises and inpatient care.

Box 40.1 Core recommendations for management and treatment of personality disorder (after NICE 2009b)

Access to services

- People with borderline personality disorder should not be excluded from any health or social care service because of their diagnosis or because they have self-harmed.

Autonomy and choice

- Work in partnership with people with borderline personality disorder to develop their autonomy and promote choice by:
  - ensuring they remain actively involved in finding solutions to their problems, including during crises
  - encouraging them to consider the different treatment options and life choices available to them, and the consequences of the choices they make.

Developing an optimistic and trusting relationship

- When working with people with borderline personality disorder:
  - explore treatment options in an atmosphere of hope and optimism, explaining that recovery is possible and attainable
  - build a trusting relationship, work in an open, engaging and non-judgemental manner, and be consistent and reliable
  - bear in mind when providing services that many people will have experienced rejection, abuse and trauma, and encountered stigma often associated with self-harm and borderline personality disorder.

Managing endings and transitions

- Anticipate that withdrawal and ending of treatments or services, and transition from one service to another, may evoke strong emotions and reactions in people with borderline personality disorder. Ensure that:

(Continued)

Box 40.1 Core recommendations for management and treatment of personality disorder (after NICE 2009b) *(Continued)*

- such changes are discussed carefully beforehand with the person (and their family or carers if appropriate) and are structured and phased

- the care plan supports effective collaboration with other care providers during endings and transitions, and includes the opportunity to access services in times of crisis

- when referring a person for assessment in other services (including for psychological treatment), they are supported during the referral period and arrangements for support are agreed beforehand with them.

Assessment

■ Community mental health services (CMHTs, related community-based services, and Tier 2/3 services in child and adolescent mental health services – CAMHS) should be responsible for the routine assessment, treatment and management of people with borderline personality disorder.

Care planning

■ Teams working with people with borderline personality disorder should develop comprehensive multi-disciplinary care plans in collaboration with the service user (and their family or carers, where agreed with the person). The care plan should:

- identify clearly the roles and responsibilities of all health and social care professionals involved

- identify manageable short-term treatment aims and specify steps that the person and others might take to achieve them

- identify long-term goals, including those relating to employment and occupation, that the person would like to achieve, which should underpin the overall long-term treatment strategy; these goals should be realistic, and linked to the short-term treatment aims

- develop a crisis plan that identifies potential triggers that could lead to a crisis, specifies self-management strategies likely to be effective and establishes how to access services (including a list of support numbers for out-of-hours teams and crisis teams) when self-management strategies alone are not enough

- be shared with the GP and the service user.

Psychological treatment

■ When providing psychological treatment for people with borderline personality disorder, especially those with multiple co-morbidities and/or severe impairment, the following service characteristics should be in place:

- an explicit and integrated theoretical approach used by both the treatment team and the therapist, which is shared with the service user

- structured care in accordance with this guideline

- provision for therapist supervision.

■ Although the frequency of psychotherapy sessions should be adapted to the person's needs and context of living, twice-weekly sessions may be considered.

Box 40.1 Core recommendations for management and treatment of personality disorder (after NICE 2009b) *(Continued)*

- Do not use brief psychotherapeutic interventions (of less than three months' duration) specifically for borderline personality disorder or for the individual symptoms of the disorder.

Drug treatment

- Drug treatment should not be used specifically for borderline personality disorder or for the individual symptoms or behaviour associated with the disorder (e.g. repeated self-harm, marked emotional instability, risk-taking behaviour and transient psychotic symptoms).
- Antipsychotic drugs should not be used for the medium- and long-term treatment of borderline personality disorder.
- Drug treatment may be considered in the overall treatment of co-morbid conditions.
- Short-term use of sedative medication may be considered cautiously as part of the overall treatment plan for people with borderline personality disorder in a crisis. The duration of treatment should be agreed with them, but should be no longer than one week.

The role of specialist personality disorder services within trusts

- Mental health trusts should develop multi-disciplinary specialist teams and/or services for people with personality disorders. These teams should have specific expertise in the diagnosis and management of borderline personality disorder and should:
  - provide assessment and treatment services for people with borderline personality disorder who have particularly complex needs and/or high levels of risk
  - provide consultation and advice to primary and secondary care services
  - offer a diagnostic service when general psychiatric services are in doubt about the diagnosis and/or management of the disorder
  - develop systems of communication and protocols for information-sharing among different services, including those in forensic settings, and collaborate with all relevant agencies within the local community including health, mental health and social services, the Criminal Justice System, CAMHS and relevant voluntary services
  - be able to provide and/or advise on social and psychological interventions, including access to peer support, and advise on the safe use of drug treatment in crises and for co-morbidities and insomnia
  - work with CAMHS to develop local protocols to govern arrangements for the transition of young people from CAMHS to adult services
  - ensure that clear lines of communication between primary and secondary care are established and maintained
  - support, lead and participate in the local and national development of treatments for people with borderline personality disorder, including multi-centre research.

Managing crises

Someone experiencing the acute disturbance of mood, perception, behaviour and identity that Moskovitz (2001) says characterizes a crisis in borderline personality disorder is likely to put nurses' communication and interpersonal skills to the test. Many of the recommendations in the NICE guidelines (NICE 2009b) are core client-centred communication skills that we use in many contexts:

- maintain a calm and non-threatening attitude;
- attempt to understand the client's point of view;
- explore their reason for distress;
- demonstrate active, empathic listening.

There are specific skills that relate to working with this client group. It is all too easy to diminish their reason for the crisis or to offer solutions before exploring what has happened and how the client feels about this. It is important to offer validating statements and encourage and stimulate reflection. Other options, which need to be realistic and achievable, should be considered before admitting the client to hospital. Short-term drug treatment may sometimes be helpful in managing crisis. Fagin (2004) considers the importance of pharmacological treatment for co-morbid psychiatric disorders but emphasizes the importance of explaining to the client that in terms of their personality disorder, medication has a modest role in their overall treatment. The NICE guidelines recommend considering the risk of abuse, dependency, interaction with illicit drugs and alcohol and the risk of overdose before agreeing, with the team involved, prescription of the minimum effective dose. Drugs such as sedative antihistamines, that have a low side-effect profile, may be used. Review and end dates must be included as part of the plan.

Follow-up after crisis should include both reduction and cessation (where appropriate) of medication, and a review, with the client, of the antecedents to the crisis. These should then be incorporated into the person's care and crisis plans for the future.

Inpatient care

The NICE guidelines are clear that emergency inpatient admission should be considered only when there is significant risk of harm to self or others which cannot be managed by a crisis resolution or home treatment team, or when someone is detained under the Mental Health Act 1983. If admission is required then health professionals must:

- ensure the decision is based on an explicit, joint understanding of the potential benefits and likely harm that may result from admission;
- agree the length and purpose of the admission in advance;
- ensure that when, in extreme circumstances, compulsory treatment is used, management on a voluntary basis is resumed at the earliest opportunity (NICE 2009b).

However, the guidelines are not clear about how someone should be nursed or treated during this crisis admission.

Crisis admission can be viewed negatively in some services. If someone has a transient, acute disturbance of mood, behaviour, identity and perception they may be admitted for crisis management of their risk of harm to themselves or others and to continue the assessment to distinguish between an acute functional psychotic illness and a chronic personality disorder. Within a day or two this assessment will be complete and the person will be discharged, possibly with further evidence to support the diagnosis of personality disorder. Unfortunately, this can be perceived as an 'inappropriate' admission, even though both goals, safety and assessment, have been achieved. The crisis admission may indeed have saved the person's life and identified that no further emergency treatment is required.

When working with someone with a borderline personality disorder in acute mental health services, nurses should consider the purpose of the admission: what would constitute a successful outcome? If unrealistic goals are set, the admission will be unsuccessful and the health professionals involved are likely to blame the client for the perceived failed or inappropriate admission, or blame other services such as emergency departments or community teams, for not managing the person in the community. This may lead to splitting teams and staff burnout.

Fagin (2004) recognizes the limitations of inpatient acute admission for people with borderline personality disorder but provides a useful overview of how to manage these if and when they occur. He argues that the multi-professional team on acute wards need the skills to manage this client group and outlines what the threshold for admission should be. His indicators for admission of patients with personality disorders are:

- crisis intervention, particularly to reduce risk of suicide or violence to others;
- co-morbid psychiatric disorder such as depression or a brief psychotic episode;
- chaotic behaviour endangering the patient and the treatment alliance;
- to stabilize existing medication regimens;
- review of the diagnosis and the treatment plan;
- full risk assessment;
- above all, the unit must have the capacity, in terms of skills, staffing and clinical pressures, to manage the admission.

These suggest a role for both planned as well as crisis admission and take into account the clinical team's ability to manage the admission successfully. Fagin also identifies the principles of management of patients with borderline personality disorder in inpatient units which are to:

- maintain flexibility;
- establish conditions to make the patient safe;
- tolerate intense anger, aggression and hate;
- promote reflection;
- set necessary limits;
- establish and maintain the therapeutic alliance;

- avoid splitting between psychotherapy and pharmacotherapy;
- avoid or understand splitting between different members of staff, either in hospital or in the community;
- monitor counter-transference feelings (Fagin 2004).

The NICE guidelines (2009b) recommend that if someone has two or more crisis admissions within a six-month period then a Care Programme Approach (CPA) review should be arranged to link together the involvement of primary, emergency, community and emergency services. Care is going to be complex for this client group so nurses need to be prepared for this complexity. This is not to suggest that acute inpatient services are the ideal place to treat people with borderline personality disorder, rather, that it is inevitable that they will use inpatient services and it is likely to be a more positive experience for clients and staff if it is viewed as an expected compromise rather than an inappropriate admission.

Antisocial personality disorder

The guidelines for treatment of people with antisocial personality disorder (NICE 2009a) contain many of the service level recommendations found in those for borderline personality disorder (NICE 2009b). The key priorities for implementation in addition to the borderline guidelines are summarized in Box 40.2.

The guidelines emphasize the importance of multi-agency risk assessment to include risk of offending, domestic violence and abuse, and of co-morbid drug and alcohol misuse. In general, acute crisis admission should be avoided and admission for co-morbid psychiatric illnesses should be to specialist forensic services. There are no pharmacological treatments recommended to manage the cognitive and behavioural aspects of antisocial personality disorder, and any treatment for co-morbid depression or anxiety should be in line with the treatment guidelines for those disorders (NICE 2009a).

Box 40.2 Guidelines for treatment of people with antisocial personality disorder in addition to those for borderline personality disorder (after NICE 2009a)

Cognitive behavioural interventions for children aged 8 years and older with conduct problems

- Cognitive problem-solving skills training should be considered for children aged 8 years and older with conduct problems if:
  - the child's family is unwilling or unable to engage with a parent training programme
  - additional factors, such as callous and unemotional traits in the child, may reduce the likelihood of the child benefiting from parent training programmes alone.

Assessment in specialist/forensic personality disorder services

- Health care professionals in forensic or specialist personality disorder services should consider, as part of a structured clinical assessment, routinely using:
  - a standardized measure of the severity of antisocial personality disorder such as the Psychopathy Checklist – Revised (PCL-R) or the Psychopathy Checklist – Screening Version (PCL-SV)
  - a formal assessment tool such as Historical, Clinical, Risk Management-20 (HCR-20) to develop a risk management strategy.

Treatment of co-morbid disorders

- People with antisocial personality disorder should be offered treatment for any co-morbid disorders in line with recommendations in the relevant NICE clinical guideline, where available. This should happen regardless of whether the person is receiving treatment for antisocial personality disorder.

Psychological interventions

- For people with antisocial personality disorder with a history of offending behaviour who are in community and institutional care, consider offering group-based cognitive and behavioural interventions (e.g. programmes such as 'reasoning and rehabilitation') focused on reducing offending and other antisocial behaviour.

Multi-agency care

- Provision of services for people with antisocial personality disorder often involves significant inter-agency working. Therefore, services should ensure that there are clear pathways for people with antisocial personality disorder so that the most effective multi-agency care is provided. These pathways should:
  - specify the various interventions that are available at each point
  - enable effective communication among clinicians and organizations at all points and provide the means to resolve differences and disagreements.
- Clearly agreed local criteria should also be established to facilitate the transfer of people with antisocial personality disorder between services. As far as is possible, shared objective criteria should be developed relating to comprehensive assessment of need and risk.

- Services should consider establishing antisocial personality disorder networks, where possible linked to other personality disorder networks. (They may be organized at the level of primary care trusts, local authorities, strategic health authorities or government offices.) These networks should be multi-agency, should actively involve people with antisocial personality disorder and should:

  - take a significant role in training staff, including those in primary care, general, secondary and forensic mental health services, and in the Criminal Justice System
  - have resources to provide specialist support and supervision for staff
  - take a central role in the development of standards for and the coordination of clinical pathways
  - monitor the effective operation of clinical pathways.

It is recognized that working with this client group poses a significant challenge for staff. They should receive training and regular supervision specifically in relation to working with people with antisocial personality disorder. It is anticipated that there will be conflict and occasions when boundaries are broken and an atmosphere needs to be created where people can talk honestly and openly about this (NICE 2009a).

Specialist services

There are a series of psychotherapeutic interventions that have been developed for use in specialist personality disorders. These include DBT, CAT, mentalization and therapeutic community models.

Dialectical behavioural therapy

DBT integrates cognitive-behavioural and mindfulness techniques and has a moderate effect in treating people with borderline personality disorder (Kliem *et al.* 2010). Developed by Linehan, the focus is on skills training to develop emotion regulation, distress tolerance, reality testing and acceptance (Linehan 1993). The treatment usually combines individual and group therapy and may be delivered in therapeutic community settings.

Cognitive-analytic therapy

CAT was developed by Ryle and colleagues as a model of brief psychotherapeutic cognitive therapy to treat National Health Service (NHS) patients with

neurotic illnesses (Denman 2001). The approach uses procedural sequencing or mapping to identify when people repeat processes without revision, even if they have negative outcomes. There are three broad types of unrevised faulty procedures that act like traps, interrupting or diverting the procedure which feed back and reinforce the negative behaviour: repetitive cycles such as the depressive thinking trap; the 'dilemma' where an individual chooses an opposing maladaptive behaviour in response to fear of checking their first action response, and the SNAG (subtle negative aspect of goals) where someone's fears of the anticipated outcome of a possible action halts the procedure. Ryle adapted this model for work with people with borderline personality disorder whose early life experiences had led to them developing a model of polarized reciprocal roles (a role for self, for others and a paradigm for the relationship) (Ryle and Kerr 2002). The result is an active, directive brief therapy that has been shown to be effective for people with borderline personality disorder, particularly when used as an early intervention that helps people recognize and revise maladaptive patterns of behaviour (Chanen *et al.* 2009).

Mentalization

Mentalization-based treatment for borderline personality disorder aims to enable clients to expand their mentalizing capacity within the context of a therapeutic attachment relationship. Batemen and Fonagy (2006) describe mentalizing as the capacity developed in childhood to 'understand oneself and others by inferring the mental states that lie behind the overt behaviour'. The ability to retain mentalizing during emotional distress needs to be recovered in people with borderline personality disorder. Without it people experience severe emotional fluctuations and impulsivity. The aim of the treatment is for the client to develop better behavioural control, increased affect regulation, more intimate and gratifying relationships and the ability to pursue life goals.

Therapeutic community models

Therapeutic communities are residential or sometimes intensive day treatment services specializing in working with people with personality disorders. Using a therapeutic milieu model, they work with the assumption that someone's recovery happens in community and is continuous throughout the day rather than just within therapy sessions (Manning 1989). Therapeutic communities aim to offer a radically different approach to treatment of severe emotional disturbance, including personality disorders, through the 'collaborative, democratic and deinstitutionalised approach to staff-patient interaction' (Royal College of Psychiatrists 2012). The focus is often on psychosocial interventions that help people develop awareness of their behaviours and interpersonal relationships with others in the community. The community provides supervision for itself and this model identifies the importance of supervision in all work with people with personality disorders.

 ## 40.6 Conclusion

People with personality disorders require highly specialist care but are more likely to receive treatment in generic primary care, acute mental health, social and criminal justice services. The care of this group is likely to be complex, but nurses' generic client-centred interpersonal skills are transferable to support the care of this client group and to outline approaches to crisis management and inpatient care for people with borderline personality disorder in acute mental health services. The NICE guidelines for antisocial and borderline personality disorders (NICE 2009a, 2009b) provide guidance in organizing services for people and identify the role for both generic and specialist services.

The key learning points from this chapter are:

■ There is no one diagnosis of 'personality disorder' and each type presents a unique set of difficulties for the person with the diagnosis that are likely to be demonstrated in their relationships with friends, family and carers.

■ Diagnoses need to be made with care to distinguish between functional mental illnesses and personality disorders.

■ People with Cluster B type personality disorders are likely to come into regular contact with mental health services and need multiagency collaboration to assess and plan care, manage crises and refer to specialist tertiary mental health services.

■ Nurses need to adapt their interpersonal skills to work collaboratively with this client group and need to be aware of the purpose of crisis admissions to guard against forming pejorative judgements about the client or colleagues.

■ A multi-disciplinary approach to care is essential and teams working with clients with personality disorders should receive regular group supervision about their work to avoid splitting and burnout within the team.

Annotated bibliography

NICE (National Institute for Health and Clinical Excellence) (2009a) *Clinical Guideline 77: Antisocial personality disorder – treatment, management and prevention*. London: NICE, available at: www.nice.org.uk/CG77; NICE (National Institute for Health and Clinical Excellence) (2009b) *Clinical Guideline 78: Borderline personality disorder: treatment and management*. London: NICE, available at: www.nice.org.uk/CG78.

The NICE guidelines are essential reading and provide detailed overviews of the principles and practice of working with people with personality disorders.

In terms of understanding the diagnosis and the nurse's role, each of the following articles gives a useful summary related to the different diagnostic clusters.

Cluster A: Hayward, B.A. (2007) Cluster A personality disorders: considering the 'odd-eccentric' in psychiatric nursing, *International Journal of Mental Health Nursing*, 16: 15–21.

Cluster B: Woods, P. and Richards, D. (2003) Effectiveness of nursing interventions in people with personality disorders, *Journal of Advanced Nursing*, 44(2): 154–72.

Cluster C: Eskedal, G.A. and Demetri, J.M. (2006) Etiology and treatment of cluster C personality disorders, *Journal of Mental Health Counseling*, 28(1): 1–17.

References

APA (American Psychiatric Association) (2000) *Diagnostic and Statistical Manual of Mental Disorders* (DSM-IV(TR)). Washington, DC: APA.

Bateman, A. and Fonagy, P. (2006) *Mentalization-based Treatment for Borderline Personality Disorder: A practical guide.* Oxford: Oxford University Press.

Bateman, A. and Tyrer, P. (2002) Effective management of personality disorder, available at: www.nimhe.org.uk/downloads/Bateman_Tyrer.doc.

Chanen, A., McCutcheon, L.K., Germano, D., Nistico, H., Jackson, H.J. and McGorry, P.M. (2009) The HYPE clinic: an early intervention for borderline personality disorder, *Journal of Psychiatric Practice*, 15: 163–72.

Denman, C. (2001) Cognitive-analytic therapy, *Advance is Psychiatric Treatment*, 7: 243–56.

Eskedal, G.A. and Demetri, J.M. (2006) Etiology and treatment of cluster C personality disorders, *Journal of Mental Health Counseling*, 28(1): 1–17.

Fagin, L. (2004) Management of personality disorders in acute in-patient settings, part 1: borderline personality disorders, *Advances in Psychiatric Treatment*, 16: 93–9.

Fazel, S. and Danesh, J. (2002) Serious mental disorder in 23,000 prisoners: a systematic review of 62 surveys, *The Lancet*, 359: 545–50.

Gelder, M. (1996) Oxford Textbook of Psychiatry, 3rd edition. Oxford: Oxford University Press.

Harrison, P. *et al.* (1998) Lecture Notes on Psychiatry, 8th edition. Oxford: Blackwell Science.

Hawton, K. *et al.* (1999) Psychological and pharmacological treatments for deliberate self-harm. The Cochrane Library Issue 3, 2006 Oxford: Update Software.

Hayward, B.A. (2007) Cluster A personality disorders: considering the 'odd-eccentric' in psychiatric nursing, *International Journal of Mental Health Nursing*, 16: 15–21.

Kliem, S., Kröger, C. and Kossfelder, J. (2010) Dialectical behavior therapy for borderline personality disorder: a meta-analysis using mixed-effects modeling, *Journal of Consulting and Clinical Psychology*, 78: 936–51.

Krawitz, R. and Watson, C. (2003) *Borderline Personality Disorder: A practical guide to treatment.* Oxford: Oxford University Press.

Linehan, M. (1993) *Skills Training Manual for Treating Borderline Personality Disorder.* New York: Guildford Press.

Manning, N. (1989) *The Therapeutic Community Movement: Charisma and Routinization.* London: Routledge.

Mind (2012) Understanding personality disorders, available at: www.mind.org.uk/help/diagnoses_and_conditions/personality_disorders.

Moran, P., Jenkins R., Tylee, A., Blizard, R. and Mann, A. (2000) The prevalence of personality disorder amongst UK primary care attenders, *Acta Psychiatrica Scandinavica*, 101: 1–6.

Moskovitz, R. (2001) *Lost in the Mirror: An inside look at borderline personality disorder*, 2nd edn. Dallas, TX: Taylor Publishing.

NICE (National Institute for Health and Clinical Excellence) (2009a) *Clinical Guideline 77: Antisocial personality disorder – treatment, management and prevention.* London: NICE, available at: www.nice.org.uk/CG77.

NICE (National Institute for Health and Clinical Excellence) (2009b) *Clinical Guideline 78: Borderline personality disorder: treatment and management.* London: NICE, available at: www.nice.org.uk/CG78.

Paris, J. (2003) *Personality Disorders Over Time: Precursors, course and outcome.* Washington, DC: APA.

Royal College of Psychiatrists (2012) Community of communities, available at: www.rcpsych.ac.uk/quality/qualityandaccreditation/therapeuticcommunities/communityofcommunities1.aspx.

Ryle, A. and Kerr, I. (2002) *Introducing Cognitive Analytic Therapy: Principles and practice.* Chichester: Wiley.

Singleton, N., Bumpstead, R., O'Brien, M., Lee, A. and Meltzer, H. (2002) *Psychiatric Morbidity Among Adults Living in Private Households 2000.* London: ONS, available at: www.ons.gov.uk/ons/rel/psychiatric-morbidity/psychiatric-morbidity-among-adults-living-in-private-households/2000/index.html.

Svartberg, M., Stiles, T. C. and Seltzer, M. H. (2004) Randomized, controlled trial of the effectiveness of short-term dynamic psychotherapy and cognitive therapy for cluster C personality disorders, *American Journal of Psychiatry*, 161: 810–17.

WHO (World Health Organization) (2010) *International Statistical Classification of Diseases and Related Health Problems* (ICD-10), 10th revision, available at: http://apps.who.int/classifications/icd10/browse/2010/en#/F50 Accessed 24/11/11.

Woods, P. & Richards, D. (2003) Effectiveness of nursing interventions in people with personality disorders, *Journal of Advanced Nursing*, 44(2): 154–72.

Chapter

41

Forensic Mental Health Care

Graham Durcan

I still get in a bit of trouble and I'm shit at organizing my life . . . but I'm nothing like what I was . . . and I can call XXX and they put me right . . . they are very calm . . . even when I'm not listening.

(A service user who had been in medium secure service, prison and mainstream mental health care. His experience had been, in the latter particularly, that he was often poorly understood and served. When I interviewed him he was being given ongoing support by a diversion and liaison team and for the first time he experienced a flexible and tolerant service)

How do [staff] work with patients if you don't speak to the people who know them best . . . the carers?

(Centre for Mental Health 2011, reproduced by kind permission of the Centre for Mental Health)

 ## 41.1 Introduction

Forensic services have a long and distinct history. The first establishment in the British Isles built specifically to house 'the criminally insane' was the asylum in Dundrum, Dublin, now the Central Mental Health Hospital. Broadmoor followed soon after in 1863 and Rampton in 1912. The history of forensic mental health care has for most part been a history of high secure hospital-based services. In the early 1960s it was recognized that there was need for less

secure provision and that many patients were being held in conditions that were too restrictive. But it was not until the 1980s and 1990s that there was substantial growth in less secure accommodation, with even greater growth in the early years of the twenty-first century. In recent times there have been reports on the speculative development of secure beds, particularly in the private sector, but there has also been some evidence of this in the public sector (Centre for Mental Health 2011). Our present financial crisis would seem to have put an end to this for now.

Kettles *et al.* (2008: 10) describe forensic mental health nursing as 'evolving'. The skills and practices of forensic mental health nursing are not unique, but the emphasis on particular aspects does distinguish it from other specialities, for example through a particular focus on risk assessment, management and offending.

A major influence on this chapter is a Sainsbury Centre for Mental Health review of secure mental health care and the pathways through it, *Pathways to Unlocking Secure Mental Health Care* (Sainsbury Centre for Mental Health 2011); referred to hitherto as the 'Pathway Review'.

This chapter is divided into three sections:

- settings;
- personality disorder;
- key practice issues.

 ## 41.2 Settings

Secure mental health care

Mullen (2000: 307) describes some of the difficulty in defining forensic psychiatry. He notes that some definitions potentially engulf mainstream psychiatry, but says

> In practice, patients often gravitate to forensic services when the nature of their offending, or the apprehension created by their behaviour, is such as to overwhelm both the tolerance and the confidence of professionals in the general mental health services.

A traditional view is that these services are for those with a severe mental illness who have offended and pose a risk to the public – i.e. they may be dangerous, and there is a link between their mental illness and their offending. The forensic service patient may also pose a risk to her or himself but this alone would not be sufficient to impose the degree of restriction involved in secure care. This view of forensic services was held by most clinicians working in secure mental health care interviewed for the

Pathway Review (Centre for Mental Health 2011). However, the review itself revealed that there were groups of patients who had, in Mullen's words, 'gravitated to forensic services' and who did not meet the above criteria. The review found a small group of patients in all the medium secure units visited who may not have had contact with criminal justice services or been charged with an offence, but who were perceived as challenging, treatment resistant, potentially violent, (sometimes described as 'new long-stay') and who had often previously been 'bed-blocking' in a mainstream psychiatric unit.

Another group are those transferred from prison whose offending is less serious and for whom there may be no link between offending and their mental illness, but who had developed an acute mental illness while in prison (prisons are not regarded as a place of safety English and Welsh mental health legislation). In some parts of the UK there has been more success in moving these people into lower secure mental health settings or psychiatric intensive care units. But, more often than not, medium security is the default transfer destination, with risk aversion of both clinicians and the Ministry of Justice playing a part in this. The emergence of prison mental health care services in recent years has reportedly led to increased transfers of this group (Rutherford 2010).

A further group within forensic services are those patients whose problems are primarily related to their personality disorder. These patients pose harm to others and therefore there is a link between their 'disorder' and their offending, but clinicians interviewed for the Pathway Review were divided in their views about whether those with personality disorder should be clients of forensic mental health care or the Criminal Justice System. Each of the above groups of patients can be divided into further subgroups, each of which may have its own unique set of needs.

The Pathway Review concluded that the population served by forensic mental health care services varies considerably across the UK and that there is a 'general lack of written and standardised entry criteria . . . which means that professionals have to propose a clinical rationale as to why an individual requires secure care' (p. 14). The Pathway Review found that while forensic mental health services deal with a comparatively small number of people, they account for a little short of 20 per cent of the annual mental health services budget. The bulk of this cost is in the secure estate. Over a period in which there was significant investment and growth in community mental health services (2002/3 to 2009/10), estimated annually at 5.9 per cent, forensic mental health care grew at 13.4 per cent a year, a growth in spending of 141 per cent (Centre for Mental Health 2011).

The secure estate comprises three types of hospital, high, medium and low security, and there is some further division within the medium and low categories.

High secure

High security hospital care is provided entirely by the UK National Health Service (NHS), across four hospital sites: Carstairs serving Scotland (and Northern Ireland), and Ashworth, Rampton and Broadmoor serving England and Wales. Rampton has the small number of women who require high secure care and also provides for those with learning disability, in addition to those with mental illness and personality disorder. The total number of beds across the three English sites is in the region of 800 and the newly developed State Hospital at Carstairs is reducing its number of beds to under 150.

Patients who are deemed to require high secure beds are those detained under the Mental Health Act 1983 who 'pose a grave and immediate danger to the public'. However, there have been a significant number of patients who have been deemed to require less restrictive regimes. A review of this in 2000 resulted in 400 people being transferred to lower secure settings (Tilt *et al.* 2000); however, this appears to be less of an issue in the high secure hospitals at the present time than previously.

Two of the high secure hospitals (Broadmoor and Rampton) host units for those with personality disorder deemed to pose the highest harm. These dangerous and severe personality disorder (DSPD)

units have been part of a network of services targeted at this group. The DSPD programme is undergoing reform at the time of writing and will be discussed further later in the chapter.

A minority of high security patients will remain in these services for life, but the average stay has reduced over time – for example, Broadmoor report the average stay is now five to six years (see: www. wlmht.nhs.uk/bm/broadmoor-hospital). While some patients may be released to community-based support, most will be 'stepped down' to medium secure and then a lower secure service before being reintegrated with the community.

Medium secure

Medium secure services provide around 3,500 beds in England and Wales. This has been one of the growth areas in forensic mental health care, not just in England and Wales, but also in Scotland, Northern Ireland and the Republic of Ireland. Most are still provided by the NHS, but a significant proportion of medium secure beds (in England particularly) are provided by the independent sector; Rutherford and Duggan estimated that this was around 35 per cent in 2007 (Rutherford and Duggan 2007) and there has been growth in both sectors since then.

Medium secure units cater for patients detained under the Mental Health Act 1983 who 'pose a serious danger to the public'. Within these services there is considerable variety of provision, examples being specialist beds for hearing impaired patients, those with personality disorder, those with learning disability or autism, and the Women's Enhanced Medium Secure Service. The latter has been developed to provide enhanced treatment and support in a gender-specific context for those women not deemed to be benefiting from other medium secure care.

Over the past 10 years I have visited many medium secure services and a consistent theme in these visits has been the significant minority of patients in each unit deemed by clinical staff to no longer require this level of security. This was also a finding of the Pathways Review. Risk aversion, lack of appropriate 'step-down' facilities, the commissioning process and an unwillingness of community mental health services to provide support were the commonly cited reasons for this.

Low secure

At the outset of the Pathways Review I was somewhat unclear about the defining features of low secure provision. At the end of the Review I was even less clear. These services are particularly ill-defined and while some are attached to forensic mental health services and form the next step down, others are provided alongside more mainstream mental health care. They are provided by both the independent sector and the NHS. Laing and Buisson (2006) commented that it was difficult to distinguish some low secure services from mental health rehabilitation services. The Pathways Review found it impossible to obtain a definitive statistic for the number of units or beds and could only estimate that low secure accounted for perhaps another 3,500 beds. The definition of those requiring any type of secure bed is particularly difficult to pin down and no more so than for low secure – i.e. those held under the Mental Health Act who 'pose a significant danger to themselves or others'. Some low secure facilities will contain a small number of voluntary patients, particularly those awaiting transfer to community care or some other form of accommodation. Clearly though there is a range of provision within this category.

The Pathway Review found that medium secure services (2008/9 estimates) have an average daily cost of £482 per patient, while the average low secure services cost £418 per bed per day. This relatively small difference in daily cost suggests that much so-called low secure provision may actually not be much less secure than medium secure, given that a significant factor in both security and cost is in staffing.

The total bed provision across all categories of adult forensic mental health care is in the region of 7,000–8,000. Many of those beds have appeared within the last decade. And yet accessing these beds is often perceived as being difficult. The Pathways Review found that transfers from prison to secure mental health care remained problematic, taking weeks and often months. Perhaps counter-intuitively the Pathways Review did not see the solution as building more medium and so-called low secure beds, but concluded that reinvesting some of the resources currently used on medium and low secure to develop 'step-down' in the form of appropriate supported accommodation and enhanced community support would lead to an unblocking of secure care.

Case Study

Shawn

Shawn is in his early thirties and is currently a patient in a low secure unit. He moved there quite recently from the medium secure facility that the unit is attached to. Six months ago he transferred from a Category B prison where he had started serving a two-year sentence for assault occasioning actual bodily harm. Shawn could not remember how many times he had been to prison, as he had been remanded on quite a number of occasions, but in fact had received five custodial sentences, the first when he was 17. He had numerous convictions and had received fines and community orders as well as serving time in custody. His offending had involved assaults, burglary, shoplifting and driving while under the influence of drink. In most cases drugs and alcohol had played a part in his offending, as he had either offended to fund taking illicit substances or had offended while under the influence of drugs and or alcohol.

Shawn had experienced what he now recognized as mental health problems for much of his life. As a toddler he had presented with marked behavioural difficulty. This had been noted by the family health visitor and doctor and this behaviour had continued throughout his childhood resulting in a disruptive schooling, multiple exclusions and finally placement in an educational referral unit at age 13. Shawn stopped attending schooling at age 14 and had been in trouble with the police regularly from age 11. Shawn states that his mother had suffered depression for much of her life.

Shawn was the second of four brothers, two of whom had also served at least one custodial sentence. His older brother was the only one who had not been in significant trouble with the police and who had never experienced problematic use of drugs or alcohol. All four brothers had by and large been raised by their single mother, but shared a biological father who they had very limited contact with. Shawn's two younger brothers had both experienced episodes in local authority care. Shawn had for the most part lived with his mother until he was 16. At that age he describes his mother as having had enough of him and from that point on having only short periods of stable housing.

Shawn has two children with two different former girlfriends, neither of which he has any contact with. He has never 'experienced' gainful employment and has instead survived through benefits, theft and occasional trading in illicit drugs.

Up until recently he has had very limited contact with mental health services. As a teenager he remembers seeing a psychiatrist on one occasion but doesn't remember the outcome. His first contact as an adult was during his previous sentence, with the prison mental health inreach team in one of the prisons he spent a few months in. 'I had been self-harming . . . cutting more seriously and having very bad thoughts . . . and I was very paranoid.' Shawn was seen by the team's psychiatrist and by one of the nurses. 'I hadn't seen myself as mentally ill before . . . so it was the first time . . . I just thought I was very moody and very angry.' Shawn felt helped for the first time and found the sessions with the nurse helpful: ' . . . it all kind of fell apart on release . . . they referred me to a mental health team where I was going to live . . . but the appointment was like 10 days away and things fell apart well before then.' Shawn returned to abusing drugs and alcohol and within eight months had returned to prison, remanded following the assault incident he was eventually convicted for.

'I asked to see the mental health team when I got there [prison] . . . but nothing really happened until I had a breakdown.' Shawn experienced what appeared to be an acute psychotic episode and this ultimately led to his transfer under the Mental Health Act to the medium secure unit. 'I have been told I have a personality disorder, depression and psychosis and of course I have abused drugs and alcohol . . . so that's quite a bit to have to deal with.'

Shawn isn't certain of his future. 'I feel a lot better and I want to be out [in the community] . . . the quickest way would be to go back to prison as I don't have too long to my earliest possible release date . . . but I'm worried it will all fall apart on release again like before . . . if I stay here then I might be stuck here for a long time but they [his current mental health team] might be able to arrange better support in the community.'

Community services

Some medium secure services provide parallel community teams for patients discharged from their units and/or outreach and consultative services designed to work with mainstream community mental health teams for ex-secure care patients. The provision of either type of service has been and remains patchy. There is limited evidence on which approach is superior – i.e. the parallel approach versus the more integrated consultative approach. Coid *et al.* (2007) found little difference between the two in one of the few studies conducted in this area. Kirby and I reported (Kirby and Durcan 2009: 579) that 'the development of integrated models of services may be a product of limited funding and therefore a necessity' and Coid *et al.* (2007) state that parallel services do not have sufficient resource to provide aftercare for all their discharged patients.

The Pathway Review recommended the development of community support and favoured the integrated approach, partially because in the absence of evidence that another approach has better outcomes this is likely to be the more economically viable option. The Pathway Review saw funding for this as needing to come from redesign of existing services and ultimately a reduction in the number of secure beds.

Young people's services

Hoare and Wilson (2010) attempted to capture the range of provision for children and adolescents. They found that, like adult services, it is an expanding field but also something of a postcode lottery with few if any areas having what could be called comprehensive provision. Hoare and Wilson found the following categories of provision:

- nationally commissioned medium secure services for young people;
- secure inpatient services (not nationally commissioned);
- Tier 4 custodial estate mental health resource for young people with complex and specialist needs;
- forensic adolescent community treatment services (FACTS);
- community based forensic teams (CBFTs);
- complex needs services.

A brief description of each follows.

Nationally commissioned medium secure service

Hoare and Wilson reported that there were 105 beds spread across seven units, which represents a significant increase in provision to that which Kirby and I reported in the second edition of this book (i.e. 68 beds across five units). Nevertheless, Hoare and Wilson reported difficulties in achieving timely admission. A small part of this commissioned provision is for those with learning disability.

Secure inpatient services (not nationally commissioned)

Hoare and Wilson identified another 100 beds divided across three units (on two locations) for those young people who fall short of the entry criteria for nationally commissioned medium secure provision. Most of the provision is provided in two units on one site by one independent sector provider based in the south Midlands, providing for both males and females and with some beds being dedicated to those young people with learning disability. The remaining beds (n = 10) are in the North East in a unit attached to an adolescent inpatient unit. The latter unit is reported to have some expertise in those with emerging personality disorder and those with autism.

Tier 4 custodial estate

There are just two such specialist units, each within a young offenders institute (i.e. a prison for those under the age of 18), but each providing to seemingly quite different groups. One unit in the North East provides 48 places for young prisoners who have mental health problems (but not severe mental illness), who are vulnerable and do not cope with the young offender institute regime. The other unit in England's North West offers intensive and individualized treatment and care for up to eight young men who are disruptive and violent to staff and other young people. One of the aims of the unit is to provide a graduated reintegration to the ordinary young offender regime.

Additionally, all young offender institutes (eight for males and three for females), secure training centres (n = 4) and secure children's homes (n = 10) have commissioned mental health services, but provision is variable.

FACTS and CBFTs

These are a few forensic mental health services providing consultation and direct care for young people outside institutional care, though some of these services also provide mental health inreach to young offenders institutes. The FACTS are those teams that have emerged from medium secure services and the CBFTs are those which are purely community services. Most FACTS appear to have closed since Hoare and Wilson reported.

Complex needs services

Hoare and Wilson describe these as 'soft' forensic services and most have similarities to Tier 3 child and adult mental health services (CAMHS) and act as parallel services that have prioritized more 'at risk' populations, such as 'looked after' children and those already in contact with criminal justice. Often the children and adolescents seen by the complex needs services have indeterminate diagnosis that may be a barrier to their entry to mainstream CAMHS.

Diversion

Adult diversion and liaison services have existed in England and Wales for over 20 years. The first service was launched in 1989 and their number reached a peak in England in 1997 with 194 such services (Spurgeon 2005). Nacro's most recent survey of adult diversion and liaison services lists 112 in England and 14 in Wales (Nacro 2011), and this listing includes some mentally disordered offender panels, which deal with referrals from court for a higher risk group. The decline in these services has been due in part to their never being a policy 'must do'; they did not, for example, feature in the National Service Framework for Mental Health or the NHS Plan (DH 1999, 2000 respectively). There is some provision in Scotland and the Scottish Office conducted research of 18 pilot schemes in the late 1990s (Scottish Government 2000). More recently the Scottish Government has invested £1.46 million in developing such schemes (L&BCJA 2011). The earliest schemes in Scotland date back to the mid-1980s and most of these are generic diversion services, diverting to social work. However, those with mental health problems and learning disabilities are regarded as a priority group. It is unclear to what extent mental health and forensic mental health care are involved with the Scottish schemes. Provision in Northern Ireland is currently negligible.

The English and Welsh schemes have worked primarily with magistrates and crown courts, screening and assessing those in the cells and making recommendations to the probation service and sentencers, and referring or signposting those they assess. Some also work at the point of arrest in police custody suites.

Provision has always been patchy with most courts and police custody suites not receiving any service. Some teams are small with limited capacity and respond to referrals rather than offering a proactive service, which is regarded as good practice (Sainsbury Centre for Mental Health 2009).

Lord Bradley, a former Home Office minister, was commissioned by the Labour government to conduct a review, across England, of mental health and learning disability diversion in 2007. Lord Bradley extended the time of the review and adopted an 'all stages' diversion approach. The result was the Bradley Report (MOJ 2009) with 82 recommendations, covering community policing, police custody suites, courts, prison mental health care, personality disorder, resettlement/re-entry, alternatives to custody and use of the mental health treatment requirement.

The coalition government is maintaining the focus on mental health diversion and has developed a programme to 'roll-out' these services to all magistrate and crown courts and all police custody suites. This programme will also develop the 'best practice' model that services should be based on. Both adults' and children's diversion services are included in the project (DH 2011a). The government has pledged up to £50 million to support the development of diversion and liaison across England.

Most adult diversion and liaison services largely provide a screening and assessment service, followed by onward referral and/or signposting to other services, but very few provide any case management, support or outreach beyond this. The MO:DEL team in the City of Manchester is an exception, providing up to six months intensive case management (for a brief description of the team see http://www.gmw.nhs.uk/dropdownlinks/documents/ModelLeaflet.pdf).

Children's mental health diversion is new. The Centre for Mental Health, in collaboration with the Department of Health (DH) and Youth Justice Board, developed the first six pilots in 2008 and 2009 and the coalition government's current development programme consists of 37 such services.

Prison

The NHS in all four nations of the UK has now taken over responsibility for prison health care. Alongside this reform is the development of new forms of prison mental health care. This is arguably most progressed in England and Wales, where since the early years of this century there has been a roll-out of dedicated secondary mental health care ('inreach') to all prisons and young offender institutes. These inreach teams have by and large been mental health nursing teams (HMIP 2007), though there is anecdotal evidence of an increase in the multi-disciplinary nature of teams in recent times.

Multiple and complex needs

While the high prevalence of mental illness in prisons has long since been established (e.g. Singleton et al. 1998), understanding of prisoners' mental health needs probably did not emerge until inreach teams were introduced to prisons. In Durcan (2008a) I write about the need to develop primary mental health care because at that time the majority of prisoners had moderate mental health problems but fell short of the threshold for most inreach teams. I argued that the primary care mental health role was every bit as much a specialist role as the secondary care mental health nurse's role. I still hold to this view and a number of prisons have now introduced dedicated primary mental health care teams or have a merged primary and secondary mental health care service. What is becoming increasingly clear is that most prisoners, and indeed clients of all forensic mental health care services,

Table 41.1 Mental illness among prisoners and the general population

Mental illness	Prisoners (%)*	General population (%)**
Schizophrenia and delusional disorder	8	0.5
Personality disorder	66	5.3
Neurotic disorder (e.g. depression)	45	13.8
Drug dependency	45	5.2
Alcohol dependency	30	11.5

* Singleton et al. (1998) ** Singleton et al. (2001)

have, as a default, multiple and complex needs. For example, in addition to having mental health problems many will have concurrent problems with substance misuse, histories of trauma, learning difficulty and/or disability, poor life and coping skills, lack of security of tenure on release and limited experience of employment. For many of those in the prison system and those in diversion and liaison their various individual problems will often fall below service entry thresholds and yet, because of the multiplicity and complexity of their problems, they suffer considerable disability.

I have profiled several secondary and primary prison mental health care caseloads and they match closely those of assertive outreach teams I have profiled in terms of severity of problems and complexity. This begs the question of whether an assertive outreach approach involving robust case management and brokering of inputs would best meet the needs of these clients. I will return to this question later.

41.3 Personality disorder

The problem of personality disorder is considered elsewhere in this book (Chapter 40), but it is also very much part of the daily business of forensic mental health care and hence will receive some consideration here. Those with personality disorder often find themselves excluded from many mainstream mental health services, and while some parts of forensic mental health care also exclude them, by and large personality disorder is part of the daily business of the forensic mental health nurse (FMHN).

Controversy has always accompanied the diagnosis of personality disorder and in spite of the firm policy directive given in *Personality Disorder: No longer a diagnosis of exclusion* (NIMH 2003), it remains on the margins in many places (e.g. see Rutherford 2010). Kendell (2002) discusses the difficulties in distinguishing personality disorder from mental illness, and links the notion of treatability with the 'acceptance' of personality disorder by British psychiatrists, suggesting that if there was

more evidence of effective treatments then there might be less tendency to exclude this group. In the late 1990s the then Home Secretary Jack Straw was extremely critical of a trend that he saw among psychiatrists to 'only take on those patients they regard as treatable' (BBC 1998) and called for psychiatrists to 'modernize' their practice. The reforms to the Mental Health Act 2007 arguably made the exclusion of those with personality disorder more difficult on treatability grounds by replacing the treatability criterion of the 1983 Act with the notion of the availability of 'appropriate treatment'. Experts contributing to a Centre for Mental Health review of policy in justice and health saw this as paving 'the way for long term incarceration of mentally disordered offenders whether they chose to engage in treatment or not' (Rutherford 2010: 65).

The Pathways Review found there was huge variability across England in the availability of personality disorder services. Some areas had no services, whereas others provided tiered care for people with personality disorder. This is also true of prison mental health inreach teams, some being willing to accept referrals for those with primary personality disorders while others list a primary diagnosis of personality disorder among their exclusion criteria. Singleton *et al.* (1998) over a decade ago found that 66 per cent of the prison population had one or more form of personality disorder, and in some prisons the proportion is higher (78 per cent in male remand prisoners). The prison population has more than doubled since that time and there is no reason to consider that personality disorder is any less of an issue now.

Personality disorder both in prisons and in secure mental health care has been subject to huge investment in recent times, primarily targeted at the group of those with personality disorders who pose the highest harm. The bulk of this investment came via the DSPD programme, launched in 2001. The programme operated across a number of centres, the prisons Frankland, Whitemoor and Low Newton (the latter having a dedicated unit for up to 12 women) and Broadmoor and Rampton hospitals. The programme had up to 300 secure beds (DH

2011c). There have also been some small-scale community re-entry programmes for those leaving prisons. The average number of people treated per year was 234, but with a relatively low turnover (range 1.6–4.2 years) (Eagle 2009). Less than 0.5 per cent of prisoners have access to the treatments provided by DSPD units (Fossey and Black 2010). The cost of the programme for 2006–7 rose to £60 million per year (Eagle 2009), and currently stands at £69 million per year (DH 2011c). By 2010 the DSPD programme had cost the public purse a little short of half a billion pounds. Rutherford (2010: 47) states that 'Evidence of the effectiveness of DSPD has been limited, and research has found little to support the high costs and treatments as a way to reduce risk of re-offending or provide effective treatment for personality disorder'.

If the diagnosis of personality disorder is controversial then what Rutherford calls the 'quasi-medical' term 'dangerous and severe personality disorder' is fraught with even more controversy. Rutherford cites Select Committee evidence given by Dr Mike Shooter of the Royal College of Psychiatrists (Rutherford 2010: 50): 'the link between personality disorder and dangerousness is extremely tenuous and poorly researched . . . most people with severe personality disorder are not dangerous and most people who are dangerous in the Government sense will not have personality disorder'.

The DSPD programme is currently undergoing reform with a view to expanding, but significantly changing, the programme both within the secure estate (primarily in prisons) and the community. The number of places proposed will be 1,300, with 800 of those in the community (DH 2011c). This will be achieved within the current cost envelope and indeed probably for considerably less.

41.4 Key practice issues

Risk assessment and management

Wood describes risk assessment (see Chapters 17 and 18) as 'determining the probability of harm to self or others or a serious unwanted event such as suicide or homicide' (2008: 207). Flewett (2010: 16) includes the following in his summary of what constitutes risk:

- risk is the likelihood of an adverse outcome;
- the likelihood of risk occurring changes over time;
- risk is a part of every decision-making process of patient care;
- risk involves not just the patient but the patient's family, the community, mental health staff and the mental health service.

Forensic mental health is the branch of mental health provision that is most concerned with public protection. Few of the treatments offered to forensic service users will be unique to this branch of mental health care, but what is unique are the settings in which they take place and the emphasis on risk reduction (i.e. risk of harm to others) and management within the overall treatment package.

Mental health practice can and never will be risk free. Rather pessimistically, Petch states that 'The stark reality is that however good our tools for risk assessments become, whether clinical or actuarial, professionals will not be able to make a significant impact on public safety' (2001:). Petch places little faith in training and measures which specifically target particular populations (at least without well resourced services in place): 'Better mental health care for all, especially for those about to relapse and irrespective of the risk of violence, would be more likely to prevent incidents occurring than simply targeting resources on those assessed as being a high risk' (p. ??).

Case management and meeting multiple need

So, good quality and well monitored care for any and all is in itself an effective risk management strategy. Many clients of mental health services will have poor mental health as part of multiple and complex needs. As already stated, this is certainly true for the clients of forensic mental health services in all settings. 'Good quality' care in this context is care that takes account of the broader need. A key role that FMHNs can play is in the case management, often assertive, of a package of care that meets all of these. One cannot expect any single mental health practitioner to have expertise in all areas and so the key skill of the FMHN case manager is in brokerage and coordinating a range of elements that meet the client's social, emotional, psychological and health needs. Part of this role will be advocating for needs to be met and often these are not the traditional domain of mental health care (such as housing, employment and leisure). The near 100 prisoners with mental health problems I interviewed for *From the Inside* (Durcan 2008b) did mention medication and psychological intervention when questioned about their mental health needs, but gave far greater prominence to more basic needs such as housing and security of tenure and access to funds, preferably through a job but certainly through accessing the right benefits. Safer care and care that is likely to reduce risk is care that addresses the whole person, and which starts with the most basic needs first.

Relapse prevention

Related to risk management is relapse prevention. Stresses in life may trigger the onset of symptoms and so well monitored and case managed care is that which has crisis management planning as part of the overall package of care. Crises will often be the result of problems a service user has in meeting their basic needs. Relapse prevention is, of course, a facet of care in which clients themselves and their carers can play a leading role. The FMHN can support this through supporting their client in learning and noting patterns of previous onset and then by providing access to further support when the client detects change.

Coffey (2003: 255) provides a useful summary of relapse prevention, particularly focused on those clients with psychosis, and lists five key features:

- it should be based on the individual service user's experience;
- it should develop skill development and mastery;

- it should be negotiated and collaborative;
- it should be informed but not restricted by empirical findings; and
- it should facilitate personal control over the illness.

Coffey also makes the link between relapse prevention and recovery, which I return to later in this chapter. I also recommend Witkiewitz and Marlatt (2007) who provide a useful general introduction to the topic of relapse prevention.

MAPPA

A specific area of risk management that many FMHNs will have a role in is Multi-agency Public Protection Arrangements (MAPPA): 'MAPPA is an excellent example of how agencies can work together on a formal basis, sharing information for mutual benefits' (DH 2009: 137). MAPPA is the multi-agency panel system, operating in any locality, for managing offenders who are deemed to pose a risk to the public. Scotland's system is also called MAPPA and like Northern Ireland's system (Public Protection Arrangements Northern Ireland – PPANI) is, with some minor differences, very close to the English and Welsh system.

The purpose of MAPPA (MOJ 2009: 31–2) is to:

- identify all relevant offenders;
- complete comprehensive risk assessments that take advantage of coordinated information-sharing across the agencies;
- devise, implement and review robust risk management plans;
- focus the available resources in a way which best protects the public from serious harm.

Under the MAPPA system all offenders within a local area are categorized into one of three categories:

- **Category 1:** registered sex offenders;
- **Category 2:** largely concerns violent offenders who have received a sentence of at least 12 months;

- **Category 3:** covers other dangerous offenders and sometimes those who have previously been Category 1 or 2 offenders.

Offenders in all three categories will include those with personality disorder and mental illness who are deemed to pose a risk to the public. In England and Wales the NHS is not a lead organization ('Responsible Authority') in the MAPPA process. This differs in Scotland for 'mentally disordered offenders' (Scottish Government Public Protection Unit 2008: 7). However, regardless of this, in many cases mental health practitioners and FMHNs in particular will play a significant part in delivering the programmes and treatments designed to reduce risk.

Treatment programmes

Service users of a forensic mental health service should have the same access to care and treatment programmes as all mental health service users. But what sets the forensic mental health care treatment programme apart is the emphasis on reducing risk. Not all patients in forensic care will have committed offences, but a significant proportion will have and many will have been transferred from prisons. Offender treatment programmes are available both in prison and in secure mental health care. The Pathway Review found there was a variety of programmes and all seeming of good quality, but like much else in this field, there was variability of provision by unit. Additionally, continuity of care was an issue, in that the variability of provision meant that transfers within a category of security (e.g. from one medium secure unit to another) or up or down a category often meant an abrupt ending to a programme or sometimes the repetition of the same programme.

The Centre for Mental Health's review of offending behaviour programmes for people with mental health problems (Sainsbury Centre for Mental Health 2008a) found that while there was emerging evidence of the benefits of these programmes (including a reduction in reoffending of between 10 and 24 per cent), there was little research concerning those programmes in secure mental health care. Many such programmes draw upon cognitive

behavioural therapy (CBT) techniques. They should also include interventions to promote relapse prevention and symptom management (see Duncan et al. 2006) which should engage both service user and carer.

The prisoner interviews for From the Inside (Durcan 2008b) found that most of those interviewed reported at least three significant traumatic events (i.e. physical and sexual abuse) in their lives and often in their childhoods. Most reported not receiving any help for this. So interventions addressing past traumas and managing the present distress from these are important. Some offender treatment programmes raise offenders' own experience of abuse victimization and some prisoners find this particularly difficult as another review learned (Sainsbury Centre for Mental Health 2008b: 45):

> Inreach team members reported that prisoners sometimes coped poorly with the issues raised in courses, such as the sex offender treatment programme. The prisoners found these courses to be intensive and gruelling, for example when they were forced to confront issues such as childhood trauma. The mental health team was often left to address the ramifications of this, for which it is not resourced.

My interviews with staff for From the Inside revealed similar findings; staff did not feel equipped to support those suffering such trauma. One factor was that prisoners were frequently transferred between prisons and this significantly impacted on issues that required longer-term psychological support. Nevertheless, while for those FMHNs working in prison settings it will probably always be difficult to provide appropriate psychological support for some clients, an awareness of trauma and skills in supporting those who have suffered it should be part of the FMHN's armoury. In some cases, prison inreach teams have negotiated with prison management for the 'medical hold' (an agreement not to transfer the prisoner for a period) of a prisoner to allow for the completion of a treatment programme.

Building motivation is another challenge, particularly so for people who are incarcerated for long periods. Techniques such as motivational interviewing (see Chapter 23) are likely to be an important adjunct to forensic mental health care. Alan Cohen has described recent incorporation of motivational interviewing to support physical care management of long-term high secure patients (Cohen 2011).

Most patients in secure mental health care will ultimately return to live in a community setting. The Sainsbury Centre for Mental Health's offending behaviour programmes report (2008a) stressed the need for preparation for stepping down from secure care, and considering educational needs, accommodation needs, daily living skills and routes to employment.

A pathways approach: continuity of care

One of the key findings from the Pathway Review was the absence of pathways for most forensic mental health care patients. Forensic mental health care has, by and large, evolved locally rather than been designed, and this includes prison inreach services, diversion and liaison teams and secure mental health care. Some people will pass through all of these branches of forensic mental health care, but will seldom experience any sense of continuity of care and sometimes with little in the way of information exchange between different branches.

The Pathway Review found that the least developed part of the secure mental health care pathway was the step-down from medium and low secure (these two supposed levels often being hard to distinguish). In other words, there was a need for routes out of secure mental health care; the majority of secure service patients will return to live in the community, but there is little understanding of how this can be achieved in a graduated way.

Recovery

'Recovery' (see Chapter 5) is increasingly to the fore in the thinking around the development of all mental health services, and it features prominently in the current English mental health strategy and indeed is a guiding principle (DH 2011b). Prominence is given particularly to the 'importance of employment and housing in the recovery process' (p. 8).

Shepherd *et al.* (2008: 1) include in their description of recovery a service user 'building a meaningful and satisfying life', which is defined by service users themselves, regardless of whether or not there are continued symptoms of mental illness. The role of the professional is to support recovery. In forensic mental health practice this means the FMHN and colleagues become mentors, coaches and partners rather than just experts. This is a challenging notion for any branch of mental health care, particularly in forensic mental health care, where most service users have considerable restriction placed on their lives, primarily through mental health legislation. Nevertheless, the Pathways Review found in all of the units it visited an interest in developing recovery-oriented practice, and the Review recommended that all forensic mental health care staff have access to training.

> *Housing, employment, education and participation in 'mainstream' community and leisure activities then become the central objectives, not just things that professionals hope will happen if the person is 'cured'. Treatments, whether physical, psychological or social, are useful only insofar as they assist with these aims. This turns the traditional priorities of mental health services 'upside down'.*
>
> (Shepherd *et al.* 2008: 4)

Pathways to employment

Access to employment for ex-offenders can reduce reoffending by as much as 50 per cent (Social Exclusion Unit 2002), and the right sort of supported employment can help improve mental well-being. There is therefore a powerful argument for all forms of forensic mental health practice to develop pathways to employment to promote service users' recovery and reduce risk of further offending.

Employment is key to the coalition government's ambition for a 'rehabilitation revolution' in the Criminal Justice System and is seen as one of the most effective ways of preventing reoffending and improving life chances (MOJ 2011). Reoffending costs the economy somewhere in the region of £11 billion per year and the Confederation of British Industry (CBI) estimates that a reduction of 10 per cent in reoffending by released prisoners nationally would save over £1 billion (CBI 2008). However, only 26 per cent of prisoners who leave prison enter some form of employment (Prison Reform Trust 2011). A little over of a third of prisoners have employment on coming into prison, but two thirds of these will lose these jobs while in prison and like most other offenders will find that most employers will not consider employing ex-offenders (Prison Reform Trust 2011). For those leaving secure care there are even greater difficulties in entering employment, including years of institutional care and perceived dangerousness linked to the double stigma of mental illness and their past offending. However, several forensic mental health services now have employment specialists, many of whom are versed in the individual placement and support (IPS) methodology.

The Centre for Mental Health's investigation of the employment of offenders with mental health problems (2010) found that people in the Criminal Justice System with mental health problems are routinely excluded from programmes that provide vocational rehabilitation. People who experience severe and enduring mental health problems have one of the lowest employment rates in the UK. Yet the great majority want to work, and with the right support many can. There is now considerable evidence that particular approaches to employment support can be successful in helping people with severe and enduring mental health problems enter real, competitive employment. Indeed, there have been 16 randomized controlled trials that have tested different 'pathway to employment' methodologies and these have supported 'place then train' approaches over 'train then place' ones. IPS has been found to be particularly effective. Across the studies an average of 61 per cent (range 50–70 per cent) of clients achieved real competitive employment (Bond *et al.* 2008). IPS involves an employment specialist working closely with the service user, their mental health team and their employer and offering indefinite support. The two critical factors in successfully obtaining employment are the service user wanting to work and believing they can; severity of symptoms and diagnosis are not significant predictors. IPS is radically different to the more traditional (both in mental health and criminal justice services) train then place approaches, which emphasize assessments of job readiness, and often involve lengthy preparation and training. In IPS job searching begins as soon as a service user expresses a desire to work and the goal is a 'real' salaried job.

In spite of the success of these programmes routes to employment and advocacy in this area are probably still not on the radar of most mental health practitioners although giving employment a greater priority has particular value to forensic mental health practice.

Accommodation

The accommodation needs of those able and ready to step down from secure mental health care are not well understood. When I visited the Dutch Ter Beschikking Stelling (TBS) system for high risk offenders a few years ago, they had established that while most of the patients of this system will ultimately live more or less independently in the community, approximately 15 per cent, while able to live in non-secure settings, remain very dependent and require staffed/supported accommodation for life (Centre for Mental Health 2011). Others require such supported accommodation as a transitional phase to independent living.

Not all those in secure mental health care have the same needs – for example, women will have different needs to men, younger people to older offenders, as may different cultural and ethnic groups, or those with learning disability. There is a need for more innovation and research that describes the different pathways out of secure care.

The Centre for Mental Health's discussion document on securing stable accommodation of offenders (Scott 2011) describes different approaches to accommodating those with multiple needs and compares and contrasts the more traditional 'treatment first' approaches to 'housing first' approaches which are emerging from the USA. The limited evidence to date supports the latter over the former. Scott sees a similarity in the evidence-based approach to employment described above and 'housing first': 'The "housing first" philosophy echoes the principles underlying Individual Placement and Support' (p. 9). This approach sees that the best place to prepare people for independent living is while they are living independently, but with well designed support. Like employment, the right accommodation (with skilled support) is seen as a treatment in its own right.

 41.5 Conclusion

This chapter has sought to provide an overview of some key issues in forensic mental health nursing. The main points are:

- Forensic mental health nursing is an expanding field. In the past it was practised almost exclusively with a group of people who posed high risk of harm to others in locked settings, but has now expanded to cover any person with a mental health problem coming into contact with criminal justice services, including diversion.

- The client group, whether posing high risk or not, tends to have multiple and complex needs and this requires the FMNH to increasingly become a case manager and broker of complex care packages.

- Forensic mental health nursing uses all the care and treatment approaches detailed in this book, but with a particular emphasis on risk assessment, management and reduction.

- Risk management is as much about providing comprehensive and holistic care is it is about applying any specialist skills in risk assessment. Crucially it is also about service user involvement in their own care.

- Forensic mental health service users are an especially socially excluded group and forensic mental health nursing needs to become more recovery focused to support clients to meet some of their basic needs, especially through support in achieving security of tenure and advocating evidence-based approaches to employment.

Annotated bibliography

Sainsbury Centre for Mental Health (2009) *Doing What Works: Individual placement and support into employment.* **London: Centre for Mental Health.**
The employment programme provides a number of resources that will be useful for the reader, but I have selected one that provides a short overview of the IPS methodology: http://www.centreformentalhealth.org.uk/pdfs/briefing37_Doing_what_works.pdf.

The Centre for Mental Health runs a recovery programme aimed at supporting organizations and practitioners within them in establishing the right structures and practices to best enable their service users to achieve their own recovery goals.
The weblink is a route to all of the Centre's publications and other resources as well as updates on its recovery projects: www.centreformentalhealth.org.uk/recovery/index.aspx.

Flewett, T. (2010) *Clinical Risk Management: An introductory text for mental health clinicians.* **Sydney: Elsevier.**
Tom Flewett's small book provides a detailed and pragmatic introduction. It covers: theory, risk assessment, risk measurement, risk documentation, risk management including chronic risk, risk of suicide, risk of violence, managing adverse outcomes and using standardized tools.

T2A Alliance (2012) *Ten Steps to a More Effective Approach for Young Adults in the Criminal Justice Process.* **London: Barrow-Cadbury Trust, available at: www.bctrust.org.uk/wp-content/uploads/2012/05/T2A_Pathways-from-Crime_online-ver2.pdf.**

This report makes a series of recommendations on establishing appropriate responses in criminal justice services to a group that may be legally children or adults, but is distinct from both. Mental Health services for this group are crucial and feature in the report.

The Joint Panel on Commissioning (JPG) will produce specific commissioning guidance for forensic mental health care for England later in 2012. For more on the JPG please visit: www.rcpsych.ac.uk/PDF/jcp%20briefing.pdf and http://www.rcpsych.ac.uk/policy/policyandparliamentary/projects/live/commissioning.aspx.

DH (Department of Health) (2012) Low Secure Services and Psychiatric Intensive Care: Consultation document, London: DH, available at: http://www.dh.gov.uk/health/files/2012/01/Low-Secure-Services-and-Psychiatric-Intensive-Care_Consultation-Document-with-IRB2.pdf.
Low secure services are deemed to be poorly defined and this consultation, which closed in April 2012, will shortly seek to address this. Associated documents and updates on the consultation are available at: www.dh.gov.uk/health/2012/01/consultation-on-low-secure-services-and-psychiatric-intensive-care.

The International Association of Forensic Mental Health Services runs an annual conference, edits the *International Journal of Forensic Mental Health*, coordinates an international research group, provides an international directory of services and will be organizing educational exchanges in the future.
For more details visit: http://www.iafmhs.org.

The Quality Network for Forensic Mental Health Services is is a multi-disciplinary group hosted by the Royal College of Psychiatrists and with representation from most providers and many forensic mental health care services.
The group looks at policy, good practice and service improvement issues. For further information see www.rcpsych.ac.uk/quality/qualityandaccreditation/forensic/forensicmentalhealth.aspx.

References

All Party Parliamentary Group on Women in the Penal System (2011) *Women in the Penal System: Second report on women with particular vulnerabilities in the criminal justice system*. The Howard League for Penal Reform. London. Available at: http://www.howardleague.org/fileadmin/howard_league/user/pdf/Publications/Women_in_the_penal_system.pdf

BBC (1998) Psychiatrists accuse Straw of ignorance, 26 October, available at: http://news.bbc.co.uk/1/hi/uk_politics/201795.stm.

Bond, G.R., Drake, R.E. and Becker, D.R. (2008) An update on randomized controlled trials of evidence-based supported employment, *Psychiatric Rehabilitation Journal*, 31: 280–9.

CBI (Confederation of British Industry) (2008) *Getting Back on the Straight and Narrow: A better criminal justice system for all.* London: CBI.

Centre for Mental Health (2010) *Beyond the Gate: Securing employment for offenders with mental health problems.* London: Centre for Mental Health, available at: www.centreformentalhealth.org.uk.

Centre for Mental Health (2011) *Pathways to Unlocking Secure Mental Health Care.* London: Centre for Mental Health, available at: www.centreformentalhealth.org.uk.

Coffey, M. (2003) Relapse prevention in psychosis, in B. Hannigan and M. Coffey (eds) *The Handbook of Community Mental Health Nursing.* London: Routledge.

Cohen, A. (2011) Ensuring good physical health for offenders, conference presentation at the Mental Health Congress, London, 30 November 2011.

Coid, J., Hickey, N. and Yang, M. (2007) Comparison of outcomes following after-care from forensic and general adult psychiatric services, *British Journal of Psychiatry*, 190: 509–14.

DH (Department of Health) (1999) *The National Service Framework for Mental Health.* London: DH.

DH (Department of Health) (2001) *The Mental Health Policy Implementation Guide.* London: DH.

DH (Department of Health) (2009) *The Bradley Report: Lord Bradley's review of people with mental health problems or learning disabilities in the criminal justice system.* London: DH.

DH (Department of Health) (2011a) Right Honourable Paul Barstow speech to the Revolving Doors conference on offender health, London: DH, available at: www.dh.gov.uk/en/MediaCentre/Speeches/DH_12526

DH (Department of Health) (2011b) *No Health Without Mental Health.* London: DH.

DH (Department of Health) (2011c) *Responses to the Offender Personality Disorder Consultation.* London: DH.

Duncan, E.A.S., Nicol, M.M., Ager, A. and Dalgleish, L. (2006) A systematic review of structured group interventions with mentally disordered offenders, *Criminal Behaviour and Mental Health*, 16: 217–41.

Durcan, G. (2008a) Mental health nursing in prisons, in National Forensic Research & Development Group (ed.) *Forensic Mental Health Nursing: Capabilities, roles and responsibilities.* London: Quay.

Durcan, G. (2008b) *From the Inside: Experience of prison mental health care.* London: Sainsbury Centre for Mental Health, available at: www.centreformentalhealth.org.uk.

Eagle, M. (2009) House of Commons Hansard written answers, 15 June: Column 66W.

Flewett, T. (2010) *Clinical Risk Management: An introductory text for mental health clinicians.* Sydney: Elsevier.

Fossey, M. and Black, G. (2010) *Under the Radar: Women with borderline personality disorder in prison.* London: Centre for Mental Health.

HMIP (Her Majesty's Inspectorate of Prisons) (2007) *The Mental Health of Prisoners: A thematic review of the care and support of prisoners with mental health needs*. London: The Stationery Office.

Hoare, T. and Wilson, J. (2010) *Directory of Services for High-risk Young People*. London: Centre for Mental Health.

Home Office (2007) *The Corston Report: A report by Baroness Jean Corston of a review of women with particular vulnerabilities in the criminal justice system*. London: Home Office.

Keating, F. (2009) African and Caribbean Men and Mental Health. *Ethnicity and Inequalities in Health and Social Care*; 2(2): 41–53.

Kendell, R. (2002) The distinction between personality disorder and mental illness, *The British Journal of Psychiatry*, 180: 110–15.

Kettles, A., Woods, P. and Byrt, R. (2008) Introduction, in A. Kettles, P. Woods and R. Byrt (eds) *Forensic Mental Health Nursing: Capabilities, roles and responsibilities*. London: Quay.

Kirby, S. and Durcan, G. (2009) Forensic mental health care, in I. Norman and I. Ryrie (eds) *The Art and Science of Mental Health Nursing: A textbook of principles and practice*, 2nd edn. Maidenhead: Open University Press.

Laing and Buisson (2006) *Mental Health and Specialist Care Services: UK market report 2006*. London: ????

L&BCJA (Lothian & Borders Community Justice Authority) (2011) *Good Practice Guidance: Diversion to social work and other agencies. Draft issued for consultation, July 2011*, available at: www.cjalb.co.uk/docs/ GuidanceDiversiontoSocialWorkandOtherAgenciesasanalternativetoProsecutionVersion3May2011.pdf.

MOJ (Ministry of Justice) (2009) *MAPPA Guidance 2009, Version 3.0*. London: MOJ.

MOJ (Ministry of Justice) (2010) *Breaking the Cycle: Effective Punishment, Rehabilitation and Sentencing of Offenders*. London: MOJ.

Mullen, P. (2000) Forensic mental health, *British Journal Of Psychiatry*, 176: 307–11.

Nacro (2011) *Nacro Directory of Criminal Justice Mental Health Liaison and Diversion Schemes in England and Wales*. London: Nacro.

NIMH (National Institute for Mental Health for England) (2003) *Personality Disorder: No longer a diagnosis of exclusion Policy implementation guidance for the development of services for people with personality disorder*. London: Department of Health.

Petch, E. (2001) Risk management in UK mental health services: an overvalued idea? *Psychiatric Bulletin*, 25: 203–5.

Prison Reform Trust (2011) *The Bromley Briefings Prison Fact File*. London: Prison Reform Trust, available at: www. prisonreformtrust.org.uk/Publications.

Rollnick, S., Miller, W.R., Butler, C. *Motivational interviewing in health care: helping patients change behavior*. Guilford Press, 2008.

Rutherford, M. (2010) *Blurring the Boundaries: The convergence of mental health and criminal justice policy, legislation, systems and practice*. London: Centre for Mental Health, available at: www.centreformentalhealth.org.uk.

Rutherford, M. and Duggan, S. (2007) *Forensic Mental Health Services: Facts and figures on current provision*. London: Sainsbury Centre for Mental Health, available at: www.centreformentalhealth.org.uk.

Sainsbury Centre for Mental Health (2008a) *A Review of the Use of Offending Behaviour Programmes for People with Mental Health Problems*. London: Sainsbury Centre for Mental Health, available at: www.centreformentalhealth.org.uk.

Sainsbury Centre for Mental Health (2008b) *In the Dark: The mental health implications of imprisonment for public protection*. London: Sainsbury Centre for Mental Health, available at: www.centreformentalhealth.org.uk.

Sainsbury Centre for Mental Health (2009) *Diversion: A better way for mental health and criminal justice*. London: Sainsbury Centre for Mental Health. Available at: www.centreformentalhealth.org.uk.

Scott, G. (2011) *A Place to Live: Securing stable accommodation for offenders with mental health problems*. London: Centre for Mental Health, available at: www.centreformentalhealth.org.uk.

Scottish Government (2000) The pilot schemes were monitored and this study was commissioned to evaluate their first 18 months of operation, available at: www.scotland.gov.uk/Publications/2000/03/851ca140-55f5-4a7e-bc7a-f6efe6c88ceb.

Scottish Government Public Protection Unit (2008) *MAPPA Guidance: Version 4*. Edinburgh: Scottish Government, available at: www.scotland.gov.uk/ Resource/Doc/ 220543/ 0059277.pdf.

Shepherd, G., Boardman, J. and Slade, M. (2008) *Making Recovery a Reality*. London: Centre for Mental Health, available at: www.centreformentalhealth.org.uk.

Singleton, N., Bumpstead, R., O'Brien, M., Lee, A. and Meltzer, H. (2001) *Psychiatric Morbidity Among Adults Living in Private Households, 2000*. London: ONS.

Singleton, N., Meltzer, H. and Gatward, R. (1998) *Psychiatric Morbidity Among Prisoners in England and Wales*. London: ONS.

Spurgeon, D. (2005) *Diversionary Tactics*. London: Nacro, available at: www.nacro.org.uk/data/files/nacro-2005062900-384.pdf.

Social Exclusion Unit (2002) *Reducing Re-offending by Ex-prisoners*. London: Social Exclusion Unit.

Tilt, R., Perry, B., Martin, C., Maguire, N. and Preston, M. (2000) *Report of the Review of Security at the High Security Hospitals*. London: DH.

Witkiewitz, K. and Marlatt, G. (2007) *Therapists' Guide to Evidence Based Relapse Prevention*. Burlington, MA: Academic Press/ Elsevier.

Wood, P. (2004) Norman I & Ryrie I. *The Art and Science of Mental Health Nursing: A textbook of Principles and Practice*. Maidenhead: Open University Press.

Acknowledgement

Thanks to Gael Scott, policy officer, Centre for Mental Health, for her invaluable help in compiling this chapter.

PART

6

Future Directions

Chapter 42

Older People are the Future: Towards an Understanding of the Quality of Mental Health Nursing Care for Older People

Ian Norman, Iain Ryrie and Samantha Coster

Without older people we would have nothing that we hold dear today; our lives, our families, our societies and security. We are indebted to them and as such it is our duty, when they can no longer care fully for themselves, to ensure they have all that they need for a safe and satisfying life, just as they had done for us when we were young

Anon

 42.1 Introduction

The main message of the final chapter of the first edition of this book (Norman and Ryrie 2004) was for mental health nurses to adopt recovery-ori-ented practice. By 2009, with the publication of the second edition, this had largely occurred. The interpersonal relations and evidence-based prac-tice traditions, the art and science of mental health nursing (see Chapter 3), were becoming reconciled within recovery-oriented practice and there was increasing agreement that mental health nursing involved delivering evidence-based interventions in a recovery-oriented way through the medium of the relationship between the nurse and service users and their carers.

By the time of the second edition in 2009 (Norman and Ryrie 2009), with recovery-oriented practice well established, mental health nursing looked poised to extend its remit; the focus of the final chapter of the second edition was how nurses could take recovery-oriented care beyond their traditional focus on the individual into the wider society to contribute to public mental health.

Writing in mid-2012, nursing appears to be under siege. Media reports in the UK suggest that standards of nursing care are in decline (e.g. Phillips 2007; Boseley 2009; Borland 2012) and public confidence in nurses as a professional group would seem to have fallen as a result of media exposés of uncaring nurses and supported by a series of recent official reports and enquiries into care failures (e.g. CQC 2010; EHRC 2011). Of course, much nursing care is of excellent quality, but our recent clinical experience and mounting evidence suggests that standards of nursing are too often unacceptably low, a view shared by the British prime minister, David Cameron, speaking on BBC Radio 4's *Today* programme on 6 January 2012. He said:

> *there is clearly a problem in some hospitals, in some settings, where we are not getting the standards of care the nation expects. I think politicians frankly have done nurses a bit of a disservice by not talking about this. Such is our respect for nursing that we've hidden away concerns about this.*

> (Topping A, Guardian online, 6 January 2012)

Media reports raise particular concern about the nursing care of older people, especially those living in hospitals and other institutions, a high proportion of whom suffer from dementia or other mental health problems. These patients are among the most vulnerable in our society and are least able to protect themselves or complain. Worrying also is the fact that those who have access to specialist mental health nursing receive care that falls far short of the ideal (Commission for Health Improvement 2003). Even organizations which represent professional nurses, such as the Royal College of Nursing (RCN), acknowledge mounting public concern about whether nursing care, particularly for older vulnerable people, is fit for purpose, and recognize that a way forward must be found to improve care standards and restore the public reputation of professional nursing (RCN 2012).

There are currently 3 million people aged more than 80 years in the UK and this is projected to almost double by 2030 and reach 8 million by 2050 (Cracknell 2010). Care of older people is possibly our greatest public health challenge for the first half of this century and mental health nurses must be part of the solution – it is our duty. *Older people are the future, not children* – this is literally true for all of us and we need to sort out our practice.

In view of these concerns we have devoted this final chapter to a consideration of what has gone wrong with nursing in some care settings for older people, many of whom may have mental health problems, and propose a model of nursing care quality for testing in future studies and as a guide to interventions to promote quality in nursing care. The chapter covers:

- the ideal of person-centred and relationship-centred care;
- what's gone wrong with nursing?;
- a workforce under strain;
- the nature of nursing work in older adult mental health services;
- organizational support;
- a conceptual model of the quality of nursing care;
- a research agenda for improving the quality of mental health nursing care.

42.2 The ideal of person- and relationship-centred care

NHS policy (DH 2000, 2001) has stipulated that optimum care for older patients should be 'person-centred', which requires that they are treated with dignity and respect; that they are valued, treated as individuals with a unique personal history and approach to life; and are provided with opportunities to form meaningful relationships which foster happiness and personal growth. This vision of high quality care is supported by reports which highlight the importance of positive, individualized approaches to caring for older adults, and set out how the philosophy of person-centred care might be realized through service delivery. In addition, frameworks have been developed by researchers that may be used to assess care quality, including 'dementia care mapping' which requires close staff observation of the patient's daily living to understand their perspective (Kitwood and Bredin 1992) and the Senses Framework (Nolan et al. 2004, 2006) which is based on a model of 'relationship'-centred care. This framework proposes that the best way to enrich care is by creating an environment where the older person experiences relationships which provide them with feelings of security, belonging, achievement, purpose, continuity and significance, and crucially within which staff and their family carers also experience these same feelings.

There is considerable consensus on the key elements of high quality care and substantial guidance on the best ways to care for vulnerable older adults, but nursing care too often falls far short of the ideal. Findings of unannounced hospital inspections by the Care Quality Commission (CQC), published in October 2011 (CQC 2011), found that in some hospitals nursing staff and aides forgot to give food and water to older patients, while dignified care was lacking in 40 per cent of hospitals. Other inquiries have found that while physical care standards are usually acceptable the psychosocial care of older patients is poor; nurses, or nursing aides working under the supervision of nurses, fail to respect patients' privacy, provide batch treatment which denies patient choice, fail to promote patient activity and provide only minimal interaction during routine care.

42.3 What's gone wrong with nursing?

Inadequate staffing is the explanation most frequently cited by nursing organizations, such as the RCN, to explain compromised care standards, based on a substantial body of research which demonstrates a positive relationship between numbers of registered nurses, increased patient safety and improved patient experience (Rafferty et al. 2007). The RCN (2012) argues that current changes in National Health Service (NHS) services triggered in England by the 'Nicholson challenge' to save £20 billion by 2014–15, have led to bed closures in older adult services and inpatient admission avoidance strategies, leading in turn to inpatient care facilities being occupied by the most frail older people who have complex physical and mental health needs. RCN research (2012) shows that older people's wards in most NHS hospitals have a more dilute skill mix than other types of ward; it is estimated that in a typical daytime shift only half the nursing staff on duty are registered nurses. The key to improving nursing care quality, argues the RCN, is increased investment by the UK government to improve nurse:patient ratios to acceptable levels. However, simply increasing numbers of staff does not necessarily lead to improvements in care for patients. For example, Sandford et al.'s (1990) observation study of nursing activities in wards where nursing numbers differed found that 15–18 per cent of nurses' time was spent with patients and 31–34 per cent was spent with other nurses and that when the number of nurses was increased, nurses spent a higher proportion of their time with other staff. Moreover, given the financial outlook, increasing the number of nurses is unlikely to be possible in most clinical settings.

Other commentators, particularly newspaper journalists, have blamed what they perceive to be declining nursing standards on nurse education reforms introduced by Project 2000 (UKCC 1986) which, in the 1990s, moved UK nurse education wholesale from the hospital training schools into the universities. They argue that nurses are now selected for their academic rather than personal qualities and that too much emphasis is placed upon classroom learning at the expense of practical experience which develops nurses' caring skills (e.g. Boycott 2009). The evidence base for this claim is weak but it appeals to a widely held view that professional nurses need little more than common sense and also a view that positive attitudes to patients and caring nursing skills are somehow incompatible with 'brains'. Common sense is important in nursing, as it is in life, and it is certainly true that nursing needs to recruit people of 'the right type'; that is, people who can put themselves in the place of a person who is ill, are aware of their reactions and emotions towards people, and who can reflect on and learn from their mistakes and experiences. However, these personal qualities, while essential, are not sufficient. Nurses today need to be educated to be 'thinking people', to take the initiative in care rather than be simply reactive, and be able to give an account of their actions based upon best evidence. It is this vision of professional mental health nursing which is supported by this book.

In sum, while it is widely accepted that the quality of professional nursing, particularly that provided currently to vulnerable older adults, many of whom are mentally ill, falls far short of expectations, the hypothesis that this is simply the result of too few nurses or the recruitment of uncompassionate nurses who are poorly trained in caring skills does not take account of the complexity of the care situation in older adult mental health services.

42.4 A workforce under strain

There is evidence that nurses working in old age psychiatric units have lower job satisfaction than those working in standard geriatric wards or care homes (Philp *et al.* 1991). Relationships between clinicians' work satisfaction and patient outcomes are complex, however research suggests that the job satisfaction and well-being of nurses is reflected in the standards of nursing care they deliver; more satisfied nurses give better patient care (Redfern *et al.* 2002; Maben *et al.* 2012). This is illustrated in research by Robertson *et al.* (1995) who found that nurses in older adult psychiatric wards with high levels of satisfaction placed greater emphasis on patient dignity and engaged in more meaningful communication with patients during personal care activities than those on low satisfaction wards. Conversely, research by Nolan and Grant (1993) reported that improved staff-patient relationships on older adult psychiatric wards led to staff benefits in terms of improved job satisfaction.

We know also that nurses who work in psychiatric settings for older people seem to experience high levels of stress (MacPherson *et al.* 1994). In particular, nurses report greater stress when caring for older people with dementia (Rodney 2000; Brodaty *et al.* 2003). The stress of caring for a person with dementia on family carers is well documented (Ballard *et al.* 2000) but less is known about the impact of caring for disoriented older people on professional nurses' levels of psychological stress and the consequences for the quality of their care. Psychological stress and job satisfaction may be mediated by nurses' ability to cope with work demands; but the coping capacity of nurses working with older adult mental health services is underresearched. What is known is that caring for older adults is not a popular career choice for newly qualified nurses (Happell and Brooker 2001) and that older adult mental health services struggle to recruit and retain nurses with good skills and positive attitudes to their work.

In sum, there is a well established relationship between high levels of psychological stress and poorer nursing care. Staff dissatisfaction also leads to high levels of absenteeism and turnover, leading to staff shortages (Larrabee *et al.* 2003; Coomber and Barriball 2007). Aside from the lack of care continuity and the emotional impact on patients of having their personal care provided by a large number of different people who are not aware of their needs or preferences, there is also a strong relationship between high staff turnover and poor patient outcomes in services for older people, including increased general hospital admissions and the overuse of psychoactive drugs (Zimmerman *et al.* 2002; Castle and Engberg 2005).

42.5 The nature of nursing work in older adult mental health services

Improving standards of nursing care require an understanding of the pressures on nursing staff and the effects of stress on quality of care and outcomes for patients. Our reviews of the research literature (Norman 1997; Hannan *et al.* 2001), supported by our clinical experience, indicate that poor nursing arises from nurses' negative cognitive appraisal of their job and ability to cope with it – specifically, their perceptions of quantitative overload (time pressures and a repetitive daily grind of routine activities), qualitative overload (concern about not doing a job well and the psychological impact of intimate contact and patients' emotional needs) or alternatively, qualitative underload (caused by boredom and unrewarding interpersonal relationships with cognitively impaired and dependent patients) which is characteristic of many continuing care settings for older people in the context of two further cognitive appraisals; poor job control (low status, unchallenging, routinized nursing work which has similarities with mass production) and poor job support (unsupportive leadership and poor work organization). These negative cognitive appraisals lead to burnout or the lesser known 'rust-out', low morale and poor job commitment, which in turn results in depersonalized, emotionally detached nursing and batch processing rather than individualized, relationship-centred care.

The central role of cognitive appraisal (i.e. perceptions and interpretations, which give meaning to events and determine whether they are viewed as threatening or positive) in determining the impact of work on nurses has been supported by research in a number of settings including care wards for older people (Nova and Chappell 1994).

Burned out care workers are emotionally exhausted, they depersonalize patients and have difficulty in accomplishing their personal goals (Maslach and Jackson 1981). Seminal work by Menzies (1960) reported that close physical care of patients generates unpleasant feelings in general nurses such as revulsion, worries about coping with intimacy and dependency, fear of failure and fear of lack of competence. To avoid these feelings nurses defend themselves from the stress of patient encounters through practices and structures to protect themselves from conflicts and anxieties related to the demands of the job. These practices are manifest in rigid routines, authoritarian attitudes and batch processing rather than individualized treatment. Supporting this, more recent research by Chiesa (1993) and Donati (1989) found that psychiatric nurses kept themselves physically busy in order to manage anxiety relating to potentially meaningful exchanges with patients. This is a particular problem among vulnerable patients, with nurses being more likely to avoid interaction with those they perceive to be 'difficult' patients, with confused or demented patients often having the least meaningful interactions of all (Armstrong-Esther and Browne 1986). Clinical experience suggests that these avoidant behaviours and dehumanized nursing practices, while exhibited by nurses in many fields of practice, including continuing care settings for older people, are particularly evident in inpatient settings for mentally ill older adults in which patients' dementia or other mental illness is expressed in passive, bizarre, aggressive or demanding behaviours, or where it hampers their ability to communicate and form relationships with other patients and nursing staff. Moreover, our experience suggests that dehumanized care practices are inadvertently reinforced by the current economic climate and resulting nursing staff shortages cited by the RCN. Staff shortages often lead to a task-orientated approach to nursing care in the interests of efficiency, which prioritizes getting through the work and delivery of adequate physical care; this, in effect, legitimates nurses' avoidance of meaningful patient interaction.

There is also evidence which highlights the contribution of two further job characteristics to poor nursing care quality in older adult mental health settings: poor job control and poor job support. Organizational theories of job strain (e.g. Karasek's 1972 demand-control theory) suggest that it is not high job demands *per se* but high demands in combination with an appraisal of low job control which creates job strain. In previous work (Norman 1997) we argue that nurses who work with mentally ill older adults in NHS care settings may often have little sense of control over the nature of their work, and point to similarities between the pressures of low social status, unchallenging routinized nursing care in long-stay wards and pressures of other types of work, including highly automated work assignments, shift work, routine office work and mass production.

42.6 Organizational support

In terms of job support, the importance of the organization cannot be underestimated, having a powerful impact on the morale and organizational commitment of staff, especially in care settings where relationships between patients and staff are distant or are disrupted by communication difficulties. Tellis-Nayak and Tellis-Nayak (1989) describe a vicious cycle of nurse discontentment and poor patient care which can occur in unsupportive organizations or what Sheridan et al. (1992) call 'laissez faire' climates where staff are not given clear objectives, not rewarded or incentivized for good work, and where long-term planning does not occur. Sheridan argues that organizational climate, regardless of adequate levels of staff supervision, will contribute to demoralized staff and poor patient care. At a more basic level, nurse managers need to clearly communicate to staff the importance of treating patients as individuals and this phi-

losophy of care should be explicit; Kitwood (1993) contends that for person-orientated care to occur, it has be embedded into the service culture, which can be created at ward level by good leadership, but crucially requires recognition and encouragement and support at the organizational level. Thus the formation of relationships between staff and patients must be seen as 'a legitimate and valued activity' (Gilloran et al. 1995). To acknowledge this, Nolan and Keady (1996) suggest that the organization needs to provide both positive feedback to staff committing to this form of work and also arrange regular clinical support or supervision for the emotional impact that this greater intimacy entails.

Maben et al. (2011) reported on the importance of having a strong visible ward leader to influence the caring and work culture. A leader working at a strategic level, but also role modelling by providing direct personal care to patients, tends to be viewed most positively. There is good evidence that a strong supportive leadership style can 'buffer' or protect staff from the effects of stress arising from challenging nursing work (Duxbury et al. 1984; Bakker et al. 2000). Effective transformational leadership, for example, can encourage staff to find innovative ways to problem-solve in the appraisal process, and is linked to higher social support perceptions, greater efficacy beliefs and lower threat appraisals. Research also suggests that transformational leadership can moderate the relationship between emotional exhaustion and turnover intention (Green et al. 2011). High levels of support from nurse supervisors can reduce feelings of emotional exhaustion and help protect staff from the poor work environments (Constable and Russell 1986).

42.7 A conceptual model of the quality of nursing care

The conceptual framework shown in Figure 42.1 draws upon the research literature outlined above and our clinical experience to explain how nurses' appraisal of their environment and of their own

Figure 42.1 Quality of nursing care: proposed conceptual framework (Norman and Coster 2012, copyright King's College London, reproduced with permission)

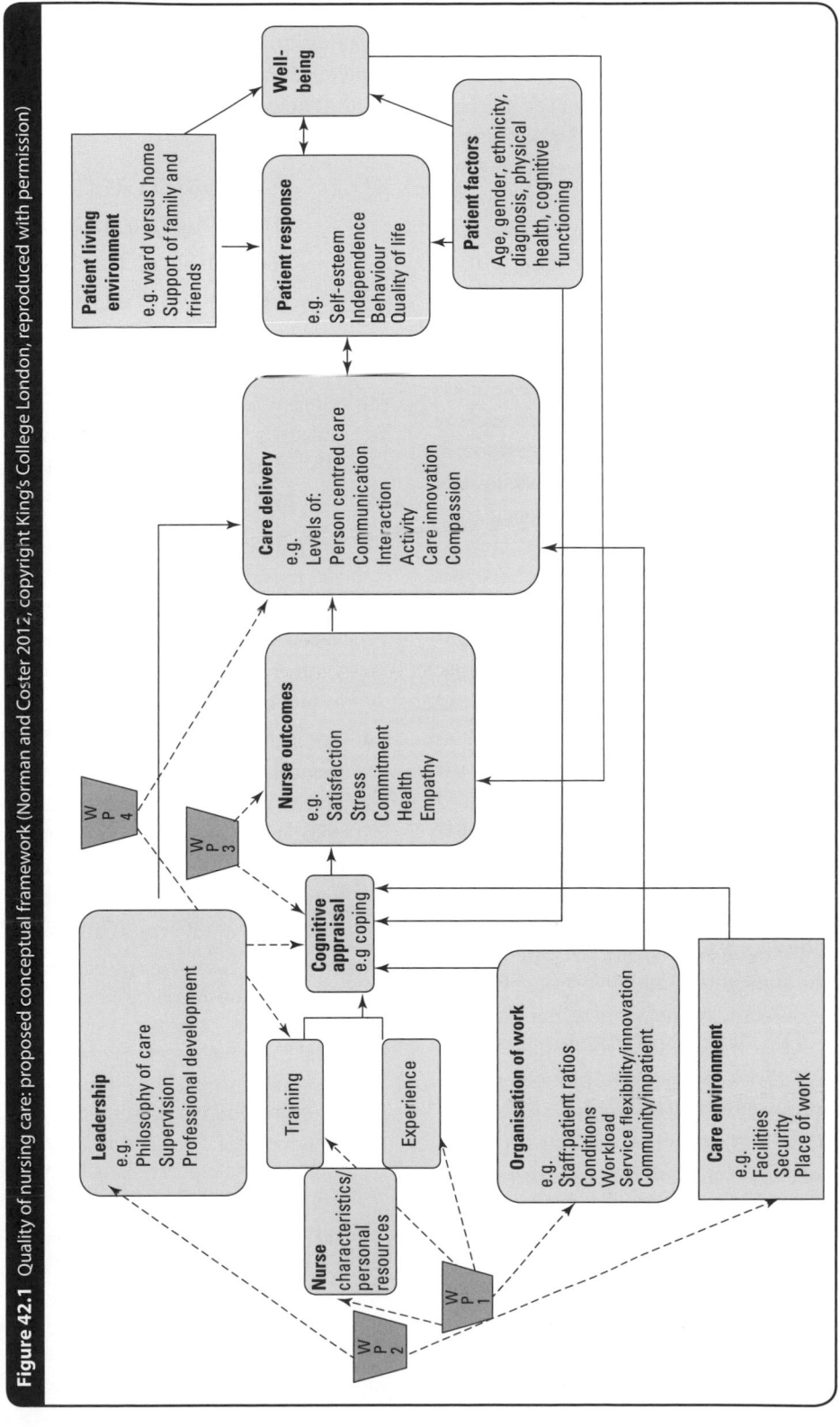

personal resources and skills, will, in turn, influence the quality of patient care. The framework hypothesizes that nurses' work performance will be the result of an appraisal influenced by their perceptions of leadership (e.g. whether there is strong nurse leadership that values caring over curing and provides positive feedback for staff), of how their work is organized (e.g. their workload, the degree to which they can innovate or control their job), of environmental factors (e.g. the security of the workplace) and their perception of their ability to deliver care, based on their personal resources, experience, previous training and knowledge. Negative appraisals are likely to lead to poor staff outcomes, such as low satisfaction, high stress, low work commitment, ill health and reduced empathy, which will in turn lead to the delivery of sub-standard nursing care. This care is unlikely to be person-centred, innovative or compassionate, and is likely to be characterized by lack of meaningful interaction or relationships with patients, block treatment and dehumanized care. This will, in turn, impact on patients' behaviour, their quality of life, their self-esteem and their ability to maintain their independence. Through a system of negative feedback loops the act and result of delivering poor nursing care may reinforce work dissatisfaction and lead to greater stress and reduced nurse motivation.

The conceptual framework also recognizes a number of patient factors such as age, gender, diagnosis and cognitive and physical functioning that will moderate the relationship between care delivery and the patient's response to the care provided. Thus, while the model is applicable to continuing care settings for older people, older inpatients suffering from mental disorder are particularly powerless and so vulnerable; for them the quality of nursing received determines their quality of life. Conversely, for example, mentally ill older people who are supported at home in the community are likely to have, or may be perceived by nurses to have, a greater sense of 'agency' or control over their life. It is likely therefore that the impact of nursing care on quality of life for those living in the community will be less than for those

living in NHS inpatient wards, and that the nurse's relationship with the older mentally ill people's families will be of particular importance for patients living at home.

42.8 A research and improvement agenda for enhancing the quality of mental health nursing care

The conceptual framework represented in Figure 42.1 raises a number of questions for future research, which we have grouped into a series of work packages (WPs).

1. **WP1:** what are the characteristics of the current UK nursing workforce for older adults with mental health problems, in terms of training, experience and background, and what are its strengths and limitations? What is needed to improve the workforce?

2. **WP2:** of what does high quality nursing care of mentally ill older people comprise? Which organizational factors and processes enable the provision of high quality nursing care to mentally ill older people? Which features, systems and styles of nursing leadership contribute to delivering high standards of nursing care?

3. **WP3:** how can nurses be best trained and supported to positively appraise their work and enhance their ability to cope more effectively with the challenges of working with older adults with mental health problems? How can they be helped to develop the confidence and skills needed to supervise health care assistants and non-professionally qualified staff to give high quality nursing care?

4. **WP4:** what skills do nurses need to reduce patients' anxiety and agitation, and also improve the quality of their relationships with patients, and what training do they need to provide them with these skills?

Finally, we would need to know what are the costs of developing the nursing workforce in this way and the anticipated short- and long-term benefits and value of these investments?

 42.9 Conclusion

This final chapter provides a conceptual model of nursing care quality to help guide practice development, stimulate debate, and for development and testing in future research. The framework has the potential, we believe, to help us understand the quality of nursing in a variety of specialties. However, it was developed drawing on the research literature and our clinical experience in response to concerns in the media about the quality of nursing for mentally and physically frail older people, particularly those living in care homes and geriatric wards. These people are our future and raising the quality of their experience of nursing care and making older people's care a desirable and rewarding career choice should be a priority for the profession now and in the decades ahead.

References

Armstrong-Esther, C. and Browne, K. (1986) The influence of elderly patients' mental impairment on nurse-patient interaction, *Journal of Advanced Nursing*, 11: 379–87.

Bakker, A., Killmer, C., Siegriest, J. and Schaufeli, W. (2000) Effort-reward imbalance and burnout among nurses, *Journal of Advanced Nursing*, 31: 884–91.

Ballard, C., Lowery, K., Powell, I., O'Brien, J. and James, I. (2000) Impact of behavioral and psychological symptoms of dementia on caregivers, *International Psychogeriatrics*, 12(1): 93–105.

Borland, S. (2012) You can't teach people compassion, *Daily Mail*.

Boseley, S. (2009) Patients 'demeaned' by poor-quality nursing care, *Guardian*.

Boycott, O. (2009) All new nurses to have degrees by 2013, *Guardian*.

Brodaty, H., Draper, B. and Low, L. (2003) Nursing home staff attitudes towards residents with dementia: strain and satisfaction with work, *Journal of Advanced Nursing*, 44: 583–90.

Castle, N. and Engberg, J. (2005) Staff turnover and quality of care in nursing homes, *Medical Care*, 43(6): 616–26.

Chiesa, M. (1993) At the border between institutionalisation and community psychiatry: psychodynamic observations of a hospital admission ward, *Free Associations*, 4(2)30: 214–63.

Commission for Health Improvement (2003) *Investigation Into Matters Arising from Care on Rowan Ward*. Manchester: Manchester Mental Health & Social Care Trust.

Constable, J. and Russell, D. (1986) The effect of social support and the work environment upon burnout among nurses, *Journal of Human Stress*, 12: 20–6.

Coomber, B. and Barriball, K.L. (2007) Impact of job satisfaction components on intent to leave and turnover for hospital-based nurses: a review of the research literature, *International Journal of Nursing Studies*, 44(2): 297–314.

CQC (Care Quality Commission) (2010) *The State of Health and Social Care in England*. London: CQC.

CQC (Care Quality Commission) (2011) *Dignity and Nutrition Inspection Programme: National overview*. London: CQC.

Cracknell, R. (2010) *The Ageing population: Key Issues for the new Parliament 2010, Value for Money in Public Services*, available at: www.parliament.uk/documents/commons/lib/research/key_issues/Key%20Issues%20The%20ageing%20population2007.pdf.

DH (Department of Health) (2000) *The NHS Plan: A plan for investment, plan for reform*. London: DH.

DH (Department of Health) (2001) *National Service Framework for Older People*. London: DH.

Donati, F. (1989) A psychodynamic observer in a chronic psychiatric ward, *British Journal of Psychotherapy*, 5: 317–29.

Duxbury, M., Armstrong, G., Drew, D. and Henley, S. (1984) Head nurse leadership style with staff nurse burnout and job satisfaction in neonatal intensive care units, *Nursing Research*, 33: 97–101.

EHRC (European Human Rights Commission) (2011) *Close to Home: An inquiry into older people and human rights in home care*. London: EHRC.

Gilloran, A., Robertson, A. and McGlew, T. (1995) Improving work satisfaction among nursing staff and quality of care for elderly patients with dementia: some policy implications, *Ageing Society*, 15: 375–91.

Green, A., Miller, E. and Aarons, G. (2011) Transformational leadership moderates the relationship between emotional exhaustion and turnover intention among community mental health providers, *Community Mental Health*, 4 November.

Hannan, S., Norman, I. and Redfern, S. (2001) Care work and quality of care for older people: a review of the research literature, *Reviews in Clinical Gerontology*, 11: 189–203.

Happell, B. and Brooker, J. (2001) Who will look after my grandmother? Attitudes of student nurses toward the care of older adults, *Journal of Gerontological Nursing*, 27: 12–17.

Karasek, R. (1979) Job demands, job decision latitude, and mental strain: implications for job redesign, *Administrative Science Quarterly*, 24: 285–308.

Kitwood, T. (1993) Person and process in dementia, *Journal of Geriatric Psychiatry International*, 8: 541–5.

Kitwood, T. and Bredin, K. (1992) A new approach to the evaluation of dementia care, *Journal of Advances in Health and Nursing Care*, 1(5): 41–60.

Larrabee, J., Janney, M., Ostrow, C. *et al.* (2003) Predicting registered nurse job satisfaction and intent to leave, *Journal of Nursing Administration*, 33(5): 271–83.

Maben, J., Adams, M., Peccei, R., Murrells, T.M. and Robert, G. (2011) Poppets and parcels: the links between staff experience of work and acutely ill older people's experience of hospital care, *International Journal of older people nursing*, 7: 83–94.

Maben, J., Peccei, R., Robert, G., Adams, M., Richardson, A. and Murrells, T. (2012) *Patients' Experiences of Care and the Influence of Staff Motivation, Affect and Wellbeing, Final Report*. London: King's College.

MacPherson, R., Easterly, R., Richards, H. and Mian, I. (1994) Psychosocial distress among workers caring for the elderly, *International Journal of Geriatric Psychiatry*, 9: 381–6.

Maslach, C. and Jackson, S. (1981) The measurement of experienced burnout, *Journal of Occupational Behavior*, 2: 99–113.

Menzies, I. (1960) Social systems as a defense against anxiety: an empirical study of the nursing service of a general hospital, *Human Relations*, 13: 95–121.

Nolan, M. and Grant, G. (1993) Rustout and therapeutic reciprocity: concepts to advance the nursing of older people, *Journal of Advanced Nursing*, 18: 1305–14.

Nolan, M. and Keady, J. (1996) Training in long-term care: the road to better quality, *Reviews in Clinical Gerontology*, 6: 333–42.

Nolan, M., Davies, S., Brown, J., Keady, J. and Nolan, J. (2004) Beyond 'person-centred' care: a new vision for gerontological nursing, *Journal of Clinical Nursing*, 13(3a): 45–53.

Nolan, M., Brown, J., Davies, S., Nolan, J. and Keady, J. (2006) *The Senses Framework: Improving care for older people through a relationship-centred approach (GRIP)*. Sheffield: University of Sheffield.

Norman, I. (1997) Supporting paid carers, in I. Norman and Redfern, S. (eds) *Mental Health Care for Elderly People*. London.

Norman, I.J. and Ryrie, I. (2004) Reflections: recovery oriented nursing in the context of the National Service Framework, in I. Norman and I. Ryrie (eds) *The Art & Science of Mental Health Nursing*. London: Open University Press.

Norman, I.J. and Ryrie, I. (2009) Future directions: taking recovery into society, in I. Norman and I. Ryrie (eds) *The Art and Science of Mental Health Nursing*, 2nd edn. Maidenhead: Open University Press.

Nova, K. and Chappell, N. (1994) Nursing assistant burnout and the cognitively impaired elderly, *International Journal of Aging and Human Development*, 39: 105–20.

Phillips, M. (2007) The real reason our hospitals are a disgrace, *Daily Mail*.

Philp, I., Mutch, W., Ballinger, B. and Boyd, L. (1991) A comparison of care in private nursing homes, geriatric nursing homes and psychogeriatric hospitals, *International Journal of Geriatric Psychiatry*, 1(6): 253–8.

Rafferty, A., Clarke, S., Coles, J. *et al.* (2007) Outcomes of variation in hospital nurse staffing in English hospitals: cross-sectional analysis of survey data and discharge records, *International Journal of Nursing Studies*, 44(2): 175–82.

RCN (Royal College of Nursing) (ed.) (2011) *Views from the Frontline RCN Employment Survey*. London: RCN.

RCN (Royal College of Nursing) (2012) *Safe Staffing for Older People's Wards*. London: RCN.

Redfern, S., Hannan, S. and Norman, I. (2002) Work satisfaction, stress, quality of care and morale of older people in a nursing home, *Health and Social Care in the Community*, 10(6): 512–17.

Robertson, A., Gilloran, A., McGlew, T., McKee, K., McKinley, A. and Wight, D. (1995) Nurses' job satisfaction and the qualtiy of care received by patients in psychogeriatric wards, *International Journal of Geriatric Psychiatry*, 10: 575–84.

Rodney, V. (2000) Nurse stress associated with aggression in people with dementia: its relationship to hardiness, cognitive appraisal and coping, *Journal of Advanced Nursing*, 31(1): 72–80.

Sandford, A., Elzinga, R. and Iversen, R. (1990) A quantitative study of nursing staff interactions in psychiatric wards, *Acta Psychiatrica Scandinavica*, 81: 46–51.

Sheridan, J., White, J. and Fairchild, T. (1992) Ineffective staff, ineffective supervision, or ineffective administration? Why some nursing homes fail to provide adequate care, *Gerontologist*, 32: 334–41.

Tellis-Nayak, V. and Tellis-Nayak, M. (1989) Quality of care and the burden of two cultures: when the world of the nurse's aides enters the world of the nursing home, *Gerontologist*, 29: 307–13.

UKCC (1986) *A New Preparation for Practice*. London: UKCC for Nursing, Midwifery and Health Visiting.

Zimmerman, S., Gruber-Baldini, A., Hebel, J., Sloane, P. and Magaziner, J. (2002) Nursing home facility risk factors for infection and hospitalization: importance of registered nurse turnover, administration, and social factors, *Journal of American Geriatric Society*, 50(12): 1987–95.

Index